S0-CPT-323

An Atlas of Histology

An Atlas of
HISTOLOGY

JOHANNES A. G. RHODIN, M.D., Ph.D.
University of Michigan Medical School

New York · OXFORD UNIVERSITY PRESS · London Toronto 1975

This book is a reprint of the atlas section of
Histology: An Atlas and Text,
Copyright © 1974 by Johannes A. G. Rhodin.

COVER
Electron micrograph of human
odoriferous sweat gland. ×1000.

Copyright © 1975 by Johannes A. G. Rhodin
Library of Congress Catalogue Card Number: 75-4107
Printed in the United States of America

This book is dedicated to my sons

ANDERS annd ERIK

—students of medicine and architecture

Preface

This reprint of the illustrations in Rhodin *Histology: A Text and Atlas* **is** made in response to requests from many teachers and students who expressed an interest in obtaining a separate collection of these illustrations to be used as laboratory guide and supplement to other texts in biology, histology, and cell biology.

The photographs are carefully selected and organized to show sequential magnifications of the same field from light microscopy to low magnification electron microscopy as well as medium and high magnification electron microscopy. To achieve superior resolution, numerous illustrations are taken from electron micrographs even though a similar magnification could have been achieved by light microscopy. These low magnification electron micrographs contain a wealth of structural information which may not be apparent immediately to the student. However, the micrographs will prove to be especially useful as reference material during discussions related to what the student should—or should not—be able to see in the light microscope.

The collection of illustrations includes analyses of many organs which earlier have not been described adequately by means of electron microscopy. This includes the development of blood cells in human bone marrow; spleen; lymph nodes; blood vessels; bone formation; male and female reproductive systems. The light microscope preparations are almost exclusively taken from human or monkey tissue. The electron microscope preparations are taken for the most part from rats and cats. Human tissues are used also for electron microscopy in instances in which they differ considerably from those of lower animals.

Numerals are used to identify structures in the illustrations. The student will, therefore, easily find a specific item in the picture, and the micrographs can readily be used by the student for testing purposes.

The illustrations were prepared by the author during his tenure as chairman and professor in the Department of Anatomy, New York Medical College, Valhalla, New York.

Ann Arbor, Michigan   Johannes A. G. Rhodin
February 1, 1975

Acknowledgments

The author is greatly indebted to his research associates, Miss Shirley Lim Sue and Mrs. Carin Silversmith, for their very skilled assistance in preparing the material through vascular perfusion, embedding, sectioning, electron microscopy, photographic printing, final mounting, and labeling of the illustrations. Without their willingness to tackle these chores, their cheerful encouragement and incredible endurance, the illustrations would not have materialized.

Dr. Yen Fen Pei, M.D., secured the material necessary to illustrate the chapter on the eye. Her knowledge of ophthalmology contributed invaluably to the careful selection and proper preservation of the specimens. Her unselfish technical assistance is gratefully acknowledged.

The maintenance of the electron microscopes by Mr. Eugene W. Minner throughout the several years of specimen preparation was of immeasurable help. Special appreciation is extended to my wife Gunvor Rhodin for preparing the drawings.

Mrs. Betsey Stiepock, Administrative Associate of the Department of Anatomy, was most helpful in typing and proofreading.

Figures 2-22, 2-23, and 31-22 are reprinted by permission of National Tuberculosis and Respiratory Diseases Association; figures 4-25, 23-8, 23-9, and 16-32 by permission of Academic Press; figures 16-35, 16-38 and 16-41 by permission of Harper and Row; and figure 32-5 is redrawn and modified by permission of Dr. L. C. Junqueira and Dr. J. Carneiro.

The cooperation and enthusiasm of Mr. William C. Halpin, Vice-President, and of his staff at Oxford University Press throughout the preparation of the text are deeply and sincerely appreciated.

Contents

1 Introduction

WHAT IS HISTOLOGY?

Histology deals with the normal microscopical appearance of the body. It is the basis for the understanding of physiological and pathological processes. The light microscope is used to observe an organ, either *in vivo* or after its removal from the body. *In vivo* observations are restricted to observing the general, coarse texture of the component parts, as well as the pattern of blood flow. After the removal of an organ, it can be examined with both the light microscope and the electron microscope following preservation by fixative solutions, dehydration, embedding, sectioning, and staining. This results in the light microscopical slides used routinely in the histological laboratory and surgical pathology. Entire organs or parts thereof can be sectioned. (Fig. 1-1) For electron microscopy, only small pieces can be preserved at a time, and the sections must be extremely thin (100 Å–1000 Å).

Light microscopy relies on the staining of the sections to bring out variations in color. This is desirable since the resolving power of the light microscope is in the order of 0.2μ (2000 Å), and differences in optical density of various organ components are enchanced by the dye, aiding in the discrimination of one component from another. The electron microscope also relies on the staining of the sections, although to a lesser degree. The theoretical limit of the resolving power of the electron microscope is in the order of 2 Å. The practical limit of resolution in ultrathin sections is about 10 Å; in thin sections about 25 Å; and in thick sections about 50–100 Å. The resolving power (resolution) is dependent, therefore, on the thickness of the section and the wave length of the source of radiation. It is a linear measure of the smallest distance at which two structures can still be distinguished from each other. The following is a table for measuring structures in histology:

1 mm = 1000 microns (μ)
1 μ = 10,000 Angstrom units (Å)
In some texts, micron (μ) is often expressed as micrometer (μm) 1 μ = 1 μm.
Average diameter of a red blood cell = 7 μ
Average diameter of a ribosome = 200 Å

ORGAN COMPONENTS

Based on light and electron microscope observations, it has been established that organs consist of four primary tissues: epithelium, connective tissue, muscle tissue, and nervous tissue. Each tissue in turn consists of **cells** and **extracellular components.** Each cell consists of a cell membrane, the nucleus, organelles, and inclusions. All organs, tissues, cells, and cell organelles of the mammalian body are described in subsequent chapters.

Knowledge of the structural architecture of living substance and its components is only one aspect of understanding the intricate mechanisms involved in the functions of organs, tissues, cells, and organelles. Many techniques are now available to identify biochemically the many varied components. During the last two decades, a combination of light microscopy, electron microscopy, histochemistry, radioautography, cell fractionation, differential centrifugation, and cytochemistry has contributed greatly to a better understanding of structural and functional interrelationships. It is considered beyond the scope of this book to describe these techniques which are accounted for in detail in standard textbooks of research methods in cell biology.

GUIDE TO ILLUSTRATIONS

The illustrations in this book were obtained by photographing sectioned specimens under light and electron microscopes. In order to bring out differences in density between organs, tissues and cellular components, stains were applied to enhance the inherent light and electron density of a given structure.

In **light microscopy** the sections are stained with a variety of colored dyes, the most common being a combination of eosin and hematoxylin. The proteins of cells and extracellular components take on a red or pink color with eosin, whereas nucleic acids of the nuclei and certain components of the cytoplasm take on a deep blue color with hematoxylin. In **electron microscopy,** a solution of osmium tetroxide is used both as a general fixative and as an electron stain. In addition, salt solutions of heavy metals (lead, phosphotungstic acid) are used to enhance the electron density of tissue components. It should be kept in mind that these metals are not bound specifically to cellular or tissue components, although a **linear arrangement** of structures enhanced by the electron stain is generally accepted to indicate the location of membranes or filaments, whereas a **granular** configuration is believed to reflect a particulate arrangement of molecules. (Fig. 1-4)

The importance of staining a light microscope section by a variation of colored dyes is often overemphasized in the study of histological and pathological slides. Since the electron microscope cannot reproduce colors but depends entirely on differences in electron density of the tissue components, the light micrographs in this book are presented in black and white to facilitate the transition from light microscopy to electron microscopy. (Figs. 1-2, 1-3)

The adjectives **ultrastructural, submicroscopic,** and **fine structural** often used in contemporary textbooks of histology and cell biology express the details resolved by the electron microscope which lie beyond the resolving power of the light microscope.

Fig. 1-1. Section of entire organ. Kidney. Rabbit. L.M. X 15.5. This demonstrates the considerable amount of structural information which can be obtained at low magnification in the light microscope, if the tissue section is of proper thickness and the colored dyes carefully selected to show differences in optical density of different structures. **1.** Capsule. **2.** Cortex. **3.** Medulla. **4.** Pyramid. **5.** Papilla. **6.** Renal pelvis. **7.** Adipose tissue in renal sinus. **8.** Ureter. This section is enlarged further in Fig. 32-2 (p. 649).

Fig. 1-2. Proximal convoluted tubule of the nephron. Cross section. Enlargement of area similar to circle in Fig. 1-1. Kidney. Rabbit. L.M. × 1100. This demonstrates the practical limit of light microscopical resolution in a routinely prepared histological specimen. The preparation included formalin fixation, paraffin emebdding, and staining with hematoxylin and eosin. **1.** Lumen. **2.** Brush border zone. **3.** Nuclei.

Fig. 1-3. Proximal convoluted tubule of the nephron. Kidney. Rat. E.M. X 1100 (as in Fig. 1-2). This demonstrates the superiority of the preparation techniques and resolving power of the electron microscope. The tissue was fixed by intravascular perfusion of glutaraldehyde followed by intravascular perfusion of osmium tetroxide, embedding in epoxy resin, thin-sectioning, and staining with lead citrate. **1.** Lumen. **2.** Microvilli. **3.** Apical vacuoles (not present in Fig. 1-2). **4.** Nucleus. **5.** Cytoplasmic granules (mitochondria and secondary lysosomes). **6.** Peritubular capillary. Section of a similar area is enlarged further in Fig. 32-13 (p. 657).

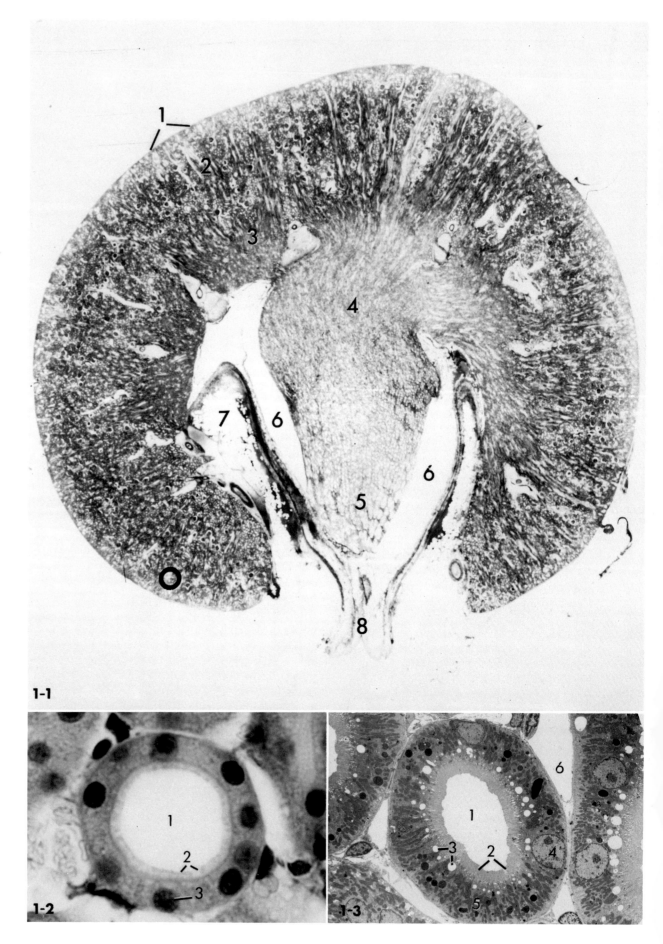

1-1

1-2

1-3

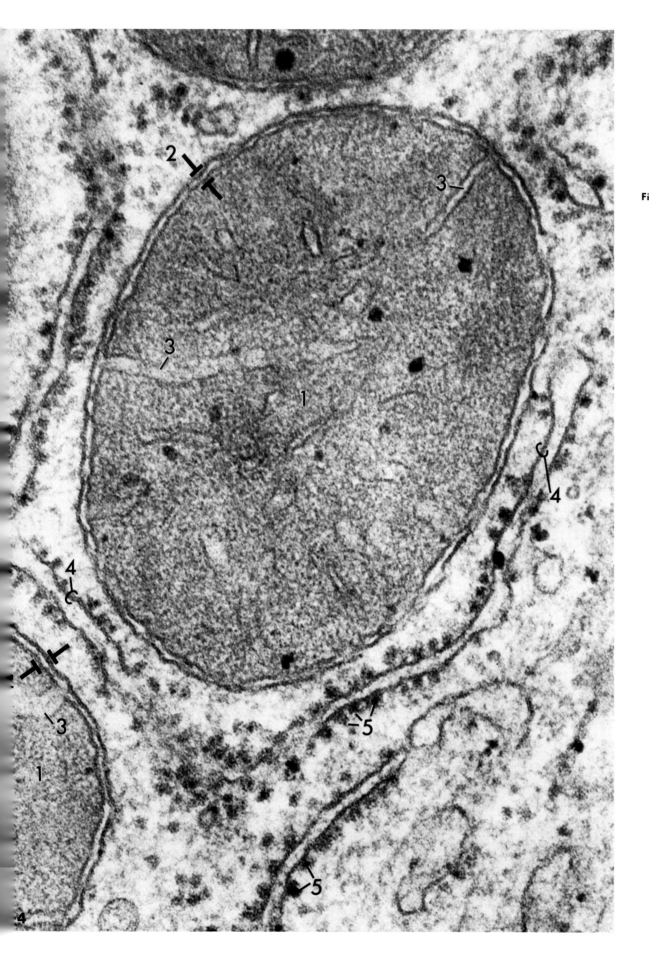

Fig. 1-4. Detail of parenchymal cell. Liver. Rat. E.M. X 160,000. This demonstrates the resolving power of the electron microscope and the enhancement of the electron density of linear and granular components of the cell by osmium tetroxide fixation and staining of the section with lead citrate. **1.** Mitochondria. **2.** Mitochondrial external envelope, total thickness 200 Å. Each dense linear component of this envelope is 60 Å thick and consists of three subunits, each averaging 20 Å in thickness. The resolution achieved in this electron micrograph is therefore approximately 20 Å. **3.** Mitochondrial cristae, each originating from the inner membranous component of the mitochondrial external envelope. **4.** Membrane of granular endoplasmic reticulum, 60 Å thick. This membrane also consists of three subunits, each 20 Å thick. **5.** Ribosomes, particles averaging 200 Å in diameter.

References

Hollenberg, M. J. and Erickson, A. M. The scanning electron microscope: potential usefulness to biologists. A review. J. Histochem. Cytochem. *21*: 109–130 (1973).

Kay, D. H. Techniques for Electron Microscopy. F. A. Davis Co., Philadelphia, 1965.

Pearse, A. G. E. Histochemistry, Theoretical and Applied. Third Edition, Little, Brown, Boston, 1968.

Pease, D. C. Histological Techniques for Electron Microscopy. Second Edition: Academic Press, New York, 1965.

Rogers, A. W. Techniques of Autoradiography. American Elsevier, New York, 1967.

Sjöstrand, F. S. Electron Microscopy of Cells and Tissues. Vol. I. Instrumentation and Techniques. Academic Press, New York, 1967.

Wied, G. L. (Ed.). Introduction to Quantitative Cytochemistry. Academic Press, New York, 1966.

2 Cells and organelles

Fig. 2-1. Macrophage. This connective tissue cell contains a fair representation of the many varied components of a mammalian cell. Interstitial tissue. Testis. Rat. E.M. X 22,000. **1.** Nuclear euchromatin. **2.** Nuclear heterochromatin. **3.** Nuclear envelope. **4.** Cell membrane. **5.** Microvilli or sheet-like cell processes. **6.** Pinocytic vesicles. **7.** Phagocytic vacuoles **8.** Phagosomes. **9.** Granular endoplasmic reticulum. **10.** Golgi apparatus. **11.** Mitochondria. **12.** Condensing vacuoles. **13.** Primary lysosomes. **14.** Secondary lysosomes. **15.** Extracellular collagenous fibrils.

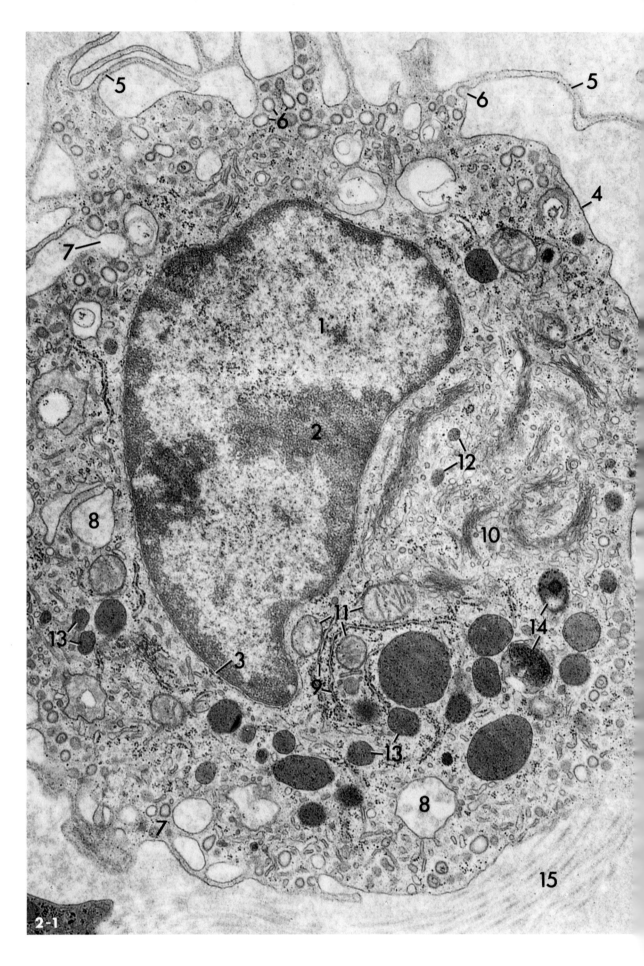

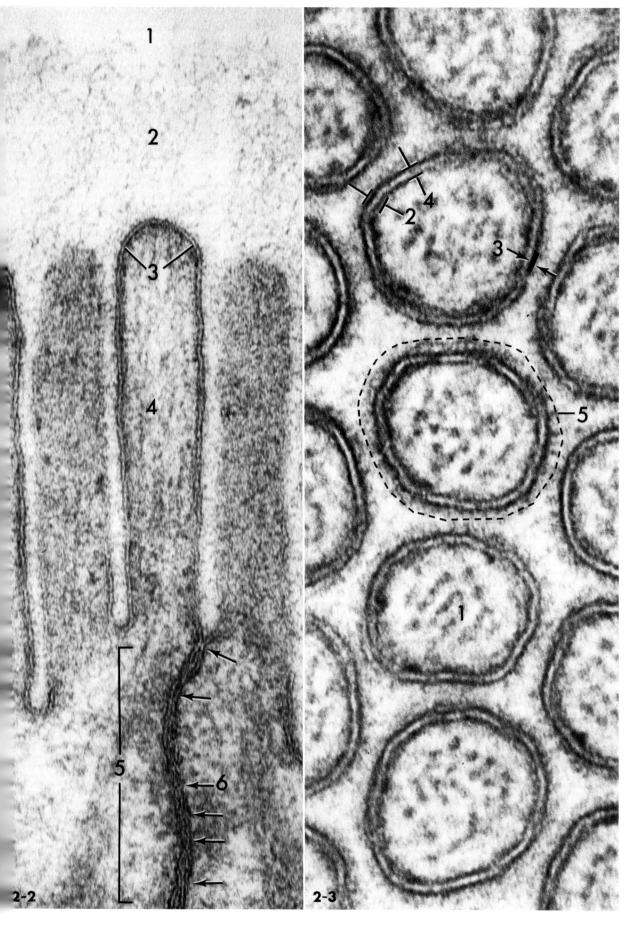

Fig. 2-2. Epithelial cell. Longitudinal section. Large intestine. Rat. E.M. X 211,000.
1. Lumen of gut. **2.** Finely filamentous glycoprotein coating (glycocalyx). **3.** Cell membrane. **4.** Microvillus. **5.** Tight junction (zonula occludens). **6.** Punctate contacts of fusion marked by **arrows**.

Fig. 2-3. Cross-sectioned microvilli. Epithelial cell. Large intestine. Rat. E.M. X 440,000. (1 mm=22 Å). **1.** Center of microvillus with core filaments, 45 Å in diameter.
2. Trilaminar cell membrane, 90 Å.
3. Electron-dense leaflet, 25 Å in diameter.
4. Electron-lucent middle layer, 35 Å in diameter. **5.** Dotted line indicates approximate height of glycoprotein surface layer (glycocalyx), 75 Å.

Fig. 2-4. Attachment devices of surface epithelial cells. Stomach. Rat. E.M. X 90,000.
1. Trilaminar cell membrane. **2.** Tight junction (zonula occludens). **3.** Intermediate junction (zonula adhaerens).

Fig. 2-5. Junctional complex of surface epithelial cells. Large intestine. Rat. E.M. X 155,000.
1. Tight junction. **2.** Intermediate junction.
3. Desmosome (macula adhaerens).

Fig. 2-6. Gap-junction. Parenchymal cells. Liver. Rat. E.M. X 124,000. **1.** Lumen of bile canaliculus. **2.** Gap-junction (nexus).
3. Intermediate junction. **4.** Agranular endoplasmic reticulum. **5.** Intercellular space of regular width.

Fig. 2-7. Gap-junction. Blood capillary. Cardiac muscle. Rat. E.M. X 128,000. **1.** Lumen of capillary. **2.** Endothelial cell cytoplasm.
3. Gap-junction. **4.** Possible punctate fusion of apposed cell membranes. **5.** Thin basal lamina.

Fig. 2-8. Surface epithelial cells, cross-sectioned at a slight angle. This demonstrates the distribution of the junctional complex in the ''horizontal'' plane. Jejunum. Rat. E.M. X 40,000. **1.** Base of microvilli. **2.** Core filaments. **3.** Tight junction between **arrows**.
4. Intermediate junction with parajunctional filamentous network. **5.** Desmosome.

Fig. 2-9. Desmosome (macula adhaerens). Epidermis. Human. E.M. × 114,000. **1.** Cell A.
2. Cell B. **3.** Intercellular space. **4.** Trilaminar cell membrane. **5.** Intercellular laminar density. **6.** Plate-like paradesmosomal material. **7.** Area of anchorage for cytoplasmic filaments.

Fig. 2-10. Stratified squamous epithelium, non-keratinized. Soft palate. Kitten. E.M. X 116,000. **1.** Cytoplasm of cell, detached in preparation for sloughing. **2.** Intercellular space. **3.** Cytoplasmic filaments (tonofilaments). **4.** Half desmosome. **5.** Inner leaflet of trilaminar cell membrane is thicker in this epithelial cell than in other cells, averaging 80 Å. **6.** Outer leaflet of cell membrane with filamentous glycocalyx.

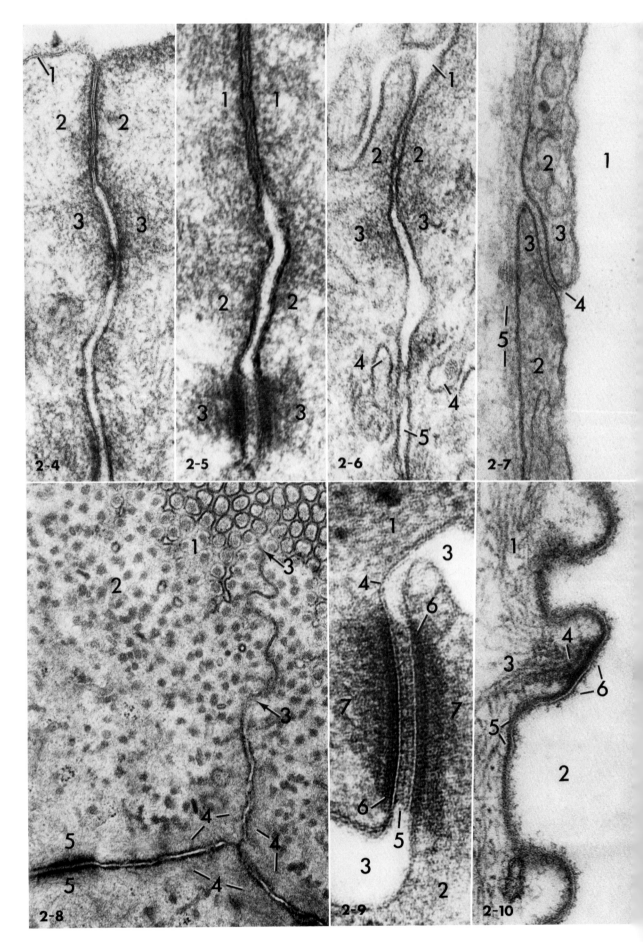

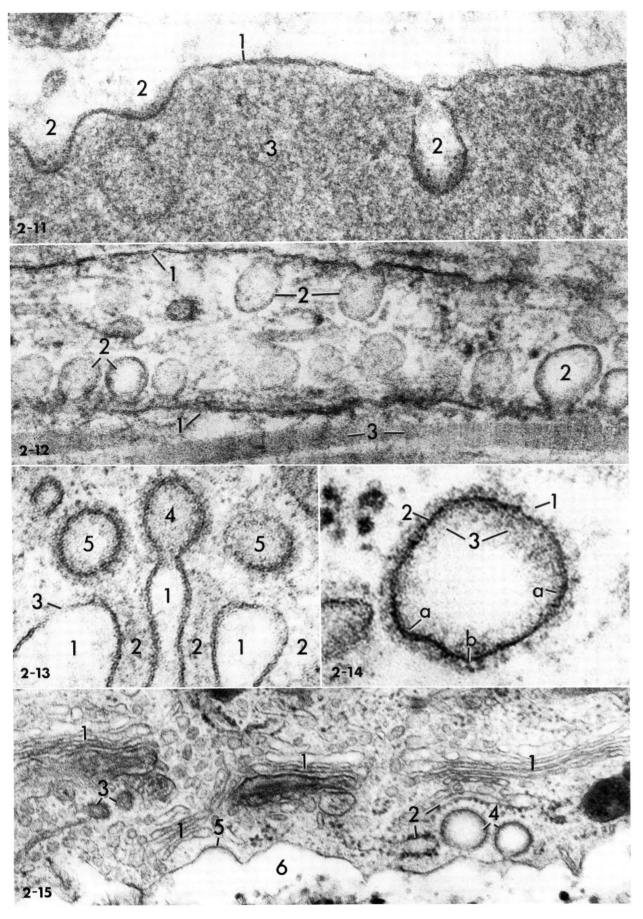

Fig. 2-11. Part of late erythroblast. Bone marrow. Human. E.M. X 128,000. **1.** Cell membrane (trilaminar structure not resolved). **2.** Different stages of **endocytosis.** Cytoplasmic aspect of pinocytic membrane is smooth, but a faint coating appears at the bottom of the invaginations. Ferritin particles appear as small, distinct dots within the coating. **3.** Hemoglobin.

Fig. 2-12. Part of cell process. Fibroblast. Urethra. Kitten. E.M. X 128,000. **1.** Cell membrane. **2.** Micropinocytic uncoated vesicles with trilaminar membranes. **3.** Collagenous fibril.

Fig. 2-13. Surface of macrophage. Interstitial tissue. Testis. E.M. X 165,000. **1.** Connective tissue space. **2.** Microvilli. **3.** Cell membrane. **4.** Coated pinocytic invagination. **5.** Coated pinocytic vesicles.

Fig. 2-14. Coated pinocytic vesicle. Macrophage. Interstitial tissue. Testis. Rat. E.M. X 240,000. **1.** External coating of spines or bristles. **2.** Boundary membrane, seen in a phase where the molecules of the membrane are rearranging from a trilaminar (a) to a unilaminar (b) structure. **3.** Internal lining of flocculent material.

Fig. 2-15. Surface of osteoblast. Diaphysis of radius. Two-day-old rat. E.M. X 66,000. **1.** Golgi zones (dictyosomes). **2.** Cisternae of granular endoplasmic reticulum. **3.** Small coated vesicles. **4.** Coated vesicles fusing with the cell membrane in a process of **exocytosis. 5.** Discharge of materials almost completed. **6.** Periosteoblastic connective tissue space.

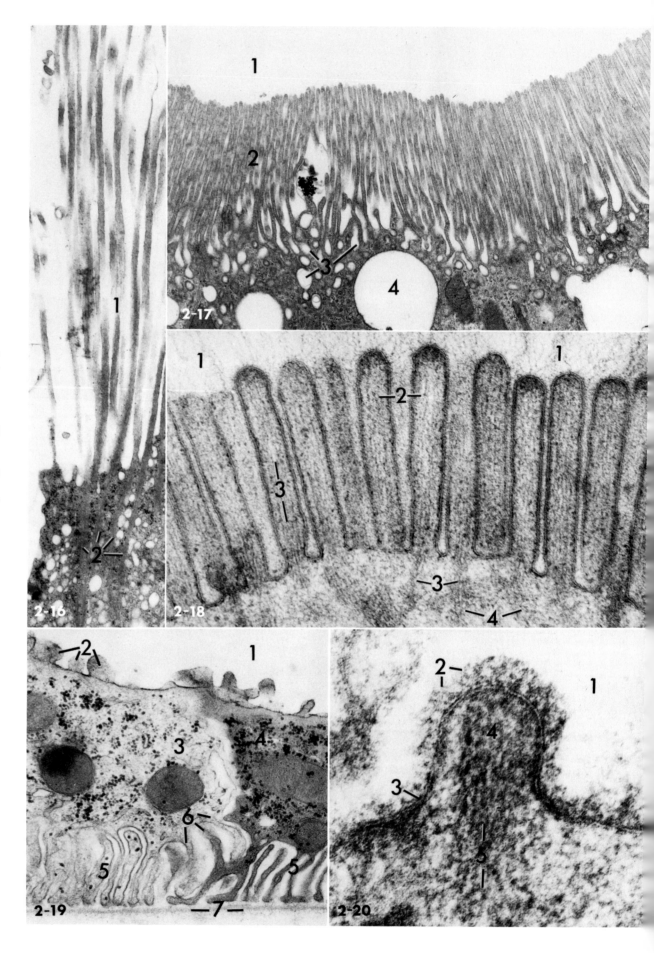

Fig. 2-16. Stereocilia. Epididymis. Rat. E.M. X 9000. **1.** Stereocilia, 10-15 μ long. **2.** Cores of filaments in apical cell cytoplasm.

Fig. 2-17. Brush border. Proximal tubule cell. Kidney. Rat. E.M. X 11,000. **1.** Lumen of tubule. **2.** Microvilli, 3 μ long. **3.** Pinocytic invaginations and vesicles. **4.** Enlarged pinocytic vesicle (apical vacuole).

Fig. 2-18. Striated border. Epithelial surface cell. Large intestine. Rat. E.M. X 92,000. **1.** Filaments of glycocalyx projecting into the gut lumen. **2.** Microvilli: length 0.6 μ; width 0.1 μ **3.** Core of filaments. **4.** Terminal web.

Fig. 2-19. Epithelial cells of distal tubule. Kidney. Rat. E.M. X 33,000. **1.** Lumen of tubule. **2.** Short microvilli. **3.** Cell with electron-lucent cytoplasm. **4.** Cell with electron-dense cytoplasm. **5.** Invagination of basal cell surface. **6.** Cytoplasmic lamellae of dark and light cells interdigitate. **7.** Basal lamina.

Fig. 2-20. Short microvillus. Epithelial surface cell. Stomach. Rat. E.M. X 189,000. **1.** Lumen of stomach. **2.** Glycocalyx. **3.** Trilaminar cell membrane. **4.** Microvillus; length 0.1 μ; width 0.1 μ. **5.** Core filaments.

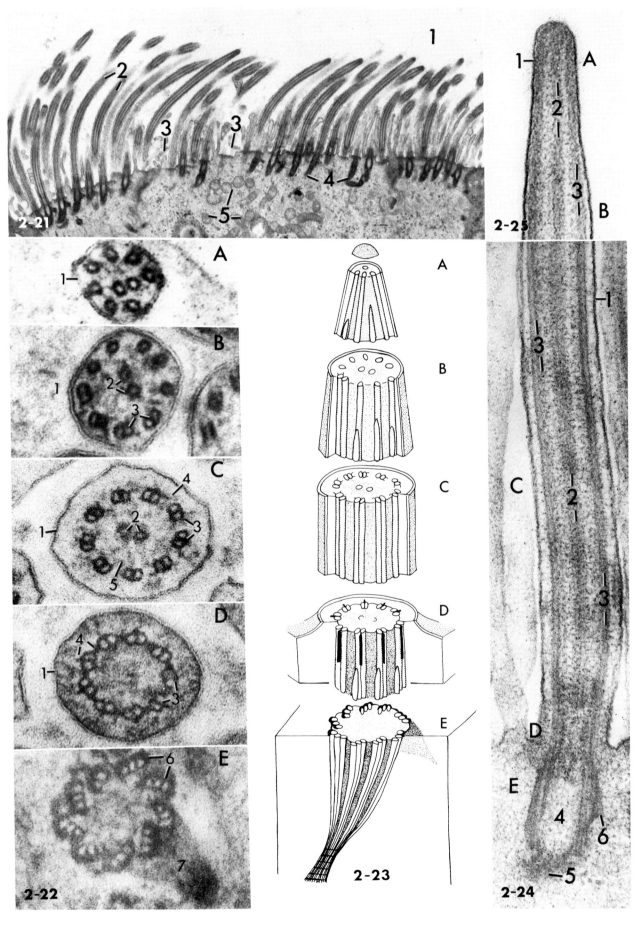

Fig. 2-21. Cilia. Epithelial cell. Oviduct. Rat. E.M. X 6200. **1.** Lumen. **2.** Cilia; length 6 μ; width 0.3 μ. **3.** Microvilli. **4.** Basal bodies, some with spurs. **5.** Mitochondria.

Fig. 2-22. Cross-sectioned cilia. Epithelial cell. Trachea. Human. E.M. X 144,000. **1.** Cell membrane. **2.** Central pair of microtubules. **3.** Peripheral doublets of microtubules. **4.** Arms. **5.** Faint radial spokes. **6.** Triplets of microtubules. **7.** Spur. **A, B, C, D,** and **E** correspond to levels of cilium indicated in Figs. 2-23, 2-24, and 2-25.

Fig. 2-23. Three-dimensional diagram of microtubular disposition in cilium and basal body. From Rhodin, Am. Rev. Respir. Dis. 93: 1 (1966). **A.** Tip of cilium. **B.** Tapering part of cilium. **C.** Middle part of cilium. **D.** Transitional, narrowed segment between cilium and basal body. **E.** Basal body.

Fig. 2-24. Longitudinally sectioned cilium. Respiratory nasal epithelium. Cat. E.M. X 68,000. **1.** Cell membrane. **2.** Central microtubules. **3.** Peripheral microtubules. **4.** Basal body. **5.** Rootlets. **6.** Spur.

Fig. 2-25. Tip of cilium. Trachea. Human. E.M. X 78,000. **1.** Cell membrane. **2.** Central microtubules. **3.** Peripheral microtubules.

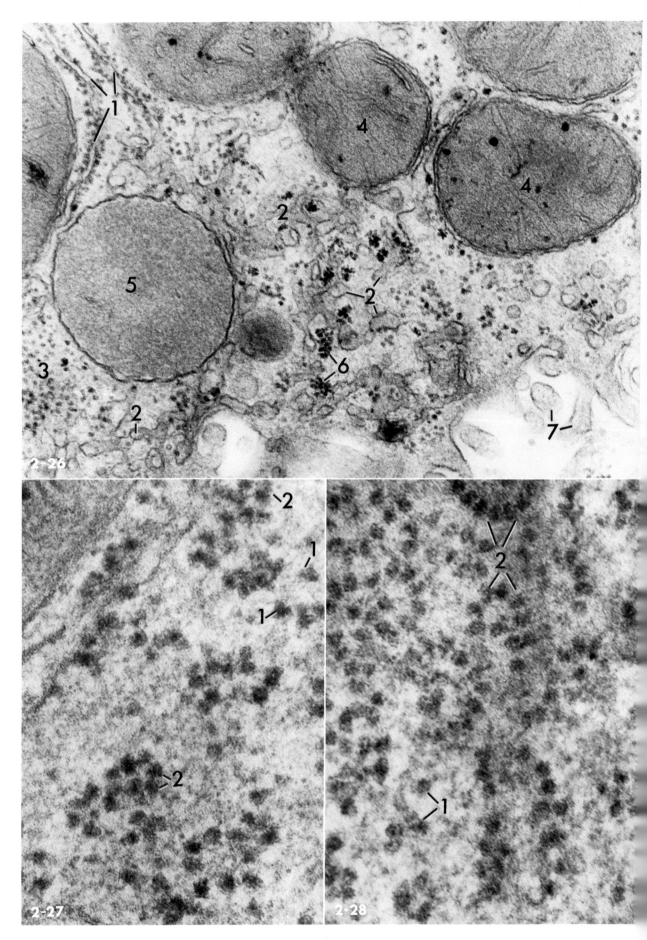

Fig. 2-26. Endoplasmic reticulum. Parenchymal cell. Liver. Rat. E.M. X 64,000. **1.** Cisternae of granular endoplasmic reticulum. **2.** Tubules of agranular endoplasmic reticulum. **3.** Free ribosomes. **4.** Mitochondria. **5.** Microbody. **6.** Glycogen particles. **7.** Surface microvilli projecting into space of Disse.

Fig. 2-27. Ribosomes. Epithelial cell of proximal tubule. Kidney. Rat. E.M. X 192,000. **1.** Free ribosomes, averaging 175 Å in diameter. **2.** Groups of ribosomes (polysomes).

Fig. 2-28. Ribosomes. Parenchymal cell. Liver. E.M. X 182,000. **1.** Free ribosomes. **2.** Groups of ribosomes (polysomes).

14

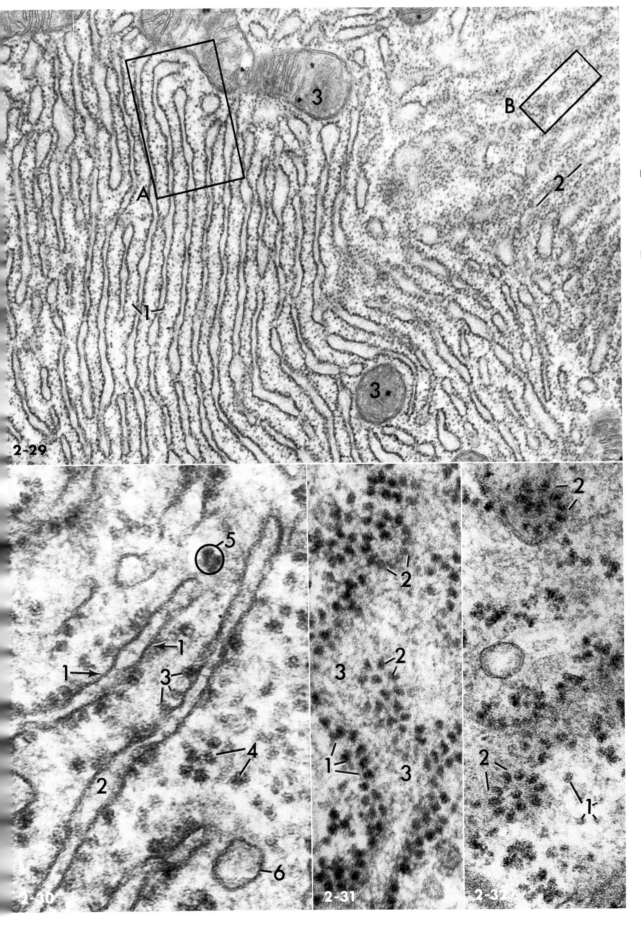

Fig. 2-29. Granular endoplasmic reticulum. Acinar cell. Pancreas. Mouse. E.M. X 35,000. **1.** Membranes and cisternae in parallel arrays, sectioned in a plane perpendicular to the membranes. **2.** Membranes sectioned tangentially. **3.** Mitochondria.

Fig. 2-30. Granular endoplasmic reticulum. Enlargement of area similar to rectangle (A) in Fig. 2-29. Parenchymal cell. Liver. E.M. X 173,000 (1 mm= 60 Å). **1.** Membranes of the granular endoplasmic reticulum, 60 Å in diameter. A trilaminar substructure is seen at arrows. **2.** Cisterna. **3.** Attached ribosomes. **4.** Free ribosomes. **5.** Circle: glycogen particles (alpha type). **6.** Cross-sectioned tubule of agranular endoplasmic reticulum.

Fig. 2-31. Tangentially sectioned membranes of granular endoplasmic reticulum. Enlargement of area similar to rectangle (B) in Fig. 2-29. Fibroblast. Urethra. Kitten. Rat. E.M. X 124,000. **1.** Ribosomes. **2.** Polysomes. **3.** Area of cisterna.

Fig. 2-32. Polysomes. Kupffer cell. Sinusoid. Liver. Rat. E.M. X 124,000. **1.** Free ribosomes. **2.** Polysome; 11 ribosomes seem to make up this particular polysome. The thin strand of connecting messenger RNA can be resolved only after cell fractionation and negative staining.

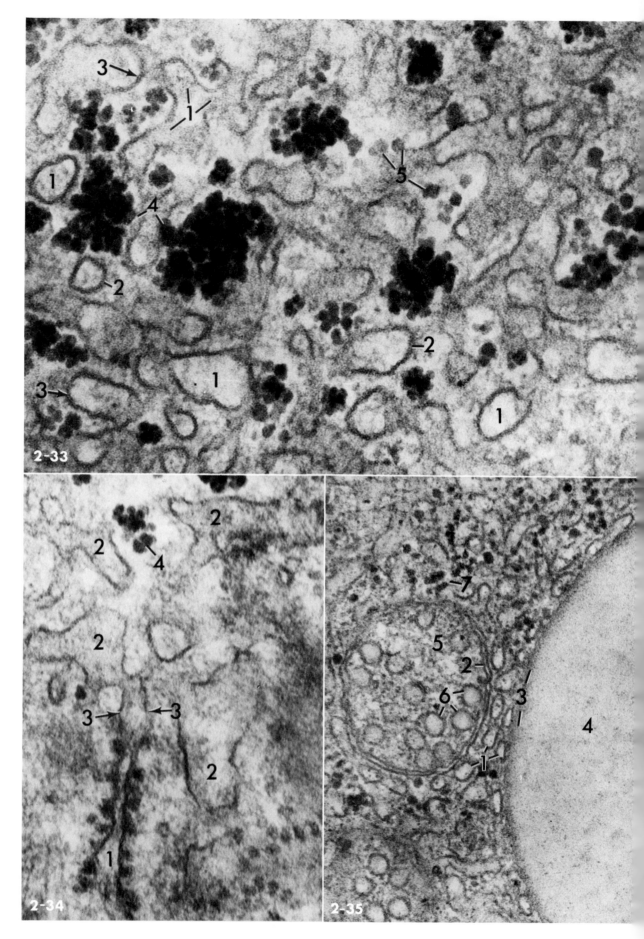

Fig. 2-33. Agranular endoplasmic reticulum. Parenchymal cell. Liver. Rat. E.M. X 166,000. **1.** Lumina of agranular, smooth tubules; average width 500 Å. **2.** Membrane of agranular endoplasmic reticulum; 60 Å in diameter. **3.** Indication of a trilaminar substructure at arrows. **4.** Glycogen particles (alpha type). **5.** Glycogen particles (beta type).

Fig. 2-34. Continuity of granular and agranular endoplasmic reticulum. Parenchyma cell. Liver. Rat. E.M. X 152,000. **1.** Cisterna and membranes of granular endoplasmic reticulum with attached ribosomes. **2.** Tubular profiles of agranular endoplasmic reticulum. **3.** Point of continuity between the two types of endoplasmic reticulum. **4.** Glycogen particles (alpha type).

Fig. 2-35. Relationship of agranular endoplasmic reticulum to other cytoplasmic components. Epithelial cell. Adrenal cortex. Zona fasciculata. Rat. E.M. X 98,000. **1.** Tubules and vesicles of agranular endoplasmic reticulum. **2.** Mitochondrial external envelope. **3.** Interface: cytoplasm/lipid droplet. **4.** Lipid droplet. **5.** Mitochondrial matrix. **6.** Vesicular cristae. **7.** Glycogen particles (beta type).

16

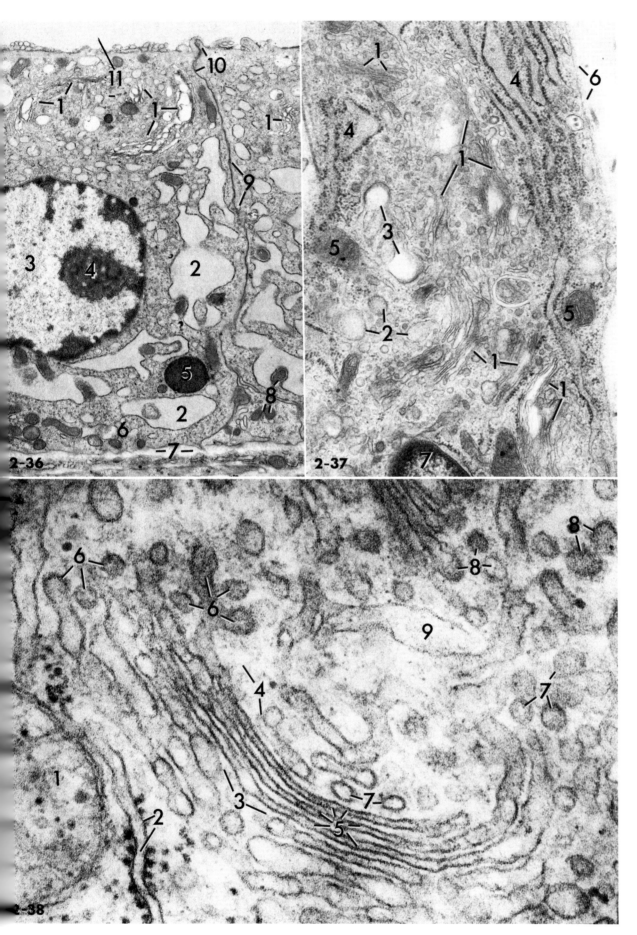

Fig. 2-36. Golgi apparatus. Epithelial cell. Prostate gland. Rat. E.M. X 9000. **1.** Golgi zones (dictyosomes). **2.** Dilated cisternae of granular endoplasmic reticulum. **3.** Nucleus. **4.** Nucleolus. **5.** Lysosome. **6.** Base of cell. **7.** Basal lamina. **8.** Mitochondria. **9.** Cell membranes. **10.** Junctional complex. **11.** Lumen of gland.

Fig. 2-37. Golgi apparatus. Fibroblast during active synthesis of tropocollagen. Dermis. Human. E.M. X 31,000. **1.** Golgi zones (dictyosomes). **2.** Condensing vacuoles. **3.** Coated vacuoles. **4.** Granular endoplasmic reticulum. **5.** Mitochondria. **6.** Cell membrane. **7.** Nucleus.

Fig. 2-38. Golgi apparatus. Macrophage. Interstitial tissue. Testis. Rat. E.M. X 120,000. **1.** Part of mitochondrion. **2.** Cisterna and membrane of granular endoplasmic reticulum. **3.** Forming, convex, face. **4.** Maturing, concave, face. **5.** Saccules. **6.** Vesicles "budding off" from saccule. **7.** Uncoated vesicles. **8.** Coated vesicles. **9.** Distended saccule.

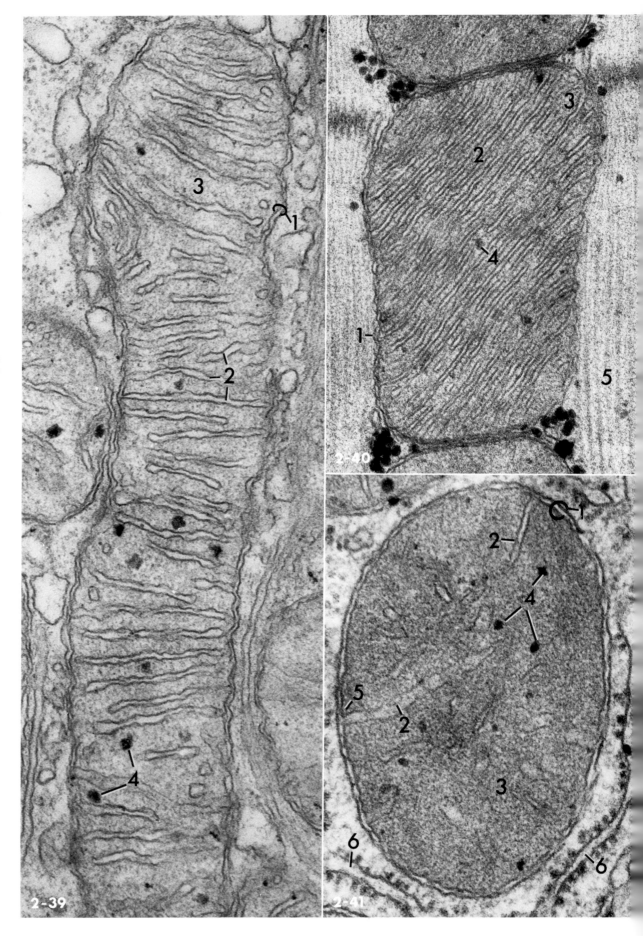

Fig. 2-39. Mitochondrion. Epithelial cell of proximal tubule. Kidney. Mouse. E.M. X 82,000. **1.** External envelope. **2.** Membranous, flat cristae. **3.** Matrix. **4.** Matrix granules.

Fig. 2-40. Mitochondrion. Muscle cell. Myocardium. Rat. E.M. X 93,000. **1.** Delicate external envelope. **2.** Densely packed membranous cristae. **3.** Sparse matrix. **4.** Matrix granule. **5.** Myofilaments.

Fig. 2-41. Mitochondrion. Parenchymal cell. Liver. Rat. E.M. X 114,000. **1.** External envelope. **2.** Small number of cristae, mostly membranous. **3.** Matrix abundant. **4.** Matrix granules. **5.** Mitochondrial crista originates from inner membranous component of external envelope. **6.** Profiles of granular endoplasmic reticulum.

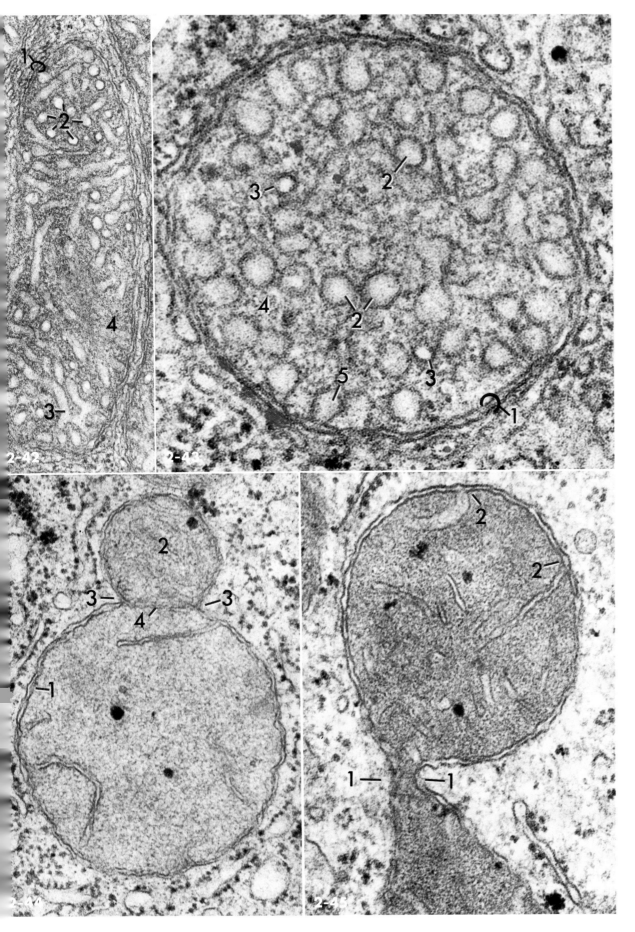

Fig. 2-42. Mitochondrion. Epithelial cell. Adrenal cortex. Zona reticularis. Rat. E.M. X 58,000. **1.** Delicate external envelope. **2.** Cross-sectioned tubular cristae. **3.** Longitudinally sectioned, interconnected tubular cristae. **4.** Sparse matrix.

Fig. 2-43. Mitochondrion. Epithelial cell. Adrenal cortex. Zona fasciculata. Rat. E.M. X 204,000. **1.** External envelope. **2.** Vesicular cristae. Their limiting membrane shows a trilaminar substructure. **3.** Cross-sectioned tubular cristae. **4.** Sparse matrix. **5.** Membrane of vesicular crista in continuity with inner membranous component of external envelope.

Fig. 2-44. Mitochondrial replication. Parenchymal cell. Liver. Rat. E.M. X 65,000. **1.** External envelope. **2.** Mitochondrial "bud." **3.** Constriction precedes separation of bud from maternal mitochondrion. **4.** Membranous cristae form separation plate.

Fig. 2-45. Mitochondrial replication. Parenchymal cell. Liver. Rat. E.M. X 96,000. **1.** Constriction and separation almost completed. **2.** Membranous cristae in continuity with inner membranous component of external envelope.

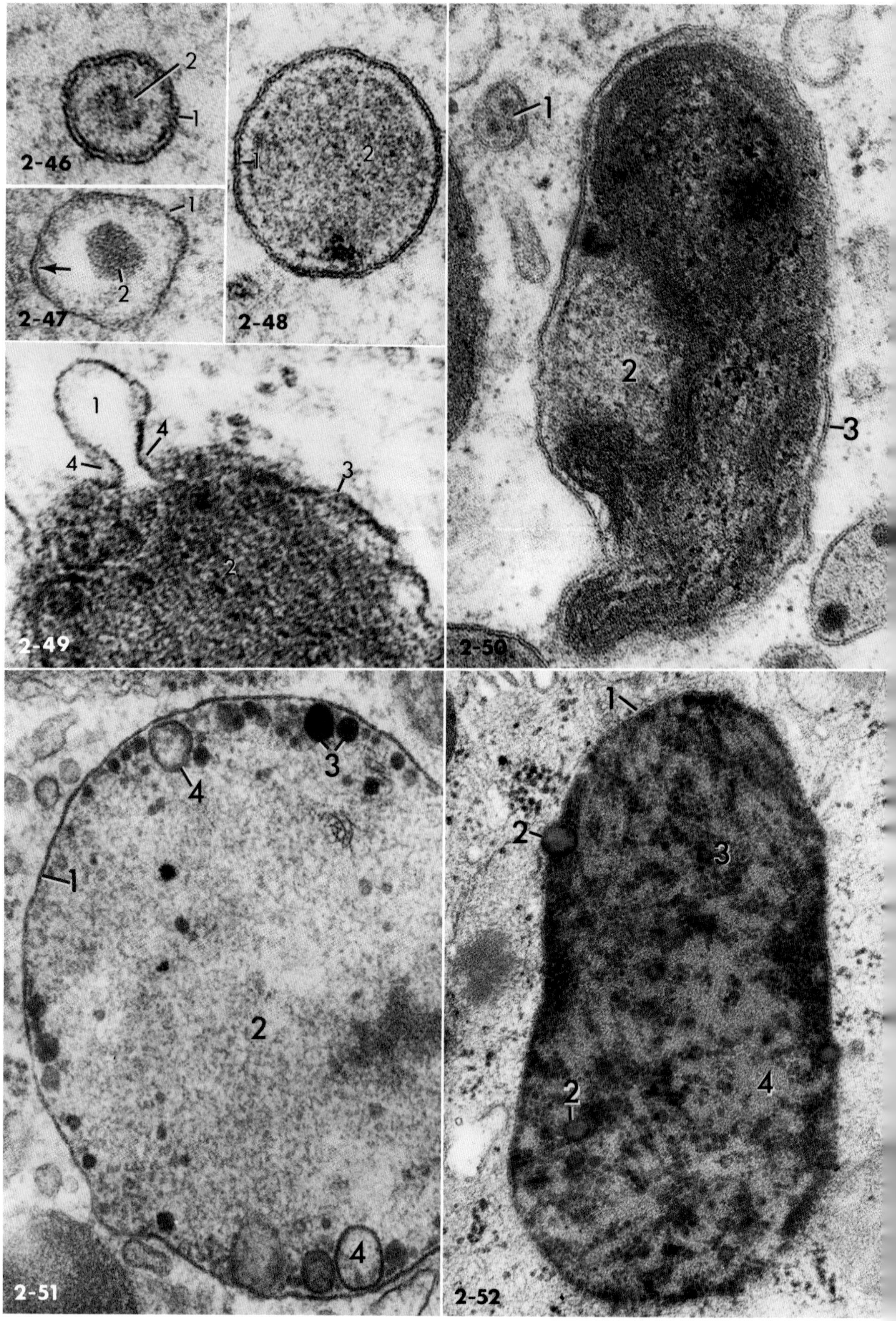

Fig. 2-46. Primary lysosome (0.1 μ wide). Kupffer cell. Liver. Rat. E.M. X 228,000.
1. Boundary membrane, 60 Å in diameter.
2. Condensing matrix.

Fig. 2-47. Phagosome. Kupffer cell. Liver. Rat. E.M. X 168,000. **1.** Boundary membrane of pinocytic vesicle appears single, except at **arrow** where it is trilaminar. **2.** Engulfed material.

Fig. 2-48. Primary lysosome (0.3 μ wide). Kupffer cell. Liver. Rat. E.M. X 140,000.
1. Boundary membrane, 60 Å in diameter.
2. Matrix.

Fig. 2-49. Fusion of pinocytic vesicle and primary lysosome, resulting in a secondary lysosome. Kupffer cell. Liver. Rat. E.M. X 156,000.
1. Pinocytic, uncoated vesicle. **2.** Matrix of primary lysosome. **3.** Boundary membrane.
4. Point of continuity between pinocytic vesicle and primary lysosome. *Note:* The possibility exists that this is a fusion between a small primary lysosome (1) and a secondary lysosome (2) at the moment when the latter receives an additional "shot" of hydrolytic enzymes.

Fig. 2-50. Lysosomes. Macrophage. Interstitial tissue. Testis. Rat. E.M. X 120,000.
1. Primary lysosome. **2.** Secondary lysosome with lipoprotein material being hydrolyzed.
3. Boundary membrane, 60 Å in diameter.

Fig. 2-51. Secondary lysosome (residual body). Kupffer cell. Liver. Rat. E.M. X 84,000.
1. Boundary membrane, 60 Å in diameter.
2. Matrix. **3.** Lipid droplets. **4.** Vesicles.

Fig. 2-52. Lipofuscin granule. Odoriferous sweat gland. Axilla. Human. E.M. X 60,000.
1. Boundary membrane (difficult to resolve because of dense granule content). **2.** Lipid droplets. **3.** Minute, highly electron-dense particles of unknown nature. **4.** Matrix.

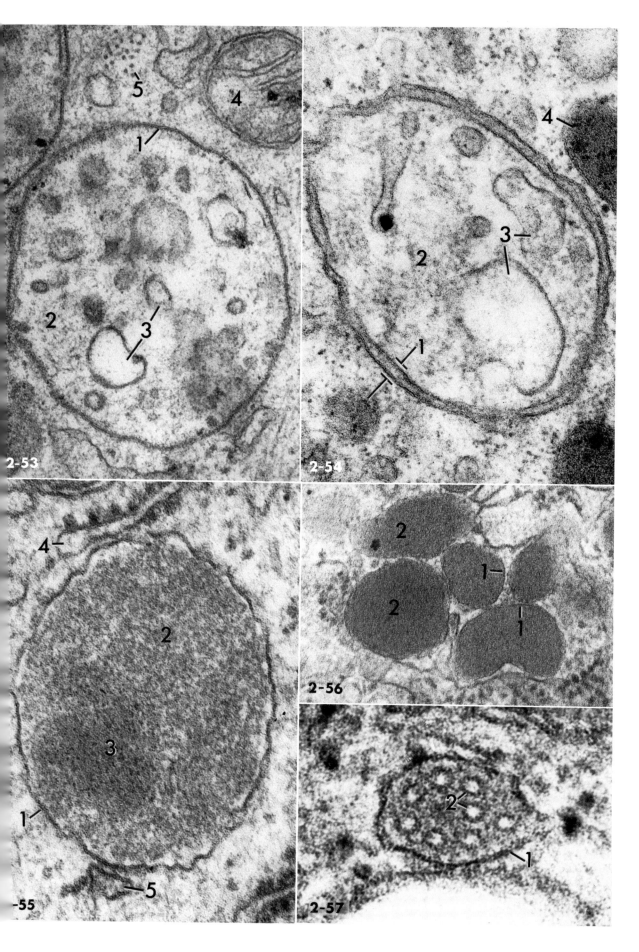

Fig. 2-53. Multivesicular body. Kupffer cell. Liver. Rat. E.M. X 96,000. **1.** Boundary membrane, 60 Å in diameter. **2.** Electron-lucent matrix. **3.** Vesicles of varied diameters. **4.** Mitochondrion. **5.** Filaments.

Fig. 2-54. Autosome (autophagic vacuole). Macrophage. Interstitial tissue. Testis. Rat. E.M. X 105,000. **1.** Boundary membrane consists of two trilaminar membranes, total diameter 270 Å. **2.** Matrix density similar to that of surrounding cytoplasm. **3.** Vesicles and membranes. **4.** Part of secondary lysosome.

Fig. 2-55. Microbody (peroxisome). Parenchymal cell. Liver. Rat. E.M. X 135,000. **1.** Boundary membrane, 60 Å in diameter. **2.** Matrix. **3.** Area of crystalloid (no substructure resolved in this illustration). **4.** Profile of granular endoplasmic reticulum. **5.** Profile of agranular endoplasmic reticulum.

Fig. 2-56. Specific endothelial granules. Pulmonary vein. Rat. E.M. X 108,000. **1.** Boundary membrane, 40 Å in diameter. **2.** Matrix.

Fig. 2-57. Specific endothelial granule. Renal vein. Rat. E.M. X 268,000. **1.** Boundary membrane. **2.** Component tubules, cross-sectioned, averaging 200 Å in diameter.

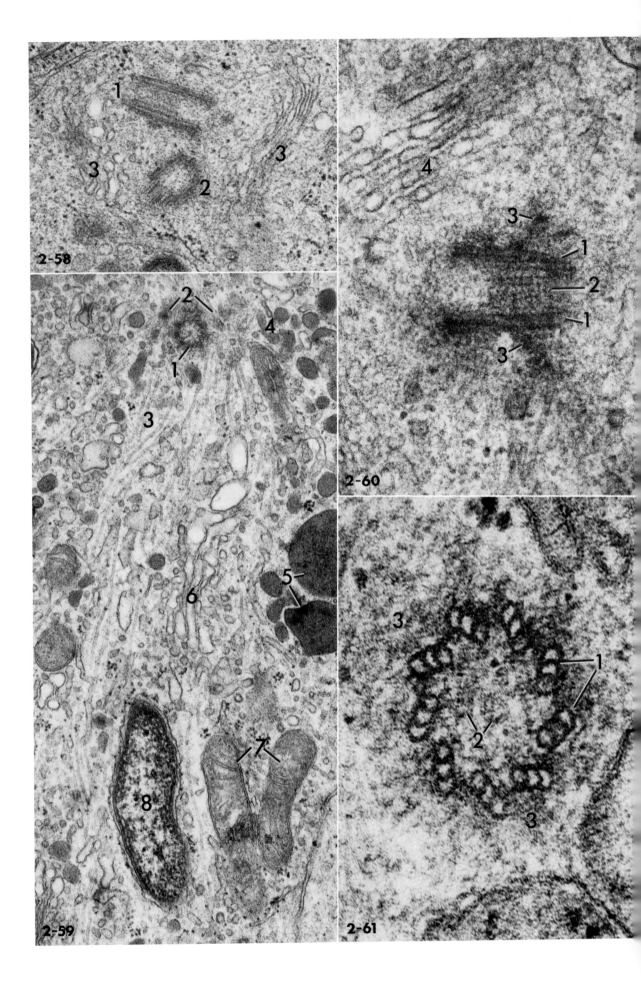

Fig. 2-58. Two centrioles (one diplosome). Macrophage. Spleen. Rat. E.M. X 54,000. **1.** Longitudinally sectioned centriole. **2.** Obliquely sectioned centriole. **3.** Golgi zones (dictyosomes).

Fig. 2-59. Macrophage. Spleen. Rat. E.M. X 38,000. **1.** Centriole. **2.** Pericentriolar satellites (centrosphere). **3.** Microtubules. **4.** Primary lysosomes. **5.** Secondary lysosomes. **6.** Golgi apparatus. **7.** Mitochondria. **8.** Lobe of nucleus.

Fig. 2-60. Longitudinally sectioned centriole. Myelocyte. Bone marrow. Human. E.M. X 94,000. **1.** Peripheral microtubules. **2.** Location of spiral filament (not resolved unequivocally). **3.** Pericentriolar satellites (centrosphere). **4.** Golgi apparatus.

Fig. 2-61. Cross-sectioned centriole. Epithelial surface cell. Large intestine. Rat. E.M. X 245,000. **1.** Triplets of fused microtubules. **2.** Faint indication of spiral filament and "cartwheel" configuration. **3.** Centrosphere.

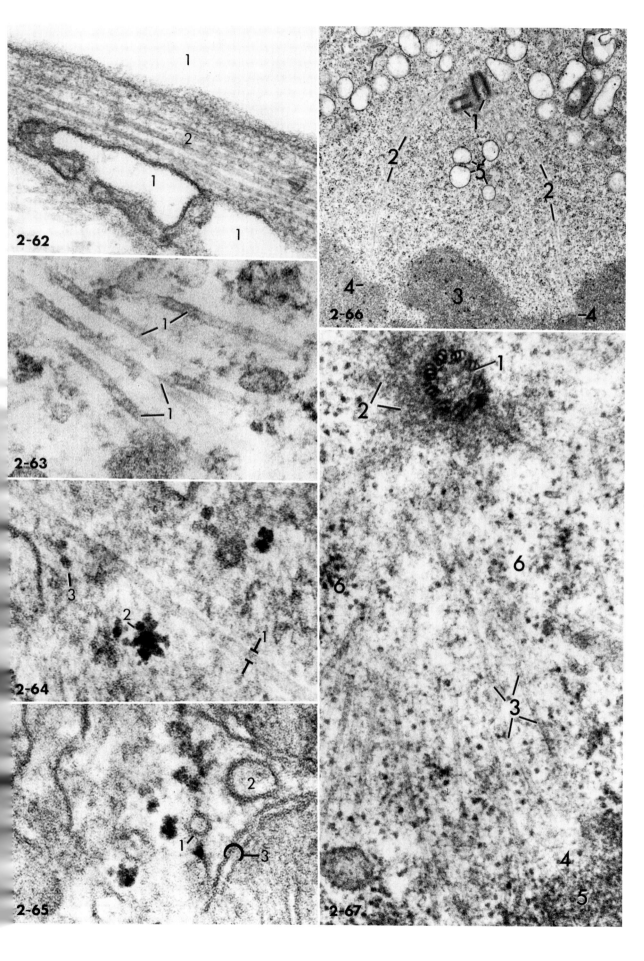

Fig. 2-62. Microtubules. Endothelial cell. Peritubular capillary. Kidney. Rat. E.M. X 70,000. **1.** Lumen of capillary. **2.** Bundle of parallel microtubules in endothelial cytoplasm.

Fig. 2-63. Microtubules. Kupffer cell. Liver. Rat. E.M. X 137,000. **1.** Microtubules, average width 250 Å.

Fig. 2-64. Parenchymal cell. Liver. Rat. E.M. X 161,000. **1.** Microtubule; width between T-bars: 270 Å. **2.** Glycogen particles (alpha type). **3.** Glycogen particles (beta type).

Fig. 2-65. Parenchymal cell. Liver. Rat. E.M. X 178,000. **1.** Cross-sectioned microtubule. **2.** Cross-sectioned tubule of agranular endoplasmic reticulum. **3.** Mitochondrial external envelope.

Fig. 2-66. Part of mitotic spindle. Metaphase of dividing membrana granulosa cell. Follicle. Ovary. Rat. E.M. X 17,000. **1.** Two centrioles (at right angles to each other). **2.** Spindle microtubules. **3.** Chromosomes in equatorial plate. **4.** Kinetochore regions. **5.** Vesicular profiles of endoplasmic reticulum.

Fig. 2-67. Metaphase. Dividing membrana granulosa cell. Follicle. Ovary. Rat. E.M. X 75,000. **1.** Centriole with central "cartwheel" configuration. **2.** Centrosphere (pericentriolar satellites). **3.** Spindle microtubules. **4.** Kinetochore region. **5.** Chromosomal material. **6.** Ribosomes.

Fig. 2-68. Tonofilaments. Superficial cell of stratified squamous, non-keratinized epithelium. Soft palate. Kitten. E.M. X 84,000. **1.** Filaments, averaging 75 Å in diameter. **2.** Fibrils (= bundle of filaments).

Fig. 2-69. Cytoplasmic filaments. Endothelial cell. Aorta. Squirrel monkey. E.M. X 93,000. **1.** Lumen of aorta. **2.** Cell membrane. **3.** Pinocytic invaginations. **4.** Specific endothelial granule. **5.** Cytoplasmic filaments, averaging 80 Å in diameter, some with a minute, electron-lucent core.

Fig. 2-70. Myofilaments. Skeletal muscle. Rat. E.M. X 66,000. **1.** Thin actin filaments, 50 Å in diameter. **2.** Zone of thin filament attachment (Z-line). **3.** Glycogen particles (beta type). **4.** Zone of interdigitating thin and thick filaments (A-band). **5.** Thick myosin filaments. **6.** Zone of laterally interconnected thick filaments (M-band).

Fig. 2-71. Myofilaments. Cross-sectioned. Skeletal muscle. Rat. E.M. X 132,000. **1.** Thin filaments. **2.** Thick filaments.

Fig. 2-72. Microtubules and filaments. Tail of spermatozoon. Cross-sectioned. Testis. Rat. E.M. X 104,000. **1.** Central pair of microtubules. **2.** Peripheral 9 doublets of fused microtubules, one of which has an electron-dense core, and therefore could be classified as filament. **3.** Minute longitudinal filaments. **4.** Longitudinal fibrous columns. **5.** Rib of fibrous sheath. **6.** Cell membrane.

Fig. 2-73. Neurofilaments. Axon of sciatic nerve fiber. Rat. E.M. X 93,000. **1.** Neurofilaments, 55 Å in diameter. **2.** Microtubules, 225 Å in diameter.

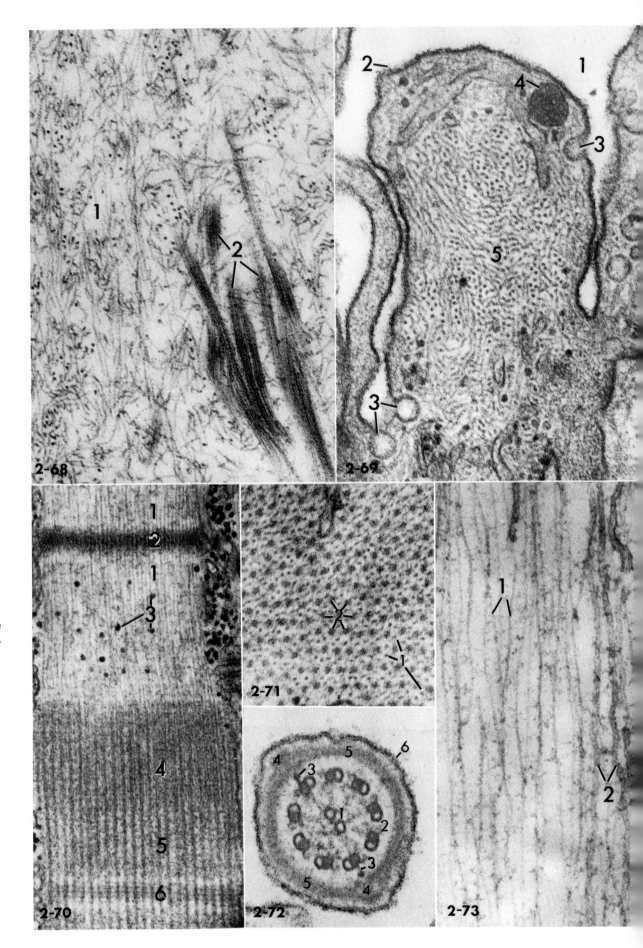

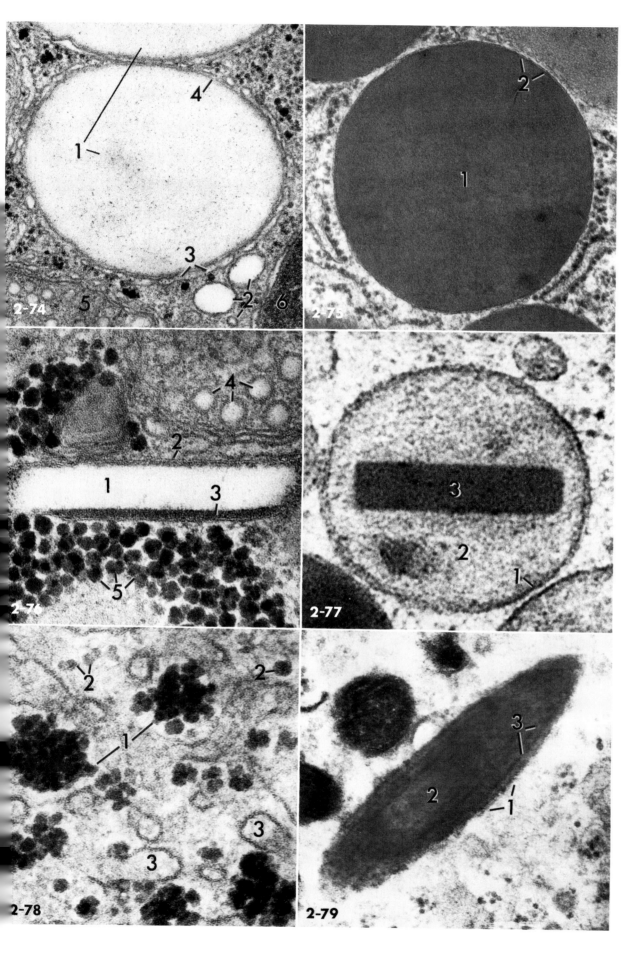

Fig. 2-74. Lipid droplets. Epithelial cell. Adrenal cortex. Zona fasciculata. Rat. E.M. X 100,000. **1.** Large lipid droplet. **2.** Developing lipid droplets. **3.** Casing of merging tubules of agranular endoplasmic reticulum. **4.** Interface membrane; cytoplasm/lipid droplet. **5.** Mitochondrion. **6.** Part of nucleus.

Fig. 2-75. Proteinaceous secretory granule. Serous gland. Tongue. Rat. E.M. X 108,000. **1.** Secretory granule. **2.** Boundary membrane.

Fig. 2-76. Cholesterol crystal in lysosome. Epithelial cell. Adrenal cortex. Zona fasciculata. Rat. E.M. X 180,000. **1.** Cholesterol crystal (dissolved). **2.** Boundary membrane (trilaminar) of lysosome. **3.** Matrix of lysosome. **4.** Vesicular mitochondrial cristae. **5.** Glycogen particles (beta type).

Fig. 2-77. Lipoprotein crystal in lysosome. Eosinophilic leukocyte. Mouse. E.M. X 134,000. **1.** Boundary membrane of lysosome (specific eosinophilic granule). **2.** Matrix. **3.** Lipoprotein crystal.

Fig. 2-78. Glycogen particles. Parenchymal cell. Liver. Rat. E.M. X 166,000. **1.** Alpha particles. **2.** Beta particles. **3.** Tubules of agranular endoplasmic reticulum.

Fig. 2-79. Pigment granules (melanosomes). Epidermal cell. Skin. Squirrel monkey. E.M. X 90,000. **1.** Delicate boundary membrane (mostly obscured). **2.** Dense core of melanosome. **3.** Filaments.

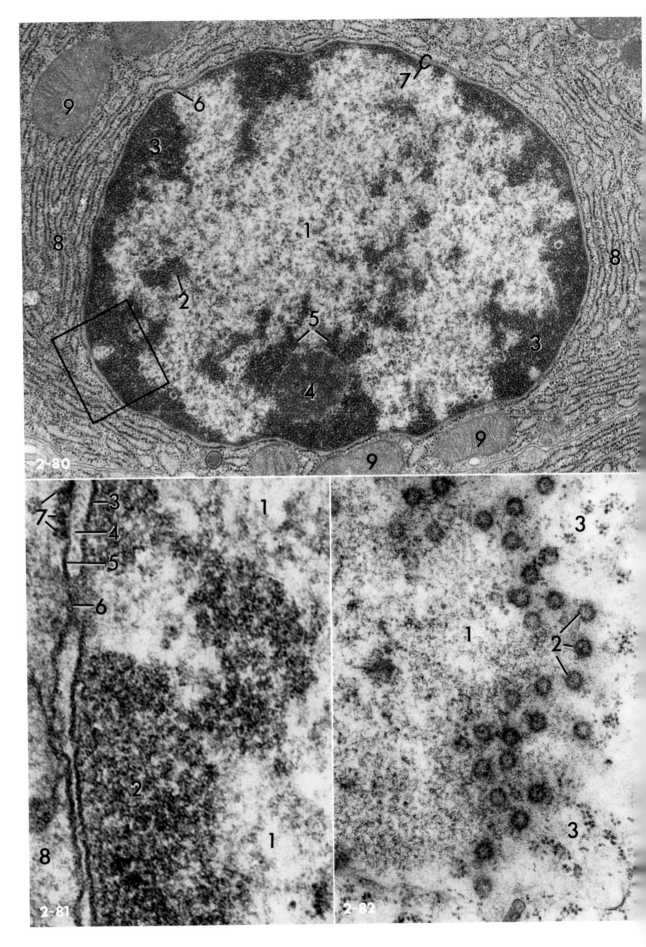

Fig. 2-80. Interphase (intermitotic) nucleus. Acinar cell. Pancreas. Rat. E.M. X 24,000. **1.** Electron-lucent euchromatin. **2.** Electron-dense heterochromatin (karyosome). **3.** Marginated heterochromatin. **4.** Nucleolus. **5.** Nucleolus-associated chromatin. **6.** Nuclear pore. **7.** Nuclear envelope. **8.** Granular endoplasmic reticulum. **9.** Mitochondria.

Fig. 2-81. Nuclear margin. Enlargement of area similar to rectangle in Fig. 2-80. Parenchymal cell. Liver. Rat. E.M. X 184,000. **1.** Euchromatin. **2.** Chromatin particles of marginated dense heterochromatin. **3.** Inner nuclear membrane. **4.** Perinuclear cisterna. **5.** Outer nuclear membrane. **6.** Nuclear pore with diffuse plug-like substance. **7.** Ribosomes attached to outer nuclear membrane. **8.** Cytoplasm.

Fig. 2-82. Tangential section of nuclear envelope. Spermatocyte Testis. Mouse. E.M. X 51,000. **1.** Chromatin particles of nucleus. **2.** Annuli of nuclear pores. **3.** Ribosomes of cytoplasm.

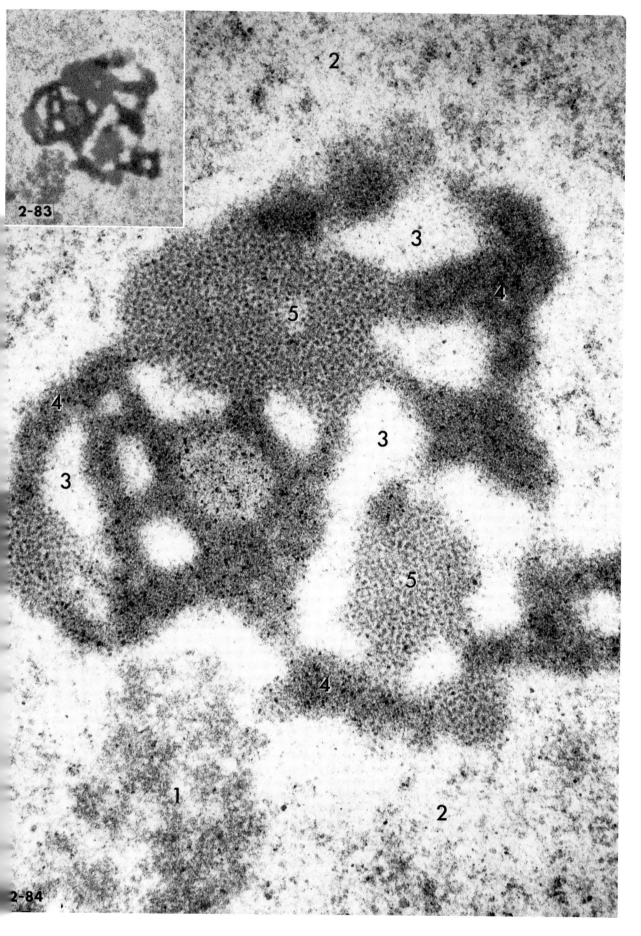

Fig. 2-83. Nucleolus. Primary oocyte. Ovary. Rat. E.M. X 22,000.

Fig. 2-84. Nucleolus. Enlargement of Fig. 2-83. E.M. X 90,000. **1.** Nucleolar-associated heterochromatin. **2.** Euchromatin. **3.** Pars amorpha of nucleolus. **4.** Filamentous part of nucleolonema. **5.** Nucleolar ribosomes of nucleolonema; particles averaging 110 Å in diameter.

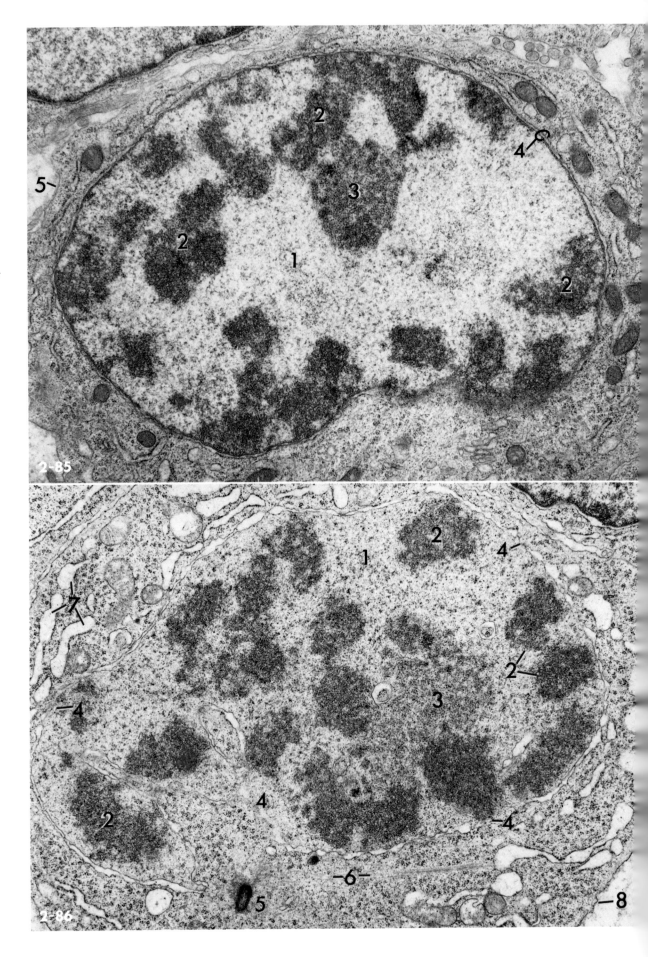

Fig. 2-85. Early prophase nucleus. Membrana granulosa cell. Follicle. Ovary. Rat. E.M. X 15,000. **1.** Euchromatin (less electron-dense than cytoplasm). **2.** Contracting (condensing) areas of heterochromatin (= chromosomes). Nuclear DNA has now replicated. **3.** Nucleolus beginning to disperse. **4.** Nuclear enveope still intact. **5.** Cell membrane.

Fig. 2-86. Late prophase nucleus. Membrana granulosa cell. Follicle. Ovary. Rat. E.M. X 15,000. **1.** Euchromatin (now same electron density as cytoplasm). **2.** Chromosomes. **3.** Nucleolus further dispersed (compared to Fig. 2-85). **4.** Nuclear envelope starts to disintegrate. **5.** Centriole. **6.** Spindle microtubules. **7.** Elements of endoplasmic reticulum. **8.** Cell membrane.

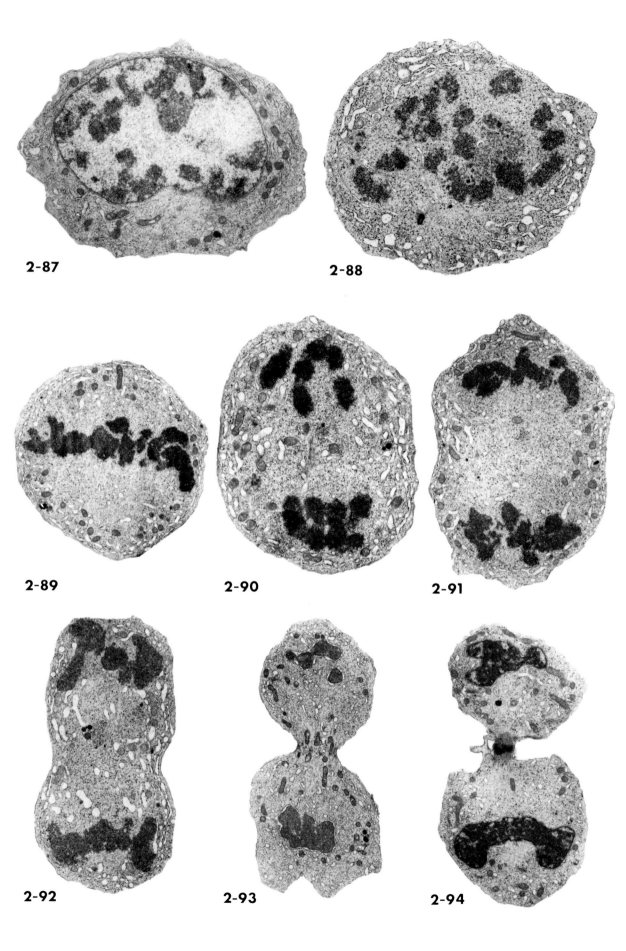

2-87

2-88

2-89

2-90

2-91

2-92

2-93

2-94

Figs. 2-87 through 2-94. Some of the more obvious stages of **mitotic division** have been selected from dividing membrana granulosa cells of the rat ovary. They have been arranged to facilitate the study of nuclear, chromosomal, and cytoplasmic changes during division of a mammalian cell. Centrioles are not seen in most of the illustrations, since these organelles are not always in the plane of section. In contrast to some plant and vertebrate cells which are anastral, centrioles are always present during cell division in mammalian cells. The cells are not shown at the same magnifications since eight dividing cells would not fit into the space allotted. The purpose of this display is to give a quick overview of mitosis as it appears with the resolving power of the electron microscope. Membrana granulosa cells. Follicle. Ovary. Rat.

Fig. 2-87. Early prophase. Enlarged in Fig. 2-85. E.M X 5600.

Fig. 2-88. Late prophase. Enlarged in Fig. 2-86. E.M. X 5600.

Fig. 2-89. Metaphase. Chromosomes lined up in the equatorial plate. Similar cell enlarged further in Fig. 2-95. E.M. X 4500.

Fig. 2-90. Late anaphase. Chromosomes have separated and almost arrived at opposite cell poles. E.M. X 5500.

Fig. 2-91. Early telophase. Cytoplasmic furrow starts to appear. E.M. X 4400.

Fig. 2-92. Early telophase. Cytoplasmic furrow deepens. E.M. X 4500.

Fig. 2-93. Mid-telophase. Nuclear envelope reappears. Cytoplasmic cleavage furrow quite deep. Enlarged further in Fig. 2-97. E.M. X 3600.

Fig. 2-94. Late telophase. Mid-body present. Enlarged further in Figs. 2-98 and 2-99. E.M. X 5200.

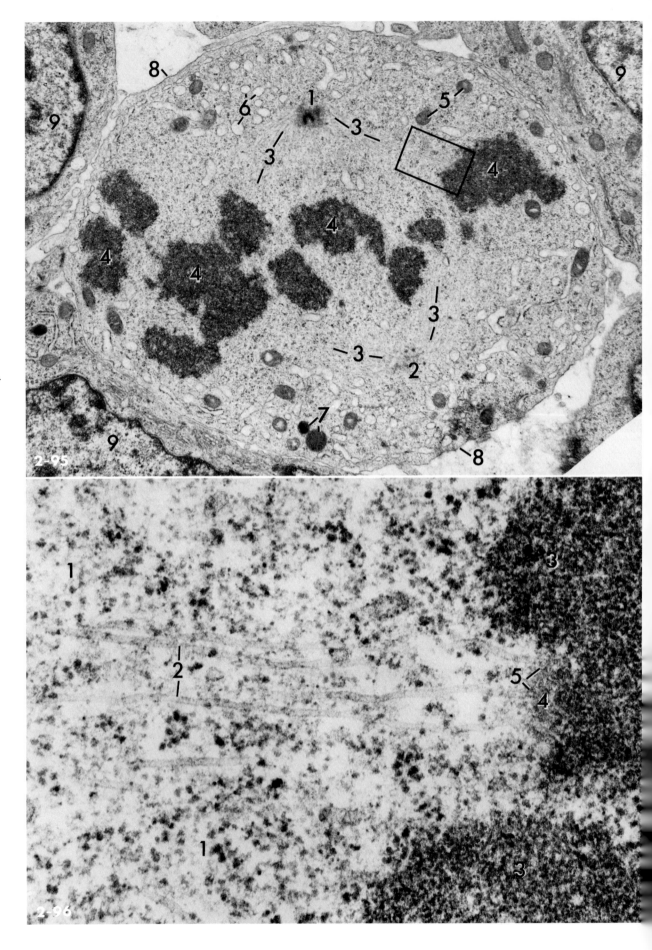

Fig. 2-95. Metaphase. Membrana granulosa cell.
Follicle. Ovary. Rat. E.M. X 15,000.
  1. Centriole with dense centrosphere.
  2. Pericentriolar satellites (centrosphere).
  3. Mitotic spindle microtubules.
  4. Chromosomes in equatorial plate.
  5. Mitochondria. **6.** Vacuolar and tubular
profiles of endoplasmic reticulum.
  7. Lysosomes. **8.** Cell membrane. **9.** Nuclei
of neighboring cells of membrana granulosa.

Fig. 2-96. Kinetochore. Enlargement of area
similar to rectangle in Fig. 2-95. **Metaphase.**
Membrana granulosa cell. Follicle. Ovary. Rat.
E.M. X 58,000. **1.** Ribosomes. **2.** Microtubules
of mitotic spindle, averaging 250 Å in width.
  3. Particulate structure of chromosomes.
  4. Amorphous structures of kinetochore.
  5. Insertion and/or penetration of mitotic
spindle microtubules.

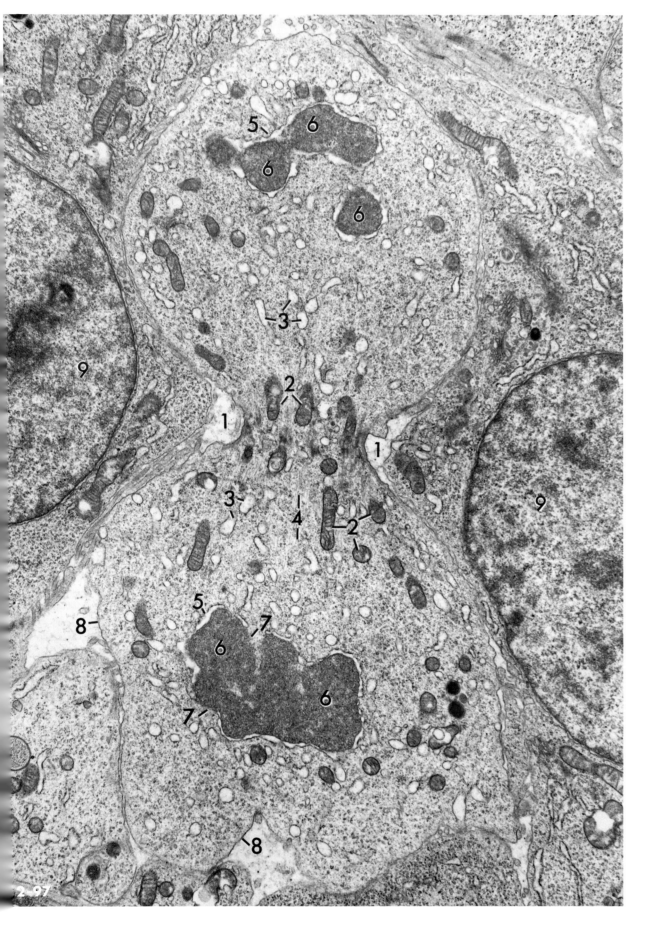

Fig. 2-97. Mid-telophase. Membrana granulosa cell. Follicle. Ovary. Rat. E.M. X 11,500.
1. Deep cytoplasmic cleavage furrow.
2. Mitochondria. **3.** Profiles of endoplasmic reticulum. **4.** Remaining spindle microtubules.
5. Formation of nuclear envelope.
6. Chromosomes. **7.** Some imperfections in nuclear envelope. **8.** Cell membrane. **9.** Nuclei of neighboring cells of membrana granulosa.

Fig. 2-98. Late telophase (immediately preceding cell separation). Membrana granulosa cell. Follicle. Ovary. Rat. E.M. X 15,000.
1. Cleavage furrow extremely deep. **2.** Midbody. **3.** Nuclear membrane completely surrounding the chromosomes.
4. Chromosomes start to become dispersed (uncoiled) and areas of electron-lucent euchromatin reappear. **5.** Remnants of spindle microtubules. **6.** Mitochondria. **7.** Endoplasmic reticulum. **8.** Cell membrane. **9.** Nuclei of neighboring cells of membrana granulosa.

Fig. 2-99. Mid-body (intermediate body). Late telophase. Membrana granulosa cell. Follicle. Ovary. Rat. E.M. X 60,000. **1.** Mitotic spindle microtubules. **2.** Electron-dense material associated with microtubules. **3.** Cell membrane.

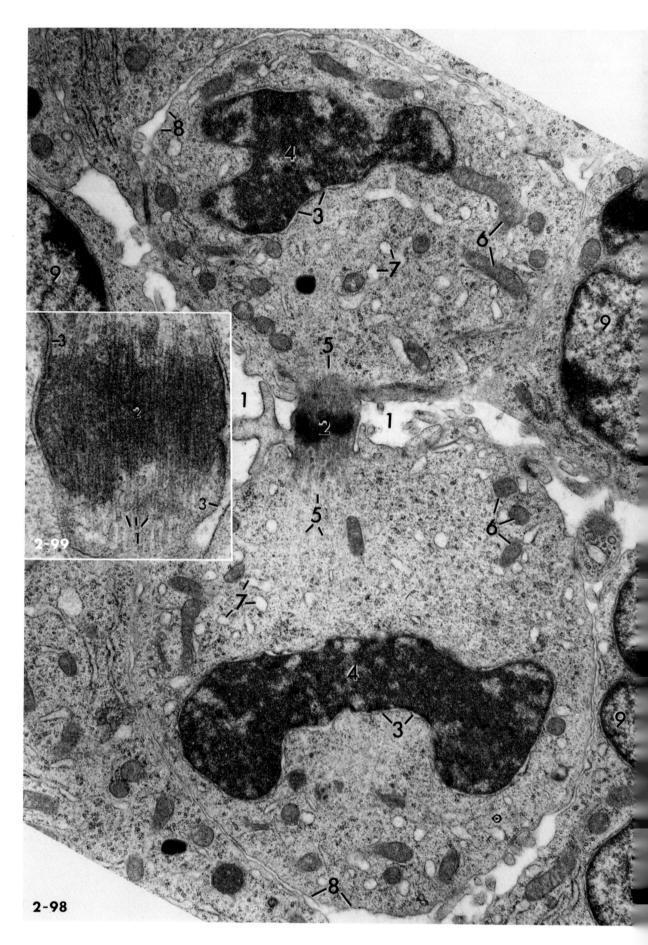

References

GENERAL

Brown, W. V. and Bertke, E. M. Textbook of Cytology. C. V. Mosby, St. Louis, 1969.

Burke, J. D. Cell Biology. Williams and Wilkins, Baltimore, 1970.

De Robertis, E. D. P., Nowinski, W. W. and Saez, F. A. Cell Biology, 5th ed. W. B. Saunders, Philadelphia, 1970.

DuPraw, E. J. Cell and Molecular Biology. Academic Press, New York, 1968.

Fawcett, D. W. An Atlas of Fine Structure. The Cell. Its Organelles and Inclusions. W. B. Saunders, Philadelphia, 1966.

Fell, D. H. and Brachet, J. L. (Eds.). A discussion on cytoplasmic organelles. Proc. Royal Soc. (London) *173*: 1–111 (1969).

Finean, J. B. Biological ultrastructure. *In* Biological Ultrastructure (Eds. A. Engström and J. B. Finean). Academic Press, New York, 1967.

Matthews, J. L. and Martin, J. H. Atlas of Human Histology and Ultrastructure. Lea & Febiger, Philadelphia, 1971.

Novikoff, A. B. and Holtzman, E. Cells and Organelles. Holt, Rinehart and Winston, New York, 1970.

Oberling, C. The structure of the cytoplasm. Int. Rev. Cytol. *8*: 1–32 (1959).

Porter, K. R. and Boneville, M. A. Fine Structure of Cells and Tissues. Lea & Febiger, Philadelphia, 1968.

Rhodin, J. A. G. An Atlas of Ultrastructure. W. B. Saunders, Philadelphia, 1963.

Sandborn, E. B. Cells and Tissues by Light and Electron Microscopy. Academic Press, New York, 1970.

Sjöstrand, F. S. The ultrastructure of cells as revealed by the electron microscope. Int. Rev. Cytol. *5*: 455–533 (1956).

Sjöstrand, F. S. Electron Microscopy of Cells and Tissues. Academic Press, New York, 1967.

Toner, P. G. and Carr, K. E. Cell Structure. Williams and Wilkins, Baltimore, 1968.

Threadgold, L. T. The Ultrastructure of the Animal Cell. Pergamon, Oxford, 1967.

CELL MEMBRANE

Benedetti, E. L. and Emmelot, P. Studies on plasma membranes. IV. The ultrastructural localization and content of sialic acid in plasma membranes isolated from rat liver and hepatoma. J. Cell Sci. *2*: 499–512 (1967).

Bretscher, M. S. Membrane structure: some general principles. Science *181*: 622–629 (1973).

Brunser, O. and Luft, J. H. Fine structure of the apex of absorptive cells from rat small intestine. J. Ultrastruct. Res. *31*: 291–311 (1970).

Fawcett, D. W. Surface specializations of absorbing cells. J. Histochem. Cytochem. *13*: 75–91 (1965).

Fishman, A. P. (Ed.). Symposium on the plasma membrane (New York Heart Association). Circulation *26*: Suppl. 983–1232 (1962).

Gesner, B. M. Cell surface sugars as sites of cellular reactions: possible role in physiological processes. Ann. N.Y. Acad. Sci. *129*: 758–766 (1966).

Groniowski, J., Biczyskowa, W. and Walski, M. Electron microscope studies on the surface coat of the nephron. J. Cell Biol. *40*: 585–601 (1969).

Hendler, R. W. Biological membrane ultrastructure. Physiol. Rev. *51*: 66–97 (1971).

Higgins, J. A., Florendo, N. T. and Barrnett, R. J. Localization of cholesterol in membranes of erythrocyte ghosts. J. Ultrastruct. Res. *42*: 66–81 (1973).

Ito, S. The enteric surface coat on cat intestinal microvilli. J. Cell Biol. *27*: 475–491 (1965).

Ito, S. Structure and function of the glycocalyx. Fed. Proc. *28*: 12–25 (1969).

Korn, E. D. Structure of biological membranes. Science *153*: 1491–1498 (1966).

Loewenstein, W. R. Permeability of membrane junctions Ann. N.Y. Acad. Sci. *137*: 441–472 (1966).

Porter, K. R., Kenyon, K. and Badenhausen, S. Specializations of the unit membrane. Protoplasma *63*: 262–274 (1967).

Rambourg, A. and Leblond, C. P. Electron microscope observations on the carbohydrate-rich cell coat present at the surface of cells in the rat. J. Cell Biol. *32*: 27–53 (1967).

Robertson, J. D. The unit membrane. *In* Electron Microscopy in Anatomy (Eds. J. D. Boyd and J. D. Lever). Arnold, London, 1961.

Robertson, J. D. The structure of biological membranes. Arch. Intern. Med. *129*: 202–228 (1972).

Sjöstrand, F. S. The ultrastructure of the plasma membrane of columnar epithelium cells of the mouse intestine. J. Ultrastruc. Res. *8*: 517–541 (1963).

Stoeckenius, W. and Engelman, D. M. Current models for the structure of biological membranes. J. Cell Biol. *42*: 613–646 (1969).

Weiss, L. The cell periphery. Int. Rev. Cytol. *26*: 63–105 (1969).

VESICLES

Bodian, D. An electron microscopic characterization of classes of synaptic vesicles by means of controlled aldehyde fixation. J. Cell Biol. *44*: 115–124 (1970).

Casley-Smith, J. R. The dimensions and numbers of small vesicles in cells, endothelial and mesothelial and the significances of these for endothelial permeability. J. Microscopy *90*: 251–269 (1969).

Friend, D. and Farquhar, M. G. Functions of coated vesicles during protein absorption in the rat vas deferens. J. Cell Biol. *35*: 357–376 (1967).

Holter, H. Pinocytosis. Int. Rev. Cytol. *8*: 481–505 (1959).

Kanaseki, T. and Kadota, K. The "vesicle in a basket." A morphological study of the coated vesicle isolated from the nerve endings of the guinea pig brain, with special reference to the mechanism of membrane movements. J. Cell Biol. *42*: 202–220 (1969).

Palade, G. E. and Bruns, R. R. Structural modulations of plasmalemmal vesicles. J. Cell Biol. *37*: 633–649 (1968).

Zucker-Franklin, D. and Hirsch, J. G. Electron microscope studies on the degranulation of rabbit peritoneal leukocytes during phagocytosis. J. Exp. Med. *120*: 569–576 (1964).

CELL JUNCTIONS

Brightman, M. W. and Reese, T. S. Junctions between intimately apposed cell membranes in the vertebrate brain. J. Cell Biol. *40*: 648–677 (1969).

Bullivant, S. and Loewenstein, W. R. Structure of coupled and uncoupled cell junctions. J. Cell Biol. *37*: 621–632 (1968).

Cobb, J. L. S. and Bennett, T. A study of nexuses in visceral smooth muscle. J. Cell Biol. *41*: 287–297 (1969).

Dewey, M. M. and Barr, L. A study of the structure and distribution of the nexus. J. Cell Biol. *23*: 553–585 (1964).

Farquahar, M. G. and Palade, G. E. Junctional complexes in various epithelia. J. Cell Biol. *17*: 375–412 (1963).

Flickinger, C. J. Extracellular specializations associated with hemidesmosomes in the fetal rat urogenital sinus. Anat. Rec. *168*: 195–202 (1970).

Friend, D. S. and Giluda, N. B. Variations in tight and gap junctions in mammalian tissues. J. Cell Biol. *53*: 758–776 (1972).

Goodenough, D. A. and Revel, J. P. A fine structural analysis of intercellular junctions in the mouse liver. J. Cell Biol. *45*: 272–290 (1970).

Kelly, D. E. Fine structure of desmosomes, hemidesmosomes, and an adepidermal globular layer in developing new epidermis. J. Cell Biol. *28*: 51–72 (1966).

McNutt, N. S. and Weinstein, R. S. The ultrastructure of the nexus. A correlated thin-sectioning and freeze-cleave study. J. Cell Biol. *47*: 666–688 (1970).

Reese, T. S. and Karnovsky, M. J. Fine structural localization of a blood-brain barrier to exogenous peroxidase. J. Cell Biol. *34*: 207–217 (1967).

Revel, J. P. and Karnovsky, M. J. Hexagonal array of subunits in intercellular junctions of the mouse heart and liver. J. Cell Biol. *33*: C7–C12 (1967).

Steere, R. L. and Sommer, J. R. Stereo ultrastructure of nexus faces exposed by freeze-fracturing. J. Microscopie *15*: 205–218 (1972).

MICROVILLI AND CILIA

Crane, R. K. Structural and functional organization of an epithelial cell brush border. Symp. Int. Soc. Cell Biol. *5*: 71–102 (1966).

Fawcett, D. W. Cilia and flagella. *In* The Cell (Eds. J. Brachet and A. E. Mirsky), 2: 217–297. Academic Press, New York, 1961.

Frisch, D. and Farbman, A. I. Development of order during ciliogenesis. Anat. Rec. *162*: 221–232 (1968).

Gibbons, I. R. The structure and composition of cilia. Symp. Int. Soc. Cell Biol. *6*: 99–114 (1967).

Grimstone, A. V. Observations on the substructure of flagellar fibres. J. Cell Sci. *1*: 351–362 (1966).

Hopkins, J. M. Subsidiary components of the flagella of *Chlamydomonas Reinhardii*. J. Cell Sci. 7: 823–839 (1970).

Kalnins, V. I. and Porter, K. R. Centriole replication during ciliogenesis in the chick tracheal epithelium. Z. Zellforsch. *100*: 1–30 (1969).

Millecchia, L. L. and Rudzinska, M. A. Basal body replication and ciliogenesis in a suctorian, *Tokophrya infusionum*. J. Cell Biol. *46*: 553–563 (1970).

Parducz, B. Ciliary movement and coordination in ciliates. Int. Rev. Cytol. *21*: 91–128 (1967).

Satir, P. Studies on cilia. II. Examination of the distal region of the ciliary shaft and the role of the filaments in motility. J. Cell Biol. *26*: 805–834 (1965).

Satir, P. Studies on cilia. III. Further studies on the cilium tip and a "sliding filament" model of ciliary motility. J. Cell Biol. *39*: 77–94 (1968).

Steinman, R. M. An electron microscopic study of ciliogenesis in developing epidermis and trachea in the embryo of *Xenopus laevis*. Am. J. Anat. *122*: 19–56 (1968).

GRANULAR ENDOPLASMIC RETICULUM

Dallner, G., Siekevitz, P. and Palade, G. E. Biogenesis of endoplasmic reticulum membranes. J. Cell Biol. *30*: 73–96 (1966).

Garrett, R. A. and Wittmann, H.-G. Structure and function of the ribosome. Endeavour *32*: 8–14 (1973).

Haguenau, F. The ergastoplasm: its history, ultrastructure and biochemistry. Int. Rev. Cytol. *7*: 425–483 (1958).

Palade, G. E. A small particulate component of the cytoplasm. J. Biophys. Biochem. Cytol. *1*: 59–68 (1955).

Palade, G. E. and Porter, K. R. Studies on the endoplasmic reticulum. I. Its identification in cells in situ. J. Exp. Med. *100*: 641–656 (1956).

Palade, G. E. and Siekevitz, P. Pancreatic microsomes. J. Biophys. Biochem. Cytol. *2*: 671–690 (1956).

Rich, A. Polyribosomes. Sci. American *209*: 44–53 (1963).

Sjöstrand, F. S. Endoplasmic reticulum *In* Cytology and Cell Physiology (Ed. G. H. Bourne), pp. 311–376 Academic Press, New York, 1964.

Spirin, A. S. and Gavrilova, L. P. The Ribosome. Springer-Verlag, New York, 1969.

AGRANULAR ENDOPLASMIC RETICULUM

Christensen, A. K. Fine structure of testicular interstitial cells in the guinea pig. J. Cell Biol. *26*: 911–935 (1965).

Emans, J. B. and Jones, A. L. Hypertrophy of liver cell smooth surfaced reticulum following progesterone administration. J. Histochem. Cytochem. *16*: 561–570 (1968).

Jones, A. L. and Fawcett, D. W. Hypertrophy of the agranular endoplasmic reticulum in hamster liver induced by phenobarbital. J. Histochem. Cytochem. *14*: 215–232 (1966).

Ito, S. The endoplasmic reticulum of gastric parietal cells. J. Biophys. Biochem. Cytol. *11*: 333–347 (1961).

Porter, K. R. The sarcoplasmic reticulum: Its recent history and present status. J. Biophys. Biochem. Cytol. *10*: 211–226 (1961).

GOLGI APPARATUS

Beams, H. W. and Kessel, R. G. The Golgi apparatus: structure and function. Int. Rev. Cytol. *23*: 209–276 (1968).

Jamieson, J. D. and Palade, G. E. Intracellular transport of secretory proteins in the pancreatic exocrine cell. I. Role of the peripheral elements of the Golgi complex. J. Cell Biol. *34*: 577–596 (1967).

Neutra, M. and Leblond, C. P. The Golgi apparatus. Sci. American *220*: 100–107 (1969).

Northcote, D. H. The Golgi apparatus. Endeavour *30*: 26–33 (1971).

Novikoff, A., Essner, E. and Quintana, N. Golgi apparatus and lysosomes. Fed. Proc. *23*: 1010–1022 (1964).

Thiéry, J.-P. Role de l'appareil de Golgi dans la synthèse des mucopolysaccharides. Etude cytochimique. I. Mise en évidence de mucopolysaccharides dans les vésicules de transition entre l'ergastoplasme et l'appareil de Golgi. J. Microsc. *8*: 689–708 (1969).

Zeigel, R. F. and Dalton, A. J. Speculations based on the morphology of the Golgi systems in several types of protein-secreting cells. J. Cell Biol. *15*: 45–54 (1962).

ANNULATE LAMELLAE

Kessel, R. G. Annulate lamellae. J. Ultrastruct. Res. Suppl. *10*: 1–82 (1968).

Maul, G. G. Ultrastructure of pore complexes of annulate lamellae. J. Cell Biol. *46*: 604–610 (1970).

Wischnitzer, S. The annulate lamellae. Int. Rev. Cytol. *27*: 65–100 (1970).

MITOCHONDRIA

Barnard T. and Afzelius, B. A. The matrix granules of mitochondria: a review. Sub-Cell. Biochem. *1*: 375–389 (1972).

Butler, W. H. and Judah, J. D. Preparation of isolated rat liver mitochondria for electron microscopy. J. Cell Biol. *44*: 278–289 (1970).

Green, D. E. The mitochondrion. Sci. American *210*: 67–74 (1964).

Hackenbrock, C. R. Ultrastructural bases for metabolically linked mechanical activity in mitochondria. II. Electron transport-linked ultrastructural transformations in mitochondria. J. Cell Biol. *37*: 345–369 (1968).

Lehninger, A. L. The Mitochondrion. Benjamin, New York, 1965.

Malhotra, S. K. and Eakin, R. T. A study of mitochondrial membranes in relation to elementary particles. J. Cell Sci. *2*: 205–212 (1967).

Palade, G. An electron microscope study of mitochondrial structure. J. Histochem. Cytochem. *1*: 188–211 (1953).

Sjöstrand, F. S. Electron microscopy of mitochondria and cytoplasmic double membranes. Nature *171*: 30–32 (1953).

Sjöstrand, F. S. and Barajas, L. A new model for mitochondrial membranes based on biochemical information. J. Ultrastruct. Res. *32*: 293–306 (1970).

Tandler, B., Erlandson, R. A., Smith, A. L. and Wynder, E. L. Riboflavin and mouse hepatic cell structure and function. II. Division of mitochondria during recovery from simple deficiency. J. Cell Biol. *41*: 477–493 (1969).

Weber, N. E. Ultrastructural studies of beef heart mitochondria. III. The inequality of gross morphological change and oxidative phosphorylation. J. Cell Biol. *55*: 457–470 (1972).

LYSOSOMES AND RELATED BODIES

Arstila, A. U., Jauregui, H. O., Chang, J. and Trump, B. F. Studies on cellular autophagocytosis. Relationship between heterophagy and autophagy in HeLa cells. Lab. Investig. *24*: 162–174 (1971).

Björkerud, S. The isolation of lipofuscin granules from bovine cardiac muscle with observations on the properties of the isolated granules on the light and electron microscopic levels. J. Ultrastruct. Res. Suppl. *5*: 1–47 (1963).

DeDuve, C. and Wattiaux, R. Functions of lysosomes. Ann. Rev. Physiol. *28*: 435–492 (1966).

Friend, D. S. Cytochemical staining of multivesicular body and Golgi vesicles. J. Cell Biol. *41*: 269–279 (1969).

Gahan, P. B. Histochemistry of lysosomes. Int. Rev. Cytol. *21*: 1–63 (1967).

Goldfischer, S. and Bernstein, J. Lipofuscin (aging) pigment granules of the newborn human liver. J. Cell Biol. *42*: 253–261 (1969).

Goldfischer, S., Novikoff, A. B., Albala, A. and Biempica, L. Hemoglobin uptake by rat hepatocytes and its breakdown within lysosomes. J. Cell Biol. *44*: 513–529 (1970).

Ma, M. H. and Biempica, L. The normal human liver cell (emphasis on lysosomes). Am. J. Path. *62*: 353–376 (1971).

Malkoff, D. and Strehler, B. The ultrastructure of isolated and in situ human cardiac age pigment. J. Cell Biol. *16*: 611–616 (1963).

Marshall, J. and Ansell, P. L. Membranous inclusions in the retinal pigment epithelium: phagosomes and myeloid bodies. J. Anat. *110*: 91–104 (1971).

Martin, B. J. and Spicer, S. S. Multivesicular bodies and related structures of the syncytiotrophoblast of human term placenta. Anat. Rec. *175*: 15–36 (1973).

Novikoff, A. B. Lysosomes in nerve cells. *In* The Neuron (Ed., H. Hydén). Elsevier, Amsterdam 1967.

Nunez, E. A. and Becker, D. V. Secretory processes in follicular cells of the bat thyroid. I. Ultrastructural changes during the pre-, early and mid-hibernation periods with some comments on the origin of autophagic vacuoles. Am. J. Anat. *129*: 369–397 (1970).

René, A. A. Darden, J. H. and Parker, J. L. Radiation-induced ultrastructural and biochemical changes in lysosomes. Lab. Investig. *25*: 230–239 (1971).

Samorajski, T., Ordy, J. M. and Rady-Reimer, P. Lipofuscin pigment accumulation in the nervous system of aging mice. Anat. Rec. *160*: 555–574 (1968).

Weissmann, G. Lysosomes (analytical review). Blood *24*: 594–606 (1964).

MICROBODIES

DeDuve, C. and Baudhuin, P. Peroxisomes (microbodies and related particles). Physiol. Rev. *46*: 323–357 (1966).

Essner, E. Endoplasmic reticulum and the origin of microbodies in the fetal mouse liver. Lab. Investig. *17*:71–87 (1967).

Fahimi, H. D. Cytochemical localization of peroxidatic activity of catalase in rat hepatic microbodies (peroxisomes). J. Cell Biol. *43*: 275–288 (1969).

Hruban, Z., Vigil, E. L., Slesers, A. and Hopkins, E. Microbodies. Constituent organelles of animal cells. Lab. Investig. *27*: 184–191 (1972).

Novikoff, A. B. and Goldfischer, S. Visualization of microbodies for light and electron microscopy. J. Histochem. Cytochem. *16*: 507 (1968).

Novikoff, P. M. and Novikoff, A. B. Peroxisomes in absorptive cells of mammalian small intestine. J. Cell Biol. *53*: 532–560 (1972).

Svoboda, D., Grady, H. and Azarnoff, D. Microbodies in experimentally altered cells. J. Cell Biol. *35*: 127–152 (1967).

Tsukada, H. Mochizuki, Y. and Konishi, T. Morphogenesis and development of microbodies of hepatocytes of rats during pre- and postnatal growth. J. Cell Biol. *37*: 231–243 (1968).

FILAMENTS AND MICROTUBULES

Behnke, O. and Forer, A. Evidence for four classes of microtubules in individual cells. J. Cell Sci. *2*: 169–192 (1967).

Brody, I. The ultrastructure of the tonofibrils in the keratinization process of normal human epidermis. J. Ultrastruct. Res. *4*: 264–297 (1960).

Carr, I. The fine structure of microfibrils and microtubules in macrophages and other lymphoreticular cells in relation to cytoplasmic movement. J. Anat. *112*: 383–389 (1972).

Gall, J. G. Microtubule fine structure. J. Cell Biol. *31*: 639–643 (1966).

Olson, L. W. and Heath, I. B. Observations on the ultrastructure of microtubules. Z. Zellforsch. *115*: 388–395 (1971).

Peters, A. and Vaughn, J. E. Microtubules and filaments in the axons and astrocytes of early post-natal rat optic nerves. J. Cell Biol. *32*: 113–119 (1967).

Wessells, N. K. How living cells change shape. Sci. American *225*: 77–82 (1971).

Wikswo, M. A. and Novales, R. R. Effect of colchicine on microtubules in the melanophores of *Fundulus heteroclitus*. J. Ultrastruct. Res. *41*: 189–201 (1972).

CENTRIOLES

Perkins, F. O. Formation of centriole and centriole-like structures during meiosis and mitosis in *Labyrinthula* Sp. (Rhizopodea Labyrinhulida). J. Cell Sci. *6*: 629–653 (1970).

Sorokin, S. P. Reconstruction of centriole formation and ciliogenesis in mammalian lungs. J. Cell Sci. *3*: 207–230 (1968).

Szollosi, D. Centrioles, centriolar satellites and spindle fibers. Anat. Rec. *148*: 343 (1964).

STORED PRODUCTS

Caro, L. G. and Palade, G. E. Protein synthesis, storage, and discharge in the pancreatic exocrine cell. J. Cell Biol. *20*: 473–495 (1964).

de Bruijn, W. C. Glycogen, its chemistry and morphologic appearance in the electron microscope. J. Ultrastruct. Res. *42*: 29–50 (1973).

Napolitano, L. The differentiation of white adipose cells. J. Cell Biol. *18*: 663–679 (1963).

Revel, J. P. Electron microscopy of glycogen. J. Histochem. Cytochem. *12*: 104–114 (1964).

PIGMENTS

Barnicot, N. A. and Birbeck, M. S. C. The electron microscopy of human melanocytes and melanin granules. *In*: The Biology of Hair Growth. (Eds. W. Montagna and R. A. Ellis). Academic Press, New York, 1958.

Drochmans, P. Melanin granules. Their fine structure, formation and degradation in normal and pathological tissues. Int. Rev. Exp. Path. *2*: 357–422 (1963).

Hearing, V. J., Phillips, P. and Lutzner, M. A. The fine structure of melanogenesis in coat color mutants of the mouse. J. Ultrastruct. Res. *43*: 88–106 (1973).

Hu, F., Endo, H. and Alexander, N. J. Morphological variations of pigment granules in eyes of the rhesus monkey. Am. J. Anat. *136*: 167–182 (1973).

NUCLEUS AND NUCLEOLUS

Abelson, H. T. and Smith, G. H. Nuclear pores: the pore-annulus relationship in thin section. J. Ultrastruct. Res. *30*: 558–588 (1970).

Busch, H. and Smetana, K. The Nucleolus. Academic Press, New York, 1970.

Dalton, A. J. and Haguenau, F. (Eds.). The Nucleus. Academic Press, New York, 1968.

Everid, A. C., Small, J. V. and Davies, H. G. Electron-microscope observations on the structure of condensed chromatin: evidence for orderly arrays of unit threads on the surface of chicken erythrocyte nuclei. J. Cell Sci. *7*: 35–48 (1970).

Fawcett, D. W. On the occurrence of a fibrous lamina on the inner aspect of the nuclear envelope in certain cells of vertebrates. Am. J. Anat. *119*: 129–146 (1966).

Hardin, J. H. and Spicer, S. S. Ultrastructure of neuronal nucleoli or rat trigeminal ganglia: comparison of routine with pyroantimonate-osmium tetroxide fixation. J. Ultrastruct. Res. *31*: 16–36 (1970).

Mitchison, J. M. Some functions of the nucleus. Int. Rev. Cytol. *19*: 97–110 (1966).

Patrizi, G. and Poger, M. The ultrastructure of the nuclear periphery. The zonula nucleum limitans. J. Ultrastruct. Res. *17*: 127–136 (1967).

Recher, L. Fine structural changes in the nucleus induced by adenosine. J. Ultrastruct. Res. *32*: 212–225 (1970).

Recher, L., Whitescarver, J. and Briggs, L. The fine structure of a nucleolar constituent. J. Ultrastruct. Res. *29*: 1–14 (1969).

Sadowski, P. D. and Steiner, J. W. Electron microscopic and biochemical characteristics of nuclei and nucleoli isolated from rat liver. J. Cell Biol. *37*: 147–161 (1968).

Shinozuka, H. Intranucleolar dense particles in rat hepatic cell nucleoli. J. Ultrastruct. Res. *32*: 430–442 (1970).

Sidebottom, E. and Harris, H. The role of the nucleolus in the transfer of RNA from nucleus to cytoplasm. J. Cell Sci. *5*: 351–364 (1969).

Wiener, J., Spiro, D. and Loewenstein, W. R. Ultrastructure and permeability of nuclear membranes. J. Cell Biol. *27*: 107–117 (1965).

MITOSIS AND MEIOSIS

Baker, T. G. and Franchi, L. L. The fine structure of oogonia and oocytes in human ovaries. J. Cell Sci. *2*: 213–224 (1967).

Brinkley, B. R. and Stubblefield, E. Ultrastructure and interaction of the kinetochore and centriole in mitosis and meiosis. *In* Advances in Cell Biology, Vol. 1 (Eds. D. M. Prescott, L. Goldstein and E. McConkey). Appleton-Century-Crofts, New York, 1971.

deHarven, E. The centriole and the mitotic spindle. *In* The Nucleus (Eds. A. J. Dalton and F. Haguenau), pp. 197–227. Academic Press, New York, 1968.

Ford, E. H. R., Thurley, K. and Woollam, D. H. M. Electron-microscopic observations on whole human mitotic chromosomes. J. Anat. *103*: 143–150 (1968).

Friedländer, M. and Wahrman, J. The spindle as a basal body distributor: a study in the meiosis of the male silkworm moth, *Bombyx mori*. J. Cell Sci. *7*: 65–89 (1970).

Hepler, P. K. and Jackson, W. T. Isopropyl N-phenylcarbamate affects spindle microtubule orientation in dividing endosperm cells of *Haemanthus Katherinae Baker*. J. Cell Sci. *5*: 727–743 (1969).

Hepler, P. K., McIntosh, J. R. and Cleland, S. Intermicrotubule bridges in mitotic spindle apparatus. J. Cell Biol. *45*: 438–444 (1970).

Jokelainen, P. T. The ultrastructure and spatial organization of the metaphase kinetochore in mitotic rat cells. J. Ultrastruct. Res. *19*: 19–44 (1967).

Journey, L. J. and Whaley, A. Kinetochore ultrastructure in vincristine-treated mammalian cells. J. Cell Sci. *7*: 49–54 (1970).

Mazia, D. How cells divide. Sci. American *205*: 100–120 (1961).

McIntosh, J. R. and Landis, S. C. The distribution of spindle microtubules during mitosis in cultured human cells. J. Cell Biol. *49*: 468–497 (1971).

Reith, E. J. and Jokelainen, P. T. Cytokinesis in the stratum intermedium of the rat molar enamel organ. J. Ultrastruct. Res. *42*: 51–64 (1973).

Robbins, E. and Gonatas, N. K. The ultrastructure of a mammalian cell during the mitotic cycle. J. Cell Biol. *21*: 429–263 (1964).

Robbins, E. and Jentzsch, G. Ultrastructural changes in the mitotic apparatus at the metaphase-to-anaphase transition. J. Cell Biol. *40*: 678–691 (1969).

Roos, U.-P. Light and electron microscopy of rat kangaroo cells in mitosis. Chromosma *40*: 43–82 (1973).

3 Epithelia

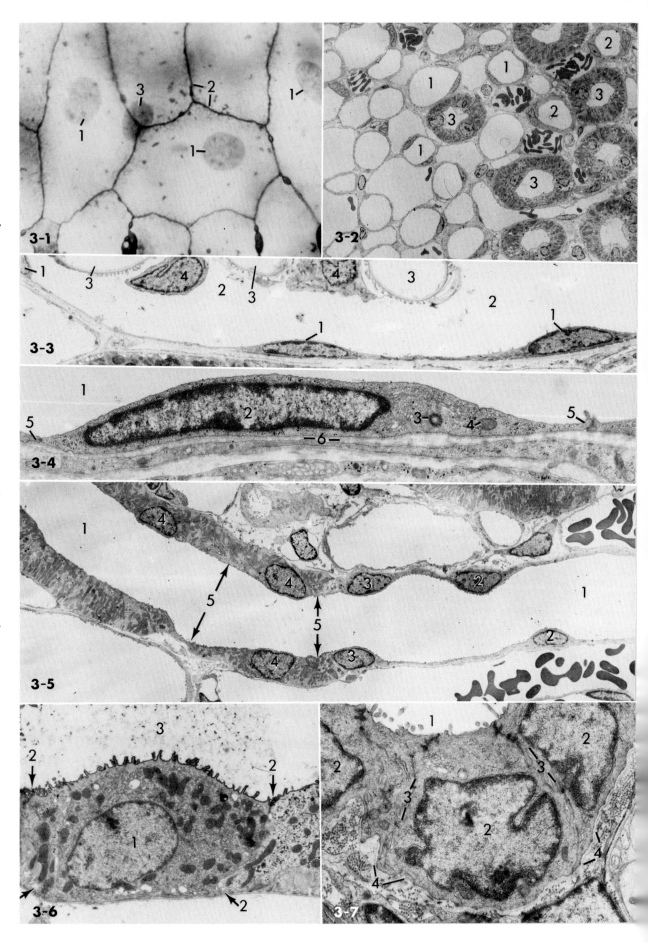

Fig. 3-1. Simple *squamous* epithelium (flat face). Mesothelium of mesentary. Silver impregnation. Rat. L.M. X 1100. **1.** Nuclei of mesothelial cells. **2.** Cell borders, enhanced by silver salts. **3.** Nucleus of connective tissue cell underneath the mesothelium.

Fig. 3-2. Simple *squamous* and *cuboidal* epithelia. Cross section of nephrons in outer medullary zone of rat kidney. The magnification is too low to show subtle differences between the two types of epithelia. It does show the difference in height of cells which line the various tubules. Kidney. Rat. E.M. X 620. **1.** Squamous epithelium. **2.** Low cuboidal epithelium. **3.** Cuboidal epithelium.

Fig. 3-3. Simple *squamous* epithelium. Parietal layer of Bowman's capsule. Renal corpuscle. Kidney. Rat. E.M. X 2100. **1.** Nuclei of squamous epithelial cells. **2.** Urinary space of Bowman's capsule. **3.** Lumina of glomerular blood capillaries. **4.** Nuclei of podocytes.

Fig. 3-4. *Squamous* epithelial cell (endothelium). Venous sinus (lacuna). Corpus cavernosum penis. Rat. E.M. X 10,000. **1.** Lumen of sinus. **2.** Nucleus. **3.** Centriole. **4.** Mitochondrion. **5.** Gap-junctions. **6.** Basal lamina.

Fig. 3-5. Transition between *low squamous* and *high squamous* simple epithelium. Hairpin turn of Henle's loop. Entire turn shown in Fig. 32-18. Nephron. Kidney. Rat. E.M. X 1300. **1.** Lumen of tubule. **2.** Nuclei of low squamous epithelial cells. **3.** Nuclei of cells changing from low to high squamous shape. **4.** Nuclei of high squamous cells. **5.** Arrows indicate approximate points of interdigitation between adjacent cells.

Fig. 3-6. *Low cuboidal* cell of simple cuboidal epithelium. Cortical collecting tubule. Kidney. Rat. E.M. X 4700. **1.** Nucleus. **2.** Cell borders. **3.** Lumen of tubule.

Fig. 3-7. *Cuboidal* cells of simple cuboidal epithelium. Bile ductule. Liver. Rat. E.M. X 10,000. **1.** Lumen of ductule. **2.** Nuclei of cuboidal cells. **3.** Cell bodies. **4.** Basal lamina.

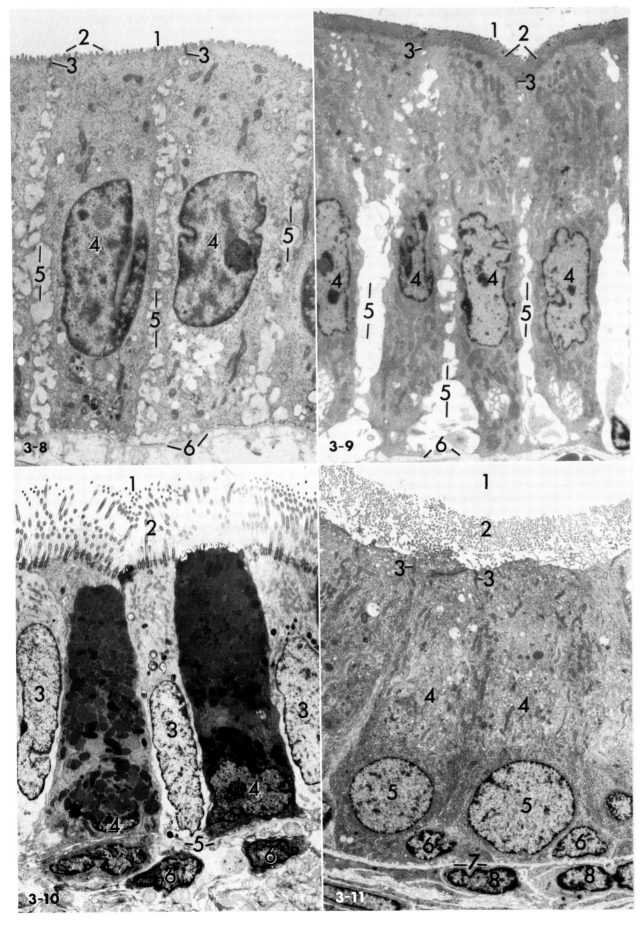

Fig. 3-8. Simple *columnar* epithelium (height 19 μ). Collecting duct. Kidney. Rat. E.M. X 5000. **1.** Lumen of tubule. **2.** Short microvilli. **3.** Junctional complexes. **4.** Nuclei of columnar epithelial cells. **5.** Intercellular space. **6.** Basal lamina.

Fig. 3-9. Simple *columnar* epithelium (height 55 μ). Absorptive epithelial cells. Small intestine. Rat. E.M. X 2300. **1.** Gut lumen. **2.** Striate border (long microvilli). **3.** Junctional complexes. **4.** Nuclei of tall columnar epithelial cels. **5.** Intercellular spaces. **6.** Basal lamina.

Fig. 3-10. Simple *columnar* ciliated epithelium (height 28 μ including cilia). Tertiary bronchus. Lung. Rat. E.M. X 3200. **1.** Lumen of bronchus. **2.** Cilia. **3.** Nuclei of ciliated columnar cells. **4.** Nuclei of mucous cells. **5.** Basal lamina. **6.** Nuclei of fibroblasts in subepithelial connective tissue.

Fig. 3-11. *Pseudostratified columnar* epithelium (height 45 μ). Duct of epididymis. Rat. E.M. X 2200. **1.** Lumen of duct. **2.** Stereocilia. **3.** Junctional complexes. **4.** Large Golgi zones. **5.** Nuclei of columnar cells. **6.** Nuclei of basal cells. **7.** Basal lamina. **8.** Nuclei of connective tissue cells.

Fig. 3-12. *Straified squamous non-keratinized* epithelium. Esophagus. Cat. L.M. X 200. **1.** Lumen of esophagus. **2.** Stratified squamous epithelium. **3.** Lamina propria. **4.** Connective tissue papillae.

Fig. 3-13. Stratified squamous non-keratinized epithelia. Enlargement of area similar to rectangle in Fig. 3-12. Esophagus. Cat. E.M. X 1600. **1.** Lumen. **2.** Superficial squamous cell being sloughed. **3.** Nuclei of squamous cells. **4.** Nucleus of cell changing from polyhedral to squamous shape. **5.** Nucleus of polyhedral cell. **6.** Nucleus of cuboidal basal cell. **7.** Basal lamina.

Fig. 3-14. *Stratified squamous keratinized* epithelium. Epidermis. Human (Negro). E.M. X 640. **1.** Skin surface. **2.** Stratified squamous epithelium **3.** Dermis.

Fig. 3-15. Stratified squamous keratinized. epithelium. Enlargement of area similar to rectangle in Fig. 3-14. Skin. Human (Negro). E.M. X 1800. **1.** Surface of skin. **2.** Stratum corneum: keratinized squamous cells. **3.** Thin stratum granulosum. **4.** Nucleus of squamous non-keratinized cell. **5.** Intercellular space with cell processes attached by desmosomes. **6.** Nuclei of polyhedral cells in stratum spinosum. **7.** Cuboidal basal cells. **8.** Basal lamina. **9.** Melanosomes (pigment granules.).

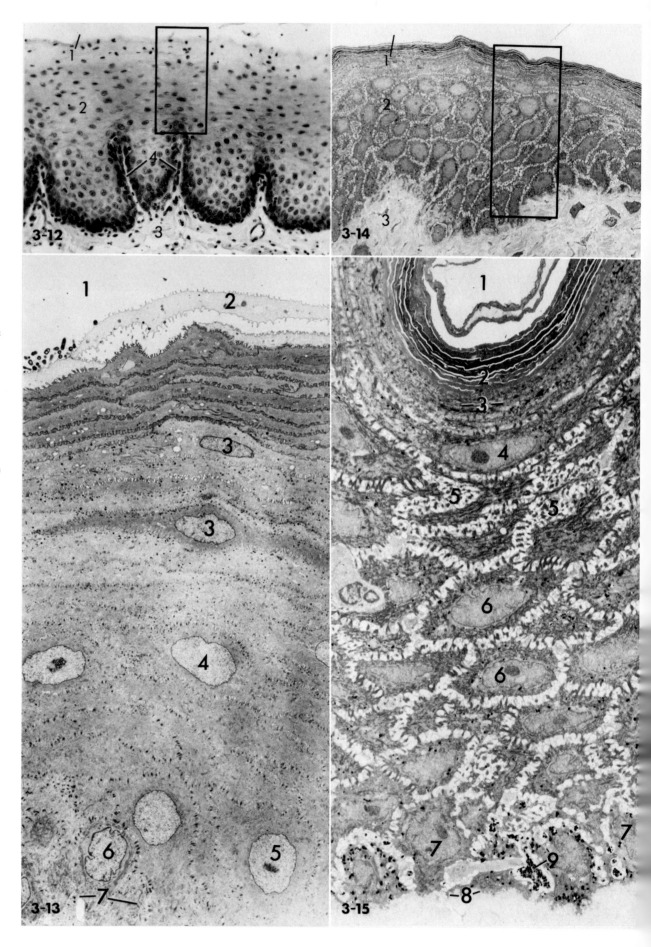

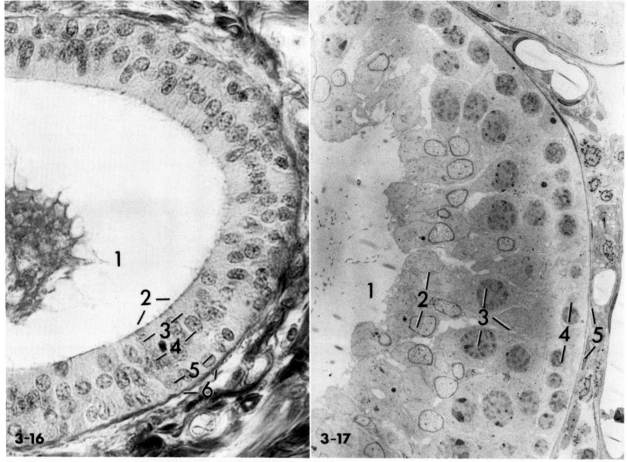

Fig. 3-16. *Stratified columnar* epithelium. Interlobular duct. Sublingual salivary gland. Monkey. L.M. X 665. **1.** Lumen of duct. **2.** Microvilli. **3.** Surface layer of columnar cells. **4.** Middle layer of cuboidal cells. **5.** Layer of basal cuboidal cells. **6.** Basement membrane.

Fig. 3-17. *Stratified cuboidal* epithelium. Seminiferous tubule. Testis. Rat. E.M. X 680. **1.** Lumen. **2.** Layer of early spermatids. **3.** Layers of primary spermatocytes. **4.** Layer of spermatogonia. **5.** Basal lamina.

Fig. 3-18. *Stratified cuboidal* epithelium. Urethra. Rat. E.M. X 5000. **1.** Lumen of urethra. **2.** Short microvilli. **3.** Nuclei of low cuboidal surface cells. **4.** Nuclei in several layers of cuboidal cells. **5.** Basal lamina. **6.** Nuclei of fibroblasts in subepithelial connective tissue.

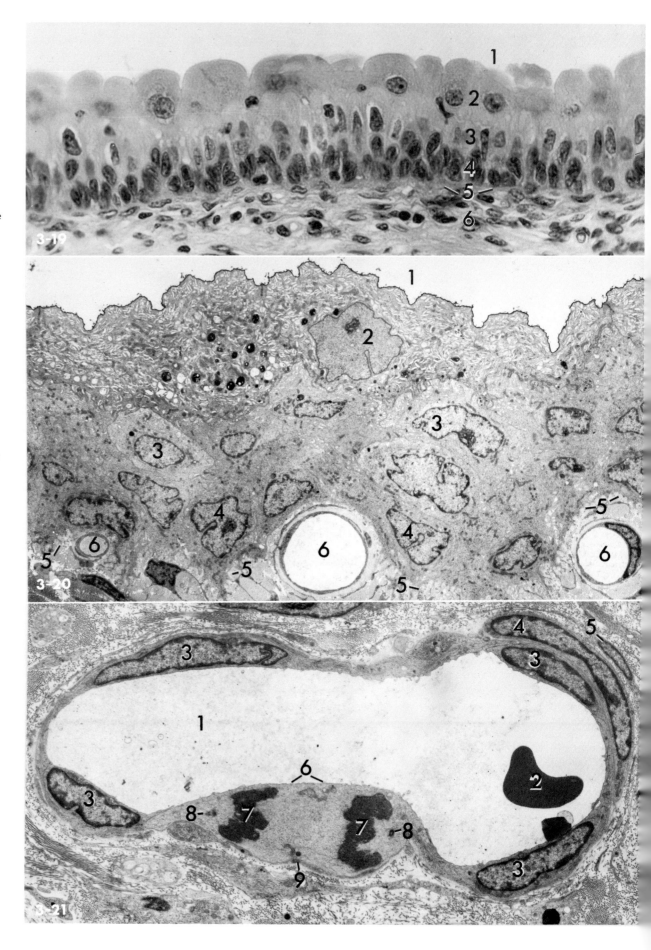

Fig. 3-19. *Transitional* epithelium. Collapsed urinary bladder. Human. L.M. X 640. **1.** Lumen. **2.** Superficial cells. **3.** Intermediate cell layers. **4.** Basal cell layer. **5.** Level of basement membrane. **6.** Subepithelial connective tissue.

Fig. 3-20. *Transitional* epithelium. Ureter. Rat. E.M. X 20,000. **1.** Lumen. **2.** Nucleus of large umbrella-like surface cell. Cytoplasm is filled with a multiude of flat, discoid vesicles. **3.** Nuclei of cuboidal cells of intermediate cell layers. **4.** Cuboidal basal cells. **5.** Level of basal lamina. **6.** Blood capillaries in subepithelial connective tissue.

Fig. 3-21. Renewal of cells in simple squamous epithelium (endothelium) during vascular growth. Postcapillary venule. Uterus. Rat. E.M. X 4000. **1.** Lumen of venule. **2.** Erythrocyte. **3.** Nuclei of endothelial cells. **4.** Nucleus of pericyte. **5.** Nucleus of fibroblast. **6.** Endothelial cell in late anaphase of mitotic division. **7.** Chromosomes. **8.** Centrioles. **9.** Cleavage furrow.

References

Adams, D. R. Olfactory and non-olfactory epithelia in the nasal cavity of the mouse. Am. J. Anat. *133*: 37–50 (1972).

Baradi, A. F. and Hope, J. Observations on ultrastructure of rabbit mesothelium. Expt. Cell Res. *34*: 33–44 (1964).

Bertalanffy, F. D. and Nagy, K. P. Mitotic activity and renewal rate of the epithelial cells of human duodenum. Acta. Anat. *45*: 362–370 (1961).

Clermont, Y. The cycle of the seminiferous epithelium in man. Am. J. Anat. *112*: 35–52 (1963).

Clyman, M. J. Electron microscopy of the human fallopian tube. Fertil. & Steril. *17*: 281–301 (1966).

Kurtz, S. M. The fine structure of the lamina densa. Lab. Investig. *10*: 1189–1208 (1961).

Leblond, C. P., Greulich, R. C. and Pereira, J. P. M. Relationship of cell formation and cell migration in the renewal of stratified squamous epithelia. *In* Advances in the Biology of the Skin. (Eds. W. Montagna and R. E. Billingham). Vol. *5*: 39–67. Pergamon Press, New York 1964.

Lipkin, M., Sherlock, P. and Bell, B. Cell proliferation kinetics in the gastrointestinal tract of man. Gastroenterology *45*: 721–729 (1963).

Monis, B. and Zambrano, D. Transitional epithelium of urinary tract in normal and dehydrated rats. Z. Zellforsch. *85*: 165–182 (1968).

Niemi, M. The fine structure and histochemistry of the epithelial cells of the rat vas deferens. Acta Anat. *60*: 207–219 (1965).

Parakkal, P. F. An electron microscopic study of esophageal epithelium in the newborn and adult mouse. Am. J. Anat. *121*: 175–196 (1967).

Pierce, G. B., Jr., Midgley, A. R. and Sri Ram, J. The histogenesis of basement membranes, J. Expt. Med. *117*: 339–348 (1963).

Piezzi, R. S., Santolaya, R. S. and Bertini, F. The fine structure of endothelial cells of toad arteries. Anat. Rec. *165*: 229–236 (1969).

Rhodin, J. A. G. Ultrastructure and function of the human tracheal mucosa. Am. Rev. Resp. Dis. *93*: 1–15 (1966).

Smith, B. G. and Brunner, E. K. The structure of the human vaginal mucosa in relation to the menstrual cycle and to pregnancy. Am. J. Anat. *54*: 27–86 (1934).

Zelickson, A. S. (ed.) Ultrastructure of Normal and Abnormal Skin. Lea & Febiger, Philadelphia, 1967.

4 Glands

Fig. 4-1. *Unicellular* exocrine mucous gland. Goblet cell. Large intestine. Rat. E.M. X 6000. **1.** Connective tissue of lamina propria. **2.** Basal lamina. **3.** Tapered base of goblet cell. **4.** Intercellular space. **5.** Nucleus of mucous (goblet) cell. **6.** Nucleus of absorptive epithelial cell. **7.** Golgi zone. **8.** Goblet (apical part of cell) filled with mucigen droplets. **9.** Apex of mucous cell. **10.** Microvilli of absorptive cell. **11.** Lumen of gut. Areas similar to rectangles (A) and (B) are enlarged in Figs. 4-21 and 4-22.

Fig. 4-2. *Simple tubular* straight, non-branching multicellular gland. Crypt of Lieberkühn. Jejunum. Rat. E.M. X 1300. **1.** Lumen of intestinal gland. **2.** Nuclei of mucous cells. **3.** Intracellular accumulation of mucigen droplets. **4.** Nucleus of Paneth cell with secretory granules (proteinaceous secretion). **5.** Nuclei of undifferentiated cells. **6.** Nuclei of apparent absorptive cells. **7.** Undifferentiated cells in varied stages of mitosis. **8.** Connective tissue of lamina propria. **9.** Lumen of capillaries.

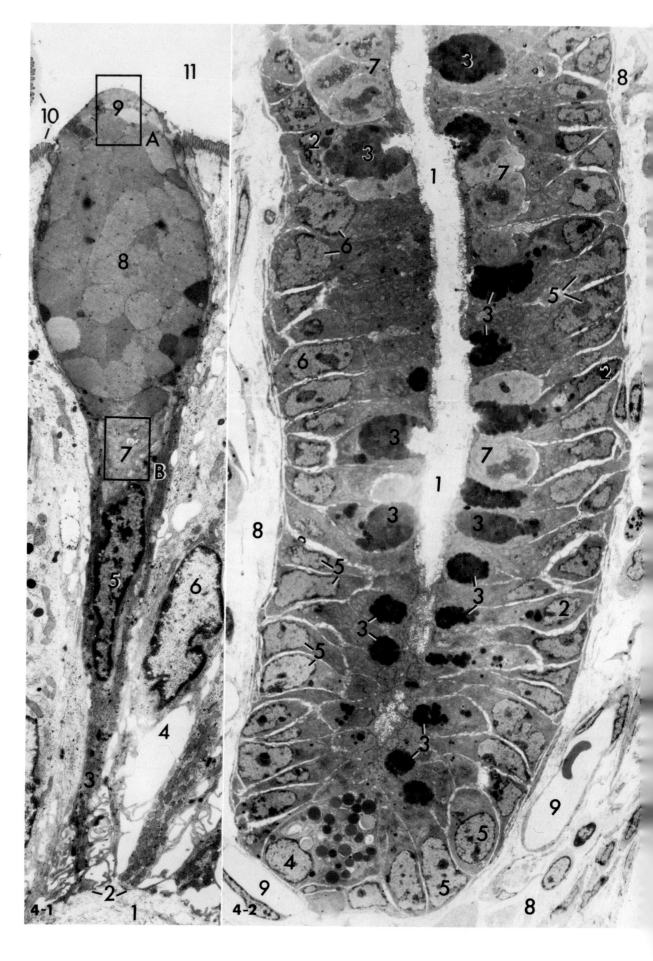

46

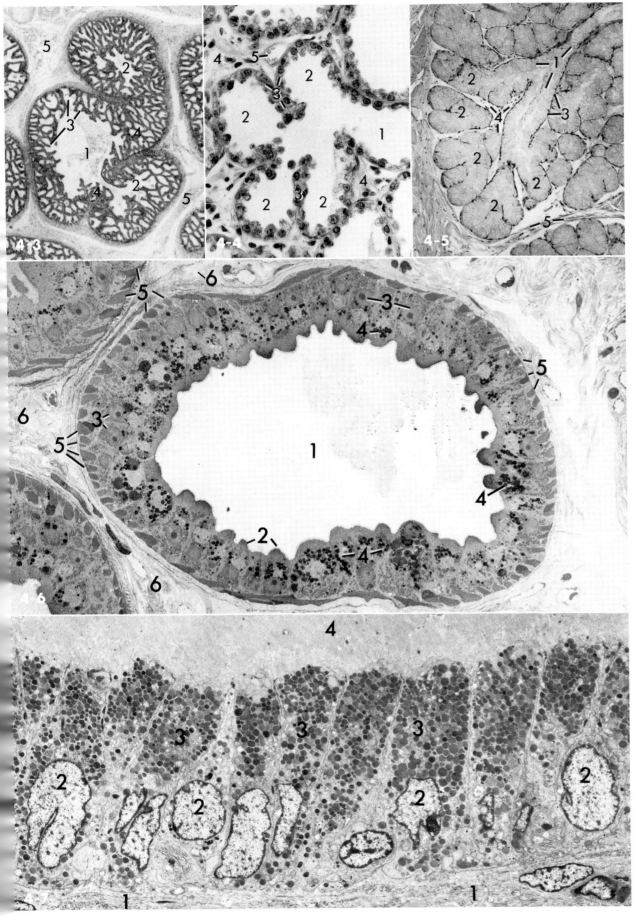

Fig. 4-3. *Simple saccular* coiled, non-branching multicellular gland. Seminal vesicle. Monkey. L.M. X 27. **1.** Main lumen of gland. **2.** Saccular dilatations. **3.** Diverticuli. **4.** Ridges covered by secretory epithelium. **5.** Connective tissue.

Fig. 4-4. *Compound saccular*, multicellular gland. Lactating mammary gland. Human. L.M. X 280. **1.** Branch of terminal duct. **2.** Saccules (distended acini; alveoli). **3.** Simple cuboidal secretory epithelium. **4.** Intralobular connective tissue. **5.** Blood capillary.

Fig. 4-5. Small *compound tubulo-acinar* multicellular gland. Mucous salivary gland. Soft palate. Monkey. L.M. X 92. **1.** Lumen of secretory tubules. **2.** Acinar end-pieces. **3.** Nuclei of mucous cells, flattened against base of cells. **4.** Intralobular connective tissue. **5.** Interlobular connective tissue.

Fig. 4-6. *Simple tubular* coiled, non-branching multicellular gland. Cross section. Odoriferous sweat gland. Human. E.M. X 600. **1.** Lumen. **2.** Simple columnar epithelium, consisting of secretory cells. **3.** Nuclei of secretory cells. **4.** Accumulations of electron-dense granules representing lysosomes (lipofuscin granules). They are not secretory granules in the classical sense. **5.** Cross-sectioned myoepithelial cells appear as regularly spaced, electron-dense profiles at the base of the epithelium. **6.** Peritubular connective tissues. This gland is enlarged further in Figs. 25-58, 25-59, and 25-60.

Fig. 4-7. Simple columnar secretory epithelium in *simple branched tubular* gland. Mucous gland. Cervix of uterus. Human. E.M. X 1800. **1.** Connective tissue elements. **2.** Nuclei of mucous cells. **3.** Mucigen droplets are most numerous in apical part of cell, but also occur below the nucleus. **4.** Lumen of tubule.

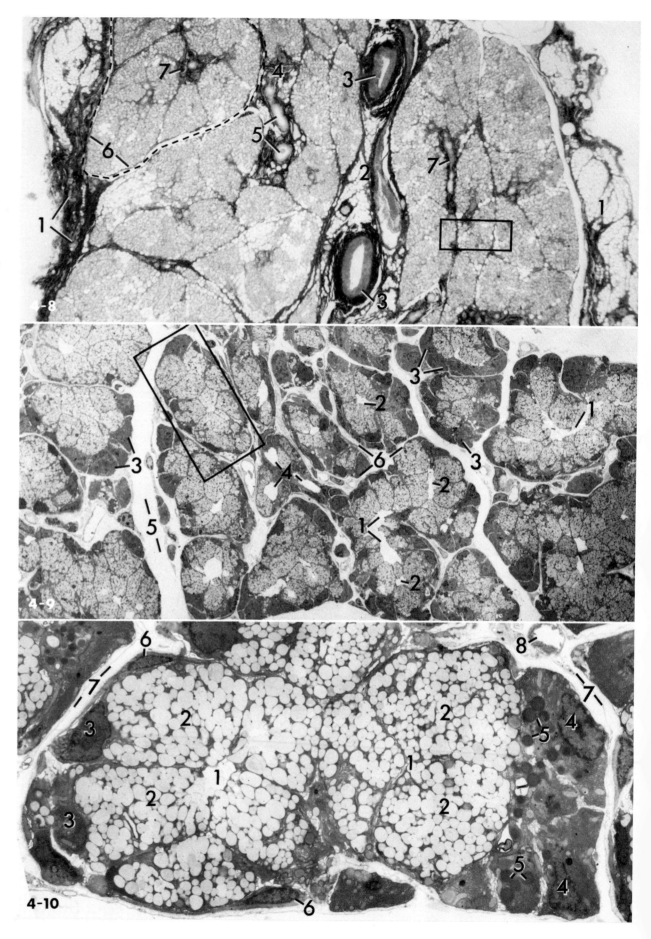

Fig. 4-8. Large *compound tubulo-acinar* gland. Sublingual salivary (mixed) gland. Human. L.M. X 22. **1.** Connective tissue capsule with some adipose tissue. **2.** Interlobar connective tissue septum. **3.** Lobar (interlobar) arteries. **4.** Interlobular connective tissue septum. **5.** Interlobular ducts. **6.** Dashed line indicates approximate limits of one lobule. **7.** Intralobular ducts.

Fig. 4-9. *Compound tubulo-acinar* gland. Enlargement of area similar to rectangle in Fig. 4-8. Sublingual salivary (mixed) gland. Rat. E.M. X 600. **1.** Lumen of secretory tubule. **2.** Lumen of acinar end-piece. **3.** Serous demilunes. **4.** Lumen of intercalated ducts at point of connection with secretory tubule. **5.** Interlobular connective tissue septum, slightly distended by tissue preparation. **6.** Delicate interacinar connective tissue septa.

Fig. 4-10. Acinar *end-piece*. Enlargement of area similar to rectangle in Fig. 4-9. Sublingual salivary (mixed) gland. Rat. E.M. X 1800. **1.** Acinar lumina. **2.** Accumulation of mucigen droplets. **3.** Nucleus of mucous cells. **4.** Nuclei of serous cells in demilunes. **5.** Secretory granules. **6.** Nucleus of myoepithelial cells. **7.** Interacinar connective tissue septa. **8.** Lumen of blood capillary.

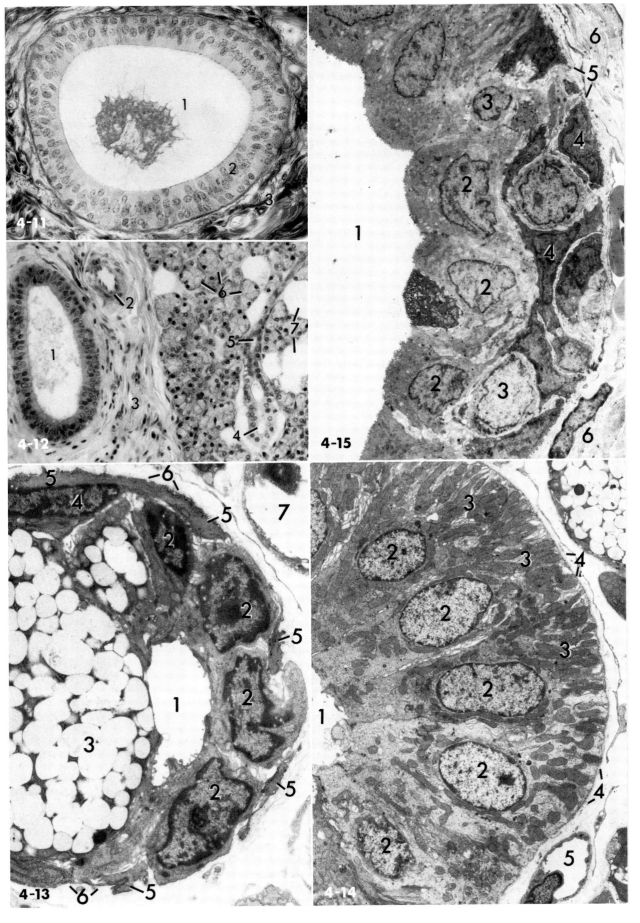

Fig. 4-11. Lobar (interlobar) duct. Sublingual salivary gland. Human. L.M. X 315. **1.** Lumen with some secretory material. **2.** Stratified columnar epithelium. **3.** Connective tissue of interlobar septum.

Fig. 4-12. Parotid (serous salivary) gland. Human. L.M. × 200. **1.** Interlobular duct with pseudostratified columnar epithelium. **2.** Arteriole. **3.** Interlobular connective tissue with low cuboidal epithelium. **4.** Intralobular duct. **5.** Intercalated duct. **6.** Serous acini. **7.** Fat cells (lipid content dissolved).

Fig. 4-13. Junction between secretory tubule and intercalated duct. Sublingual salivary (mixed) gland. Rat. E.M. X 4800. **1.** Lumen of duct. **2.** Nuclei of cuboidal duct cells. **3.** Mucigen droplets of secretory acinar cells. **4.** Nucleus of myoepithelial cell. **5.** Cytoplasmic processes of myoepithelial cell. **6.** Location of basal lamina (not resolved). **7.** Lumen of blood capillary.

Fig. 4-14. Striated (intralobular) duct. Sublingual salivary (mixed) gland. Rat. E.M. X 1600. **1.** Lumen of duct. **2.** Nuclei of columnar duct cells. **3.** Basal striations (mitochondria and infoldings of cell membrane). **4.** Location of basal lamina (not resolved). **5.** Lumen of capillary.

Fig. 4-15. Interlobular duct. Stratified cuboidal epithelium. Sublingual gland. Rat. E.M. X 1900. **1.** Lumen of duct. **2.** Nucleus of cuboidal surface cells. **3.** Nuclei of cells in intermediate epithelial layer. **4.** Nuclei of basal cells. **5.** Location of basal lamina (not resolved). **6.** Connective tissue of interlobular septum.

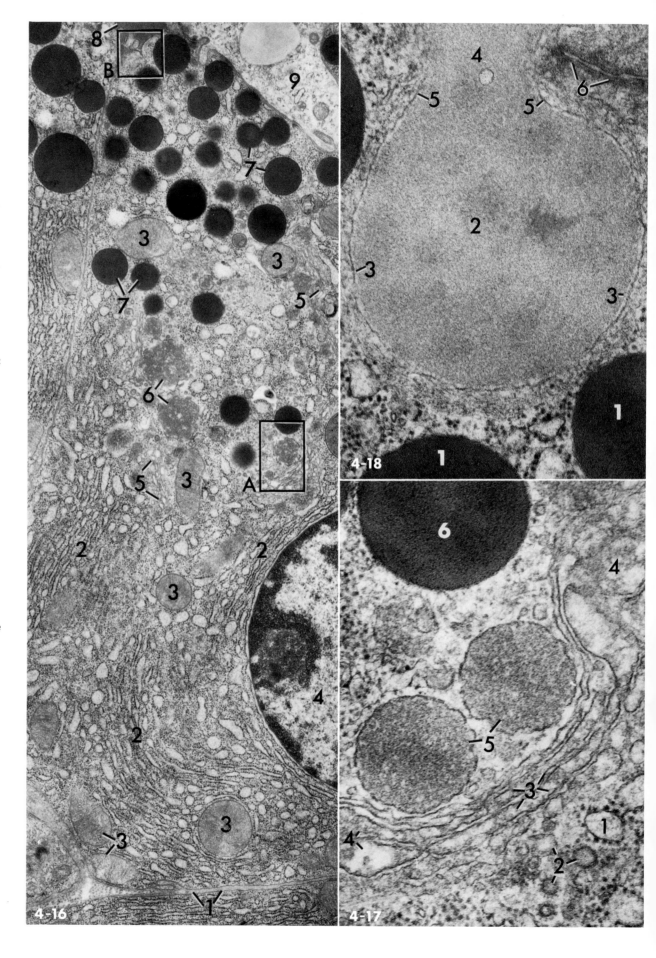

Fig. 4-16. Proteinaceous secretion. Exocrine gland. Acinar cell. Pancreas. Rat. E.M. X 13,000. **1.** External (basal) lamina. **2.** Granular endoplasmic reticulum. Cisternae are both saccular and vesicular. **3.** Mitochondria. **4.** Nucleus. **5.** Golgi zone. **6.** Condensing vacuoles and presecretory granules. **7.** Mature secretory granule. **8.** Acinar lumen with expelled secretory material. **9.** Cytoplasm of centroacinar cell.

Fig. 4-17. Golgi zone. Enlargement of area similar to rectangle (A) in Fig. 4-16. Acinar cell. Pancreas. Rat. E.M. X 66,000. **1.** Spherical cisterna of granular endoplasmic reticulum with attached ribosomes. **2.** Transfer vesicles. **3.** Golgi saccules. **4.** Bulbous ends of Golgi saccules with medium electron-dense material. **5.** Condensing vacuoles and/or presecretory granules bounded by a distinct membrane. **6.** Mature secretory granules with highly electron-dense material.

Fig. 4-18. Discharge of exocrine secretory granule. *Merocrine* secretion. Apical part of serous acinar cell. Enlargement of area similar to rectangle (B) in Fig. 4-16. Lingual salivary (mixed) gland. Rat. E.M. X 96,000. **1.** Mature secretory granules. **2.** Secretory granule at the moment of discharge through the process of *exocytosis*. Matrix of granule is now less electron-dense than in the unexpelled mature granules. **3.** Boundary membrane of discharging granule. **4.** Lumen of acinus. **5.** Points of fusion between surface cell membrane and granule boundary membrane. **6.** Junctional area of apposed acinar cell membranes.

50

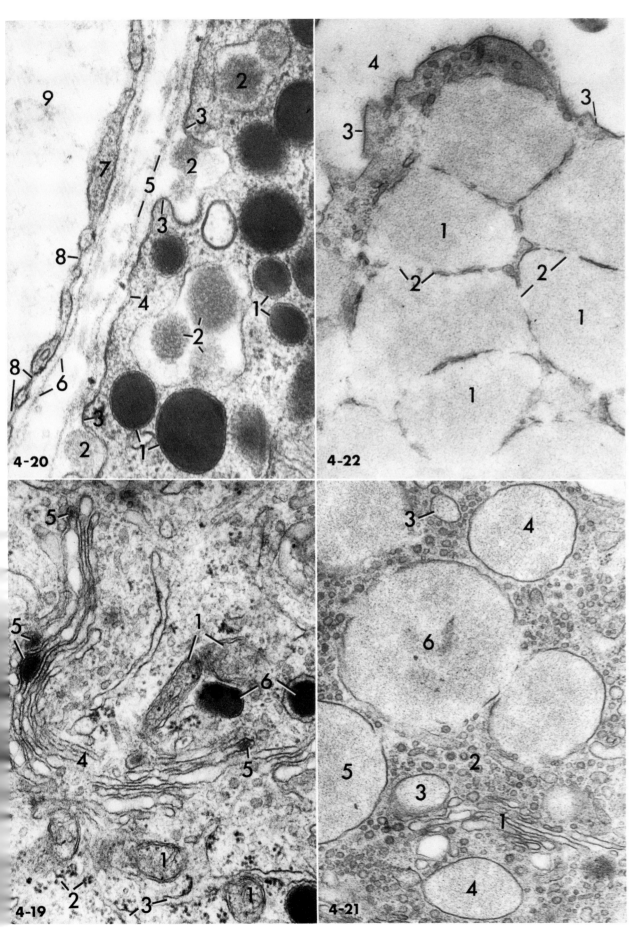

Fig. 4-19. Proteinaceous secretion. Endocrine gland. Gonadotroph cell. Adenohypophysis. Rat. E.M. X 51,000. **1.** Mitochondria. **2.** Ribosomes. **3.** Cisternae of granular endoplasmic reticulum. **4.** Golgi zone. **5.** Condensing presecretory material within Golgi saccules. **6.** Mature secretory granules with boundary membrane.

Fig. 4-20. Discharge of endocrine secretory granules. Gonadotroph cell. Adenohypophysis. Rat. E.M. X 93,000. **1.** Mature secretory granules. **2.** Discharging secretory granules. **3.** Points of fusion between boundary membrane of secretory granule and cell membrane. **4.** Cell membrane. **5.** External (basal) lamina of endocrine cell cords. **6.** Basal (external) lamina of blood capillary. **7.** Capillary (sinusoidal) endothelium. **8.** Fenestrations closed by a thin diaphragm. **9.** Capillary lumen.

Fig. 4-21. Mucoid secretion. Mucous (goblet) cell. Enlargement of area similar to rectangle (B) in Fig. 4-1. Tracheal epithelium. Human. E.M. X 33,000. **1.** Golgi zone with saccules. **2.** Transfer vesicles. **3.** Condensing vacuoles. **4.** Presecretory mucigen droplets. **5.** Mucigen droplets. **6.** Mature mucigen droplet with disintegrating boundary membrane.

Fig. 4-22. Discharge of mucoid secretion. Mucous (goblet) cell. Enlargement of area similar to rectangle (A) in Fig. 4-1. Tracheal epithelium. Human. E.M. X 33,000. **1.** Merging mucigen droplets. **2.** Disintegrating boundary membranes. **3.** Surface cell membrane of goblet cell. **4.** Lumen of trachea.

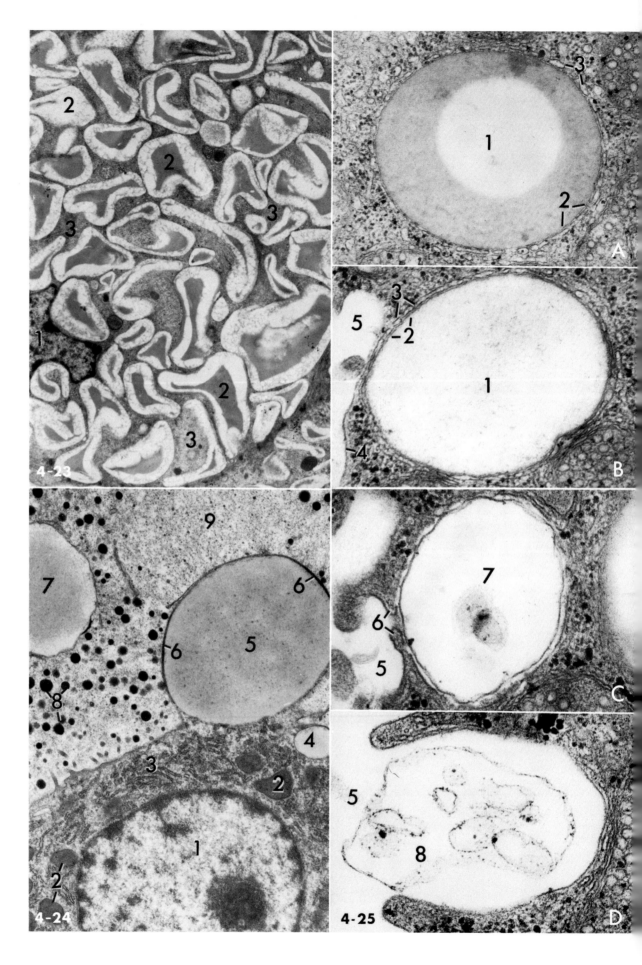

Fig. 4-23. *Holocrine* secretion. Sebaceous gland. Monkey. E.M. X 5000. **1.** Nucleus of secretory cell, highly compressed. **2.** Irregularly shaped and densely packed sebaceous lipid droplets. **3.** Narrow strands of cytoplasm. This cell is ready to be expelled by a process of holocrine excretion. The entire cell represents a small drop of sebum.

Fig. 4-24. *Apocrine* secretion. Discharge of lipid droplet. Lactating mammary gland. Mouse. E.M. X 10,000. **1.** Nucleus of secretory cell. **2.** Mitochondria. **3.** Granular endoplasmic reticulum. **4.** Small intracellular lipid droplet. **5.** Large lipid droplet at the moment of apocrine discharge. **6.** Thin rim of cell membrane and cytoplasm surrounds the lipid droplet. **7.** Discharged lipid droplet. **8.** Milk protein particles. These are discharged from the secretory cells by a process of merocrine secretion (exocytosis). **9.** Lumen of saccular acinus with finely granular proteinaceous secretion.

Fig. 4-25. *Endoplasmocrine* secretion. Cells of zona fasciculata. Adrenal cortex. Rat. The sequence A–D is arranged to simulate an assumed mechanism of lipid droplet discharge concurrent with steroid hormone release under normal and experimental conditions. (From: Rhodin J. Ultrastruct. Res. 34:23-71 (1971).) Magnifications: A) X 42,000; B) X 62,000; C) X 68,000; D) X 64,000. **1.** Lipid droplet. **2.** Interface membrane: lipid droplet/cytoplasm. **3.** Membranous casing of merging tubules of agranular endoplasmic reticulum. **4.** Cell membrane. **5.** Extracellular (interstitial) space. **6.** Fusion of cell membrane and peripheral lamina of agranular endoplasmic reticulum casing. **7.** Content of lipid droplet has disappeared, leaving behind a membranous ghost. **8.** Membranous ghost enters extracellular space, leaving behind a pit-like invagination of the cell surface. Stages similar to Fig. 4-25 B and C are seen in figs. 23-8 and 23-9 at higher magnification.

References

Freeman, J. A. Goblet cell fine structure. Anat. Rec. *154*: 121–148 (1966).

Hand, A. R. The fine structure of von Ebner's gland of the rat. J. Cell Biol. *44*: 340–353 (1970).

Hokin, L. E. Dynamic aspects of phospholipids during protein secretion. Int. Rev. Cytol. *23*: 187–208 (1968).

Kurosumi, K. Electron microscopic analysis of the secretion mechanism. Int. Rev. Cytol. *XI*: 1–124 (1961).

Moe, H. On goblet cells, especially of the intestine of some mammalian species. Int. Rev. Cytol. *IV*: 299–334 (1955).

Neutra, M. and Leblond, C. P. Synthesis of the carbohydrate of mucus in the Golgi complex as shown by electron microscope radioautography of goblet cells from rats injected with glucose-H[3]. J. Cell Biol. *30*: 119–136 (1966).

Palay, S. The morphology of secretion. *In* Frontiers in Cytology (Ed. S. Palay), pp. 305–342, Yale University Press, New Haven, 1958.

Peterson, M. and Leblond, C. Synthesis of complex carbohydrates in the Golgi region, as shown by radioautography after injection of labeled glucose. J. Cell Biol. *21*: 964–974 (1959).

Rhodin, J. A. G. The ultrastructure of the adrenal cortex of the rat under normal and experimental conditions. J. Ultrastruct. Res. *34*: 23–71 (1971).

5 Blood and lymph

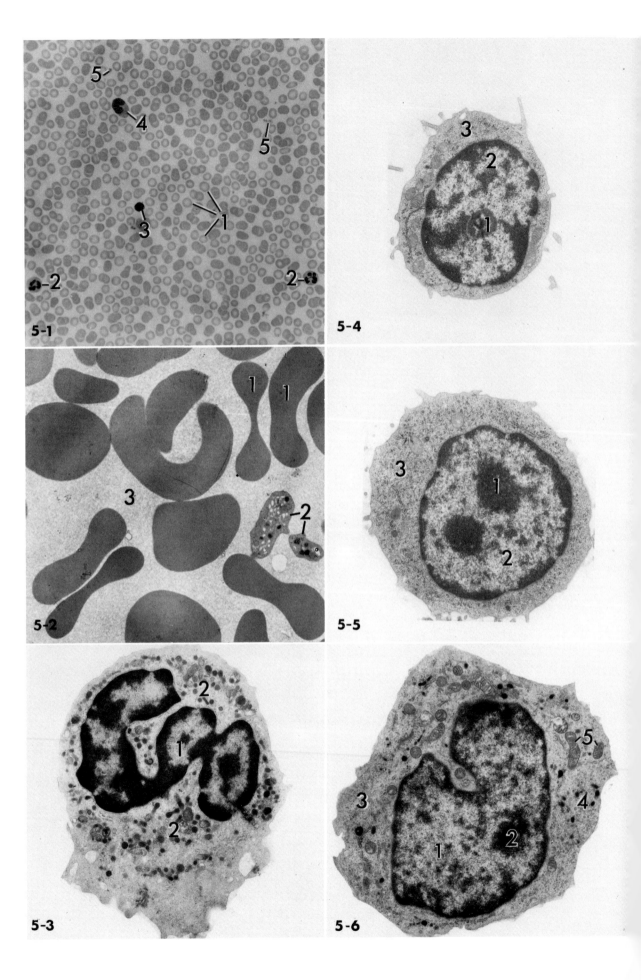

Fig. 5-1. Smear preparation of circulating blood cells. Human. L.M. X 350. **1.** Erythrocytes. **2.** Polymorphonuclear leukocytes (neutrophils). **3.** Small lymphocyte. **4.** Monocyte. **5.** Platelets.

Fig. 5-2. Sectioned blood cells in the lumen of blood vessel. Rabbit. E.M. X 4500. **1.** Erythrocytes (biconcave disks, 7 μ in diameter). **2.** Thrombocytes (platelets). **3.** Blood plasma (finely precipitated).

Fig. 5-3. Polymorphonuclear leukocyte (neutrophil), 9 μ in diameter. Bone marrow. Human. E.M. X 9000. **1.** Lobated nucleus. **2.** Specific and azurophilic granules. This neutrophil is further enlarged in Fig. 5-10.

Fig. 5-4. Small lymphocyte (4 μ in diameter) in medullary sinus of lymph node. Cat. E.M. X 10,500. **1.** Nucleolus. **2.** Nucleus. **3.** Cytoplasm. This lymphocyte is further enlarged in Fig. 5-16.

Fig. 5-5. Medium-sized lymphocyte (5.5 μ in diameter) in medullary sinus of lymph node. Cat. E.M. X 10,500. **1.** Nucleoli. **2.** Nucleus. **3.** Cytoplasm. This lymphocyte is enlarged further in Fig. 17-24.

Fig. 5-6. Monocyte (8 μ in diameter). Bone marrow. Human. E.M. X 10,000. **1.** Nucleus. **2.** Nucleolus. **3.** Cytoplasm. **4.** Azurophilic granules. **5.** Mitochondria.

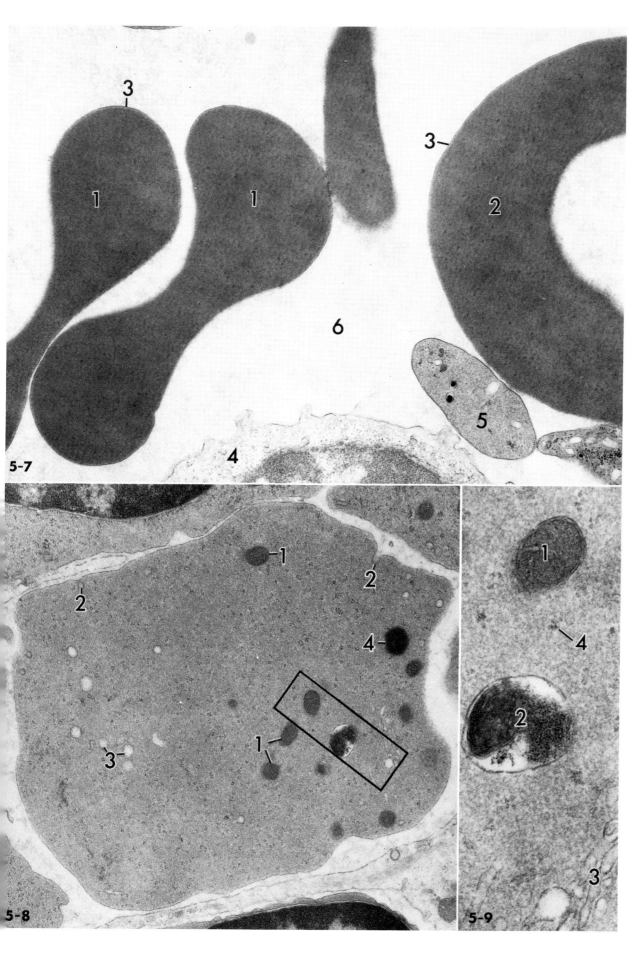

Fig. 5-7. Sectioned blood cells in lumen of blood vessel. Rabbit. E.M. X 21,000.
1. Erythrocytes sectioned perpendicularly to equatorial plane. **2.** Erthrocyte sectioned through equatorial plane. **3.** Cell membrane of erythrocyte. **4.** Part of small lymphocyte. **5.** Platelet. **6.** Blood plasma.

Fig. 5-8. Reticulocyte. Bone marrow. Human. E.M. X 24,000. **1.** Mitochondria. **2.** Pinocytotic invaginations. **3.** Vesicles. **4.** Siderosomes. **5.** Part of macrophage.

Fig. 5-9. Enlargement of rectangle in Fig. 5-8. E.M. X 60,000. **1.** Mitochondrion. **2.** Siderosome, containing ferritin particles. **3.** Membranous sacs of Golgi zone. **4.** Polyribosomes.

Fig. 5-10. Polymorphonuclear leukocyte (neutrophil). Bone marrow. Human. E.M. X 24,000. **1.** Heterochromatin of lobated nucleus. **2.** Euchromatin. **3.** Nuclear membrane. **4.** Short profile of granular endoplasmic reticulum. **5.** Azurophilic (primary) granules. **6.** Specific (secondary) granules. **7.** Cytoplasm with free monoribosomes and glycogen particles. **8.** Hyaloplasm of pseudopod. **9.** Phagocytic vacuoles. **10.** Cell membrane.

Fig. 5-11. Detail of neutrophil polymorphonuclear leukocyte. Bone marrow. Human. E.M. X 90,000. **1.** Azurophilic (primary) granules. **2.** Specific (secondary) granules. **3.** Granules with extracted core ("degranulated"). **4.** Particulate glycogen (beta-particles).

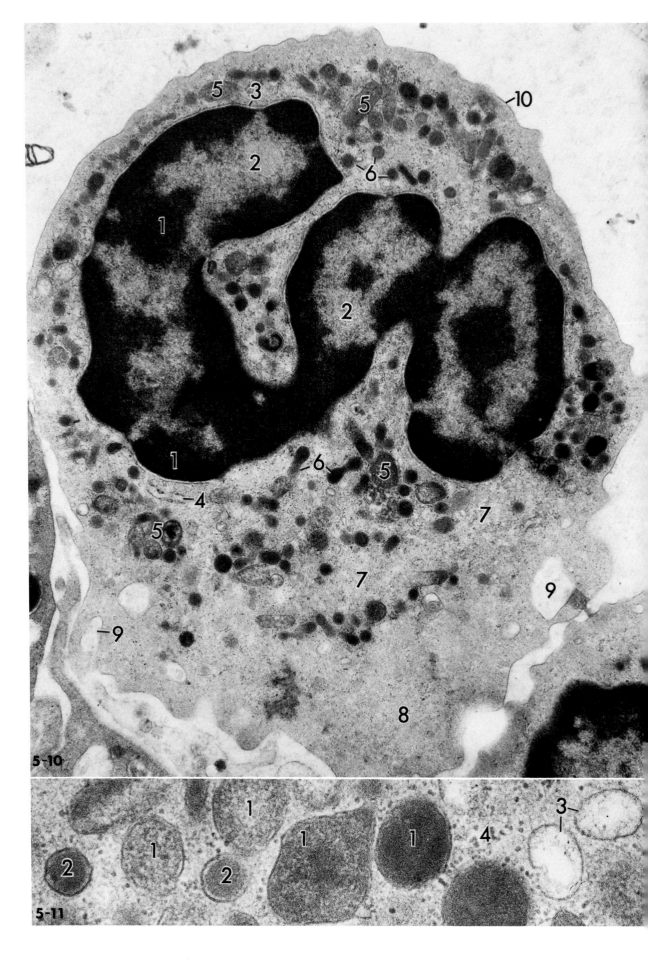

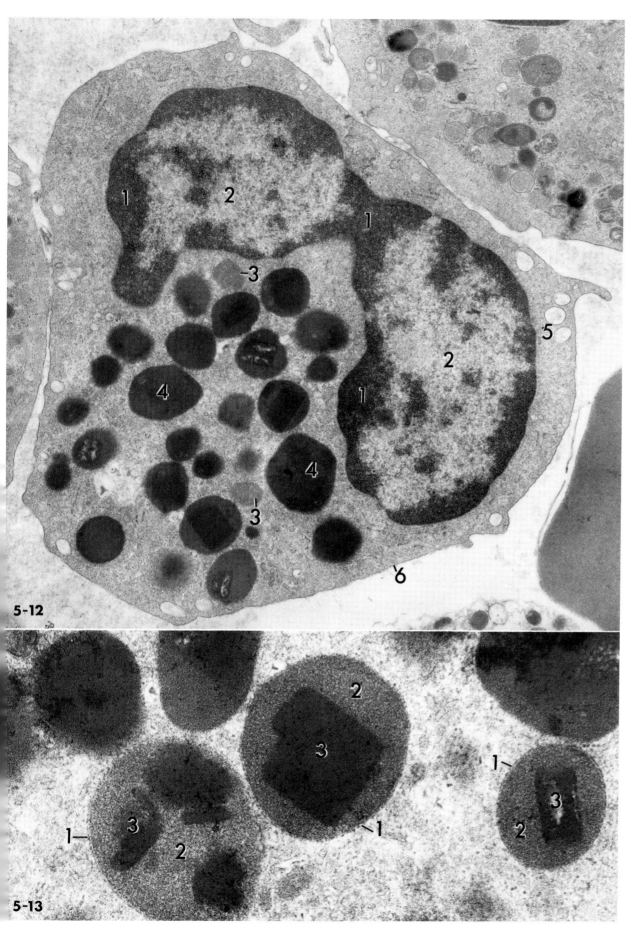

Fig. 5-12. Eosinophil polymorphonuclear leukocyte. Bone marrow. Human. E.M. X 24,000. **1.** Heterochromatin of bilobed nucleus. **2.** Euchromatin. **3.** Mitochondria. **4.** Specific granules. **5.** Phagocytic vacuoles. **6.** Cell membrane.

Fig. 5-13. Detail of eosinophil polymorphonuclear leukocyte. Bone marrow. Human. E.M. X 60,000. **1.** Boundary membrane of specific granules. **2.** Fine granular matrix of specific granules. **3.** Crystalloids.

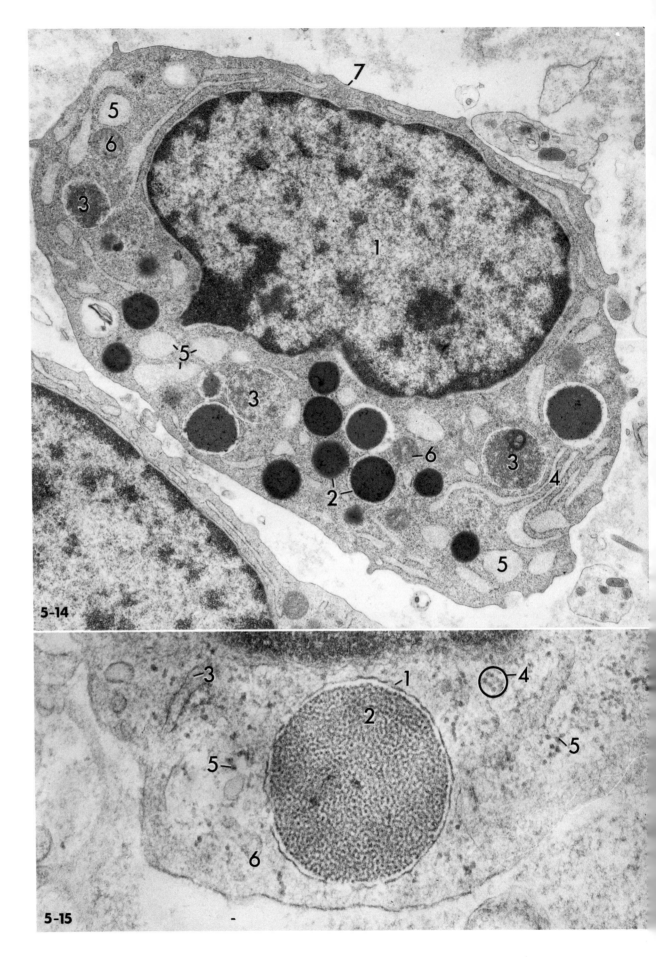

Fig. 5-14. Slightly immature basophilic polymorphonuclear leukocyte (late basophilic metamyelocyte). Bone marrow. Human. E.M. X 15,000. Since basophilic leukocytes are rare in normal human blood and marrow, and difficult to preserve adequately, a late basophilic metamyelocyte is included here. **1.** Nucleus. **2.** Granules with dense core (probably immature). **3.** Granules with light core (probably mature). **4.** Profiles of granular endoplasmic reticulum. **5.** Short dilated cisternae of granular endoplasmic reticulum. **6.** Mitochondria. **7.** Cell membrane.

Fig. 5-15. Detail of mature basophilic polymorphonuclear leukocyte. Bone marrow. Human. E.M. X 60,000. **1.** Boundary membrane of granule. **2.** Core of 150 Å particles. **3.** Short profile of granular endoplasmic reticulum. **4.** Free monoribosomes. **5.** Particulate glycogen (beta particles). **6.** Cell membrane.

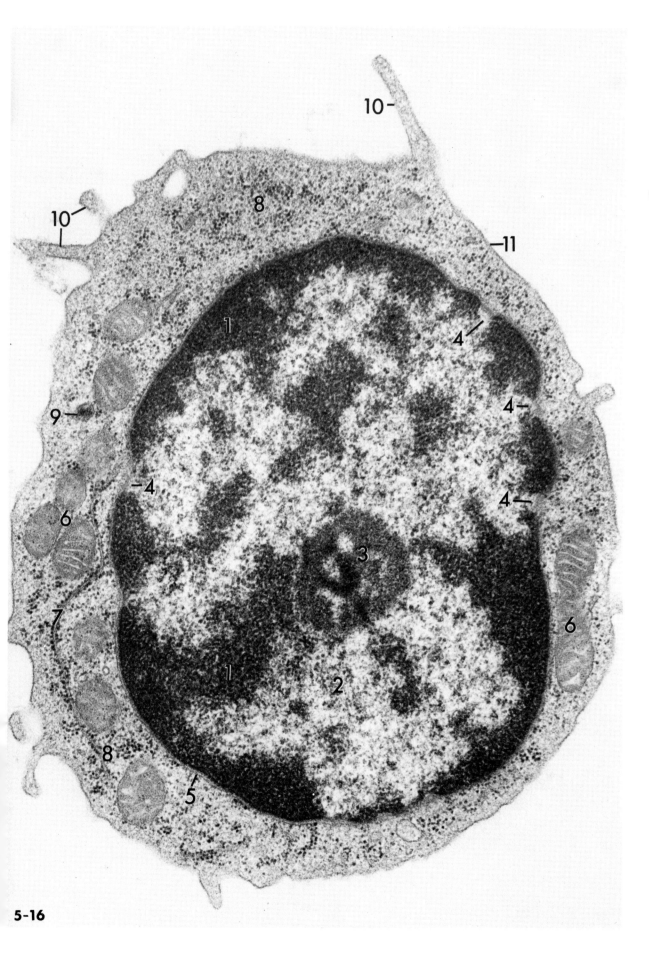

Fig. 5-16. Small lymphocyte in medullary sinus of lymph node. Cat. E.M. X 40,000.
1. Heterochromatin of nucleus.
2. Euchromatin. **3.** Nucleolus. **4.** Nuclear pore areas. **5.** Nuclear membrane.
6. Mitochondria. **7.** Profile of granular endoplasmic reticulum. **8.** Free monoribosomes.
9. Small (azurophilic) granule. **10.** Microvilli.
11. Cell (surface) membrane.

5-16

Fig. 5-17. Monocyte. Bone marrow. Human. E.M. X 18,000. **1.** Euchromatin of nucleus. **2.** Heterochromatin. **3.** Nucleolus. **4.** Mitochondria. **5.** Golgi zone. **6.** Short profiles of granular endoplasmic reticulum. **7.** Azurophilic granules. **8.** Cell membrane.

Fig. 5-18. Detail of monocyte. Bone marrow. Human. E.M. X 60,000. **1.** Golgi sacs. **2.** Golgi vesicles, probably precursors of azurophilic granules. **3.** Mitochondria. **4.** Cisternae of granular endoplasmic reticulum. **5.** Free monoribosomes. **6.** Boundary membrane of azurophilic granules. **7.** Finely stippled core of azurophilic granules.

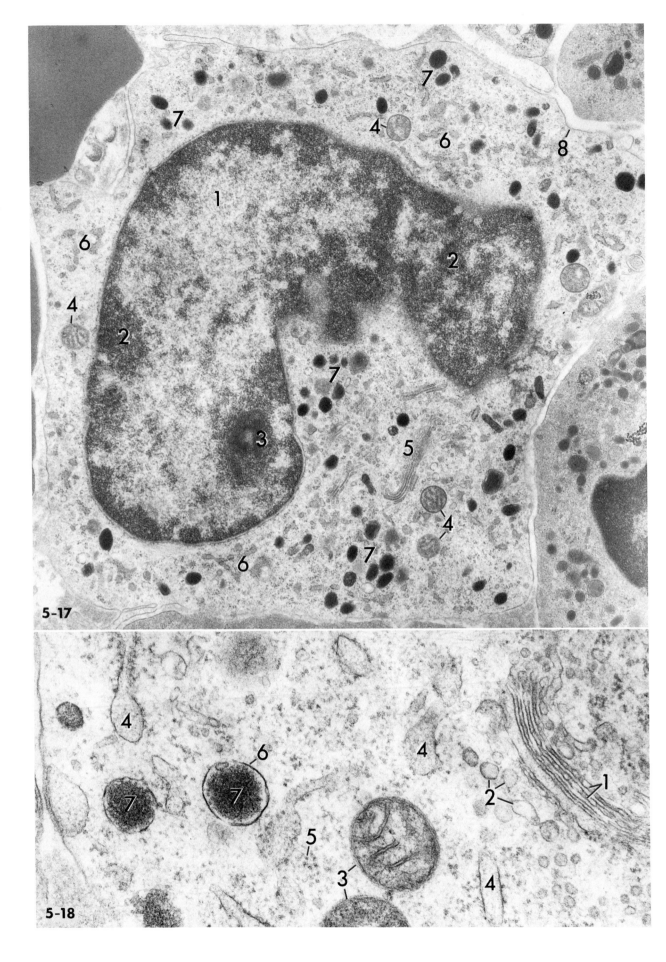

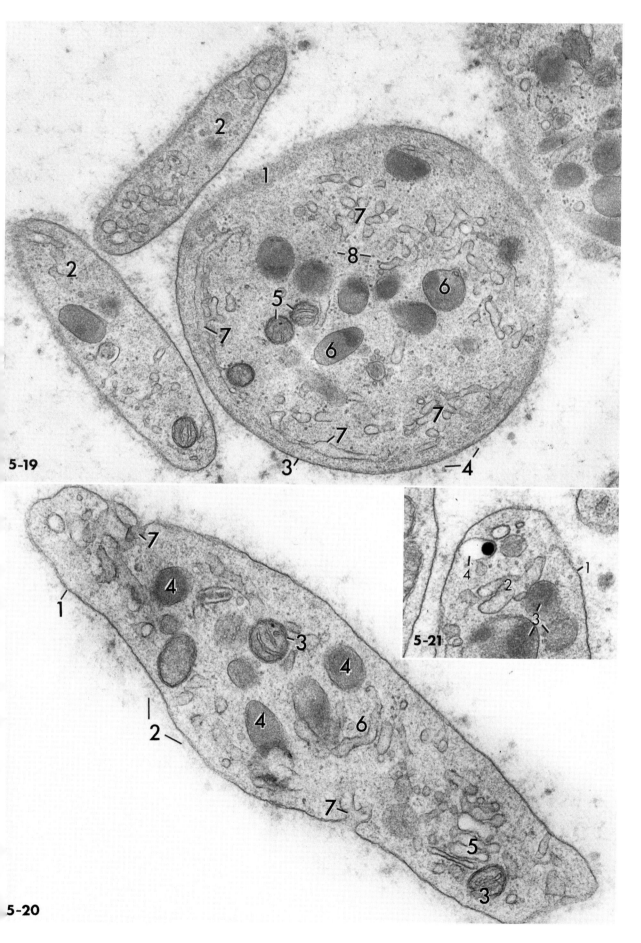

Fig. 5-19. Platelets (thrombocytes) from lumen of artery. Mouse. E.M. X 30,000. **1.** Platelet sectioned through equatorial plane.
2. Biconvex platelets, cross-sectioned.
3. Surface membrane. **4.** Fuzzy coat.
5. Mitochondria. **6.** Alpha granules.
7. System of smooth interconnected tubules.
8. Glycogen particles.

Fig. 5-20. Thrombocyte. Mouse. E.M. X 47,000.
1. Surface membrane. **2.** Fuzzy coat.
3. Mitochondria. **4.** Alpha granules. **5.** Golgi complex. **6.** Smooth tubules. **7.** Smooth tubules connected to surface membrane.

Fig. 5-21. Thrombocyte. Rabbit. E.M. X 45,000.
1. Surface membrane. **2.** Smooth tubules.
3. Alpha granules. **4.** Very dense granules with small eccentrically placed, extremely dense core.

5-19

5-20

5-21

References

Anderson, D. R. Ultrastructure of normal and leukemic leukocytes in human peripheral blood. J. Ultrastruct. Res. Suppl. *9*: 5–42 (1966).

Behnke, O. Electron microscopic observations on the membrane systems of the rat blood platelet. Anat. Rec. *158*: 121–137 (1967).

Behnke, O. Electron microscopical observations on the surface coating of human blood platelets. J. Ultrastruct. Res. *24*: 51–69 (1968).

Born, G. V. R. The functional physiology of blood platelets. Symp. Zool. Soc. Lond. *27*: 75–89 (1970).

Cohn, Z. A. The structure and function of monocytes and macrophages. Adv. Immunol. *9*: 163–214 (1968).

Daems, W. Th. On the fine structure of human neutrophilic leukocyte granules. J. Ultrastruct. Res. *24*: 343–348 (1968).

David-Ferreira, J. F. The blood platelet: electron microscopic studies. Int. Rev. Cytol. *17*: 99–148 (1964).

Fedorko, M. E. and Hirsch, J. G. Structure of monocytes and macrophages. Seminars in Hematology 7: 109–124 (1970).

Gardner, H. A., Simon, G. and Silver, M. D. The fine structure of rabbit platelets fixed in acetaldehyde. Anat. Rec. *163*: 509–516 (1969).

Lowenstein, L. M. The mammalian reticulocyte. Int. Rev. Cytol. *8*: 136–174 (1959).

Miller, F., deHarven, E. and Palade, G. E. The structure of eosinophil leukocyte granules in rodents and in man. J. Cell. Biol. *31*: 349–362 (1966).

Scott, R. E. and Horn, R. G. Ultrastructural aspects of neutrophil granulocyte development in humans. Lab. Investig. *23*: 202–215 (1970).

Silver, M. D. and Gardner, H. A. The very dense granule in rabbit platelets. J. Ultrastruct. Res. *23*: 366–377 (1968).

Spicer, S. S. and Hardin, J. H. Ultrastructure, cytochemistry and function of neutrophil leukocyte granules. A review. Lab. Investig. *20*: 488–497 (1969).

White, J. G. Interaction of membrane systems in blood platelets. Am. J. Path. *66*: 295–312 (1972).

Wivel, N. A., Mandel, M. A. and Asofsky, R. M. Ultrastructural study of thoracic duct lymphocytes of mice. Am. J. Anat. *128*: 57–72 (1970).

Zucker-Franklin, D. The ultrastructure of cells in human thoracic duct lymph. J. Ultrastruct. Res. *9*: 325–339 (1963).

Zucker-Franklin, D. Electron microscopic study of human basophils. Blood *29*: 878–890 (1967).

Zucker-Franklin, D. Electron microscopic studies of human granulocytes: structural variations related to function. Seminars in Hematology *5*: 109–133 (1968).

Zucker-Franklin, D. and Hirsch, J. G. Electron microscope studies on the degranulation of rabbit peritoneal leukocytes during phagocytosis. J. Expt. Med. *120*: 569–576 (1964).

6 Blood cell formation

Fig. 6-1. Section of red bone marrow. Human. L.M. X 150. **1.** Bone trabecula. **2.** Fat cells. **3.** Myeloid tissue (individual cell types cannot be identified at this magnification). **4.** Arteriole. **5.** Circle: sinusoidal capillary filled with blood cells. **6.** Megakaryocyte.

Fig. 6-2. Smear-preparation of bone marrow cells. Human. L.M. X 380. At this magnification some cells can easily be identified. Other cells cannot, particularly since this is a black and white illustration. **1.** Myeloblast. **2.** Promyelocyte. **3.** Neutrophil myelocyte. **4.** Eosinophil myelocyte. **5.** Neutrophil metamyelocyte. **6.** Neutrophil metamyelocyte (band cell). **7.** Neutrophil polymorph. **8.** Basophil erythroblast. **9.** Polychromatic erythroblast. **10.** Orthochromatic erythroblast. **11.** Erythrocyte.

Fig. 6-3. Section of red bone marrow fixed *in situ*. Human. E.M. X 1900. At this magnification most cells can be identified with accuracy. **1.** Hemocytoblast or very early myeloblast. **2.** Late promyelocyte. **3.** Myelocyte. **4.** Metamyelocyte. **5.** Neutrophil polymorph. **6.** Eosinophil metamyelocyte. **7.** Late proerythroblast. **8.** Basophil erythroblast. **9.** Erythrocyte. **10.** Promonocyte. **11.** Small lymphocyte. **12.** Nucleus of promegakaryocyte.

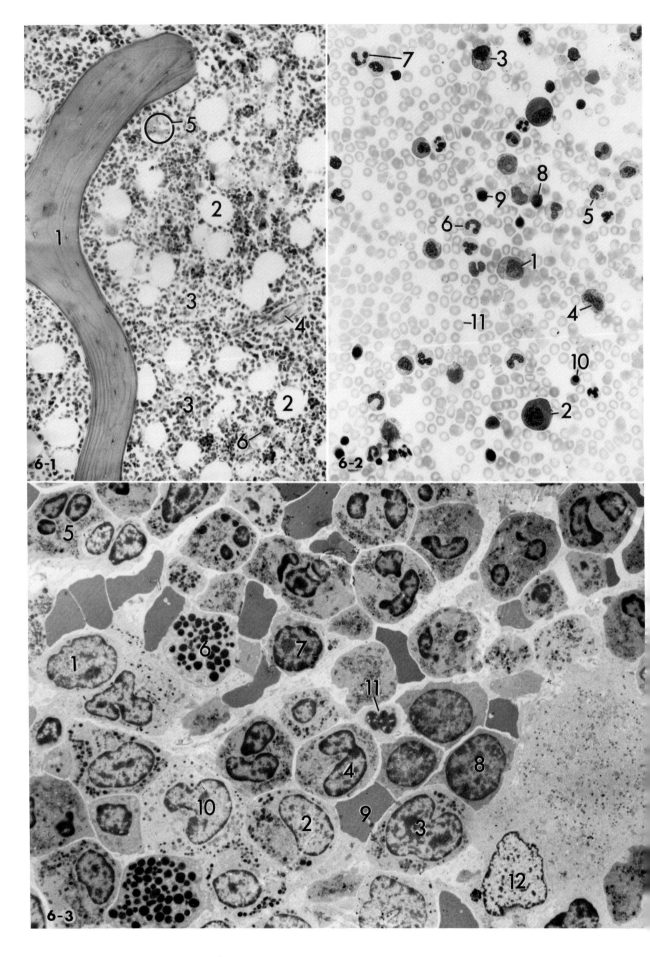

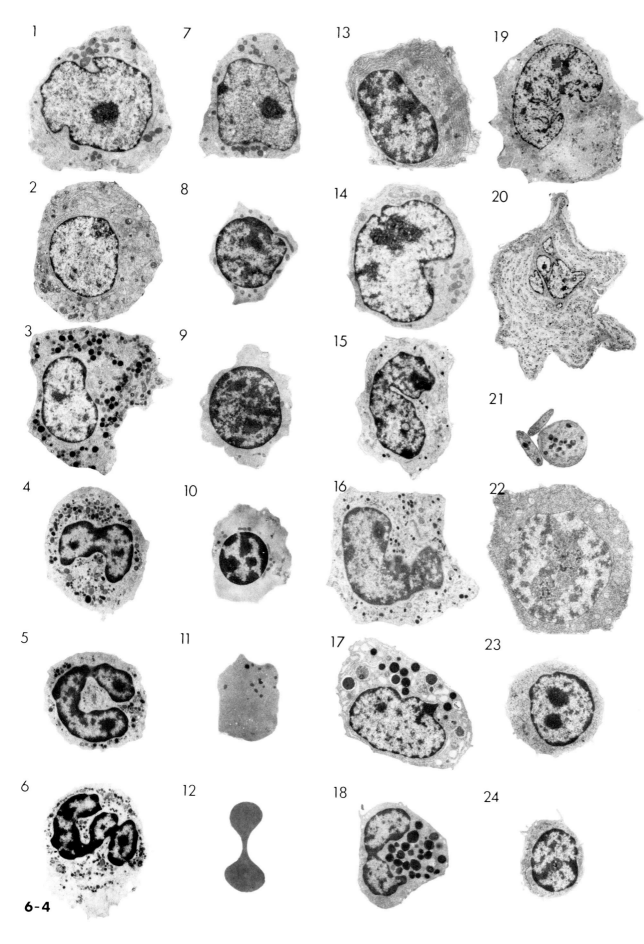

Fig. 6-4. Blood cells, their precursors in myeloid and lymphoid tissues, and some closely related cells have been selected and arranged to facilitate the study of nuclear and cytoplasmic ratios, shapes, sizes, and other characteristics. With few exceptions, the cells are presented at approximately the same magnification. Most cells or parts thereof have been further magnified for detailed study on subsequent pages or elsewhere in this book. Human (except as indicated). E.M. X 4500 (except as indicated).

Neutrophilic leukocyte series
1. Late hemocytoblast or early myeloblast. See Fig. 6-9.
2. Early promyelocyte. See Fig. 6-10.
3. Late promyelocyte. X 4000. See Fig. 6-11.
4. Late myelocyte. See Fig. 6-12.
5. Metamyelocyte (band cell). See Fig. 6-13.
6. Neutrophil polymorph. See Fig. 5-10.

Erythrocytic series
7. Late hemocytoblast or early proerythroblast. See Fig. 6-21.
8. Basophilic erythroblast. See Fig. 6-24.
9. Polychromatic erythroblast. See Fig. 6-23.
10. Orthochromatic erythroblast. See Fig. 6-26.
11. Reticulocyte. See Fig. 5-8.
12. Erythrocyte. Rabbit. See Fig. 5-7.

Plasma cell
13. Plasma cell. Bone marrow. See Fig. 7-29.

Monocytic series
14. Late monoblast. See Fig. 6-18.
15. Promonocyte. See Fig. 6-19.
16. Monocyte. See Fig. 5-17.

Basophilic polymorph
17. Basophilic polymorph. X 3500. See Fig. 5-14.

Eosinophilic polymorph
18. Eosinophilic polymorph. See Fig. 5-12.

Megakaryocytic series
19. Promegakaryocyte. X 1500. See Fig. 6-28.
20. Megakaryocyte. Spleen. Rat. X 930. See Fig. 6-31.
21. Thrombocytes/platelets. Mouse. See Fig. 5-19.

Lymphocytic series
22. Lymphoblast/large lymphocyte. Spleen. Rat. X 3500. See Fig. 17-26.
23. Medium-sized lymphocyte. Lymph node. Rat. See Fig. 17-24.
24. Small lymphocyte. Lymph node. Rat. See Fig. 5-16.

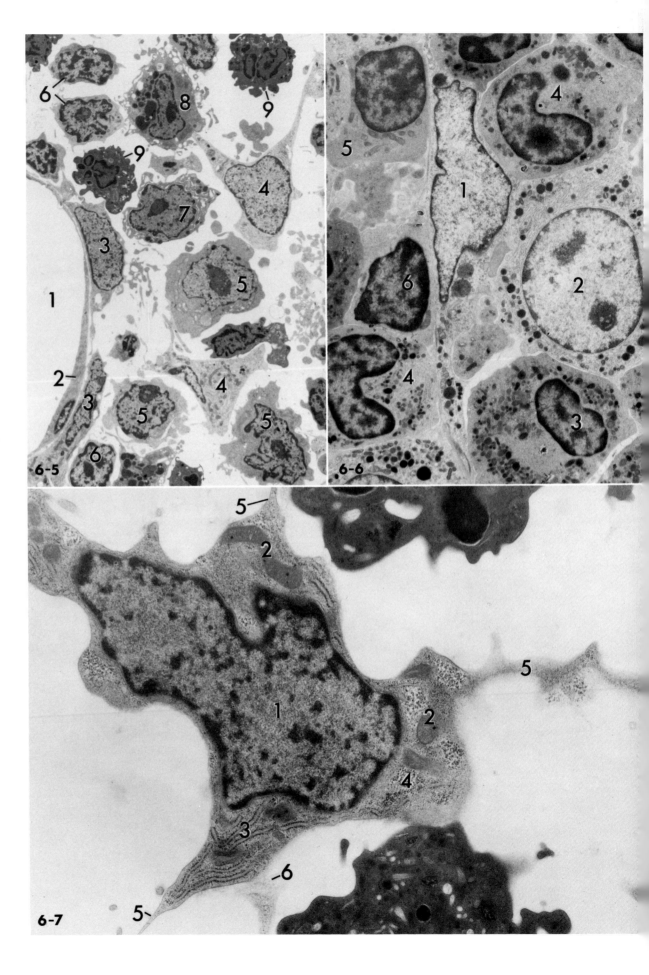

Fig. 6-5. Section of red bone marrow fixed by arterial perfusion *in situ*. Cells are slightly separated, probably because of too high perfusion pressure, but this phenomenon facilitates the study of the reticular cells of the marrow. Newborn rat. Femur. E.M. X 1800. **1.** Lumen of sinusoidal capillary. **2.** Endothelium. **3.** Pericapillary cells. **4.** Reticular cells. **5.** Hemocytoblasts or myeloblasts. **6.** Small lymphocytes. **7.** Myelocyte. **8.** Free macrophage. **9.** Polymorphs.

Fig. 6-6. Section of red bone marrow fixed *in situ*. Human. E.M. X 4200. **1.** Nucleus of reticular cell. This cell is also a fixed macrophage since its cytoplasm contains lysosomes. **2.** Nucleus of late neutrophil promyelocyte. **3.** Nucleus of late neutrophil myelocyte. **4.** Band cells. **5.** Polychromatic erythroblast. **6.** Nucleus of small lymphocyte.

Fig. 6-7. Bone marrow. Same preparation as in Fig. 6-5. Femur. Newborn rat. E.M. X 23,000. **1.** Nucleus of reticular cell. **2.** Mitochondria. **3.** Granular endoplasmic reticulum. **4.** Particulate glycogen. **5.** Slender cytoplasmic extensions give this cell a stellate shape. **6.** Fine reticular fibrils.

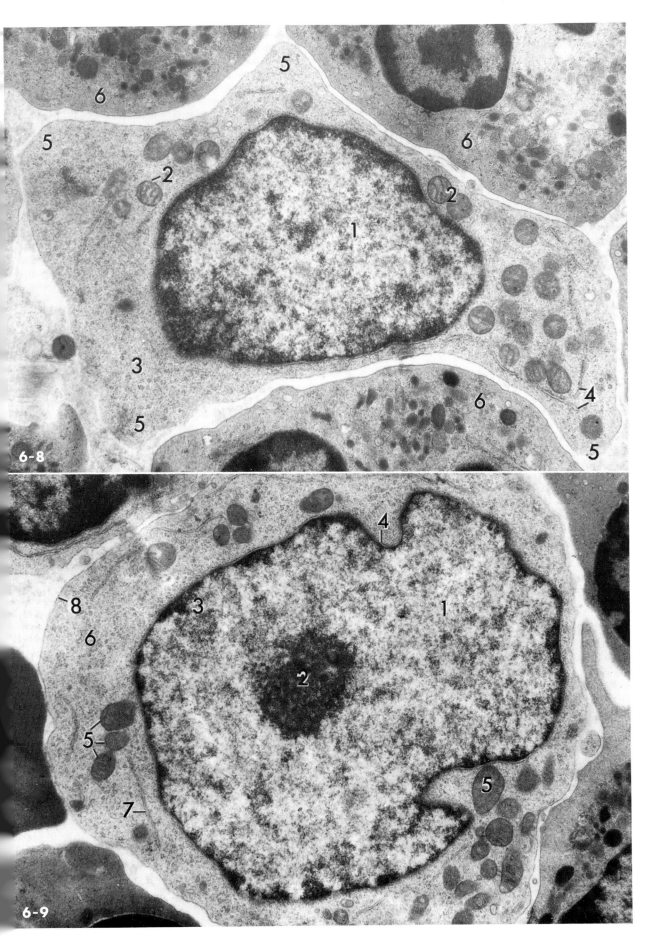

Fig. 6-8. Hemocytoblast. Although not identified by radioautography, but based on its ultrastructural characteristics, this cell could very well represent a free hemopoietic stem cell. Bone marrow. Human. E.M. X 21,000.
1. Nucleus. **2.** Mitochondria. **3.** Ribosomes. **4.** Granular endoplasmic reticulum. **5.** Blunt cytoplasmic extensions give this cell an angular shape. **6.** Cytoplasm of myelocytes.

Fig. 6-9. Early myeloblast or late hemocytoblast. Bone marrow. Human. E.M. X 18,000.
1. Abundant euchromatin. **2.** Nucleolus. **3.** Narrow rim of heterochromatin. **4.** Nuclear membrane. **5.** Mitochondria. **6.** Ribosomes. **7.** Granular endoplasmic reticulum. **8.** Smooth surface gives this cell a rounded shape.

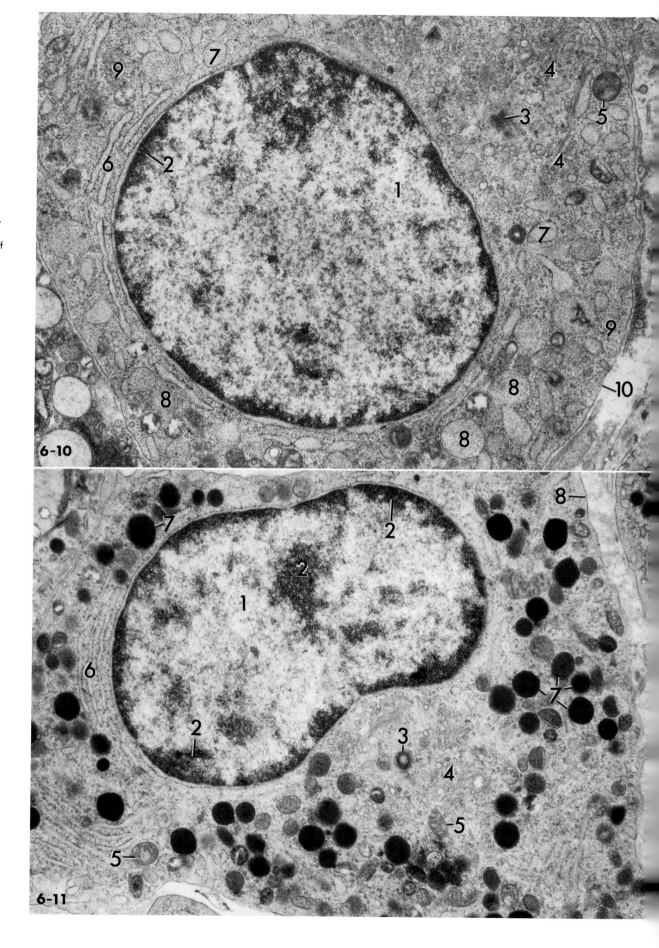

Fig. 6-10. Early neutrophilic promyelocyte. Bone marrow. Human. E.M. X 21,000. **1.** Round nucleus with abundant euchromatin. **2.** Heterochromatin. **3.** Centriole. **4.** Golgi zone. **5.** Mitochondrion. **6.** Granular endoplasmic reticulum. **7.** Dilated cisternae of granular endoplasmic reticulum. **8.** Early light azurophilic (primary) granules. **9.** Ribosomes. **10.** Cell membrane. Enlarged detail of this cell in Fig. 6-14.

Fig. 6-11. Late neutrophilic promyelocyte. Bone marrow. Human. E.M. X 18,000. **1.** Slightly indented, oval nucleus with decreasing amounts of euchromatin. **2.** Heterochromatin. Nucleolus not in plane of section. **3.** Centriole. **4.** Golgi zone. **5.** Mitochondria. **6.** Granular endoplasmic reticulum. **7.** Late dense azurophilic (primary) granules. **8.** Cell membrane. Enlarged detail of this cell in Fig. 6-15.

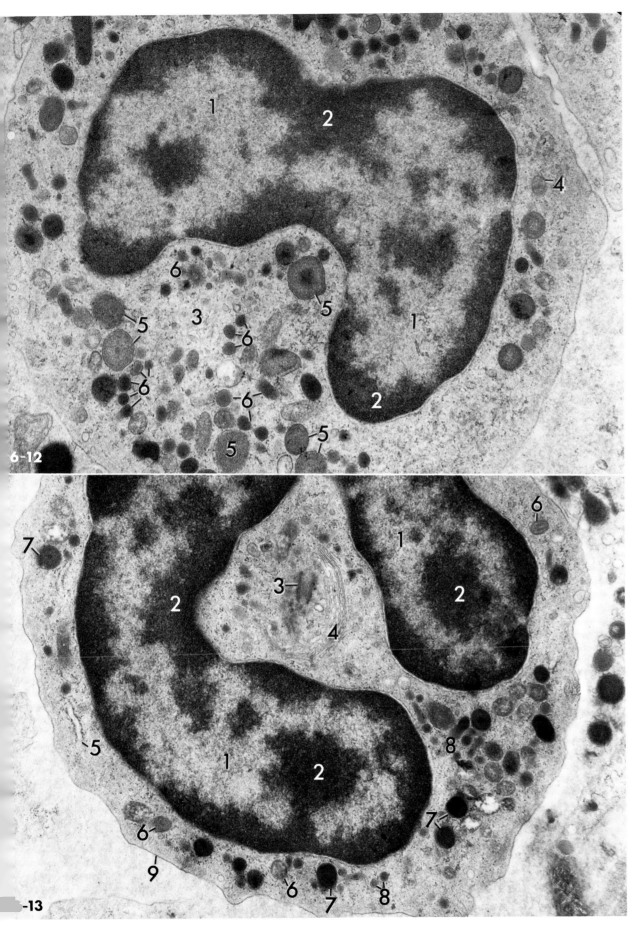

Fig. 6-12. Late neutrophilic myelocyte. Bone marrow. Human. E.M. X 24,000. **1.** Kidney-shaped nucleus with small amounts of euchromatin. **2.** Greatly increased amounts of heterochromatin. **3.** Golgi zone (mostly out of plane of section). **4.** Mitochondrion. **5.** Azurophilic (primary) granules. **6.** Specific (secondary) granules. Enlarged detail of this cell in Fig. 6-16.

Fig. 6-13. Late neutrophilic metamyelocyte (band cell). Bone marrow. Human. E.M. X 24,000. **1.** Horse-shoe shaped nucleus with small amounts of euchromatin. **2.** Heterochromatin. **3.** Centriole. **4.** Golgi zone. **5.** Granular endoplasmic reticulum. **6.** Mitochondria. **7.** Azurophilic (primary granules). **8.** Specific (secondary) granules. **9.** Cell membrane. Enlarged detail of this cell in Fig. 6-17.

Fig. 6-14. Detail of early neutrophilic promyelocyte. Bone marrow. Human. E.M. X 60,000. 1. Cisternae of granular endoplasmic reticulum. 2. Ribosomes. 3. Early azurophilic (primary) granules. These develop from small Golgi vesicles (a), enlarge and accumulate a flocculent material (b) which gradually is condensed (c & d). 4. Boundary membrane of azurophilic granule.

Fig. 6-15. Detail of late neutrophilic promyelocyte. Bone marrow. Human. E.M. X 60,000. 1. This stage is characterized by an increase in number and core density of the azurophilic (primary) granules. 2. Ribosomes. 3. Circle: Glycogen particles.

Fig. 6-16. Detail of neutrophilic myelocyte. Bone marrow. Human. E.M. X 60,000. 1. Azurophilic (primary) granules. 2. Specific secondary) granules. 3. Extracted ("degranulated") granule. 4. Circle: glycogen particles.

Fig. 6-17. Detail of neutrophilic metamyelocyte. Bone marrow. Human. E.M. X 60,000. 1. Azurophilic (primary) granules. 2. Specific (secondary) granules. 3. Extracted ("degranulated") granules. 4. Glycogen particles.

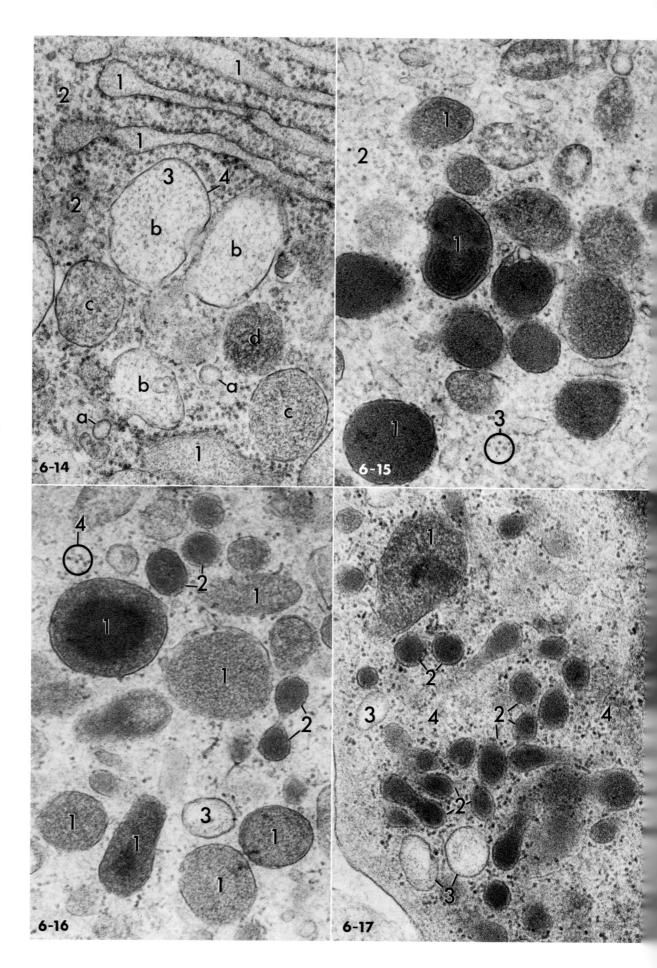

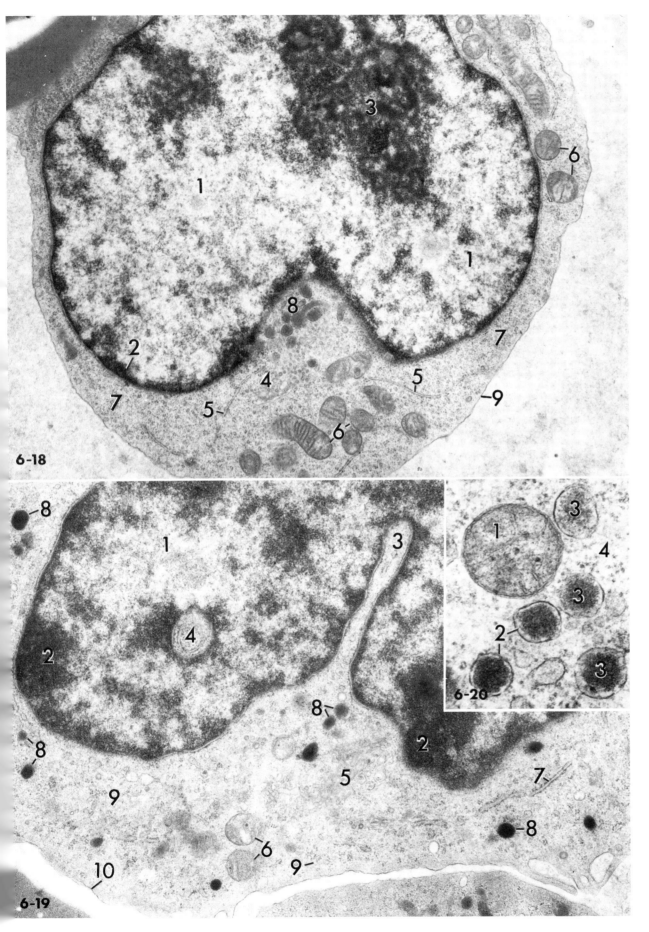

Fig. 6-18. Early monoblast. Bone marrow. Human. E.M. X 18,000. **1.** Large indented nucleus with large amounts of euchromatin. **2.** Small amounts of heterochromatin. **3.** Nucleolus. **4.** Small Golgi zone. **5.** Granular endoplasmic reticulum. **6.** Mitochondria. **7.** Ribosomes. **8.** Small azurophilic granules. **9.** Cell membrane.

Fig. 6-19. Promonocyte. Bone marrow. Human. E.M. X 25,000. **1.** Deeply indented nucleus with relatively large amounts of euchromatin. **2.** Heterochromatin. **3.** Cytoplasmic indentation, sectioned longitudinally. **4.** Cytoplasmic indentation, cross-sectioned. **5.** Golgi zone. **6.** Mitochondria. **7.** Granular endoplasmic reticulum. **8.** Azurophilic granules. **9.** Ribosomes. **10.** Cell membrane.

Fig. 6-20. Detail of promonocyte. Bone marrow. Human. E.M. X 62,000. **1.** Mitochondrion. **2.** Boundary membrane of azurophilic granules. **3.** Dense core. **4.** Ribosomes.

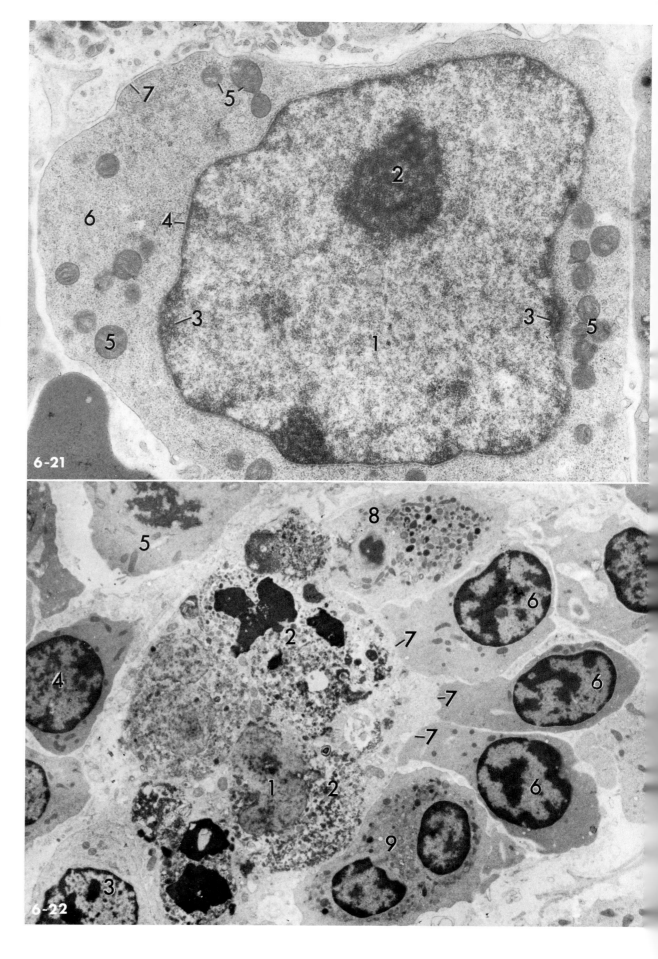

Fig. 6-21. Early proerythroblast or late hemocytoblast. Bone marrow. Human. E.M. X 21,000. **1.** Abundant euchromatin. **2.** Nucleolus. **3.** Narrow rim of heterochromatin. **4.** Nuclear membrane. **5.** Mitochondria. **6.** Ribosomes. **7.** Cell membrane.

Fig. 6-22. Colony of erythroid elements. Bone marrow. Human. E.M. X 4500. **1.** Nucleus of macrophage. **2.** Cytoplasm containing a variety of secondary lysosomes. **3.** Nucleus of proerythroblast. **4.** Nucleus of basophilic erythroblast. **5.** Basophilic erythroblast in mitosis. **6.** Nuclei of polychromatic erythroblasts. **7.** Area where cytoplasmic extensions of erythroblast make contact with the macrophage. Similar area is enlarged in Fig. 6-24. **8.** Neutrophilic myelocyte. **9.** Neutrophilic metamyelocyte.

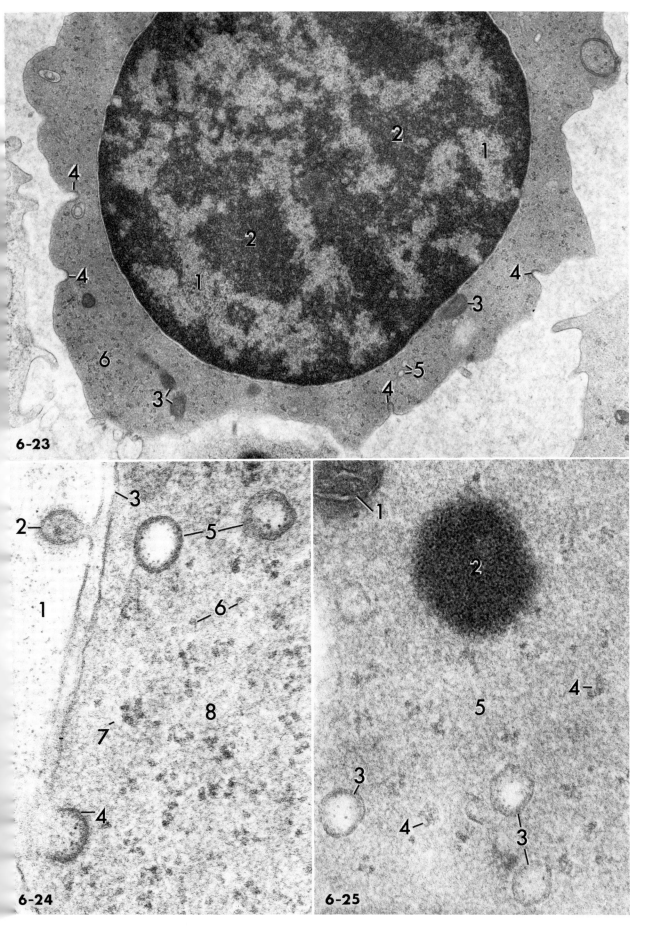

6-23

6-24

6-25

Fig. 6-23. Polychromatic erythroblast. Bone marrow. Human. E.M. X 24,000. **1.** Round nucleus with reduced amount of euchromatin. **2.** Heterochromatin. **3.** Mitochondria. **4.** Micropinocytotic invaginations of cell membrane. **5.** Micropinocytotic vesicles. **6.** Polyribosomes.

Fig. 6-24. Detail of contact between macrophage and basophilic erythroblast. Bone marrow. Human. E.M. X 90,000. **1.** Cytoplasm of macrophage with numerous 80 Å ferritin particles. **2.** Invagination of macrophage cell membrane. The direction of membrane movement can be either inward (pinocytosis) or outward (exocytosis). **3.** Cell membrane of basophilic erythroblast. **4.** Micropinocytotic invagination of cell membrane containing some ferritin particles. **5.** Micropinocytotic vesicles with ferritin particles. **6.** Monoribosomes. **7.** Polyribosomes. **8.** The low background density of the cytoplasm is caused by a small concentration of hemoglobin.

Fig. 6-25. Detail of orthochromatic erythroblast. Bone marrow. Human. E.M. X 90,000. **1.** Mitochondrion. **2.** Siderosome, packed with ferritin particles. **3.** Micropinocytotic vesicles with ferritin particles. **4.** Polyribosomes. **5.** The high background density is caused by a large concentration of hemoglobin.

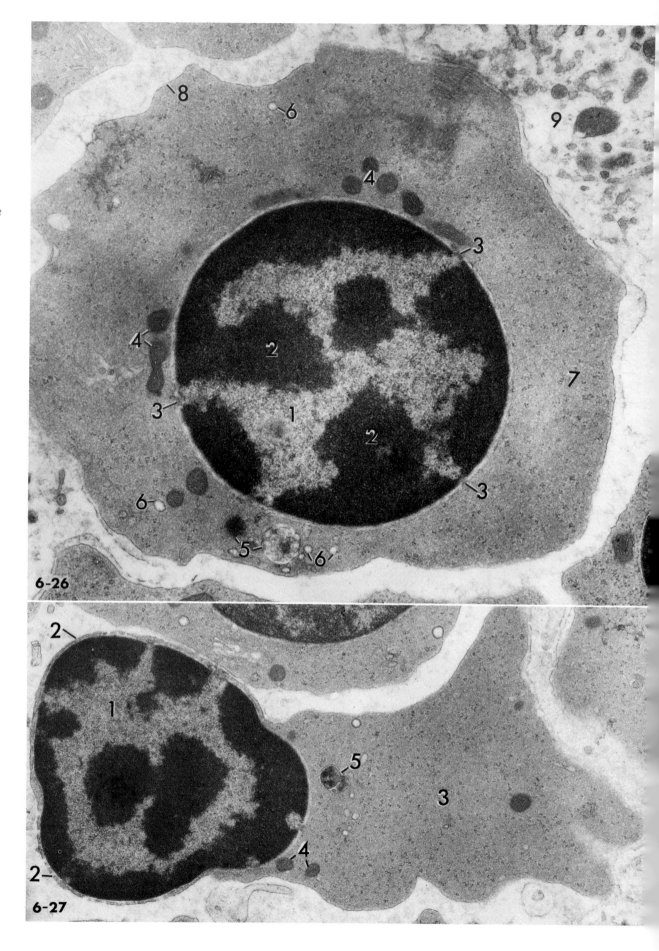

Fig. 6-26. Orthochromatic erythroblast. Bone marrow. Human. E.M. X 28,000. **1.** Small, round nucleus with greatly reduced amount of euchromatin. **2.** Heterochromatin. **3.** Areas of nuclear pores. **4.** Mitochondria. **5.** Siderosomes. **6.** Micropinocytotic vesicles. **7.** Ribosomes. **8.** Cell membrane. **9.** Macrophage cytoplasm.

Fig. 6-27. Nuclear extrusion in orthochromatic erythroblast. Bone marrow. Human. E.M. X 15,000. **1.** Nucleus. **2.** Thin rim of cytoplasm. **3.** Incumbent reticulocyte. **4.** Mitochondria. **5.** Siderosome.

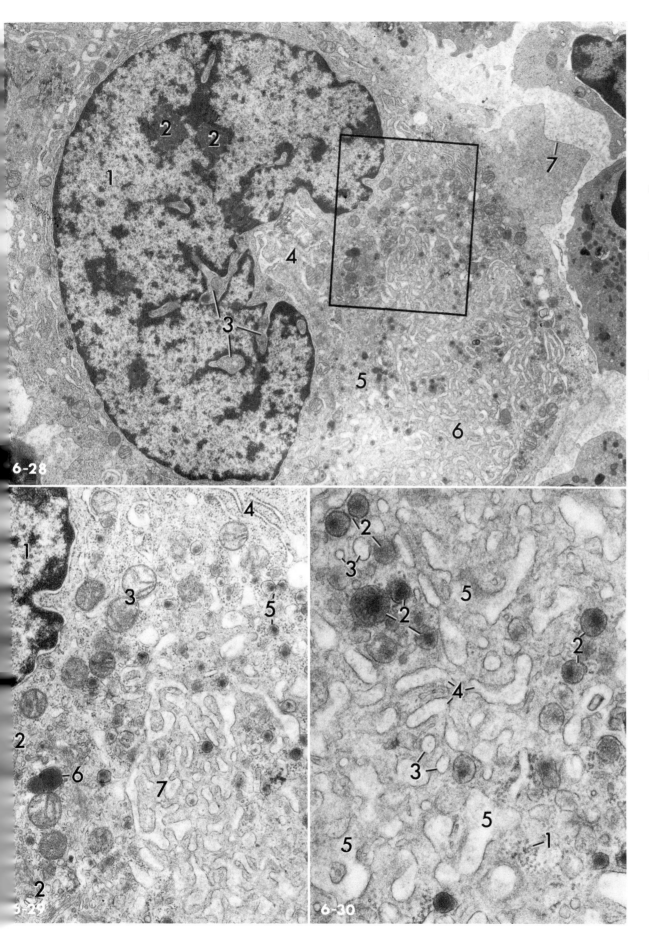

Fig. 6-28. Promegakaryocyte. Bone marrow. Human. E.M. X 6000. **1.** Nucleus. **2.** Nucleoli. **3.** Deep indentations of nuclear surface. **4.** Golgi zone. **5.** Central cytoplasm. **6.** Peripheral cytoplasm. **7.** Cell membrane.

Fig. 6-29. Promegakaryocyte. Enlargement of rectangle in Fig. 6-28. Bone marrow. Human. E.M. X 21,000. **1.** Nucleus **2.** Golgi zones. **3.** Mitochondria. **4.** Granular endoplasmic reticulum. **5.** Alpha granules. **6.** Lysosome. **7.** System of interconnected vesicles, tubules and flat membranous sacs referred to as platelet demarcation membranes and channels.

Fig. 6-30. Detail of promegakaryocyte. Bone marrow. Human. E.M. X 41,000. **1.** Ribosomes. **2.** Alpha granules. **3.** Vesicles. **4.** Tubules. **5.** Interconnected flat membranous sacs.

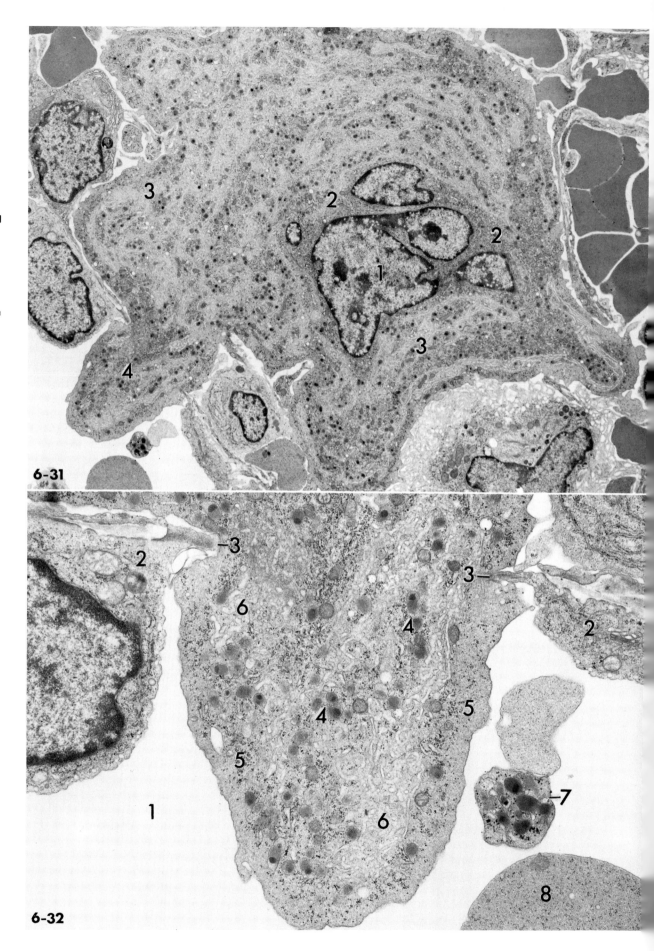

Fig. 6-31. Megakaryocyte. Diameter about 35 μ. Spleen. Rat. E.M. X 3600. **1.** Lobulated nucleus. **2.** Central cytoplasm. **3.** Peripheral cytoplasm with numerous azurophilic granules. **4.** Pseudopod protruding into the lumen of splenic venous sinus.

Fig. 6-32. Enlargement of megakaryocyte pseudopod seen in Fig. 6-31. Spleen. Rat. E.M. X 15,000. **1.** Lumen of venous sinus. **2.** Cytoplasm of lining (littoral) cells. **3.** Stoma (opening) between lining cells, penetrated by megakaryocyte pseudopod. **4.** Alpha granules (azurophilic). **5.** Cytoplasm rich in glycogen particles. **6.** Platelet demarcation channels and membranes. **7.** Free platelet (thrombocyte). **8.** Reticulocyte.

References

Ackerman, G. A. Ultrastructure and cytochemistry of the developing neutrophil. Lab. Investig. *19*: 290–302 (1968).

Ackerman, G. A. The human neutrophilic promyelocyte. Z. Zellforsch. *118*: 467–481 (1971).

Ackerman, G. A. The human neutrophilic myelocyte. Z. Zellforsch. *121*: 153–170 (1971).

Bainton, D. F. and Farquhar, M. G. Segregation and packaging of granule enzymes in eosinophilic leukocytes. J. Cell Biol. 45: 54–73 (1970).

Bainton, D. F., Ullyot, J. L. and Farquhar, M. G. The development of neutrophilic polymorphonuclear leukocytes in human bone marrow. J. Exp. Med. *134*: 907–934 (1971).

Dekkum, D. W. van, Noord, M. J. van, Maat, B. and Dicke, K. A. Attempts at identification of hemopoietic stem cell in mouse. Blood *38*: 547–558 (1971).

Berman, I. The ultrastructure of erythroblastic islands and reticular cells in mouse bone marrow. J. Ultrastruct. Res. *17*: 291–313 (1967).

Bessis, M. and Thiery, J. Electron microscopy of human white blood cells and their stem cells. Int. Rev. Cytol. *12*: 199–214 (1961).

Caffrey, R. W., Everett, N. B. and Rieke, W. O. Radioautographic studies of reticular and blast cells in the hemopoietic tissues of the rat. Anat. Rec. *155*: 41–58 (1966).

Capone, R. J., Weinreb, E. L. and Chapman, G. B. Electron microscopic studies on normal human myeloid elements. Blood 23: 300–320 (1964).

Fedorko, M. Formation of cytoplasmic granules in human eosinophilic myelocytes: an electron microscopic autoradiographic study. Blood *31*: 188–194 (1968).

Hardin, J. H. and Spicer, S. S. An ultrastructural study of human eosinophil granules: maturation stages and pyroantimonate reactive cation. Am. J. Anat. *128*: 283–310 (1970).

Hesseldahl, H. and Falck-Larsen, J. Hemopoiesis and blood vessels in human yolk sac. Acta Anat. 78: 274–294 (1971).

King, J. E. and Ackerman, G. A. Erythropoiesis in the bone marrow of the fetal rabbit. Anat. Rec. *157*: 589–606 (1967).

Lennert, K. Bildung und Differenzierung der Blutzellen, insbesondere der Lymphocyten. Verh. deutsch. Ges. Pathol. *50*: 163–213 (1966).

Marks, P. A. and Rifkind, R. A. Protein synthesis: its control in erythropoiesis. Science *175*: 955–961 (1972).

Murphy, M. J., Bertles, J. R. and Gordon, A. S. Identifying characteristics of the hematopoietic precursor cell. J. Cell Sci. *9*: 23–47 (1971).

Nichols, B. A., Bainton, D. F. and Farquhar, M. G. Differentiation of monocytes. Origin, nature, and fate of their azurophilic granules. J. Cell Biol. *50*: 498–515 (1971).

Nowell, P. C. and Wilson, D. B. Lymphocytes and hemic stem cells. Am. J. Pathol. *65*: 641–652 (1971).

Orlic, D. Ultrastructural analysis of erythropoiesis. *In* Regulation of Hematopoiesis. (Ed. A. S. Gordon), Vol. *1*: 271–296. Appleton-Century-Crofts, New York, 1970.

Orlic D., Gordon, A. S. and Rhodin, J. A. G. An ultrastructural study of erythropoietin-induced red cell formation in mouse spleen. J. Ultrastruct. Res. *13*: 516–542 (1965).

Orlic, D., Gordon, A. S. and Rhodin, J. A. G. Ultrastructural and autoradiographic studies of erythropoietin-induced red cell production. Ann. N.Y. Acad. Sci. *149*: 198–216 (1968).

Pease, D. C. An electron microscope study of red bone marrow. Blood *11*: 501–526 (1956).

Richter, G. W. A study of hemosiderosis with the aid of electron microscopy, with observations on the relationship between hemosiderin and ferritin. J. Exp. Med. *106*: 203–217 (1957).

Rifkind, R. A., Danon, D. and Marks, P. A. Alterations in polyribosomes during erythroid cell maturation. J. Cell Biol. *22*:599–611 (1964).

Scott, R. E. and Horn, R. G. Fine structural features of eosinophile granulocyte development in human bone marrow. J. Ultrastruct. Res. *33*: 16–28 (1970).

Simpson, C. F. and Kling, J. M. The mechanism of denucleation in circulating erythroblasts. J. Cell Biol. *35*: 237–245 (1967).

Simpson, C. F. and Kling, J. M. The mechanism of mitochondrial extrusion from phenylhydrazine-induced reticulocytes in the circulating blood. J. Cell Biol. *36*: 103–109 (1968).

Skutelsky, E. and Danon, D. An electron microscope study of nuclear elimination from the late erythroblast. J. Cell Biol. *33*: 625–635 (1967).

Yamada, E. The fine structure of the megakaryocyte in the mouse spleen. Acta Anat. *29*: 267–290 (1957).

Zucker-Franklin, D. The ultrastructure of megakaryocytes and platelets. *In* Regulation of Hematopoiesis. (Ed. A. S. Gordon), Vol. *2*: 1533–1586. Appleton-Century-Crofts, New York, 1970.

7 Connective tissue

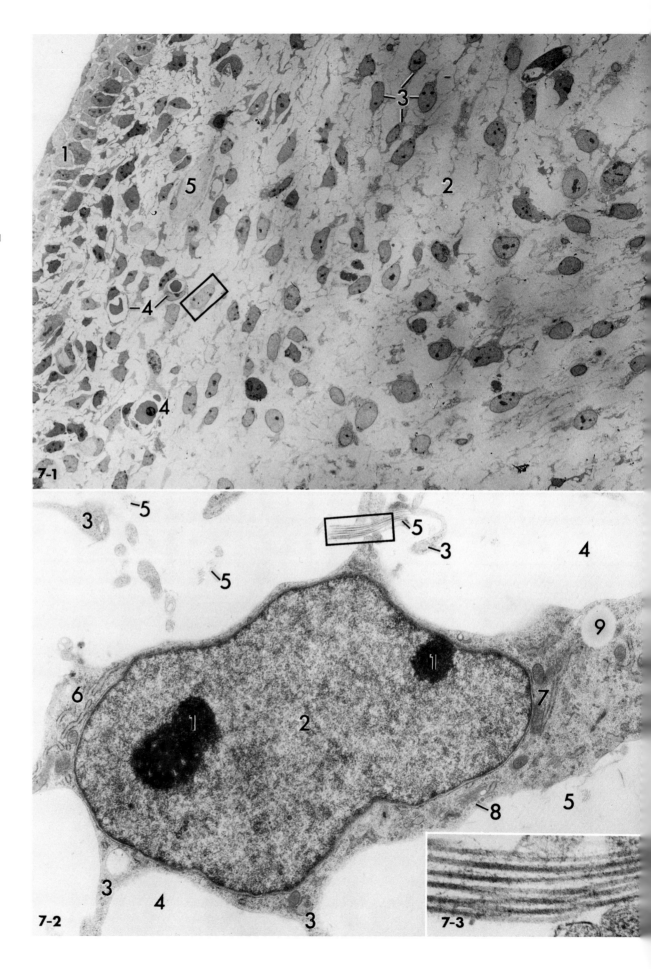

Fig. 7-1. Mesenchymal connective tissue. Hindleg. Rat fetus; 14th day of gestation. E.M. X 620. **1.** Epidermis. **2.** Ground substance of mesenchyme. **3.** Undifferentiated mesenchymal cells. **4.** Small blood vessels. **5.** Small nerve bundle.

Fig. 7-2. Mesenchymal cell. Enlargement of area similar to rectangle in Fig. 7-1. Rat fetus. E.M. X 9000. **1.** Nucleoli. **2.** Mixture of dense heterochromatin and light euchromatin. **3.** Cytoplasmic processes. **4.** Ground substance (semifluid). **5.** Thin fiber bundles. **6.** Granular endoplasmic reticulum. **7.** Mitochondria. **8.** Golgi zone. **9.** Lipid droplet.

Fig. 7-3. Fiber bundle. Enlargement of rectangle in Fig. 7-2. E.M. X 62,000. The individual fibrils average 250 Å in width. Axial banding is not clearly seen in this preparation.

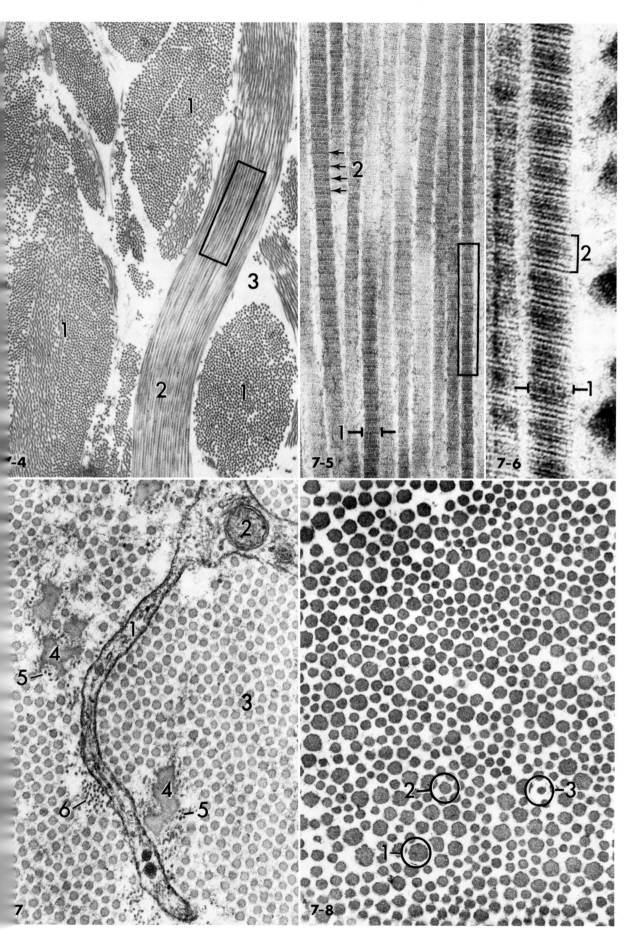

Fig. 7-4. Collagenous fibers of dense fibrous connective tissue. Ligament. Knee joint. Rat. E.M. X 9000. **1.** Cross-sectioned collagenous fibers. **2.** Longitudinally sectioned collagenous fiber. Width averages 1.6 μ. Individual collagenous fibrils appear as small dots. **3.** Ground substance. Note absence of fibroblasts.

Fig. 7-5. Collagenous fibrils sectioned longitudinally. Enlargement of area similar to rectangle in Fig. 7-4. Tunica albuginea testis. Rat. E.M. X 62,000. **1.** Width of individual fibril averages 650 Å. **2.** Spacing between arrows averages 600 Å.

Fig. 7-6. Single collagenous fibril. Enlargement of area similar to rectangle in Fig. 7-5. Sclera. Mouse. E.M. X 200,000. **1.** Width: 600 Å. **2.** Axial periodicity: 500 Å.

Fig. 7-7. Chorda tendinea. Cross section. Heart. Rat. E.M. X 51,000. **1.** Narrow cytoplasmic process of fibroblast. **2.** Mitochondrion. **3.** Collagenous fibrils, average width 500 Å. **4.** Amorphous substance of elastic fiber. **5.** Microfibrils of elastic fiber. **6.** Microfibrils unassociated with elastic amorphous substance.

Fig. 7-8. Cross-sectioned collagenous fibrils. Ligament. Knee joint. Rat. E.M. X 50,000. In this part of the ligament, the collagenous fibrils vary greatly in width. **1.** Width 1000 Å. **2.** Width: 600 Å. **3.** Width: 400 Å.

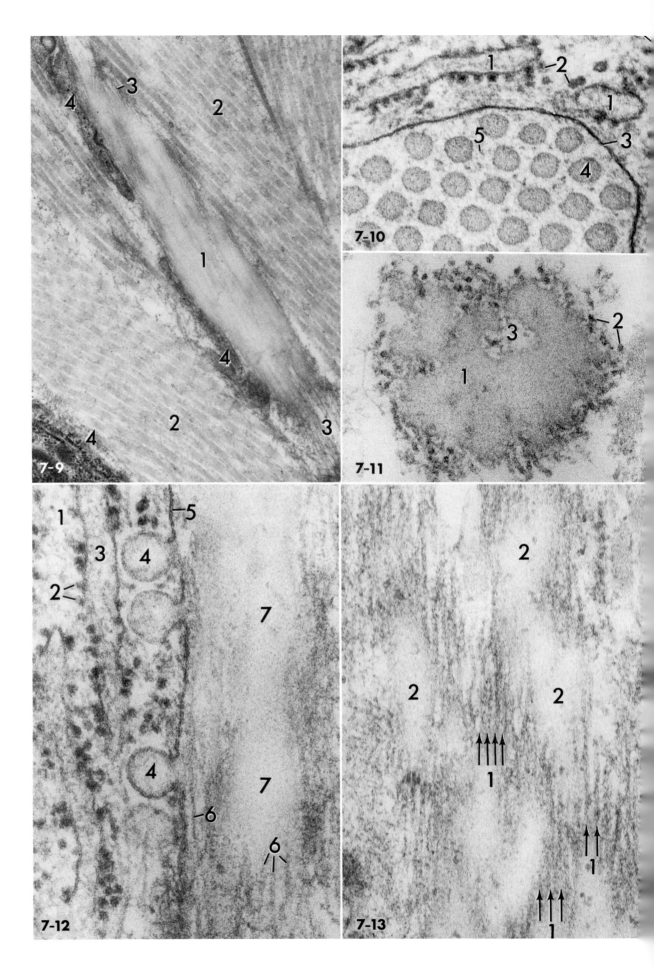

Fig. 7-9. Elastic and collagenous fibers. Tunica albuginea testis. Rat. E.M. X 32,000. **1.** Elastic fiber, sectioned longitudinally; width 0.5 μ; central amorphous substance. **2.** Collagenous fibrils. **3.** Peripheral microfibrils of elastic fiber. **4.** Cytoplasmic strands of fibroblasts.

Fig. 7-10. Part of fibroblast and collagenous fibrils. Chorda tendinea. Heart. Rat. E.M. X 120,000. **1.** Cisternae of granular endoplasmic reticulum. **2.** Ribosomes. **3.** Cell membrane of fibroblast. **4.** Cross-sectioned collagenous fibrils; width 600 Å. **5.** Ground substance of connective tissue contains some minute filaments which average 80 Å in width. They may represent double-beaded collagenous filaments or immature collagenous fibrils.

Fig. 7-11. Cross-sectioned elastic fiber (width 0.5 μ). Chorda tendinea. Heart. Rat. E.M. X 120,000. **1.** Central amorphous substance. **2.** Peripheral mantle of microfibrils; width of microfibrils averages 130 Å. **3.** Some microfibrils within amorphous substance.

Fig. 7-12. Part of fibroblast and longitudinally sectioned elastic fiber. Tunica albuginea testis. E.M. X 120,000. **1.** Cytoplasmic matrix of fibroblast. **2.** Ribosomes. **3.** Cisternae of granular endoplasmic reticulum. **4.** Central cavity of smooth surfaced micropinocytotic invaginations. **5.** Trilaminar cell membrane. **6.** Microfibrils. **7.** Amorphous substance.

Fig. 7-13. Periphery of elastic fiber sectioned longitudinally. Tunica albuginea testis. E.M. X 120,000. **1.** Arrows point to peripheral microfibrils of elastic fiber. **2.** Parts of central amorphous substance of elastic fiber.

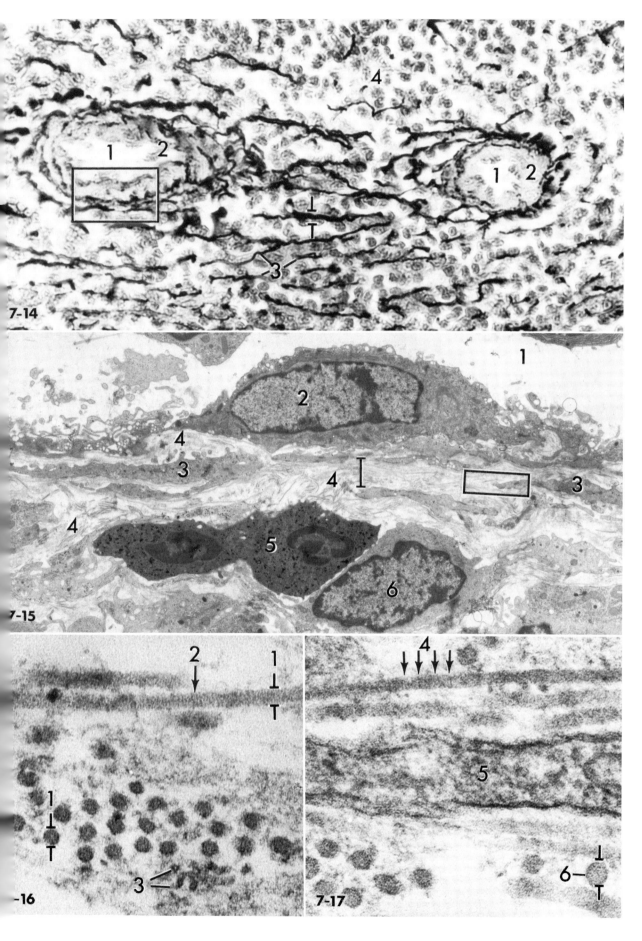

Fig. 7-14. Reticular fibers in red pulp. Silver impregnation. Spleen. Rat. L.M. X 665. **1.** Lumen of blood vessel. **2.** Wall of blood vessel. **3.** Reticular fibers; width between bars 1.5μ. **4.** Individual cells of red pulp cannot be categorized at this magnification.

Fig. 7-15. Wall of venule. Medullary cord. Lymph node. Enlargement of area similar to rectangle in Fig. 7-14. Rat. E.M. X 4800. **1.** Lumen of venule. **2.** Nucleus of endothelial cell. **3.** Cytoplasmic strands of pericytes. **4.** Reticular fibrils form a loose network in the vascular wall. Bar is 1.5 μ. **5.** Nucleus of granular leukocyte. **6.** Lymphocyte.

Figs. 7-16 & 7-17. Details of reticular fibrils. Synovial membrane. Knee joint. Enlargement of area similar to rectangle in Fig. 7-15. Rat. E.M. X 156,000. **1.** Reticular fibrils: width between bars 250 Å. **2.** Arrow: axial banding with no apparent regular periodicity. **3.** Elastic microfibrils with light core: width 90 Å. **4.** Apparent axial periodicity in this reticular fibril: distance between arrows 250 Å. **5.** Thin cytoplasmic strand of fibroblast. **6.** Delicate collagenous fibril; width 400 Å.

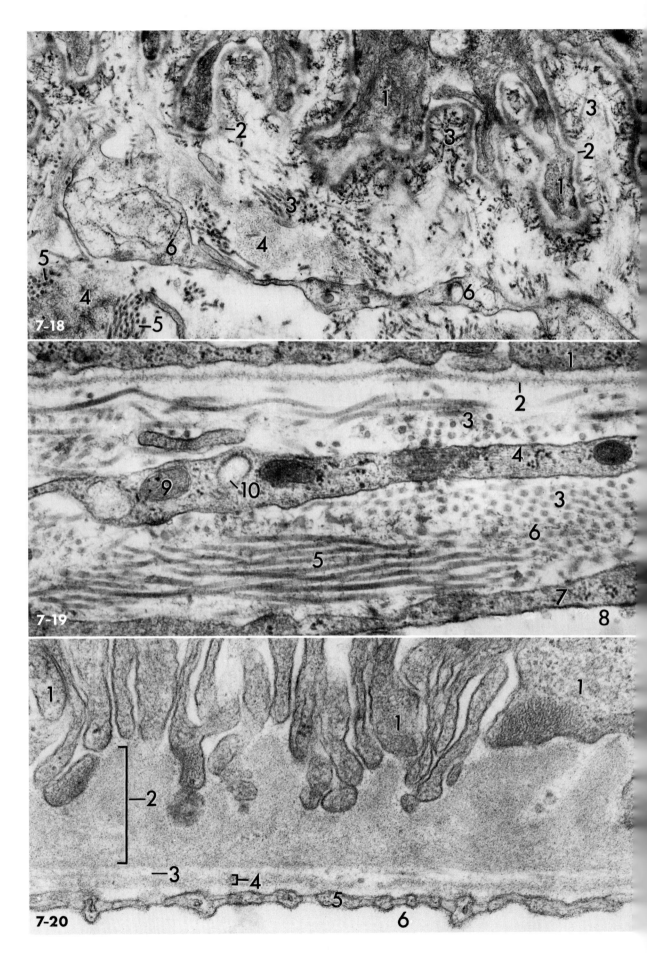

Fig. 7-18. Basement membrane. Epidermis. Human. E.M. X 18,000. **1.** Basal processes of basal cells. **2.** Basal lamina; width 1000 Å. **3.** Reticular fibrils. **4.** Aggregations of elastic microfibrils. **5.** Delicate collagenous fibrils. **6.** Cytoplasmic strand of fibroblast.

Fig. 7-19. Basement membrane. Intestine. Rat. E.M. X 48,000. **1.** Base of epithelial cells in crypt of Lieberkühn. **2.** Basal lamina; width 400 Å. **3.** Reticular fibrils; width 300 Å. **4.** Cytoplasmic strand of fibroblast. **5.** Delicate collagenous or reticular fibrils; width 300 Å. **6.** Elastic microfibrils, unassociated with amorphous elastic substance, form a finely filamentous network. **7.** Endothelial cell of lymph capillary. Note absence of basal lamina underneath lymphatic endothelium. **8.** Lumen of capillary. **9.** Mitochondrion. **10.** Coated vesicle.

Fig. 7-20. Comparison of two basal laminae. Kidney. Rat. E.M. X 60,000. **1.** Basal processes of proximal tubule cell. **2.** Basal lamina of proximal tubule. This is exceptionally thick in rat (width 5000 Å) and some of the basal cell processes are lodged partly in the basal lamina. **3.** Small interstitial space. **4.** Basal lamina of peritubular blood capillary; width 330 Å. **5.** Fenestrated capillary endothelium. **6.** Capillary lumen.

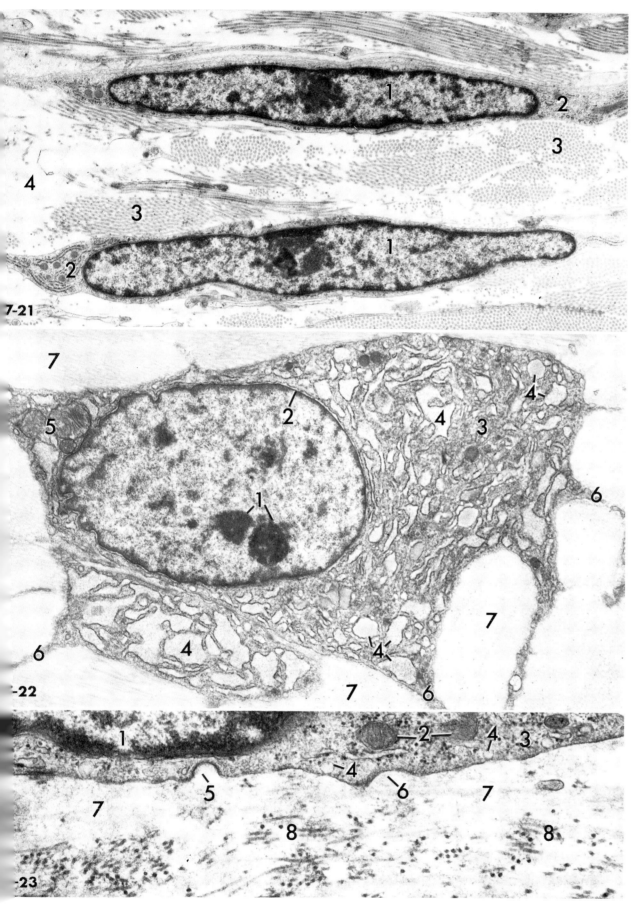

Fig. 7-21. Fibrocytes. Enlargement of rectangle in Fig. 7-32. Submucosa. Tertiary bronchus. Cat. E.M. X 9500. **1.** Nuclei of fibrocytes. **2.** Cytoplasm is sparse and the cells spindle-shaped. There is only a small amount of granular endoplasmic reticulum, indicating that this is a resting fibrocyte rather than an active fibroblast. **3.** Collagenous fibers, each made up of numerous collagenous fibrils. **4.** Ground substance of connective tissue.

Fig. 7-22. Fibroblast (tendon cell). Enlargement of area similar to rectangle in Fig. 7-35. Tendon. Tail. Rat. E.M. X 9500. **1.** Nucleoli of fibroblast. **2.** Nuclear membrane. **3.** Golgi zone (small). **4.** Dilated cisternae of granular endoplasmic reticulum. **5.** Mitochondria. **6.** Sheet-like cytoplasmic processes. **7.** Collagenous fibers.

Fig. 7-23. Fibroblast. Synovial membrane. Knee joint. E.M. X 37,000. **1.** Nucleus of fibroblast. **2.** Mitochondria. **3.** Ribosomes. **4.** Smooth surfaced micropinocytotic invaginations. **5.** Coated invagination. **6.** Coated invagination (flattening out or starting to invaginate). **7.** Flocculent ground substance. **8.** Reticular and delicate collagenous fibrils; width 300 Å.

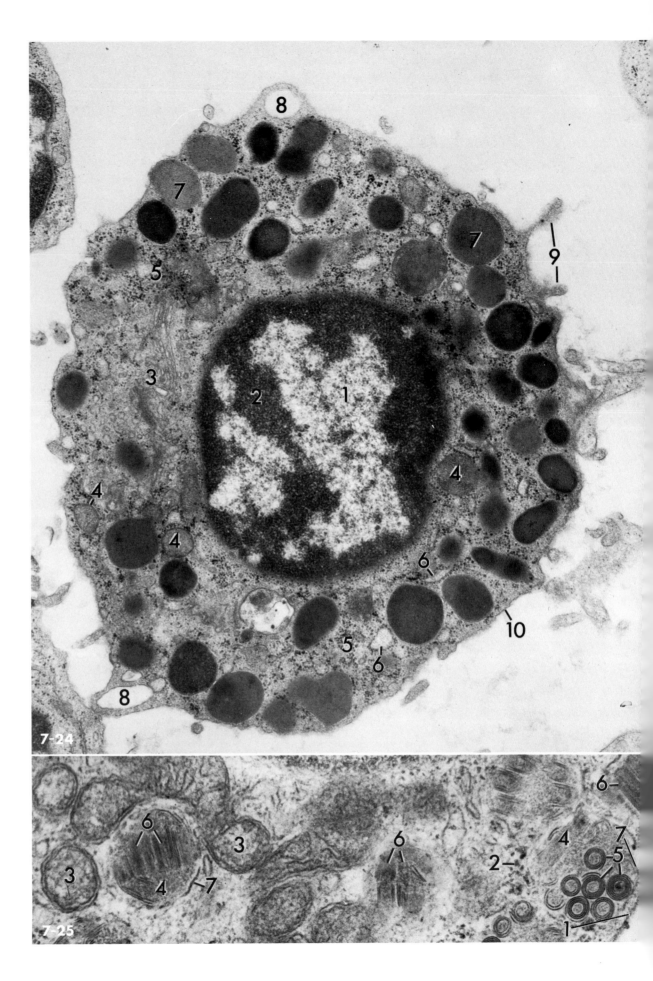

Fig. 7-24. Mast cell. Lymph node. Rat. E.M. X 24,000. **1.** Nuclear euchromatin. **2.** Heterochromatin. **3.** Golgi zone. **4.** Mitochondria. **5.** Ribosomes. **6.** Short profiles of granular endoplasmic reticulum. **7.** Secretory granules. **8.** Vacuoles, possibly remnants of discharged secretory granules. **9.** Microvilli. **10.** Cell membrane.

Fig. 7-25. Detail of mast cell. Tracheal submucosa. Human. E.M. X 54,000. **1.** Cell membrane. **2.** Ribosomes. **3.** Mitochondria. **4.** Matrix of secretory granules. **5.** "Scrolls" cross-sectioned. **6.** "Scrolls" sectioned longitudinally. **7.** Poorly preserved boundary membrane of secretory granule.

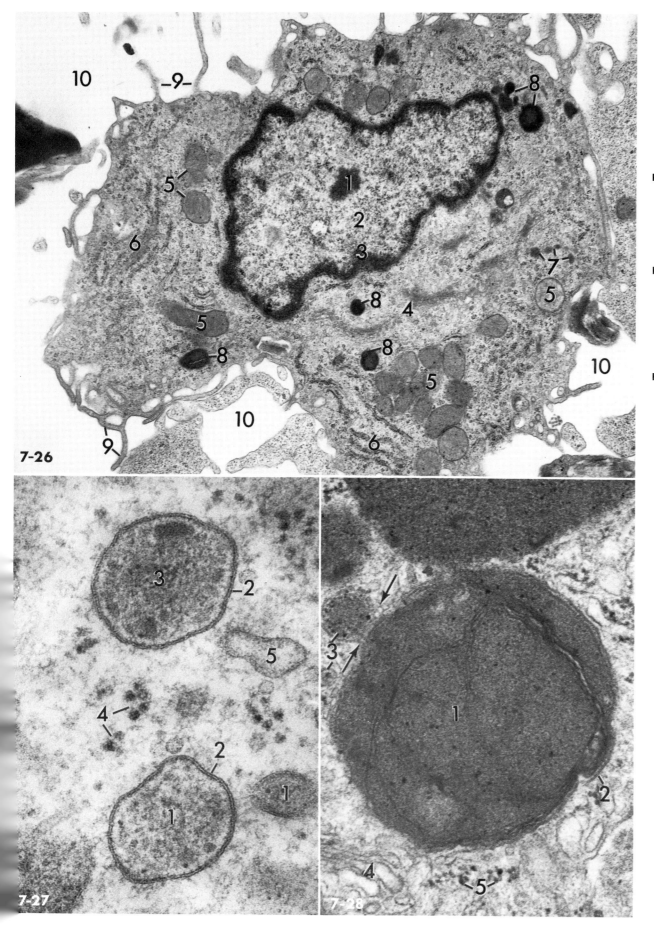

Fig. 7-26. Free macrophage. Spleen. Rat. E.M. X 19,000. **1.** Nucleolus. **2.** Euchromatin. **3.** Heterochromatin. **4.** Golgi zone. **5.** Mitochondria. **6.** Granular endoplasmic reticulum. **7.** Small primary lysosomes. **8.** Secondary lysosomes. **9.** Microvilli. **10.** Interstitial space of red splenic pulp.

Fig. 7-27. Primary lysosomes. Kupffer cell. Liver. Rat. E.M. X 120,000. **1.** Matrix of primary lysosomes. **2.** Trilaminar lysosomal boundary membrane; width 70 Å. **3.** Matrix of this primary lysosome is denser, possibly indicating ingested material. **4.** Ribosomes. **5.** Small vesicle, possibly part of nearby Golgi zone.

Fig. 7-28. Secondary lysosome. Macrophage. Spleen. Rat. E.M. X 60,000. **1.** Interior of secondary lysosome filled with dense matrix and layered structures. **2.** Lysosomal boundary membrane. **3.** Two small primary lysosomes, one of which apparently merges (arrows) with secondary lysosome. **4.** Part of Golgi zone. **5.** Ribosomes.

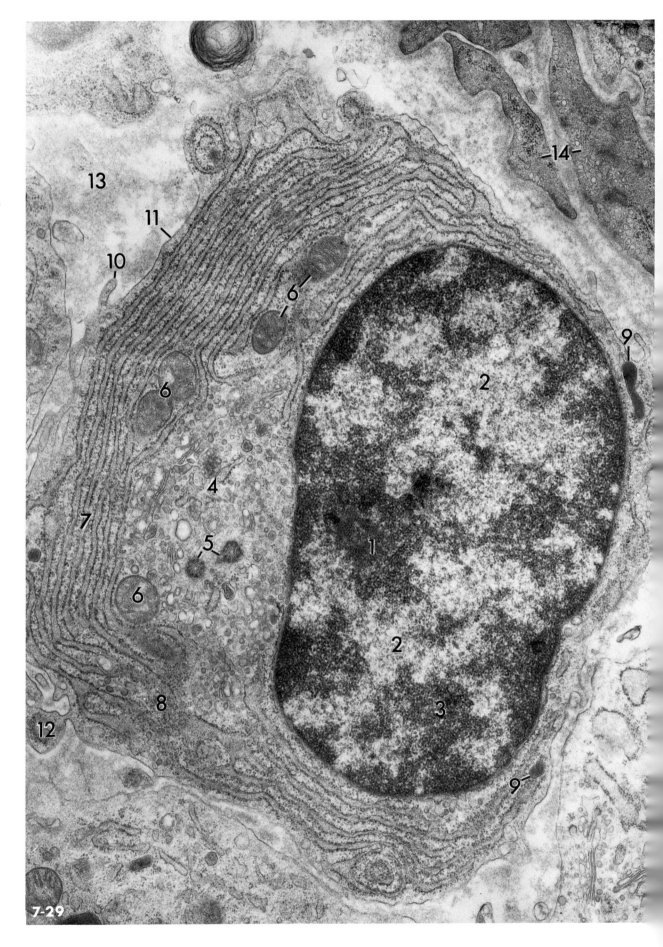

Fig. 7-29. Plasma cell. Bone marrow. Human. E.M. X 16,000. **1.** Nucleolus. **2.** Euchromatin. **3.** Heterochromatin. **4.** Golgi zone. **5.** Centrioles. **6.** Mitochondria. **7.** Granular endoplasmic reticulum. **8.** Ribosomes. **9.** Primary lysosomes. **10.** Microvillus. **11.** Cell membrane. **12.** Pseudopod. **13.** Flocculent intercellular matrix of bone marrow cavity. **14.** Part of arteriolar smooth muscle cells.

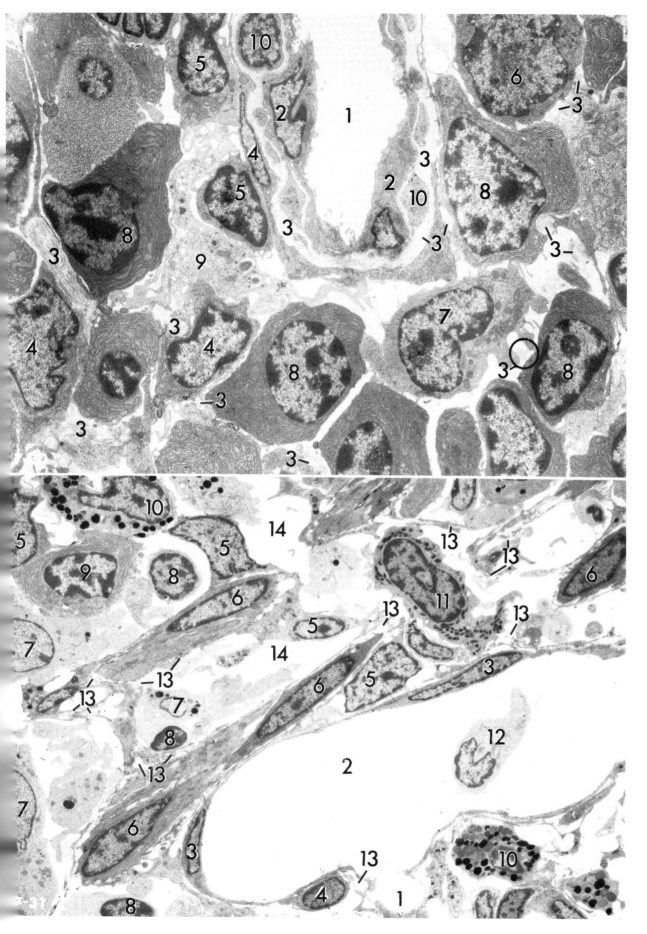

Fig. 7-30. Reticular connective tissue. Medullary cord. Lymph node. Rat. E.M. X 4500.
1. Lumen of arteriole. **2.** Endothelium.
3. Reticular fibers. **4.** Reticular cells. In this location, these cells are only phagocytic to a limited extent and resemble fibroblasts.
5. Small lymphocytes. **6.** Large lymphocyte (lymphoblast). **7.** Monocyte. **8.** Plasma cells.
9. Cytoplasmic strand of macrophage.
10. Smooth muscle cells.

Fig. 7-31. Loose connective tissue. Core of villus. Small intestine. Rat. E.M. X 17,000.
1. Venous capillary. **2.** Lumen of postcapillary venule. **3.** Endothelial cells. **4.** Pericyte.
5. Fibroblasts. **6.** Smooth muscle cells.
7. Macrophages. **8.** Lymphocytes. **9.** Plasma cell. **10.** Mast cells. **11.** Eosinophil polymorphonuclear leukocyte. **12.** Monocyte.
13. Reticular and delicate collagenous fibers are *scarce*. **14.** Interstitial spaces (areolae) filled with tissue fluid. *Note:* The identifcation of cell types and location of fibers is based on analysis of this field of view at higher magnifications.

Fig. 7-32. Comparison of loose and dense connective tissues. Lamina propria and submucosa of tertiary bronchus. Lung. Cat. E.M. X 1800. **1.** Lumen of tertiary bronchus. **2.** Ciliated respiratory epithelium. **3.** Lamina propria (loose connective tissue). **4.** Submucosa (irregular dense fibrous connective tissue). **5.** Lumen of bronchial gland. **6.** Fibroblasts and fibrocytes. Rectangle enlarged in Fig. 7-17. **7.** Loosely arranged collagenous fibers. **8.** Cross-sectioned elastic fibers. **9.** Densely arranged collagenous fibers. **10.** Plasma cells. **11.** Mast cells. **12.** Macrophages. **13.** Nerve bundle. **14.** Perineural cell nucleus. **15.** Nucleus of Schwann cell. **16.** Fat cell with two fat globules. **17.** Blood capillary. **18.** Tangentially sectioned bronchial glands. *Note:* The identification of cell types, fibers and other structures is based on analysis at higher magnifications.

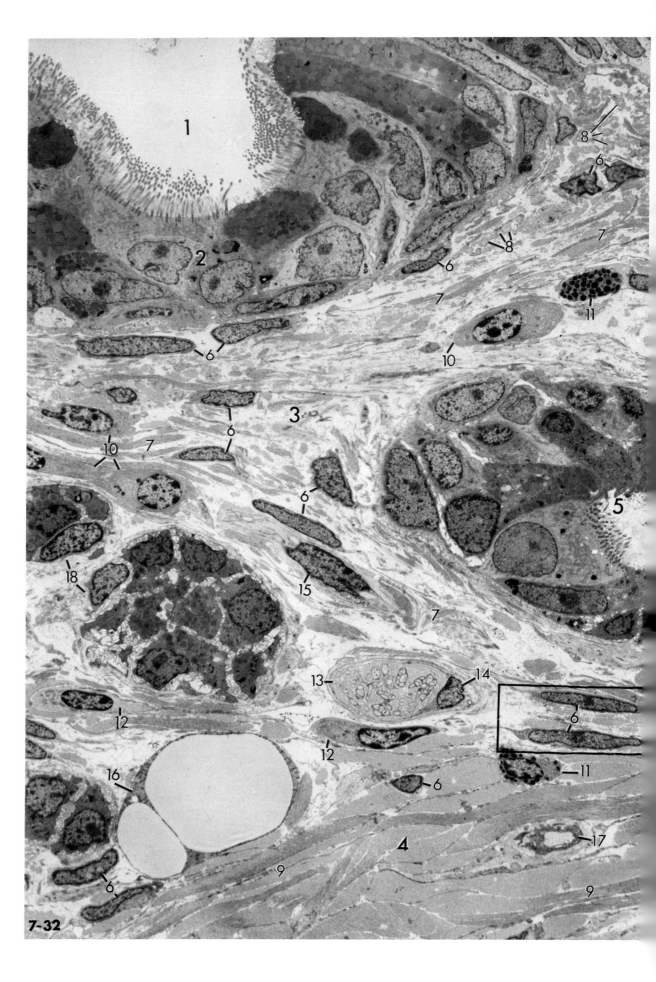

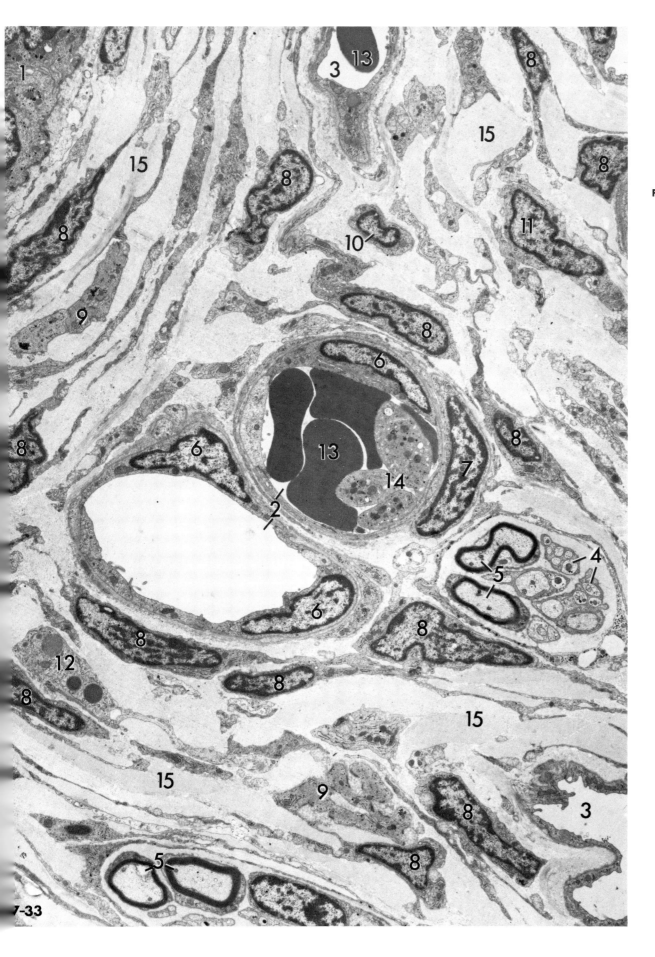

Fig. 7-33. Subepithelial connective tissue. This is an example of a cell-rich tissue which represents an intermediate type between loose and dense connective tissue. Pars cavernosa of male urethra. Rat. E.M. X 5000.
1. Base of urethral epithelium. **2.** Lumina of postcapillary venules. **3.** Lumina of capillaries. **4.** Cross-sectioned non-myelinated nerve fibers. **5.** Axons of myelinated nerves. **6.** Nuclei of endothelial cells. **7.** Nucleus of pericyte. **8.** Nuclei of fibroblasts. **9.** Cytoplasmic strands of smooth muscle cells. Smooth muscle cells are abundant in the cavernous tissue which lies under this connective tissue. **10.** Nucleus of smooth muscle cell. **11.** Nucleus of macrophage. **12.** Part of macrophage cytoplasm. **13.** Erythrocytes. **14.** Platelets. **15.** Irregularly arranged collagenous fibers completely fill the intercellular spaces.

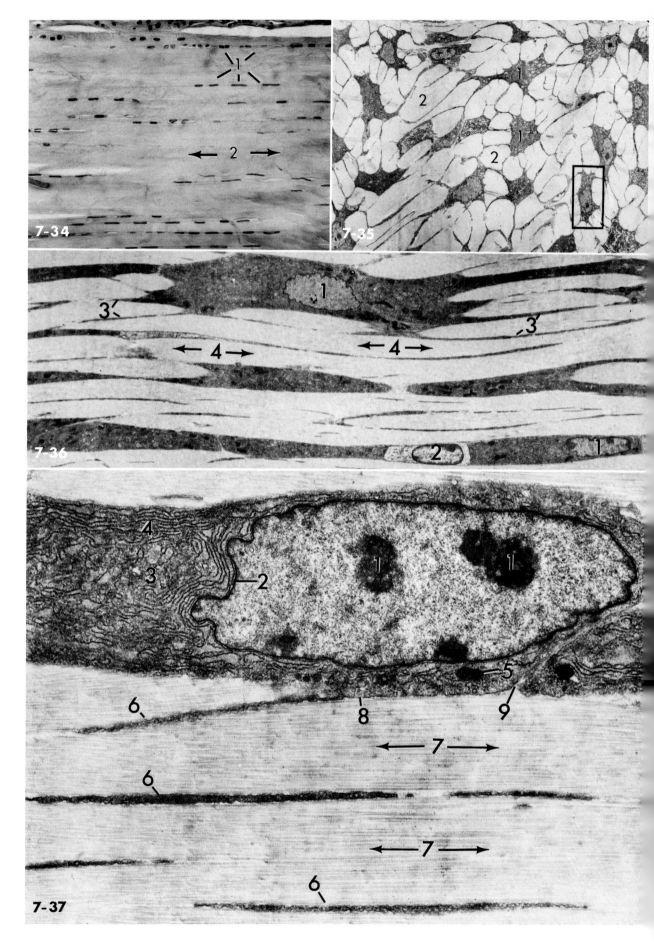

Fig. 7-34. Tendon. Longitudinal section. Rabbit. L.M. X 185. **1.** Nuclei of fibroblasts. **2.** Collagenous fibers.

Fig. 7-35. Tendon. Cross section. Tail. Rat. E.M. X 1000. **1** Fibroblasts (tendon cells). **2.** Collagenous fibers. Rectangle enlarged in Fig. 7-22.

Fig. 7-36. Tendon. Longitudinal section. Tail. Rat. E.M. X 1600. **1.** Nuclei of fibroblasts (tendon cells). **2.** Nucleus of unidentified cell. **3.** Cytoplasmic processes of fibroblasts. **4.** Collagenous fibers.

Fig. 7-37. Detail of fibroblast (tendon cell). Tendon. Longitudinal section. Tail. Rat. E.M. X 9500. **1.** Nucleoli. **2.** Nuclear membrane. **3.** Golgi zone. **4.** Granular endoplasmic reticulum. **5.** Mitochondrion. **6.** Sheet-like cytoplasmic processes. **7.** Collagenous fibers composed of numerous collagenous fibrils. **8.** Cell membrane. **9.** Narrow cleft between two adjoining fibroblasts.

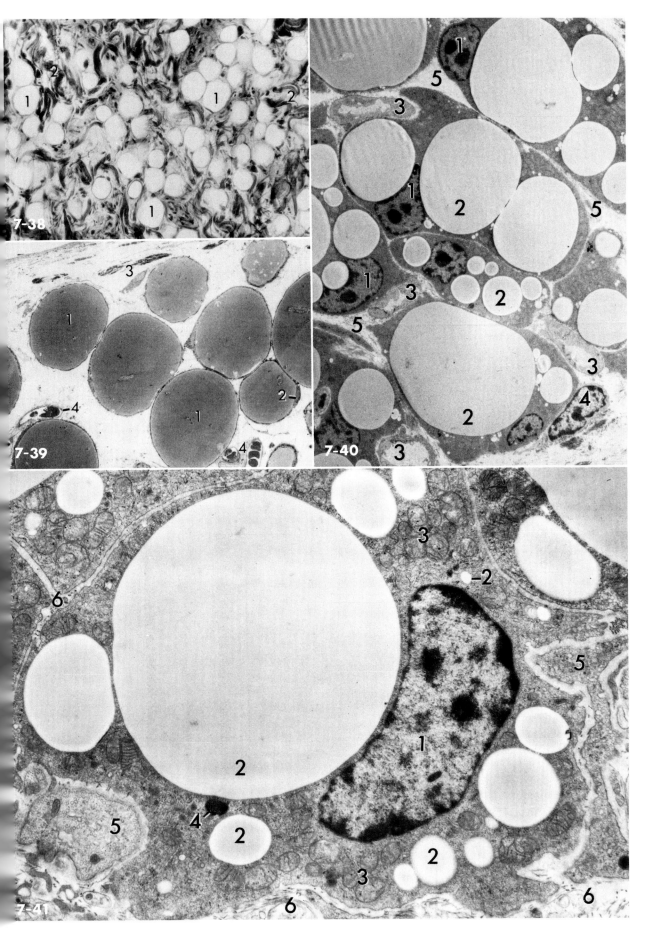

Fig. 7-38. Adipose tissue. Hypodermis. Lip. Human. L.M. X 121. **1.** Fat cells. Lipid dissolved. **2.** Collagenous fiber bundles.

Fig. 7-39. Adipose tissue. Hypodermis. Thigh. Rabbit. E.M. X 600. **1.** Fat cells. Lipid preserved by osmic acid fixation. **2.** Nucleus of fat cell. **3.** Loose connective tissue. **4.** Capillaries.

Fig. 7-40. Developing adipose tissue. Newborn kitten. E.M. X 1750. **1.** Nuclei of fat cells. **2.** Lipid droplets. **3.** Capillaries. **4.** Nucleus of fibroblast. **5.** Interstitial space.

Fig. 7-41. Developing fat cell. Newborn kitten. E.M. X 9000. **1.** Nucleus. **2.** Lipid droplets in various stages of development. **3.** Mitochondria. **4.** Lysosome. **5.** Parts of capillary endothelium. **6.** Narrow interstitial space with reticular and delicate collagenous fibrils. A thin external (basal) lamina invests each fat cell.

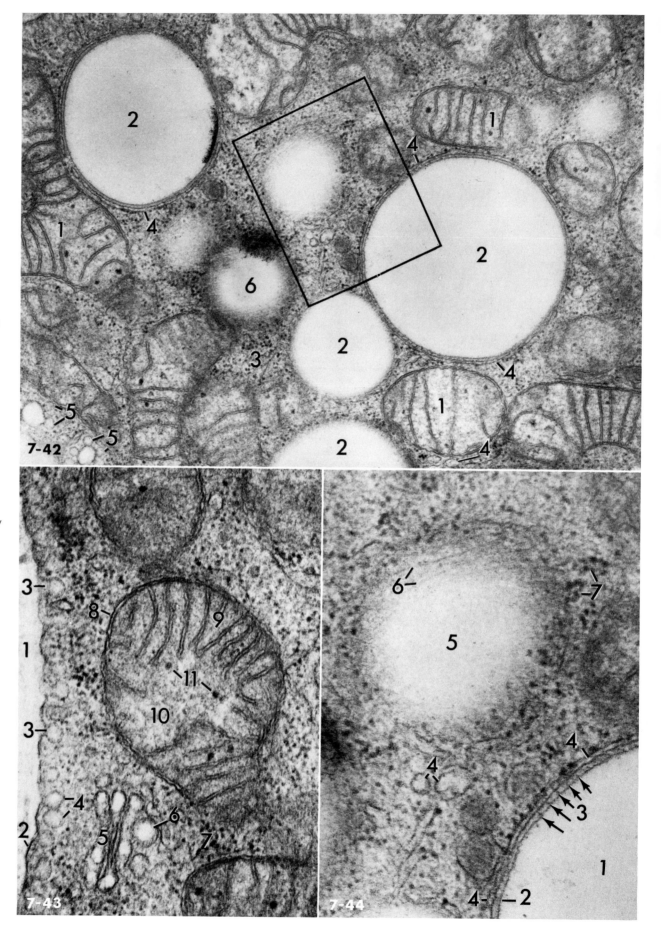

Fig. 7-42. Detail of developing fat cell. Newborn kitten. E.M. X 54,000. **1.** Mitochondria. **2.** Lipid droplets. **3.** Ribosomes. **4.** Agranular endoplasmic reticulum. **5.** Micropinocytotic invaginations of cell membrane merging to form rosette-like configurations. **6.** Parallel microfilaments are seen in this tangential section of a lipid droplet.

Fig. 7-43. Part of developing fat cell. Newborn kitten. E.M. X 90,000. **1.** External (basal) lamina. **2.** Cell membrane. **3.** Micropinocytotic invaginations. **4.** Merging vesicles. **5.** Small Golgi zone. **6.** Enlarging Golgi vesicle. **7.** Ribosomes. **8.** Outer mitochondrial membrane. **9.** Membranous cristae. **10** Matrix of mitochondrion. **11.** Intramitochondrial dense granules.

Fig. 7-44. Detail of developing fat cell. Enlargement of rectangle in Fig. 7-37. Newborn kitten. E.M. X 120,000. **1.** Center of lipid droplet. **2.** Interface membrane. **3.** Arrows point to cross-sectioned, equally spaced filaments outside of the interface membrane. **4.** Agranular endoplasmic reticulum. **5.** Tangential section of lipid droplet. **6.** Peripheral filaments, longitudinally cut. **7.** Ribosomes.

References

FIBERS

Bairati, A., Petruccioli, M. G. and Torri Tarelli, L. Studies on the ultrastructure of collagen fibrils. 1. Morphological evaluation of the periodic structure. J. Submicr. Cytol. *1*: 113–141 (1969).

Bruns, R. R. A symmetrical, extracellular fibril. J. Cell Biol. *42*: 418–430 (1969).

Fernando, N. V., von Erkel, G. A. and Movat, H. Z. The fine structure of connective tissue. IV. The intercellular elements. Exp. Molec. Path. *3*: 529–545 (1964).

Gomori, G. Silver impregnation of reticulum in paraffin sections. Am. J. Path. *13*: 993–1002 (1937).

Grant, R. A., Horne, R. W. and Cox, R. W. New model for the tropocollagen macromolecule and its mode of aggregation. Nature *207*: 822–826 (1965).

Greenlee, T. K., Jr., Ross, R. and Hartman, J. L. The fine structure of elastic fibers. J. Cell Biol. *30*: 59–71 (1966).

Gross, J. The behavior of collagen units as a model in morphogenesis. J. Biophys. Biochem. Cytol. (Suppl.) *2*: 261–274 (1956).

Hall, D. A. The fibrous components of connective tissue with special reference to the elastic fiber. Int. Rev. Cytol. *8*: 212–252 (1959).

Haust, M. D. Fine fibrils of extracellular space (microfibrils): their structure and role in connective tissue organization. Am. J. Path. *47*: 1113–1137 (1965).

Hayes, R. L. and Allen, E. R. Electron microscopic studies on a double-stranded beaded filament of embryonic collagen. J. Cell Sci. *2*: 419–434 (1967).

Low, F. N. Extracellular connective tissue fibrils in the chick embryo. Anat. Rec. *160*: 93–108 (1968).

Rhodin, J. and Dalhamn, T. Electron microscopy of collagen and elastin in lamina propria of the tracheal mucosa of rat. Exp. Cell Res. *9*: 371–375 (1955).

Ross, R. and Bornstein, P. The elastic fiber. I. The separation and partial characterization of its macromolecular components. J. Cell Biol. *40*: 366–381 (1969).

Ross, R. and Bornstein, P. Elastic fibers in the body. Sci. American *224*: 44–59 (1971).

Taylor, J. J. and Yeager, V. L. The fine structure of elastic fibers in the fibrous periosteum of the rat femur. Anat. Rec. *156*: 129–142 (1966).

Torri Tarelli, L. and Petruccioli, M. G. Studies on the ultrastructure of collagen fibrils. II. Filamentous structure with negative staining. J. Submicr. Cytol. *3*: 153–170 (1971).

Wassermann, F. Fibrillogenesis in the regenerating rat tendon with special reference to growth and composition of the collagenous fibril. Am. J. Anat. *94*: 399–438 (1954).

GROUND SUBSTANCE

Briggaman, R. A., Dalldorf, F. G. and Wheeler, C. E., Jr. Formation and origin of basal lamina and anchoring fibrils in adult human skin. J. Cell Biol. *51*: 384–395 (1971).

Gersh, I. and Catchpole, H. R. The nature of ground substance of connective tissue. Perspectives in Biology and Medicine *3*: 282–319 (1969).

Goel, S. C. and Jurand, A. Electron microscopic observations on the basal lamina of chick limb buds after trypsin and EDTA treatment. J. Cell Sci. *3*: 373–389 (1968).

Low, F. N. and Burkel, W. E. A boundary membrane concept of ultrastructural morphology. Anat. Rec. *151*: 489–490 (1965).

Meyer, K. The chemistry of the mesodermal ground substance. Harvey Lectures *51*: 88–112 (1955).

Pierce, G. B. and Nakane, P. K. Basement membranes, synthesis and deposition in response to cellular injury. Lab. Investig. *21*: 27–41 (1969).

Scalleta, L. J. and MacCallum, D. K. A fine structural study of divalent cation-mediated epithelial union with connective tissue in human oral mucosa. Am. J. Anat. *133*: 431–454 (1972).

FIBROBLASTS

Alpert, E. N. Developing elastic tissue. Am. J. Path. *69*: 89–102 (1972).

Fahrenbach, W. H., Sandberg, L. D. and Cleary, E. G. Ultrastructural studies on early elastogenesis. Anat. Rec. *155*: 563–576 (1966).

Fernando, N. V. and Movat, H. Z. Fibrillogenesis in regenerating tendon. Lab. Investig. *12*: 214–229 (1963).

Goldberg, B. and Green, H. An analysis of collagen secretion by established mouse fibroblast lines. J. Cell Biol. *22*: 227–258 (1964).

Greenlee, T. K., Jr. and Ross, R. The development of the rat flexor digital tendon, a fine structure study. J. Ultrastruct. Res. *18*: 354–376 (1967).

Haust, M. D. and More, R. H. Electron microscopy of connective tissue and elastogenesis. *In* The Connective Tissue (Eds. B. M. Wagner and B. E. Smith), pp. 352–376. Williams & Wilkins, Baltimore, 1967.

Haust, M. D., More, R. H., Bencosme, S. A. and Balis, J. V. Elastogenesis in human aorta: an electron microscopic study. Exp. Molec. Path. *4*: 508–524 (1965).

Movat, H. Z. and Fernando, N. V. The fine structure of connective tissue. I. The fibroblast. Exp. Molec. Path. *1*: 509–534 (1962).

Parry, E. W. Some electron microscope observations on the mesenchymal structures of full-term umbilical cord. J. Anat. *107*: 505–518 (1970).

Porter, K. R. and Pappas, G. C. Collagen formation by fibroblasts of the chick embryo dermis. J. Biophys. Biochem. Cytol. *5*: 153–166 (1959).

Reith, E. J. Collagen formation in developing molar teeth of rat. J. Ultrastruct. Res. *21*: 383–414 (1968).

Rhodin, J. A. G. Organization and ultrastructure of connective tissue. *In* The Connective Tissue (Eds. B. M. Wagner and D. E. Smith), pp. 1–16. Williams & Wilkins, Baltimore, 1968.

Ross, R. The connective tissue fiber forming cell. *In* Treatise on Collagan (Ed.: B. S. Gould) *2*: 1–75 (1968) Academic Press, New York.

Ross, R. and Benditt, E. P. Wound healing and collagen formation. V. Quantitative electron microscope radioautographic observations of proline-H^3 utilization by fibroblasts. J. Cell Biol. *27*: 83–106 (1965).

Van Winkle, W., Jr. The fibroblast in wound healing. Surg., Gynec. Obstet. *124*: 369–386 (1967).

Weinstock, M. Collagen formation. Observations on its intracellular packaging and transport. Z. Zellforsch. *129*: 455–470 (1972).

MAST CELLS

Combs, J. W. Maturation of rat mast cells. An electron microscope study. J. Cell Biol. *31*: 563–575 (1966).

Fernando, N. V. and Movat, H. Z. The fine structure of connective tissue. III. The mast cell. Exp. Molec. Path. *2*: 450–463 (1963).

Kobayasi, T., Midtgard, K. and Asboe-Hansen, G. Ultrastructure of human mast cell granules. J. Ultrastruct. Res. *23*: 153–165 (1968).

Padawer, J. The reaction of rat mast cells to polylysine. J. Cell Biol. *47*: 352–372 (1970).

Röhlich, P., Anderson, P. and Uvnäs, B. Electron microscope observations on compound 48/80-induced degranulation in rat mast cells. Evidence for sequential exocytosis of storage granules. J. Cell Biol. *51*: 465–483 (1971).

Smith, D. E. The tissue mast cell. Int. Rev. Cytol. *14*: 327–386 (1963).

Weinstock, A. and Albright, J. T. The fine structure of mast cells in normal human gingiva. J. Ultrastruct. Res. *17*: 245–256 (1967).

MACROPHAGES

Pearsall, N. N. and Weiser, R. S. The Macrophage. Lea & Febiger, Philadelphia, 1970.

PLASMA CELLS

dePetris, S., Karlsbad, G. and Connolly, J. M. Localization of antibodies in plasma cells by electron microscopy. J. Exp. Med. *117*: 849–862 (1963).

Leduc, E. H., Avrameas, S. and Bouteille, M. Ultrastructural localization of antibody in differentiating plasma cells. J. Exp. Med. *127*: 109–118 (1968).

Movat, H. Z. and Fernando, N. V. The fine structure of connective tissue. II. The plasma cell. Exp. Molec. Path. *1*: 535–553 (1962).

FAT CELLS

Barnard, T. The ultrastructural differentiation of brown adipose tissue in the rat. J. Ultrastruct. Res. *29*: 311–332 (1969).

Cushman, S. W. Structure-function relationship in the adipose cell. I. Ultrastructure of the isolated adipose cell. J. Cell Biol. *46*: 326–341 (1970).

Dyer, R. F. Morphological features of brown adipose cell maturation in vivo and in vitro. Am. J. Anat. *123*: 255–282 (1968).

Napolitano, L. The differentiation of white adipose cells. An electron microscope study. J. Cell Biol. *18*: 663–679 (1963).

Napolitano, L. The fine structure of adipose tissue. *In* Handbook of Physiology. Section *5*: 109–124 (1965).

Sheldon, H. The fine structure of the fat cell. *In* Fat as a Tissue (Eds. K. Rodahl and B. Issekutz), pp. 41–68. McGraw-Hill, New York, 1964.

Slavin, B. G. The cytophysiology of mammalian adipose cells. Int. Rev. Cytol. *33*: 297–334 (1972).

Wood, E. M. An ordered complex of filaments surrounding the lipid droplets in developing adipose cells. Anat. Rec. *157*: 437–448 (1967).

8 Cartilage

Fig. 8-1. Hyaline cartilage. Pulmonary bronchus. Cat. L.M. X 225. **1.** Perichondrium. **2.** Matrix of hyaline cartilage. **3.** Chondrocytes.

Fig. 8-2. Hyaline cartilage. Pulmonary bronchus. Cat. Enlargement of area similar to rectangle in Fig. 8-1. E.M. X 2600. **1.** Nucleus of fibroblast in perichondrium. **2.** Collagenous fibrils of perichondrium. **3.** Fibroblasts differentiating into chondrocytes. **4.** Nuclei of young chondrocytes. **5.** Nuclei of mature chondrocytes. **6.** Matrix. **7.** Lipid droplets.

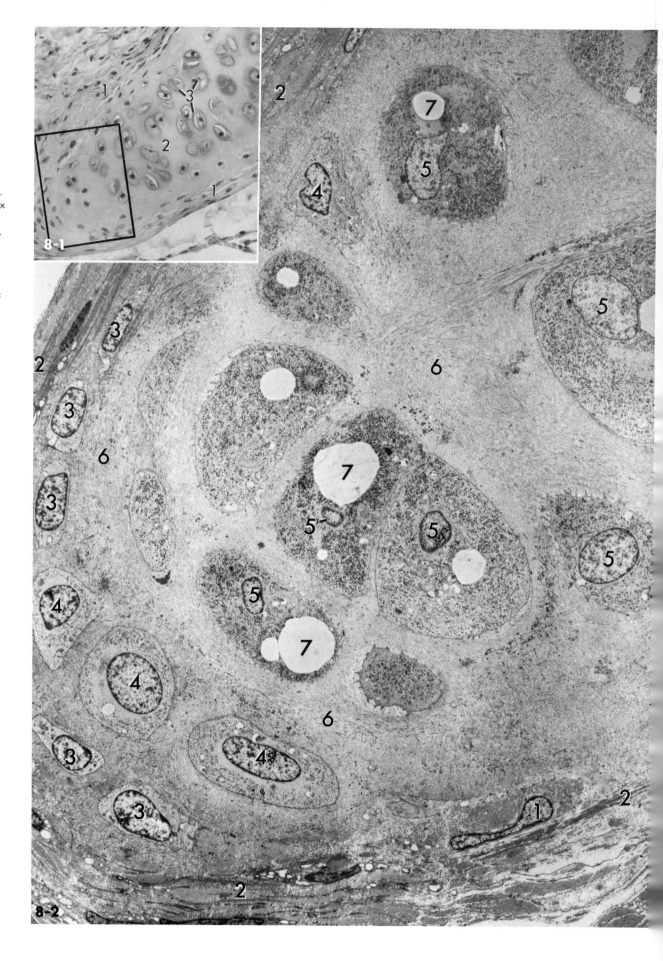

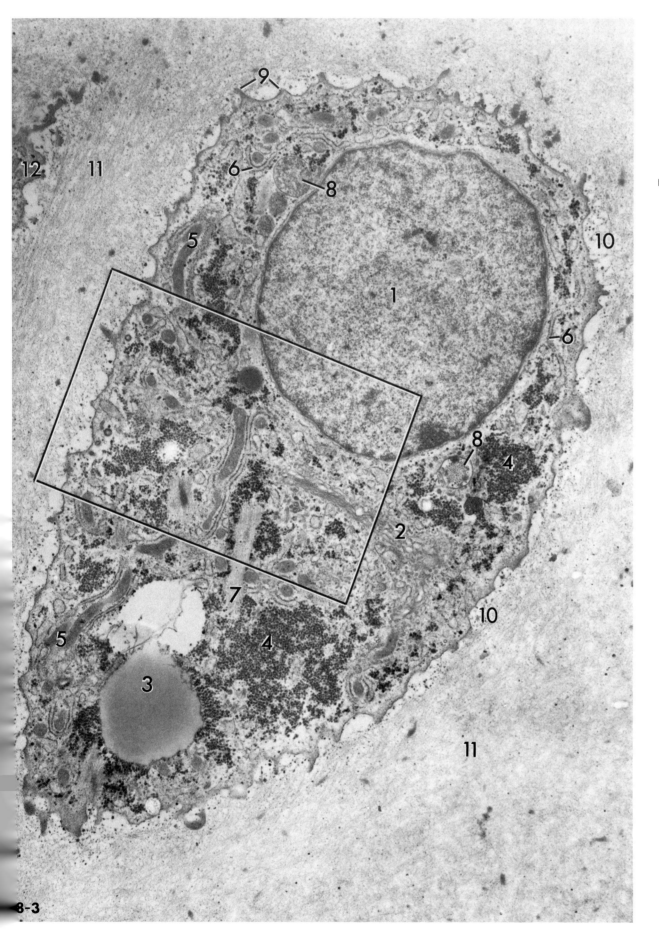

Fig. 8-3. Chondrocyte. Hyaline cartilage. Pulmonary bronchus. Cat. E.M. X 12,300. **1.** Nucleus. **2.** Golgi zone. **3.** Lipid droplet. **4.** Accumulations of particulate glycogen. **5.** Mitochondria. **6.** Profiles of granular endoplasmic reticulum. **7.** Bundle of cytoplasmic filaments. **8.** Vacuoles with some flocculent content. **9.** Scalloped cell surface. **10.** Capsular region. **11.** Cartilage matrix. **12.** Part of neighboring chondrocyte.

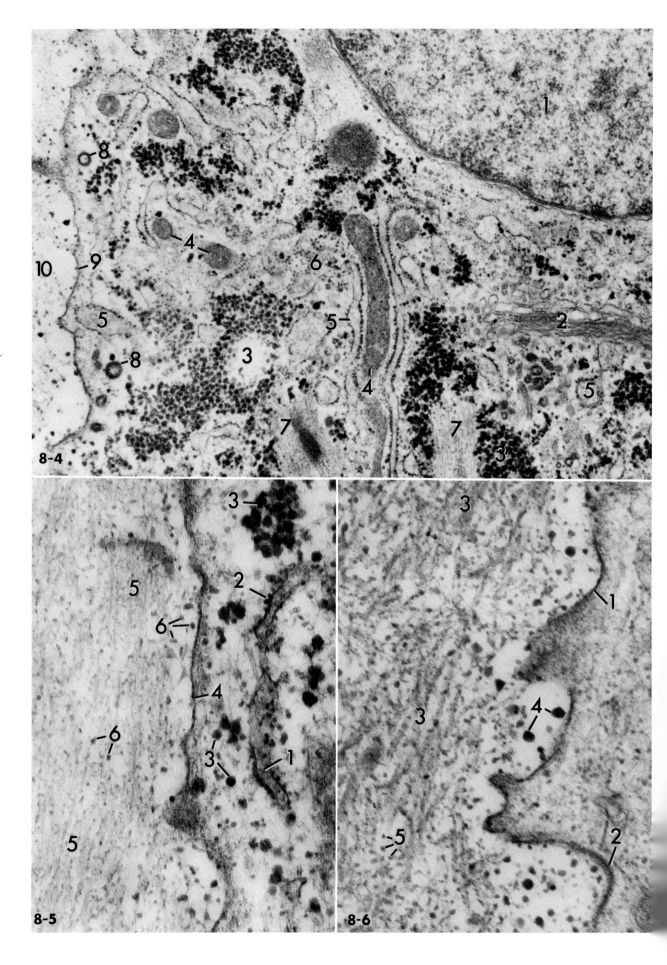

Fig. 8-4. Detail of chondrocyte in hyaline cartilage. Enlargement of rectangle in Fig. 8-3. E.M. X 33,000. **1.** Nucleus. **2.** Golgi zone. **3.** Particulate glycogen. **4.** Mitochondria. **5.** Granular endoplasmic reticulum. **6.** Ribosomes. **7.** Cytoplasmic filaments. **8.** Coated vesicles. **9.** Cell membrane. **10.** Pericellular region (capsule).

Fig. 8-5. Detail of chondrocyte. Hyaline cartilage. Same preparation as in Fig. 8-4. E.M. X 66,000. **1.** Cisterna of granular endoplasmic reticulum. **2.** Ribosomes. **3.** Particulate glycogen; average width 400 Å. **4.** Cell membrane. **5.** Dense feltwork of delicate fibrils; average width 100 Å. **6.** Matrix granules; average width 150 Å.

Fig. 8-6. Detail of chondrocyte. Hyaline cartilage. Same preparation as in Fig. 8-4. E.M. X 66,000. **1.** Cell membrane. **2.** This region represents a coated vesicle which just fused with the cell membrane. **3.** Dense feltwork of fibrils; average width 300 Å. No axial periodicity. **4.** Large matrix granules; average width 500 Å. **5.** Small matrix granules; average width 150 Å.

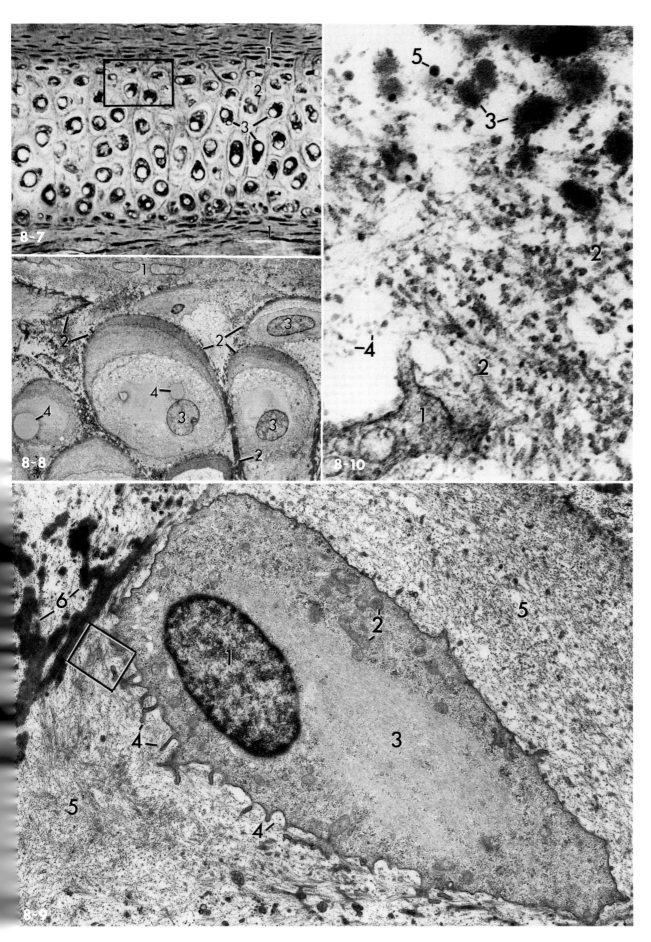

Fig. 8-7. Elastic cartilage. External ear (pinna). Mouse. L.M. X 200. **1.** Perichondrium. **2.** Matrix of elastic cartilage. **3.** Chondrocytes.

Fig. 8-8. Elastic cartilage. Pinna. Mouse. Enlargement of area similar to rectangle in Fig. 8-7. E.M. X 1100. **1.** Fibroblasts of perichondrium. **2.** Elastic fibers in cartilage matrix. **3.** Nuclei of chondrocytes. **4.** Lipid droplets in cytoplasm of chondrocytes.

Fig. 8-9. Chondrocyte. Elastic cartilage. Same preparations as in Fig. 8-8. E.M. X 9600. **1.** Nucleus. **2.** Mitochondria. **3.** Large accumulation of cytoplasmic filaments. **4.** Scalloped cell surface with microvilli. **5.** Fibrillar cartilage matrix. **6.** Elastic fibers.

Fig. 8-10. Detail of elastic cartilage. Enlargement of area similar to rectangle in Fig. 8-9. E.M. X 68,000. **1.** Part of chondrocyte cytoplasm. **2.** Feltwork of delicate fibrils; average width 200 Å. **3.** Elastic fibrils. **4.** Small matrix granules; average width 200 Å. **5.** Large matrix granule; width 500 Å.

Fig. 8-11. Fibrous cartilage. Annulus fibrosus. Intervertebral disk. Human. L.M. X 250. **1.** Rows of chondrocytes. **2.** Layers of collagenous fibers.

Fig. 8-12. Fibrous cartilage. Annulus fibrosus. Intervertebral disk. Mouse. Enlargement of area similar to rectangle in Fig. 8-11. E.M. X 2000. **1.** Nuclei of chondrocytes. **2.** Collagenous fibers.

Fig. 8-13. Chondrocyte. Fibrous cartilage. Enlargement of rectangle in Fig. 8-12. E.M. X 11,100. **1.** Nucleus. **2.** Granular endoplasmic reticulum. **3.** Golgi zone. **4.** Centrioles. **5.** Pericellular capsule of cartilage matrix. **6.** Longitudinally sectioned collagenous fibrils. **7.** Cross-sectioned collagenous fibrils.

Fig. 8-14. Detail of fibrous cartilage. Annulus fibrosus. Intervertebral disk. Mouse. Enlargement of area similar to rectangle in Fig. 8-13. E.M. X 68,000. **1.** Part of chondrocyte cytoplasm. **2.** Cell membrane. **3.** Feltwork of delicate fibrils make up the pericellular capsule of cartilage matrix. Width of fibrils averages 80 Å. **4.** Cross-sectioned collagenous fibrils: A) width 800 Å; B) width 300 Å.

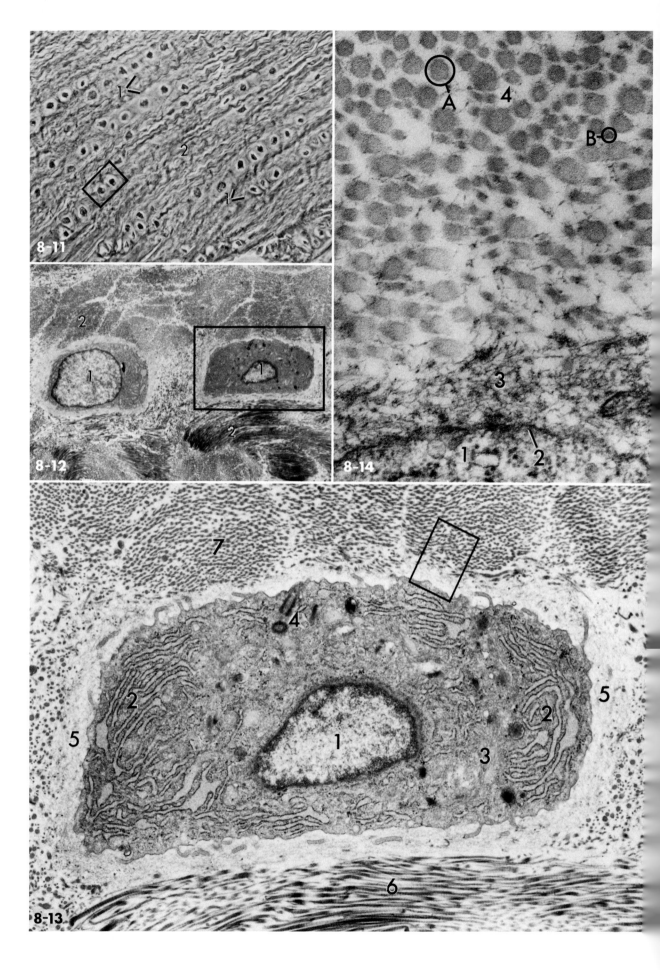

References

Anderson, D. R. Ultrastructure of hyaline and elastic cartilage of the rat. Am. J. Anat. *114*: 403–434 (1964).

Anderson, H. C. Electron microscopic studies on induced cartilage development and calcification. J. Cell Biol. *35*: 81–101 (1967).

Anderson, H. C. Vesicles associated with calcification in the matrix of epiphyseal cartilage. J. Cell Biol. *41*: 59–72 (1969).

Anderson, H. C. and Matsuzawa, T. Membranous particles in calcifying cartilage matrix. Trans. N.Y. Acad. Sci. Series II, *22*: 619–630 (1970).

Bonucci, E. Fine structure of early cartilage calcification. J. Ultrastruct. Res. *20*: 33–50 (1967).

Cooper, G. W. and Prockop, D. J. Intracellular accumulation of protocollagen and extrusion of collagen by embryonic cartilage cells. J. Cell Biol. *38*: 523–537 (1968).

Godman, G. C. and Lane, N. On the site of sulfation in the chondrocyte. J. Cell Biol. *21*: 353–366 (1964).

Godman, G. C. and Porter, K. R. Chondrogenesis, studied with the electron microscope. J. Biophys. Biochem. Cytol. *8*: 719–760 (1960).

Goel, S. C. Electron microscopic studies on developing cartilage. I. The membrane system related to the synthesis and secretion of extracellular materials. J. Embryol. Exp. Morph. *23*: 169–184 (1970).

Horwitz, A. L. and Dorfman, A. Subcellular sites for synthesis of chondromucoprotein of cartilage. J. Cell Biol. *38*: 358–368 (1968).

Matukas, V. J., Panner, B. J. and Orbison, J. L. Studies on ultrastructural identification and distribution of protein polysaccharide in cartilage matrix. J. Cell Biol. *32*: 365–378 (1964).

Minor, R. R. Somite chondrogenesis. A structural study. J. Cell Biol. *56*: 27–50 (1973).

Palfrey, A. J. and Davies, D. V. The fine structure of chondrocytes. J. Anat. *100*: 213–226 (1966).

Revel, J. P. and Hay, E. D. An autoradiographic and electron microscopic study of collagen synthesis in differentiating cartilage. Z. Zellforsch. *61*: 110–144 (1963).

Seegmiller, R., Ferguson, C. C. and Sheldon, H. Studies on cartilage. IV. A genetically determined defect in tracheal cartilage. J. Ultrastruct. Res. *38*: 288–301 (1972).

Sheldon, H. Cartilage. *In* Electron Microscopic Anatomy (Ed. S. M. Kurtz), pp. 295–313. Academic Press, New York, 1964.

Sheldon, H. and Kimball, F. B. Studies on cartilage. III. The occurence of collagen within vacuoles of the Golgi apparatus. J. Cell Biol. *12*: 599–613 (1962).

Sheldon, H. and Robinson, R. A. Studies on cartilage: electron microscope observations on normal rabbit ear cartilage. J. Biophys. Biochem. Cytol. *4*: 401–406 (1958).

Silberberg, R. Ultrastructure of articular cartilage in health and disease. Clin. Orthop. *57*: 233–257 (1968).

Silva, D. G. and Hart, J. A. L. Ultrastructural observations on the mandibular condyle of the guinea pig. J. Ultrastruct. Res. *20*: 227–243 (1967).

Silva, D. G. Further ultrastructural studies on the temporo-mandibular joint in the guinea pig. J. Ultrastruct. Res. *26*: 148–162 (1969).

Smith, J. W. and Serafini-Fracassini, A. The distribution of the protein-polysaccharide complex in the nucleus pulposus matrix in young rabbits. J. Cell Sci. *3*: 33–40 (1968).

Smith, J. W., Peters, T. J. and Serafini-Fracassini, A. Observations on the distribution of the protein-polysaccharide complex and collagen in bovine articular cartilage. J. Cell Sci. *2*: 129–136 (1967).

Thyberg, J. Ultrastructural localization of aryl sulfatase activity in epiphyseal plate. J. Ultrastruct. Res. *38*: 332–342 (1972).

Thyberg, J. and Friberg, U. Ultrastructure and acid phosphatase activity of matrix vesicles and cytoplasmic dense bodies in the epiphyseal plate. J. Ultrastruct. Res. *33*: 554–573 (1970).

9 Bone

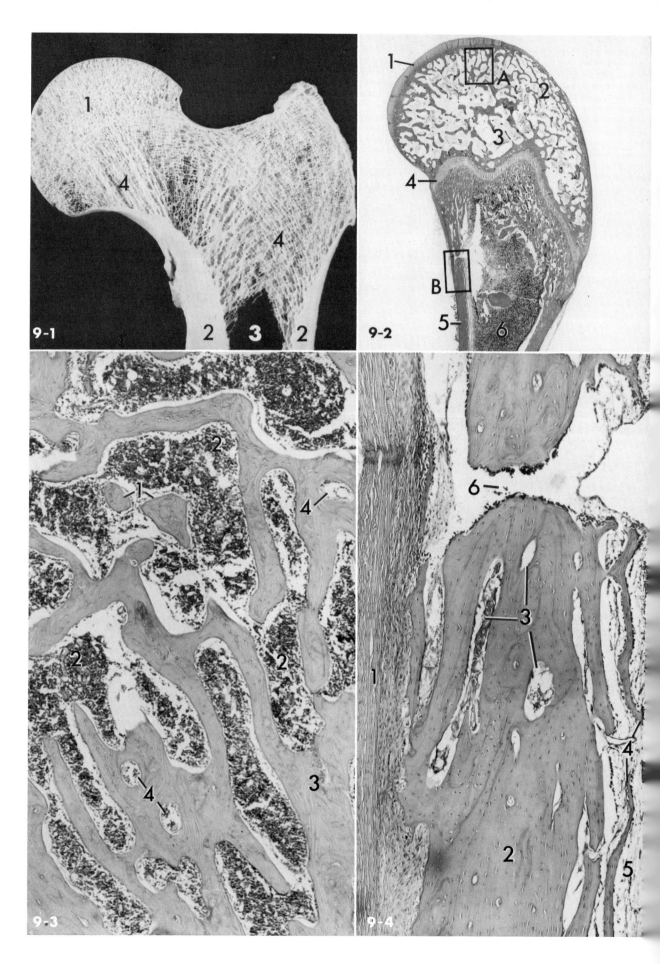

Fig. 9-1. Section of upper end of dry femur. Adult. Human. L.M. X 1.0. **1.** Spongy bone of epiphysis. **2.** Compact bone of distal part of diaphysis. **3.** Marrow cavity. **4.** Trabeculae follow major lines of stress. Note absence of epiphyseal cartilage plate.

Fig. 9-2. Sagittal section of femoral condyle. Young rabbit. L.M. X 4.2. **1.** Articular cartilage. **2.** Spongy bone of epiphysis. **3.** Marrow cavity. **4.** Narrow epiphyseal cartilage plate. **5.** Compact bone of diaphysis. **6.** Bone marrow.

Fig. 9-3. Survey of spongy bone. Enlargement of area similar to rectangle (A) in Fig. 9-2. Epiphysis. Femur. Young cat. L.M. X 72. **1.** Spicules. **2.** Bone marrow. **3.** Trabeculae. **4.** Marrow spaces simulating Haversian canals.

Fig. 9-4. Compact cortical bone. Enlargement of rectangle (B) in Fig. 9-2. L.M. X 88. **1.** Periosteum. **2.** Compact bone. **3.** Haversian canals. **4.** Trabeculae. **5.** Bone marrow. **6.** Nutrient foramen and canal.

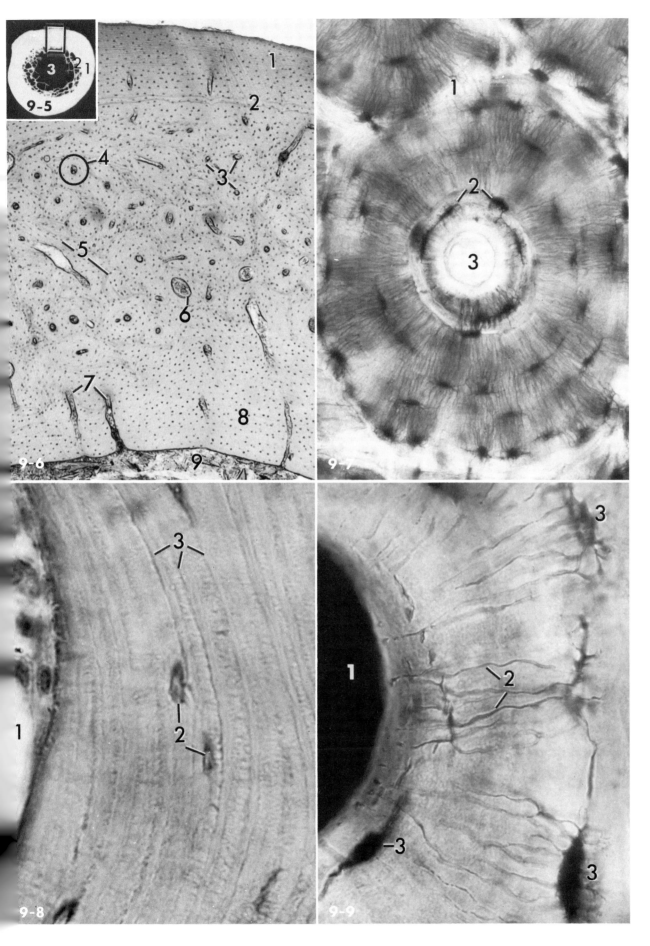

Fig. 9-5. Cross section through diaphysis of dry femur. Human. L.M. X 0.8. **1.** Compact bone. **2.** Trabeculae. **3.** Marrow cavity.

Fig. 9-6. Cross section of tibia. Enlargement of area similar to rectangle in Fig. 9-5. Human. L.M. X 70. **1.** Periosteum (removed). **2.** External circumferential lamellae. **3.** Haversian canals. **4.** Circle: osteon. **5.** Traces of interstitial lamellae. **6.** Erosion tunnel. **7.** Volkmann's canals. **8.** Internal circumferential lamellae. Each small dot represents an osteocyte in a lacuna. **9.** Bone marrow.

Fig. 9-7. Osteon (Haversian system). Ground cross section through compact bone of diaphysis. Femur. Human. L.M. X 1000. **1.** Cementing line. **2.** Lacunae. **3.** Haversian canal.

Fig. 9-8. Central part of osteon. Decalcified preparation to demonstrate bony lamellae. Rib. Human. L.M. X 360. **1.** Haversian canal. **2.** Osteocytes in lacunae. **3.** Bony circular lamellae.

Fig. 9-9. Central part of osteon. Ground section. Same preparation as in Fig. 9-7. L.M. X 1300. **1.** Haversian canal. **2.** Canaliculi; some reach the Haversian canal. **3.** Lacunae.

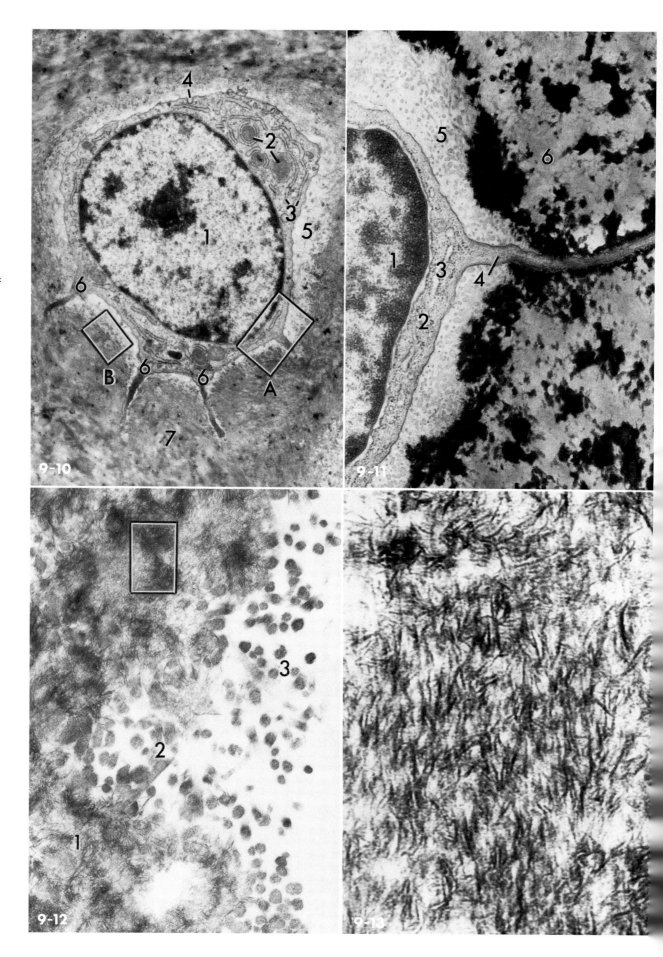

Fig. 9-10. Osteocyte in lacuna. Mandible. Decalcified preparation. Newborn rat. E.M. X 7000. **1.** Nucleus of osteocyte. **2.** Mitochondria. **3.** Granular endoplasmic reticulum. **4.** Coated vesicle. **5.** Pericellular zone of lacuna. **6.** Cytoplasmic processes. **7.** Bone matrix.

Fig. 9-11. Detail of osteocyte. Enlargement of area similar to rectangle (A) in Fig. 9-10. Diaphysis of radius. Partly decalcified preparation. Two-day-old rat. E.M. X 34,000. **1.** Nucleus of osteocyte. **2.** Ribosomes. **3.** Granular endoplasmic reticulum. **4.** Cytoplasmic process without ribosomes, entering canaliculus. **5.** Collagenous fibrils in pericellular zone of lacuna. **6.** Bone matrix: apatite crystals removed in white areas, remaining in black areas.

Fig. 9-12. Detail of osteocyte lacuna and bone matrix. Enlargement of area similar to rectangle (B) in Fig. 9-10. Diaphysis of radius. Partly decalcified preparation. Two-day-old rat. E.M. X 72,000. **1.** Bone matrix dominated by hydroxyapatite crystals which obscure the collagenous fibrils. **2.** Cross-sectioned collagenous fibrils immediately before mineralization. **3.** Periosteocytic space of the lacuna with collagenous fibrils.

Fig. 9-13. Detail of bone matrix. Enlargement of area similar to rectangle in Fig. 9-12. Head of humerus. Two-day-old rat. E.M. X 200,000. Hydroxyapatite crystals (15 Å X 300 Å) dominate in the matrix, completely obscuring the collagenous fibrils.

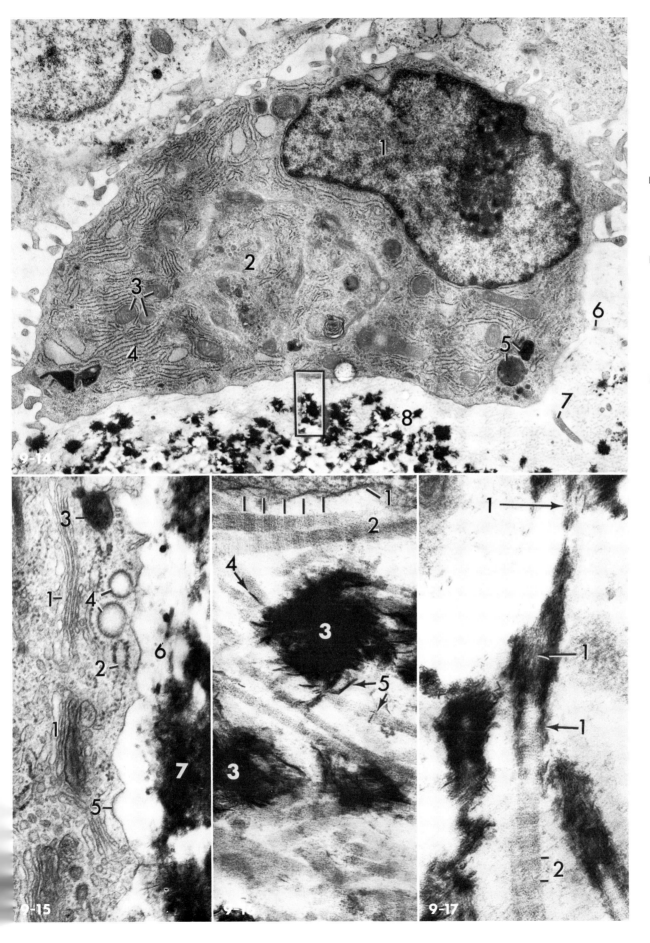

Fig. 9-14. Osteoblast. Diaphysis of radius. Two-day-old rat. E.M. X 9000. **1.** Nucleus of osteoblast. **2.** Golgi zone. **3.** Mitochondria. **4.** Granular endoplasmic reticulum. **5.** Lysosomes. **6.** Short microvillus. **7.** Long microvillus. **8.** Osteoid.

Fig. 9-15. Detail of osteoblast. Same preparation as in Fig. 9-14. E.M. X 46,000. **1.** Components of Golgi zone. **2.** Granular endoplasmic reticulum. **3.** Lysosome. **4.** Coated vesicles, the uppermost just fusing with the cell membrane. **5.** Coated vesicle completing its fusion with the cell membrane. **6.** Periosteoblastic space with some collagenous fibrils. **7.** Bone matrix.

Fig. 9-16. Detail of osteoid. Enlargement of area similar to rectangle in Fig. 9-14. Head of humerus. Two-day-old rat. E.M. X 99,000. **1.** Osteoblast cell membrane. **2.** Collagenous fibrils with 610 Å axial periodicity (between each bar). **3.** Initial calcification loci. **4.** Hydroxyapatite crystal, parallel to long axis of collagenous fibril. **5.** Crystals perpendicular to long axis of collagenous fibril.

Fig. 9-17. Detail of mineralized collagenous fibril. Same preparation as in Fig. 9-16. E.M. X 111,000. **1.** Arrows indicate sites where the hydroxyapatite crystals are oriented parallel to the long axis of the collagenous fibril. They seem to be both at the surface and within the fibril. **2.** The lower part of the fibril shows clear axial periodicity without crystals.

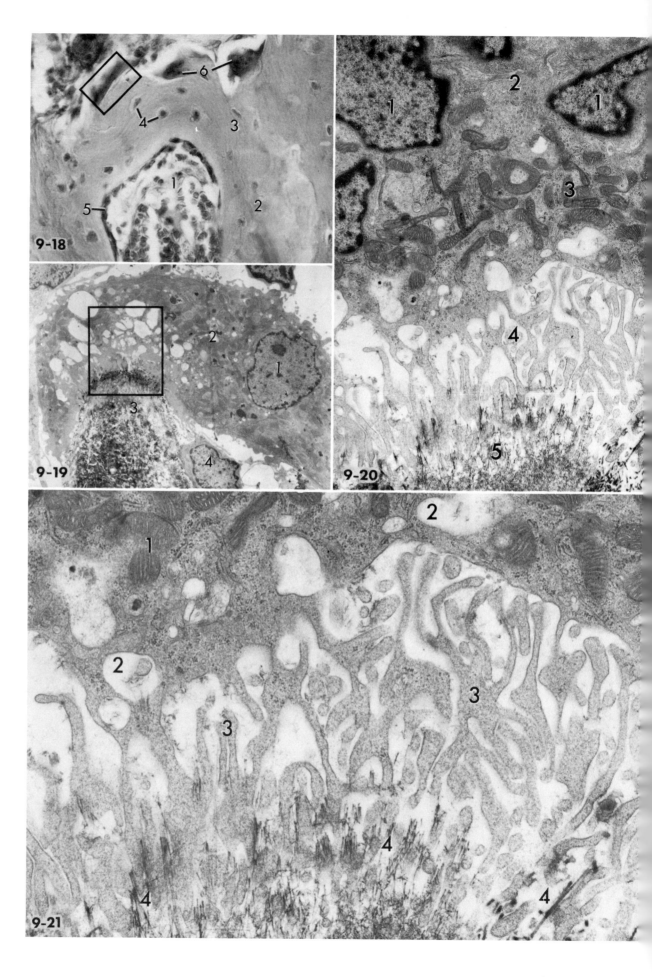

Fig. 9-18. Remodeling of spongy bone. Rib. Human. L.M. X 350. **1.** Bone marrow. **2.** Trabeculum. **3.** Bone matrix. **4.** Osteocytes. **5.** Osteoblasts. **6.** Osteoclasts.

Fig. 9-19. Osteoclast. Enlargement of area simiar to rectangle in Fig. 9-18. Head of humerus. Two-day-old rat. E.M. X 2300. **1.** Nucleus of osteoclast. **2.** Extensive cytoplasm. **3.** Bone matrix. **4.** Nucleus of neighboring osteoblast.

Fig. 9-20. Part of osteoclast. Enlargement of area similar to rectangle in Fig. 9-19. Same preparation as in Fig. 9-19. E.M. X 9000. **1.** Nuclei of osteoclast. **2.** Golgi zone. **3.** Mitochondria. **4.** Ruffled border. **5.** Bone matrix.

Fig. 9-21. Detail of osteoclast ruffled border. Enlargement of lower half of Fig. 9-20. E.M. X 17,000. **2.** Phagocytic vacuoles containing small, needle-shaped crystals. **3.** Microvilli of ruffled border. **4.** Delicate mineralized collagenous fibrils of bone matrix.

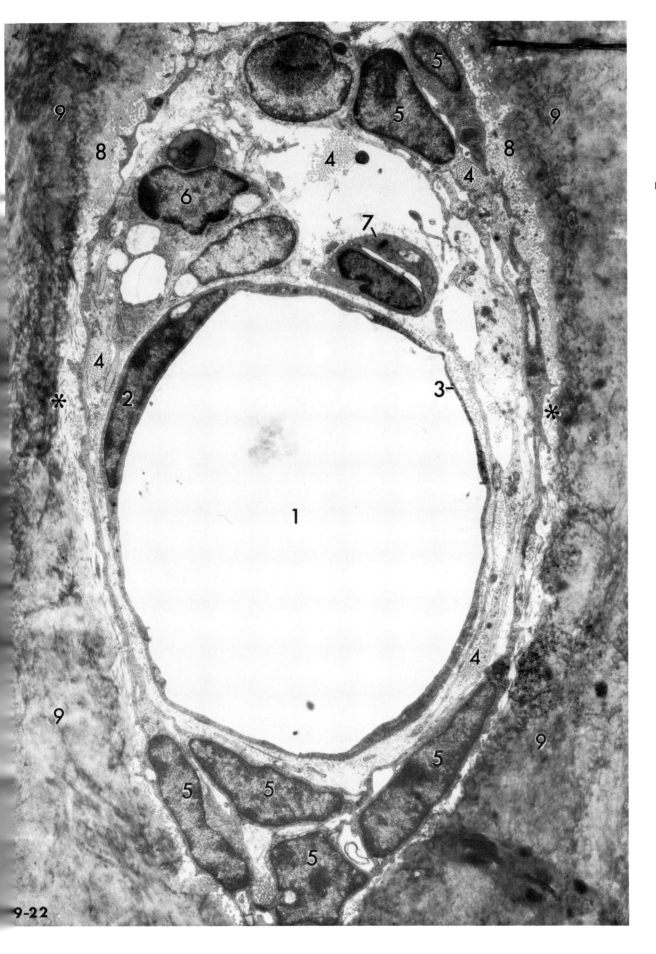

Fig. 9-22. Cross section of a 23 μ-wide Haversian canal in frontal bone of a four-week-old kitten. Specimen fixed by vascular perfusion with subsequent decalcification. E.M. X 6000. **1.** Lumen of venous capillary. **2.** Endothelial nucleus. **3.** Continuous thin endothelium; basal lamina incomplete. **4.** Collagenous fibrils. **5.** Nuclei of osteoprogenitor cells and resting, flat osteoblasts. These cells form an endosteal lining of the Haversian canal. Distance between asterisks is 23 μ. **6.** Nucleus of macrophage. **7.** Cross section of small capillary, probably in a state of sprouting growth, judging from the narrow, slit-like lumen. **8.** Osteoid. **9.** Calcified bone matrix.

9-22

Fig. 9-23. Survey of bone marrow. Diaphysis. Two-day-old rat. E.M. X 600. **1.** Wide sinusoids. **2.** Narrow blood capillaries. **3.** Remnants of bone trabeculae with core of calcified cartilage. **4.** Layer of osteoblasts (endosteum). **5.** Reticular cells (fixed macrophages). **6.** Megakaryoblasts. **7.** Osteoclasts. **8.** Circles: cells in mitosis. *Note:* Identification of cells is based on analysis of this field at higher magnifications. No attempt has been made to identify the varied stages of cells in hemopoietic development.

Fig. 9-24. Detail of bone marrow sinusoid. Enlargement of area similar to rectangle in Fig. 9-23. Same preparation. E.M. X 15,000. **1.** Lumen of sinusoid. **2.** Nucleus of endothelial (lining) cell. **3.** Coated vesicles. **4.** Phagocytic vacuole. **5.** Thin attenuated continuous endothelial cytoplasm.

Fig. 9-25. Detail of endothelial cell in bone marrow sinusoid. E.M. X 49,000. **1.** Lumen of sinusoid. **2.** Endothelial cells. **3.** Cell junction. **4.** Perisinusoidal space. Note absence of basal lamina.

Fig. 9-26. Detail of endothelial cell in bone marrow sinusoid. Same preparation as in Fig. 9-24. E.M. X 72,000. **1.** Lumen of sinusoid. **2.** Nucleus of endothelial (lining) cell. **3.** Phagocytic vacuole. **4.** Small Golgi zone. **5.** Mitochondria. **6.** Perisinusoidal space.

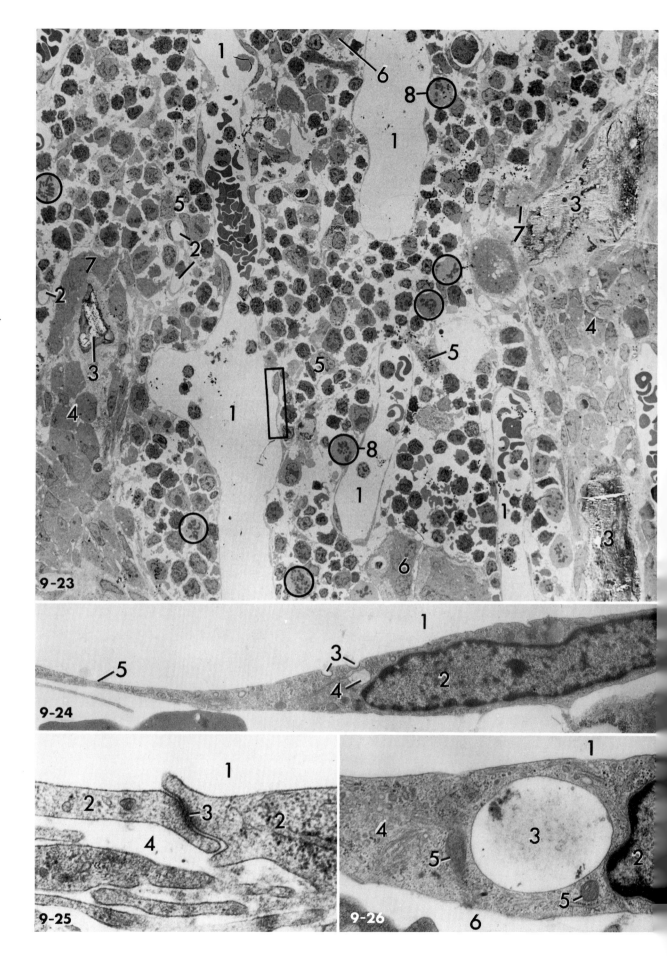

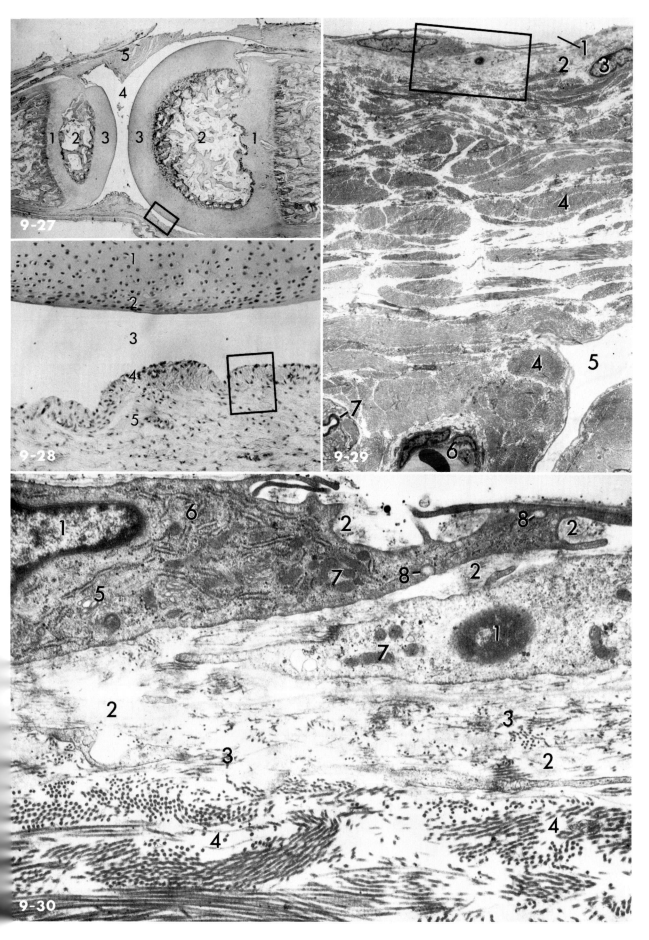

Fig. 9-27. Survey of synovial joint. Finger. Monkey. Four months old. L.M. X 10.5. **1.** Epiphyseal growth plate. **2.** Spongy bone of epiphysis. **3.** Epiphyseal and articular cartilages. **4.** Joint cavity. **5.** Articular capsule.

Fig. 9-28. Detail of joint. Enlargement of rectangle in Fig. 9-27. L.M. X 163. **1.** Epiphyseal cartilage. **2.** Articular cartilage. **3.** Joint cavity. **4.** Synovial membrane. **5.** Articular capsule.

Fig. 9-29. Articular capsule. Knee joint. Enlargement of area similar to rectangle in Fig. 9-28. Rat. E.M. X 1800. **1.** Joint cavity. **2.** Synovial membrane. **3.** Nucleus of fibroblast. **4.** Collagenous fiber bundles in articular capsule. **5.** Lymph vessel. **6.** Blood capillary. **7.** Nerve.

Fig. 9-30. Synovial membrane. Enlargement of rectangle in Fig. 9-29. E.M. X 18,000. **1.** Nuclei of synovial cells. **2.** Basement membrane-like material. **3.** Reticular fibrils. **4.** Collagenous fibrils. **5.** Golgi zone. **6.** Granular endoplasmic reticulum. **7.** Mitochondria. **8.** Coated vesicles.

References

Barland, P., Novikoff, A. B. and Hamerman, D. Electron microscopy of the human synovial membrane. J. Cell Biol. *14*: 207–220 (1962).

Baud, C. G. Submicroscopic structure and functional aspects of the osteocyte. Clin. Orthop. *56*: 227–236 (1968).

Brookes, M. The vascular architecture of tubular bone in the rat. Anat. Rec. *132*: 25–41 (1958).

Cabrini, R. L. Histochemistry of ossification. Int. Rev. Cytol. *11*: 283–306 (1961).

Cameron, D. A. The fine structure of osteoblasts in the metaphysis of the tibia of young rat. J. Biophys. Biochem. Cytol. *9*: 583–595 (1961).

Cameron, D. A. The fine structure of bone and calcified cartilage. Clin. Orthop. *26*: 199–228 (1963).

Cohen, J. and Harris, W. H. The three-dimensional anatomy of Haversian systems. J. Bone and Joint Surg. *40-A*: 419–434 (1958).

Cooper, R. R., Milgram, J. W. and Robinson, R. A. Morphology of the osteon. An electron microscopic study. J. Bone and Joint Surg. *48-A*: 1239–1271 (1966).

Drinker, C. K., Drinker, K. R. and Lund, C. C. The circulation in the mammalian bone marrow. Am. J. Physiol. *62*: 1–92 (1922).

Dudley, H. R. and Spiro, D. The fine structure of bone cells J. Biophys. Biochem. Cytol. *11*: 627–649 (1961).

Engström, A. Structure of bone from the anatomical to the molecular level. Ciba Foundation Symposium on Bone Structure and Metabolism. (Eds. G. E. W. Wolstenholme and C. M. O'Connor), pp. 3–10. Churchill, London, 1956.

Ghadially, F. N. and Roy, S. Ultrastructure of Synovial Joints in Health and Disease. Butterworths, London, 1969.

Glimcher, M. J. Molecular biology of mineralized tissues with particular reference to bone. Rev. Mod. Phys. *31*: 359–393 (1959).

Glimcher, M. J. and Krane, S. M. The organization and structure of bone, and the mechanism of calcification. *In* Treatise on Collagen (Ed. B. S. Gould), Vol. 2, part B. Academic Press, New York, 1968.

Herring, G. M. A review of recent advances in the chemistry of calcifying cartilage and bone matrix. Calc. Tiss. Res. *4*, Suppl. 17 (1970).

Hohling, H. J., Kreilos, R., Neubauer, G. and Boyde, A. Electron microscopy and electron microscopical measurements of collagen mineralization in hard tissue. Z. Zellforsch. *122*: 36–52 (1971).

Jande, S. S. Fine structural study of osteocytes and their surrounding bone matrix with respect to their age in young chicks. J. Ultrastruct. Res. *37*: 279–300 (1971).

Jande, S. S. and Belanger, L. F. Electron microscopy of osteocytes and the pericellular matrix in rat trabecular bone. Calc. Tiss. Res. *6*: 280–289 (1971).

Kallio, D. M., Garant, P. R. and Minkin, C. Evidence of coated membranes in the ruffled border of the osteoclast. J. Ultrastruct. Res. *37*: 169–177 (1971).

Lacroix, P. Bone and cartilage. *In* The Cell (Eds. J. Brachet and A. E. Mirsky) Vol. 5: 219–266. Academic Press, New York, 1961.

Mjör, I. A. The bone matrix adjacent to lacunae and canaliculi. Anat. Rec. *144*: 327–339 (1962).

Robinson, R. A. and Cameron, D. A. Bone. *In*: Electron Microscopic Anatomy (Ed. S. M. Kurtz), pp. 315–340. Academic Press, New York, 1964.

Rohr, H. Die Kollagensynthese in ihrer Beziehung zur submikroskopischen Struktur des Osteoblasten. Virchows Arch. Path. Anat. *338*: 342–354 (1965).

Roy, S. and Ghadially, F. N. Ultrastructure of normal rat synovial membrane. Ann. Rheum. Dis. *26*: 26–38 (1967).

Scherft, J. P. The lamina limitans of the organic matrix of calcified cartilage and bone. J. Ultrastruct. Res. *38*: 318–331 (1972).

Scott, B. L. The occurrence of specific cytoplasmic granules in the osteoclast. J. Ultrastruct. Res. *19*: 417–431 (1967).

Scott, B. L. and Glimcher, M. J. Distribution of glycogen in osteoblasts of the fetal rat. J. Ultrastruct. Res. *36*: 565–586 (1971).

Talmage, R. V. Morphological and physiological considerations in a new concept of calcium transport in bone. Am. J. Anat. *129*: 467–476 (1970).

Vaughan, J. M. The Physiology of Bone. Oxford University Press, London, 1970.

Wassermann, F. and Yaeger, J. A. Fine structure of the osteocyte capsule and the wall of the lacunae in bone. Z. Zellforsch. *67*: 636–652 (1965).

Yoffey, J. M. Structural peculiarities of the blood vessels of the bone marrow. Bibl. Anat. (Basel) 7: 298–303 (1965).

Zamboni, L. and Pease, D. C. The vascular bed of red bone marrow. J. Ultrastruct. Res. *5*: 65–85 (1961).

10 Bone development

Fig. 10-1. Intramembranous bone formation. Calvaria. Rat fetus. L.M. X 560. **1.** Fusiform mesenchymal cells of future periosteum. **2.** Mesenchymal cells, proliferating, aggregating, and becoming spherical. **3.** Osteoblasts. **4.** Osteocytes. **5.** Spicules of osteoid and bone matrix forming primitive trabeculae and primary spongy bone. **6.** Capillaries. **7.** Mesenchymal cells aggregating to form future dura mater (endosteum).

Fig. 10-2. Intramembranous bone formation. Enlargement of area similar to rectangle in Fig. 10-1. Mandible. Newborn rat. Decalcified preparation. E.M. X 1900. **1.** Nuclei of osteocytes. **2.** Osteoid. **3.** Bone matrix, partly mineralized.

Fig. 10-3. Osteocyte. Same preparation as in Fig. 10-2. E.M. X 9000. **1.** Nucleus. **2.** Golgi zone. **3.** Granular endoplasmic reticulum. **4.** Mitochondria. **5.** Lysosomes. **6.** Coated vesicles. **7.** Cell processes. **8.** Pericellular space with non-mineralized osteoid. **9.** Fully mineralized bone matrix.

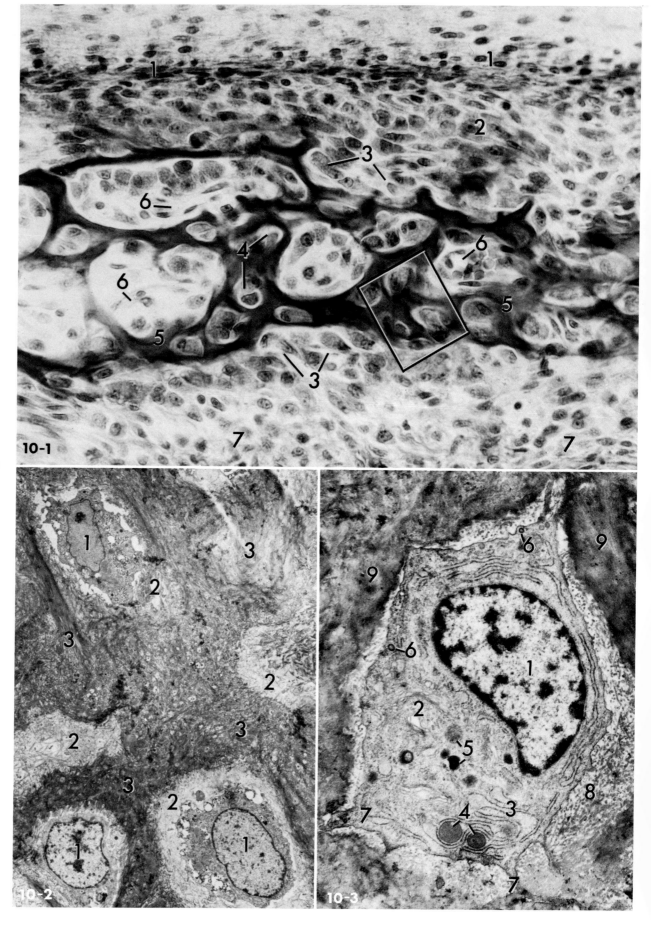

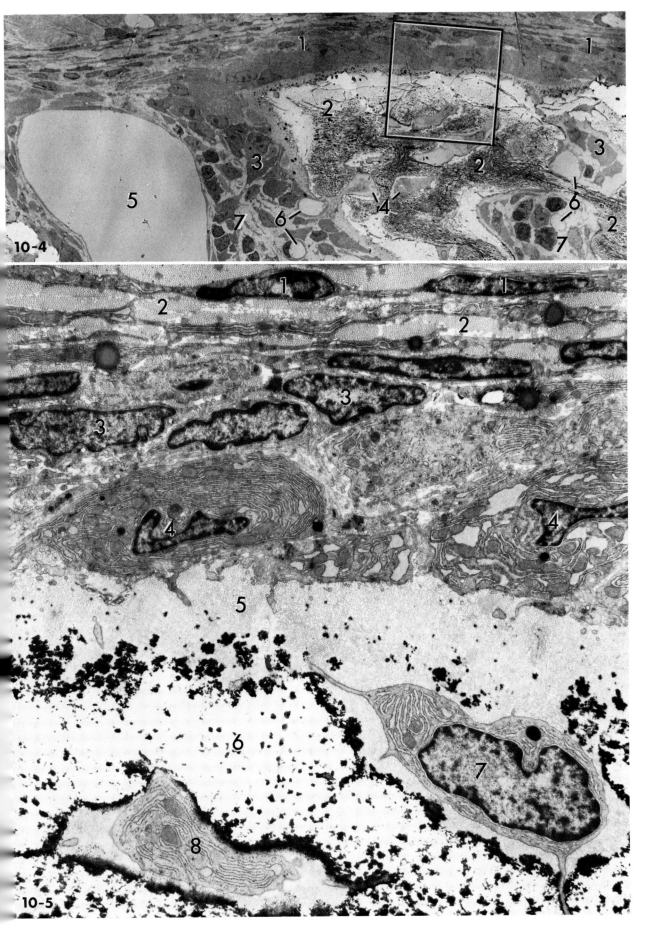

Fig. 10-4. Cross section at the level of the diaphysis of the radius. Two-day-old rat. E.M. X 660. **1.** Periosteum. **2.** Primary spongy bone. **3.** Single layer of osteoblasts forming endosteum. **4.** Osteocytes. **5.** Venule, part of periosteal sprout. **6.** Capillaries. **7.** Primary bone marrow cells.

Fig. 10-5. Periosteum. Diaphysis of radius. Enlargement of area similar to rectangle in Fig. 10-4. Two-day-old rat. E.M. X 5600. **1.** Nuclei of fibroblasts. **2.** Collagenous fibers. **3.** Nuclei of osteoprogenitor cells. **4.** Nuclei of osteoblasts. **5.** Osteoid. **6.** Mineralized bone matrix (some minerals partly removed during preparation process). **7.** Osteoblast in the process of being completely surrounded by mineralized bone matrix. **8.** Osteocyte in bone lacuna.

Fig. 10-6. Periosteum. Diaphysis of radius. Two-day-old rat. E.M. X 12,000. **1.** Nuclei of fibroblasts in superficial layers of periosteum. **2.** Bundles of collagenous fibrils. **3.** Cytoplasmic strands of fibroblasts. **4.** Nuclei of osteoprogenitor cells in middle part of periosteum. **5.** Cytoplasm of osteoblasts. **6.** Osteoid. **7.** Fully calcified bone matrix (some mineral salts removed during preparation of specimen).

Fig. 10-7. Detail of fibroblast layer of periosteum. Enlargement of area similar to rectangle (A) in Fig. 10-6. Same preparation. E.M. X 50,000. **1.** Cytoplasm of fibroblast. **2.** Cross-sectioned collagenous fibrils; average width 400 Å. **3.** Elastic fibrils.

Fig. 10-8. Details of osteoprogenitor layers of periosteum. Enlargement of area similar to rectangle (B) in Fig. 10-6. Same preparation. E.M. X 48,000. **1.** Granular endoplasmic reticulum of osteoprogenitor cells. **2.** Mitochondrion. **3.** Accumulation of particulate glycogen. **4.** Cross-sectioned delicate collagenous (reticular) fibrils; average width 200 Å. **5.** Cross-sectioned cell processes.

Fig. 10-9. Detail of osteoid. Enlargement of area similar to rectangle (C) in Fig. 10-6. Same preparation. E.M. X 48,000. **1.** Cross-sectioned cell processes. **2.** Collagenous fibrils near surface of osteoblast are delicate, newly formed. **3.** Collagenous fibrils further away from osteoblast cell surface increase in size. **4.** Collagenous fibrils still further away are coarse and tend to fuse laterally. **5.** Loci of initial calcification.

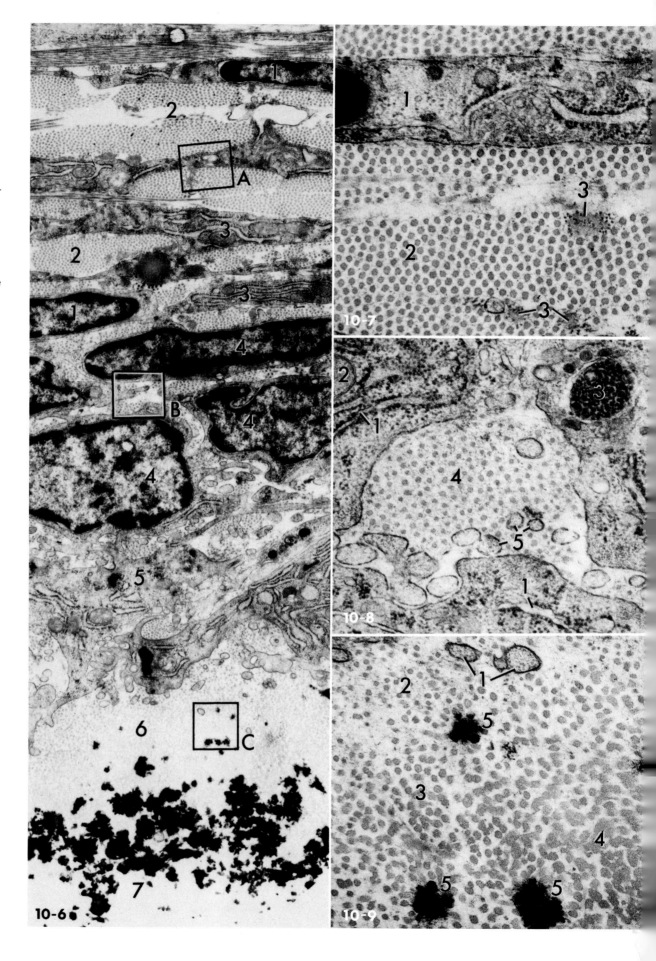

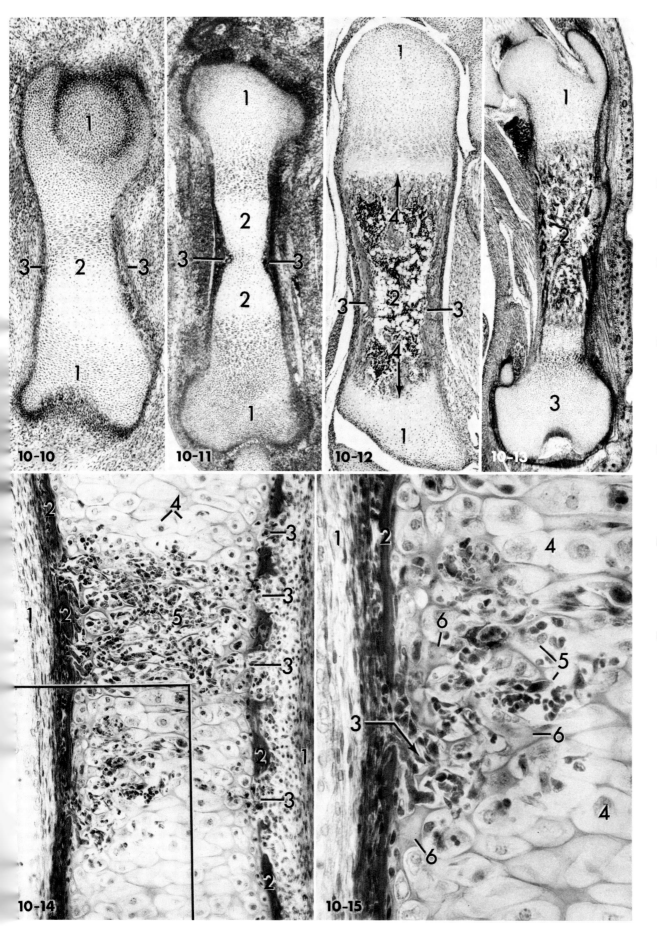

Fig. 10-10. Cartilage model. Longitudinal section. Os coxae. Mouse embryo. L.M. X 55. **1.** Hyaline cartilage of epiphysis. **2.** Diaphysis. **3.** Perichondrium: enlarging chondrocytes signify onset of endochondral ossification.

Fig. 10-11. Cartilage model. Longitudinal section. Humerus. Mouse embryo. L.M. X 43. **1.** Epiphysis. **2.** Enlarging chondrocytes in center of diaphysis. **3.** Subperichondrial (periosteal) sleeve of bone starting to form by intramembranous ossification.

Fig. 10-12. Endochondral ossification. Longitudinal section. Metatarsal bone. newborn rat. L.M. X 36. **1.** Epiphysis. **2.** Primitive bone marrow of primary ossification center. **3.** Enlarging subperiosteal bone sleeve. **4.** Endochondral ossification progresses in opposite directions (arrows) towards the epiphyses.

Fig. 10-13. Progressing endochondral ossification. Longitudinal section. Femur. Newborn mouse. L.M. X 20. **1.** Epiphysis with future head and major trochanter of femor clearly outlined. **2.** Primary ossification of entire diaphysis. **3.** Epiphysis with future condyles of femur.

Fig. 10-14. Early stages of endochondral ossification. Sphenoid bone. Rat fetus. L.M. X 168. **1.** Periosteum. **2.** Subperiosteal bone collar. **3.** Bone eroded by periosteal sprouts. **4.** Hypertrophied chondrocytes. **5.** Periosteal sprouts invading cartilage lacunae.

Fig. 10-15. Endochondral ossification. Enlargement of rectangle in Fig. 10-14. L.M. X 290. **1.** Periosteum. **2.** Subperiosteal bone collar. **3.** Periosteal sprout growing into cartilage. **4.** Hypertrophied cartilage lacunae. **5.** Capillaries and osteoprogenitor cells in enlarged cartilage lacunae. **6.** Calcified cartilage matrix.

121

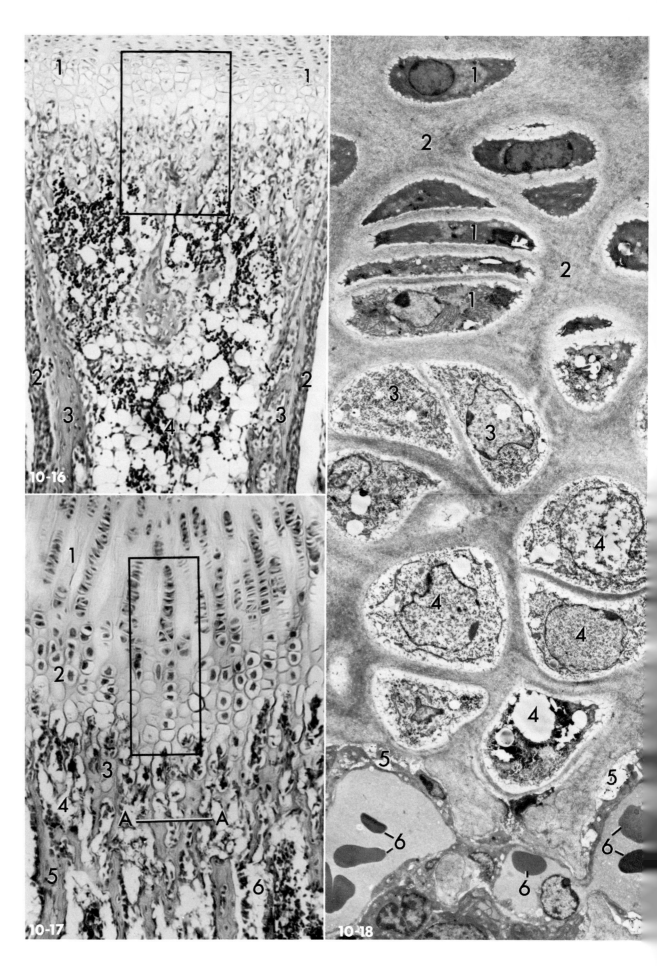

Fig. 10-16. Endochondral ossification extending toward epiphysis. Longitudinal section. Metatarsal bone. Newborn rat. L.M. X 116.
1. Epiphyseal cartilage. **2.** Periosteum.
3. Subperiosteal bone collar of diaphysis.
4. Primary bone marrow.

Fig. 10-17. Endochondral ossification. Enlargement of area similar to rectangle in Fig. 10-16. Femur. Rabbit. L.M. X 127.
1. Zone of chondrocyte multiplication with parallel rows of cells. **2.** Zone of chondrocyte hypertrophy. **3.** Zone of cartilage matrix calcification. **4.** Capillaries invade lacunar spaces. **5.** Spicules and trabeculae of calcified cartilage covered with bone. **6.** Primary bone marrow.

Fig. 10-18. Endochondral ossification. Enlargement of area similar to rectangle in Fig. 10-17. Epiphyseal growth plate. Humerus. Two-day-old rat. E.M. X 1800.
1. Chondrocytes proliferating. **2.** Matrix of hyaline cartilage. **3.** Hypertrophying chondrocytes. **4.** Degenerating and dying chondrocytes. **5.** Nodules of calcified cartilage matrix. **6.** Erythrocytes in lumina of capillaries invading cartilage lacunae.

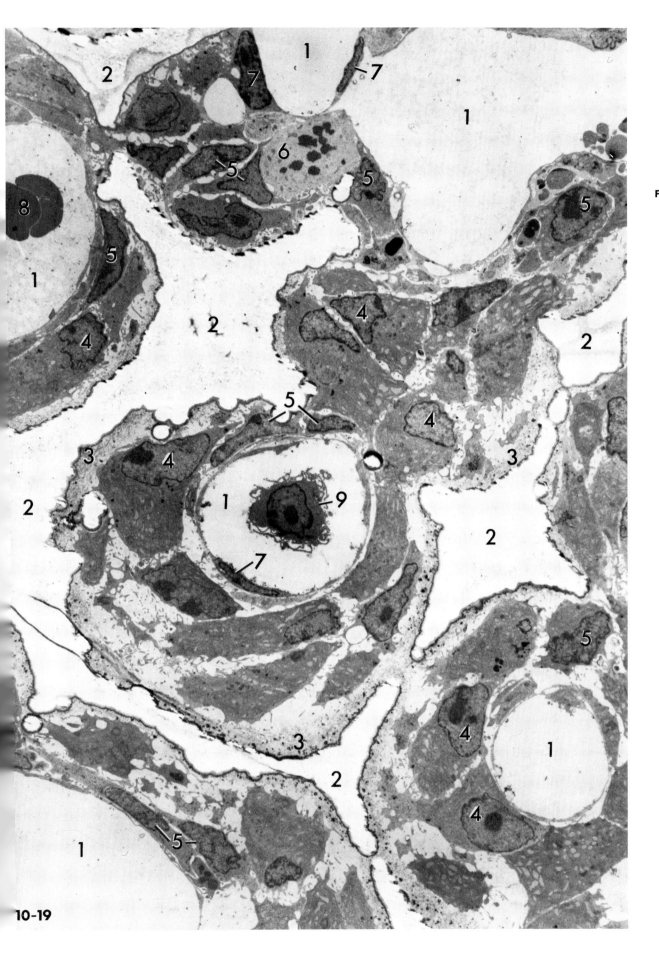

Fig. 10-19. Endochondral ossification. Zone of cartilage calcification and early bone deposition. This survey demonstrates the invading capillary sprouts as they bring in osteoprogenitor cells and osteoblasts to the cartilage lacunae. Cross section of bone at the level indicated by the line A—A in Fig. 10-17. Specimen fixed by vascular perfusion with subsequent decalcification. Upper epiphysis of humerus. Two-day-old rat. E.M. X 1800. **1.** Lumina of invading capillaries. **2.** Ragged spicules of calcified cartilage matrix. The decalcification process of specimen preparation has removed the calcium crystals, causing the white unstained background. **3.** Thin layer of osteoid deposited on the surface of the calcified cartilage matrix. **4.** Nuclei of osteoblasts. **5.** Nuclei of osteoprogenitor cells. **6.** Osteoprogenitor cell in mitosis. **7.** Nuclei of endothelial cells. **8.** Erythrocytes. **9.** Lymphocyte. *Note:* Identification of cells and other structures in this survey is based on analysis of this field at higher magnification.

10-19

Fig. 10-20. Longitudinal section of tibia. Newborn rat. L.M. × 41. **1.** Rectangle: epiphyseal ingrowth of perichondrial sprout, indicating beginning of a secondary ossification center. **2.** Zone of chondrocyte multiplication. **3.** Zone of chondrocyte hypertrophy. **4.** Primary ossification center extending toward the epiphysis. **5.** Bone marrow of diaphysis.

Fig. 10-21. Perichondrial sprout. Enlargement of rectangle in Fig. 10-20. L.M. × 218. **1.** Ordinary chondrocytes. **2.** Capillaries. **3.** Osteoprogenitor cells. **4.** Slightly calcified cartilage matrix. **5.** Hypertrophied cartilage lacunae with degenerating chondrocytes.

Fig. 10-22. Longitudinal section of phalanx. Monkey. Four months old. L.M. × 17. **1.** Articular capsule. **2.** Joint cavity. **3.** Articular and epiphyseal cartilage. **4.** Secondary ossification center with spongy bone. **5.** Epiphyseal growth plate. **6.** Primary ossification center extending toward the epiphysis. **7.** Bone marrow cavity of diaphysis. **8.** Compact cortical bone. **9.** Nutrient blood vessels.

Fig. 10-23. Epiphyseal growth plate. Enlargement of rectangle in Fig. 10-22. L.M. × 120. **1.** Marrow cavity. **2.** Bone and calcified cartilage matrix. **3.** Zone of resting cartilage cells. **4.** Vascular sprout establishing connection between primary and secondary ossification centers. **5.** Zone of chondrocyte proliferation. **6.** Zone of chondrocyte hypertrophy. **7.** Trabeculae of endochondral bone with center of calcified cartilage matrix.

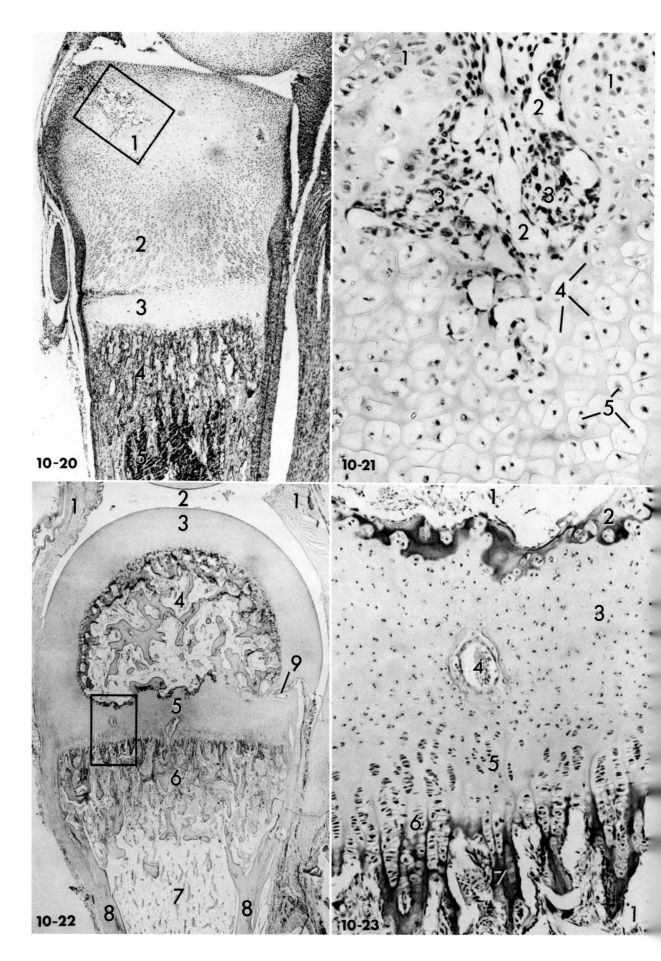

References

Amprino, R. On the growth of cortical bone and the mechanism of osteon formation. Acta. Anat. *52*: 177–187 (1963).

Anderson, C. E. and Parker, J. Invasion and resorption in endochondrial ossification. An electron microscopic study. J. Bone and Joint Surg. *48-A*: 899–914 (1966).

Ascenzi, A. and Bendetti, E. L. An electron microscopic study of the foetal membranous ossification. Acta Anat. *37*: 370–385 (1959).

Ascenzi, A., Bonucci, E. and Bocciarelli, D. S. An electron microscope study on the primary periosteal bone. J. Ultrastruct. Res. *18*: 605–618 (1967).

Bernard, G. W. and Pease, D. C. An electron microscopic study of initial intramembranous osteogenesis. Am. J. Anat. *125*: 271–290 (1969).

Bonucci, E. Further investigations on the organic/inorganic relationships in calcifying cartilage. Calc. Tiss. Res. *3*: 38–64 (1968).

Decker, J. D. An electron microscopic investigation of osteogenesis in the embryonic chick. Am. J. Anat. *118*: 591–641 (1966).

Engfeldt, B. Studies on the epiphysial growth zone. III. Electronmicroscopic studies on the normal epiphysial growth zone. Acta Path. Microbiol. Scand. *75*: 201–219 (1969).

Fitton-Jackson, S. The fine structure of the developing bone in the embryonic fowl. Proc. Roy. Soc. Lond. *146B*: 270–280 (1957).

Gonzales, F. and Karnovsky, M. J. Electron microscopy of osteoclasts in healing fractures of rat bone. J. Biophys. Biochem. Cytol. *9*: 299–316 (1961).

Knese, K. H. and Knoop, A. M. Elektronenoptische Untersuchungen über die periostale Osteogenese. Z. Zellforsch. *48*: 455–478 (1958).

Knese, K.-H. Osteoklasten, Chondroklasten, Mineraloklasten, Kollagenoklasten. Acta Anat. *83*: 275–288 (1972).

Owen, M. Uptake of (^{3}H) uridine into precursor pools and RNA in osteogenic cells. J. Cell Sci. *2*: 39–56 (1967).

Owen, M. The origin of bone cells. Int. Rev. Cytol. *28*: 213–238 (1970).

Schenk, R. K., Spiro, D. and Wiener, J. Cartilage resorption in the tibial epiphyseal plate of growing rats. J. Cell Biol. *34*: 275–291 (1967).

Schenk, R. K., Wiener, J. and Spiro, D. Fine structural aspects of vascular invasion of the tibial epiphyseal plate of growing rats. Acta Anat. *69*: 1–17 (1968).

Scott, B. L. Thymidine-^{3}H electron microscope radioautography of osteogenic cells in the fetal rat. J. Cell Biol. *35*: 115–126 (1967).

Scott, B. L. and Pease, D. C. Electron microscopy of the epiphyseal apparatus. Anat. Rec. *126*: 465–495 (1956).

Smith, J. W. The disposition of proteinpolysaccharide in the epiphysial plate cartilage of the young rabbit. J. Cell Sci. *6*: 843–864 (1970).

Thyberg, J. and Friberg, U. Ultrastructure and acid phosphatase activity of matrix vesicles and cytoplasmic dense bodies in the epiphyseal plate. J. Ultrastruct. Res. *33*: 554–573 (1970).

Young, R. W. Cell proliferation and specialization during endochondral osteogenesis in young rats. J. Cell Biol. *14*: 357–370 (1962).

Urist, M. R. Origins of current ideas about calcification. Clin. Orthop. Rel. Res. *44*: 13–39 (1966).

11 Muscular tissue

Fig. 11-1. Skeletal muscle. Longitudinal section. Human. L.M. X 290. **1.** Arrow: longitudinal axis of a skeletal muscle fiber (cell). **2.** Width of muscle fiber between bars: 25 μ. **3.** Muscle cell nuclei. **4.** Intercellular space. **5.** Transverse striations.

Fig. 11-2. Skeletal muscle. Cross section. Tongue. Monkey. L.M. X 460. **1.** Width of muscle fiber between bars: 20 μ. **2.** Muscle cell nuclei. **3.** Capillaries. **4.** Intercellular space with endomysium. **5.** Perimysium around muscle fascicle.

Fig. 11-3. Skeletal muscle. Longitudinal section. Rat. E.M. X 600. **1.** Arrow: longitudinal axis of muscle fiber. **2.** Width of muscle fiber: 38 μ. **3.** Muscle cell nuclei. **4.** Intercellular space and endomysium. **5.** Capillaries. **6.** Transverse striations.

Fig. 11-4. Skeletal muscle, fixed by intravascular perfusion. Cross section of nerve-vascular bundle and muscle cells. Rat. E.M. X 600. **1.** Myelinated nerves. **2.** Small artery; width of lumen 55 μ; wall thickness 2 μ. **3.** Small veins. **4.** Periaxial space of neuromuscular spindle with intrafusal muscle fibers. **5.** Small lymphatic vessel. **6.** Arteriole. **7.** Venule. **8.** Blood capillaries. **9.** Muscle fibers. **10.** Width of muscle fiber 37 μ. **11.** Loose connective tissue.

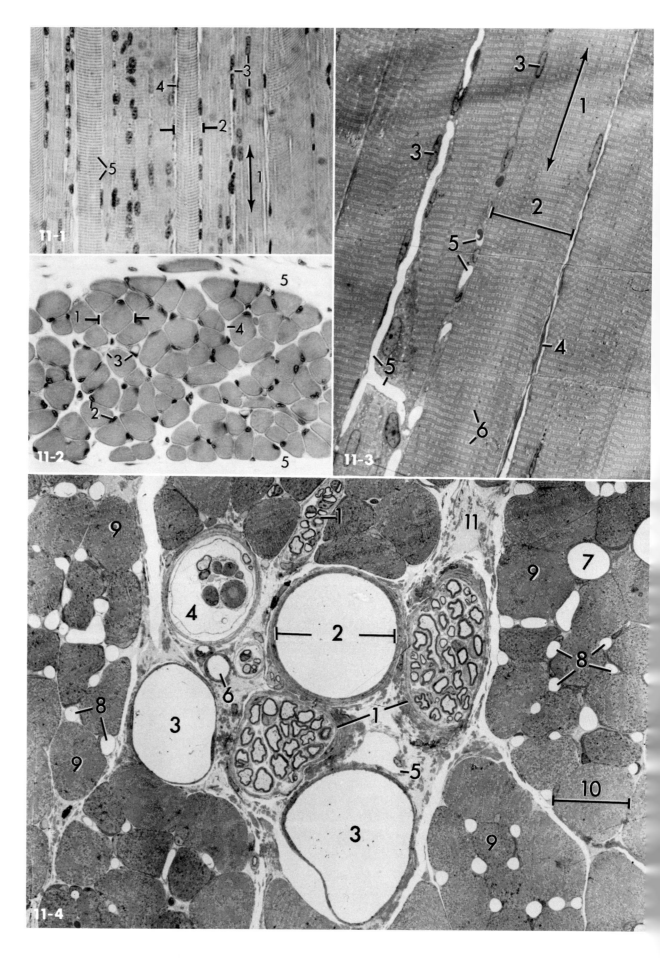

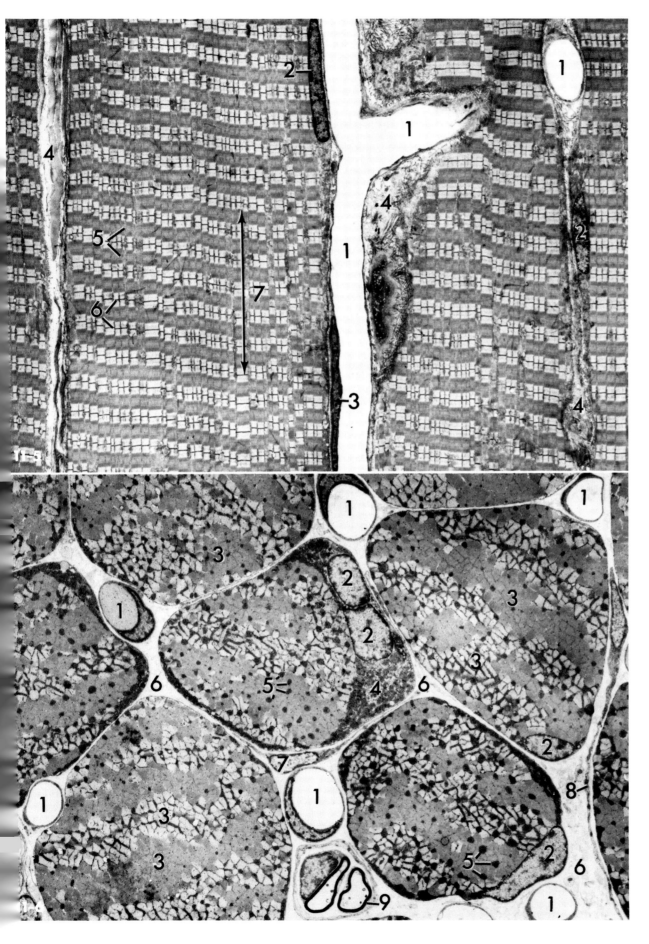

Fig. 11-5. Skeletal muscle. Longitudinal section. Rat. E.M. X 2100. **1.** Lumina of capillaries. **2.** Nuclei of muscle cells. **3.** Nucleus of endothelial cell. **4.** Intercellular space and endomysium. **5.** A-bands of transverse striations. **6.** I-bands with bisecting Z-line. **7.** Arrow: longitudinal axis of muscle cell.

Fig. 11-6. Skeletal muscle. Cross section. Rat. E.M. X 2100. **1.** Lumina of blood capillaries. **2.** Nuclei of muscle cells. **3.** Myofibrils. **4.** Extrafibrillar sarcoplasm. **5.** Mitochondria. **6.** Intercellular space with endomysium. **7.** Nucleus of fibroblast. **8.** Cytoplasm of fibroblast. **9.** Small myelinated nerve.

Fig. 11-7. Skeletal muscle. Cross section demonstrating the close relationship between muscle cells and blood capillaries. Rat. E.M. × 4800. 1 mm=0.2 μ. **1.** Lumina of blood capillaries. Width indicated by bars: 5.5 μ. **2.** Nuclei of endothelial cells. **3.** Nuclei of muscle cells. **4.** Width of muscle fiber: 19 μ. **5.** Narrow intercellular space.

Fig. 11-8. Detail of edges of two skeletal muscle cells in cross section. Rat. E.M. × 19,000. **1.** Nucleus of muscle cell. **2.** Nucleolus. **3.** Mitochondria in paranuclear sarcoplasm. **4.** Sarcolemma. **5.** Intercellular space with reticular and delicate collagenous fibrils of endomysium. **6.** Cytoplasmic process of fibroblast. **7.** Nucleus of satellite cell. **8.** Cytoplasm of satellite cell. **9.** Cell membrane of satellite cell borders on the sarcolemma of the host muscle cell. **10.** Myofilaments of host cell. **11.** External (basal) lamina encloses host cell and satellite cell.

Fig. 11-9. Detail of cross-sectioned skeletal muscle cell. Enlargement of rectangle in Fig. 11-7. Rat. E.M. × 27,000. **1.** Narrow intercellular space with apposing external (basal) laminae alone forming the endomysium. **2.** Sarcolemma. **3.** Mitochondria (sarcosomes). **4.** Myofibrils sectioned at level of I-band. **5.** Myofibril sectioned at level of A-band. **6.** Sarcoplasmic reticulum. **7.** Lipid droplet. After studying this enlargement, go back to Fig. 11-7 and try to identify details of other parts of that field of view.

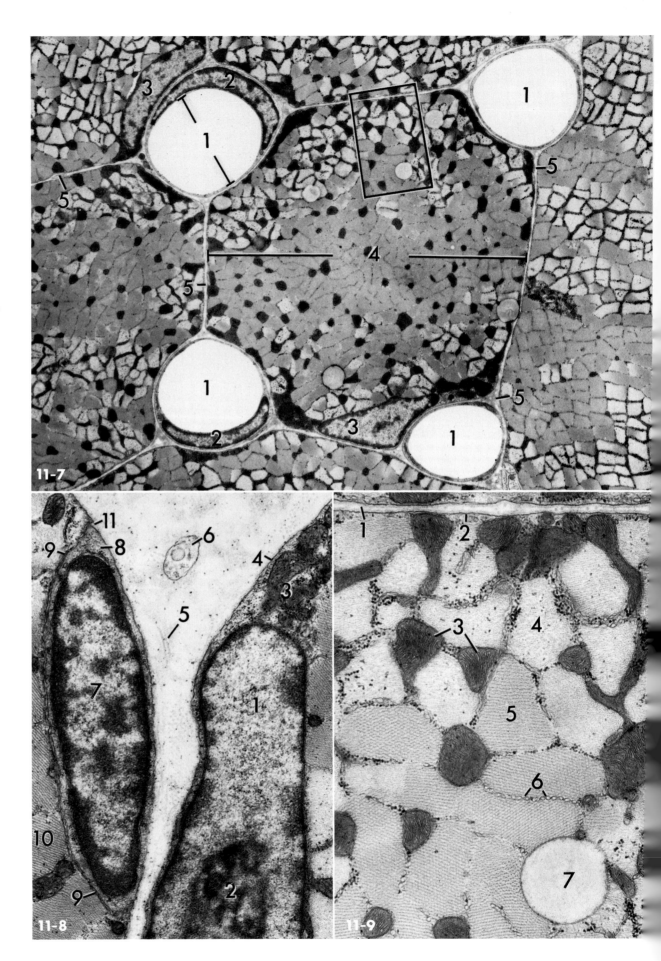

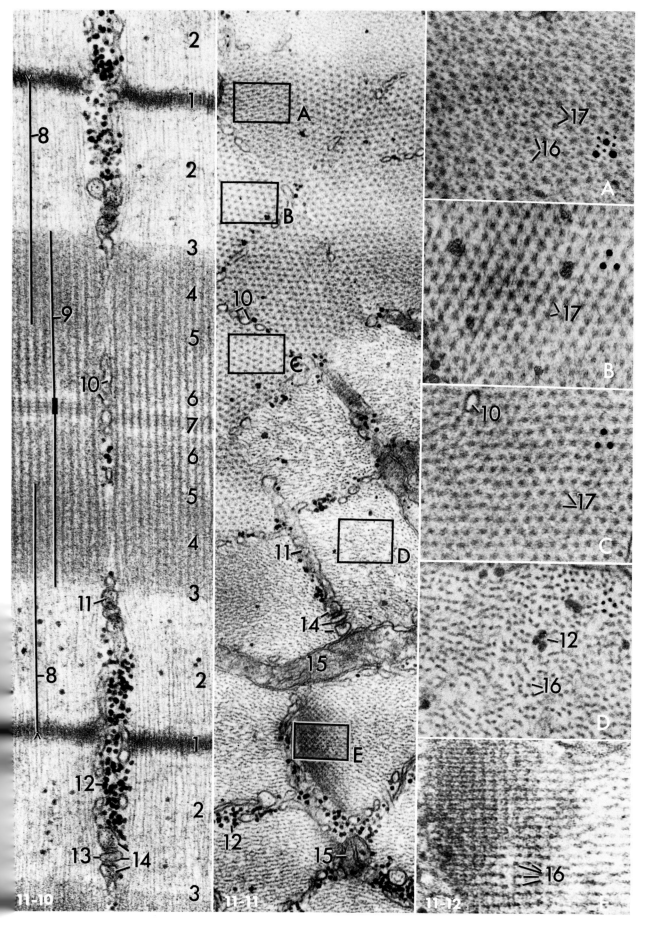

Fig. 11-10. Detail of myofibrils and myofilaments. Relaxed skeletal muscle. Longitudinal section. Rat. E.M. X 62,000. 1 mm = 161 Å. See legend Fig. 11-12.

Fig. 11-11. Relaxed skeletal muscle. Cross section. Rat. E.M. × 62,000. See legend Fig. 11-12.

Fig. 11-12. A, B, C, D and E are enlargements of areas similar to rectangle A–E in Fig. 11-11. Relaxed skeletal muscle. Cross section. Rat. E.M. × 120,000. 1 mm = 83 Å. **1.** Z-line. Distance between two Z-lines equals one sarcomere. **2.** I-band with only thin filaments. **3.** Ends of thick myofilaments; also border between I-band and A-band. **4.** Zone of interdigitating thin and thick myofilaments. **5.** Ends of thin filaments. **6.** H-band with only thick myofilaments. **7.** M-band: local swelling of thick myofilaments with cross-linking filaments. **8.** Extent of two thin myofilaments, indicated by lines (1 μ). **9.** Extent of one thick myofilament, indicated by line, marks extent of A-band (1.5 μ). **10.** Profiles of sarcoplasmic reticulum. **11.** Terminal cisterna of sarcoplasmic reticulum. **12.** Glycogen particles. **13.** Transverse tubule of T-system. **14.** Triad. **15.** Mitochondria. **16.** Thin myofilaments. **17.** Thick myofilaments. **A.** Cross section of interdigitating thin and thick filaments (level 4 in Fig. 11-10). Six thin filaments surround one thick filament; one thin filament shared by three thick filaments. **B.** Cross section of M-band. (level 7 in Fig. 11-10). **C.** Cross section of H-band (level 6 in Fig. 11-10). **D.** Cross section of I-band (level 2 in Fig. 11-10). **E.** Cross section of Z-line with square pattern of thin filaments (level 1 in Fig. 11-10).

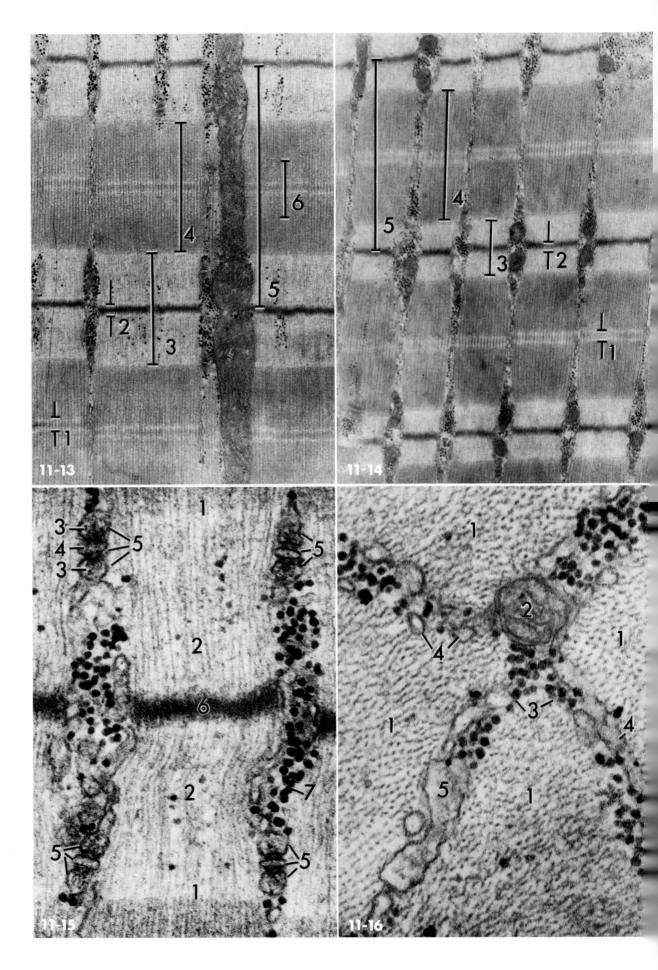

Fig. 11-13. *Relaxed* skeletal muscle. Longitudinal section. Rat. E.M. X 24,000. 1 mm = 0.0417 μ. **1.** M-band 0.13 μ. **2.** Z-line 0.08 μ. **3.** I-band 1.3 μ. **4.** A-band 1.5 μ. **5.** Sarcomere (Z-Z) 2.7 μ. **6.** H-band 0.63 μ.

Fig. 11-14. *Contracted* skeletal muscle. Longitudinal section. Mouse. E.M. X 24,000. Comparison of lengths of bands in contracted myofibrils with those of relaxed myofibrils. **1.** M-band 0.13 μ. **2.** Z-line 0.08 μ. **3.** I-band 0.63 μ. **4.** A-band 1.5 μ. **5.** Sarcomere (Z-Z) 2.1 μ. *Note:* H-band obliterated at maximum contraction.

Fig. 11-15. Topography of I-band and related structures. Skeletal muscle. Longitudinal section. Rat. E.M. X 90,000. **1.** Ends of thick filaments. **2.** I-band with thin filaments. **3.** Terminal cisternae of sarcoplasmic reticulum. **4.** T-tubule. **5.** Triads. **6.** Z-line. **7.** Particulate glycogen.

Fig. 11-16. Detail of I-band and related structures. Skeletal muscle. Cross section. E.M. X 126,000. **1.** Myofilaments of four adjacent myofibrils. **2.** Mitochondrion. **3.** Particulate glycogen. **4.** Tubular elements of sarcoplasmic reticulum. **5.** Terminal cisterna of sarcoplasmic reticulum.

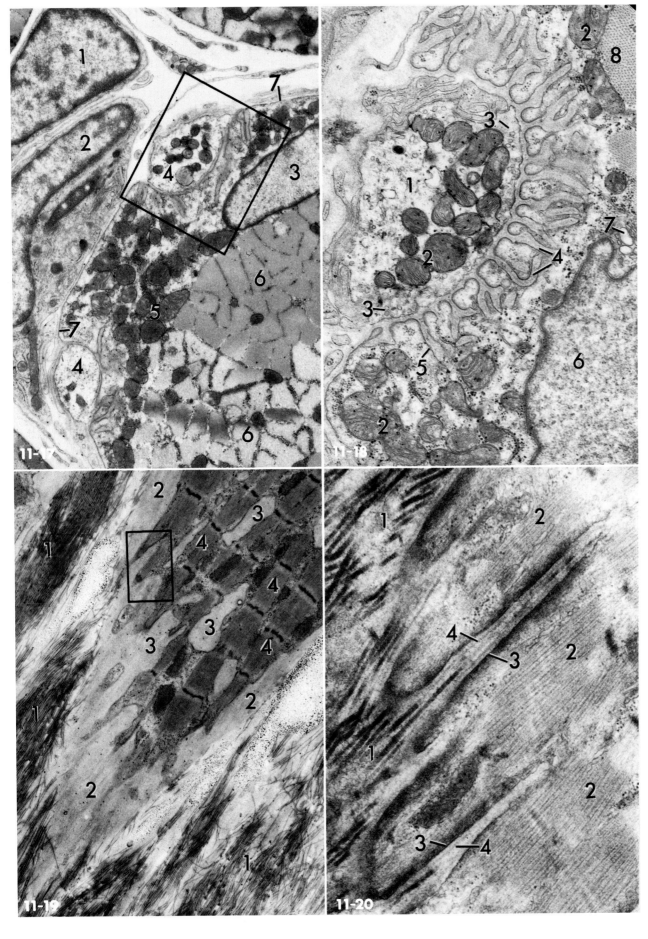

Fig. 11-17. Topography of motor end plate. Skeletal muscle. Cross section. Rat. E.M. X 9000. **1.** Nucleus of fibroblast. **2.** Nucleus of Schwann cell (teloglial cell). **3.** Nucleus of muscle cell. **4.** Terminal nerve branches. **5.** Muscle cell mitochondria (sarcosomes). **6.** Myofibrils. **7.** Sarcolemma.

Fig. 11-18. Motor end plate. Slight enlargement of area similar to rectangle in Fig. 11-17. Skeletal muscle. Rat. E.M. X 22,000. **1.** Nerve axon terminal in synaptic trough. **2.** Mitochondria. **3.** Synaptic vesicles. **4.** Subneural clefts filled with external (basal) lamina. **5.** Sarcolemma. **6.** Nucleus of muscle cell. **7.** Golgi zone. **8.** Myofilaments.

Fig. 11-19. Myotendinal junction. Papillary muscle. Heart. Rat. E.M. X 6900. **1.** Bundles of collagenous fibrils. **2.** Network of delicate collagenous fibrils, reticular fibrils, and elastic microfibrils. **3.** Invaginations of sarcolemma. **4.** Myofibrils.

Fig. 11-20. Detail of myotendinal junction. Enlargement of area similar to rectangle in Fig. 11-19. Skeletal muscle. Mouse. E.M. X 30,000. **1.** Delicate collagenous fibrils. **2.** Myofilaments. **3.** Sarcolemma with attached dense cytoplasm. Myofilaments seem to anchor in this region. **4.** External (basal) lamina.

Fig. 11-21. Cardiac muscle. Longitudinal
section. Interventricular septum of steer
heart. L.M. × 115. **1.** Myocardium. **2.** Part of
right branch of common bundle of impulse
conducting system. Width between bars:
97 μ. **3.** Endocardial connective tissue.
4. Lumen of ventricle.

Fig. 11-22. Enlargement of rectangle in Fig.
11-21. L.M. X 350. **1.** Nuclei of cardiac
muscle cells. **2.** Erythrocytes in capillary.
3. Width of cardiac muscle cell: 12 μ.
4. Connective tissue. **5.** Myofibrils of
Purkinje fibers. **6.** Nuclei.

Fig. 11-23. Cross section of a branch of the
common bundle. Interventricular septum of
steer heart. L.M. X 350. **1.** Sheath of
connective tissue. **2.** Nuclei of Purkinje
fibers (cells). **3.** Cell borders of Purkinje
fibers enhanced by accumulations of
peripheral myofibrils. **4.** Nuclei of fibroblasts.

Fig. 11-24. Cardiac muscle cells. Cross section.
Left ventricle of steer heart. L.M. X 350.
1. Nuclei of cardiac muscle cells. **2.** Cardiac
muscle cell; width 14 μ. **3.** Endomysium.
4. Perimysium enclosing muscle fascicle.
5. Fine stippling of sarcoplasm represents
cross-sectioned myofibrils. **6.** Rectangle
enlarged in Fig. 11-28.

Fig. 11-25. Cardiac muscle cells. Longitudinal
section. Enlargement of area similar to
rectangle in Fig. 11-22. Heart. Rat. E.M. X
1900. **1.** Erythrocytes in lumina of blood
capillaries. **2.** Nuclei of endothelial cells.
3. Nucleus of fibroblast. **4.** Nuclei of cardiac
muscle cells. **5.** Width of cardiac muscle cell:
19 μ. **6.** Myofibrils. **7.** Rows of mitochondria.
8. Intercalated disks.

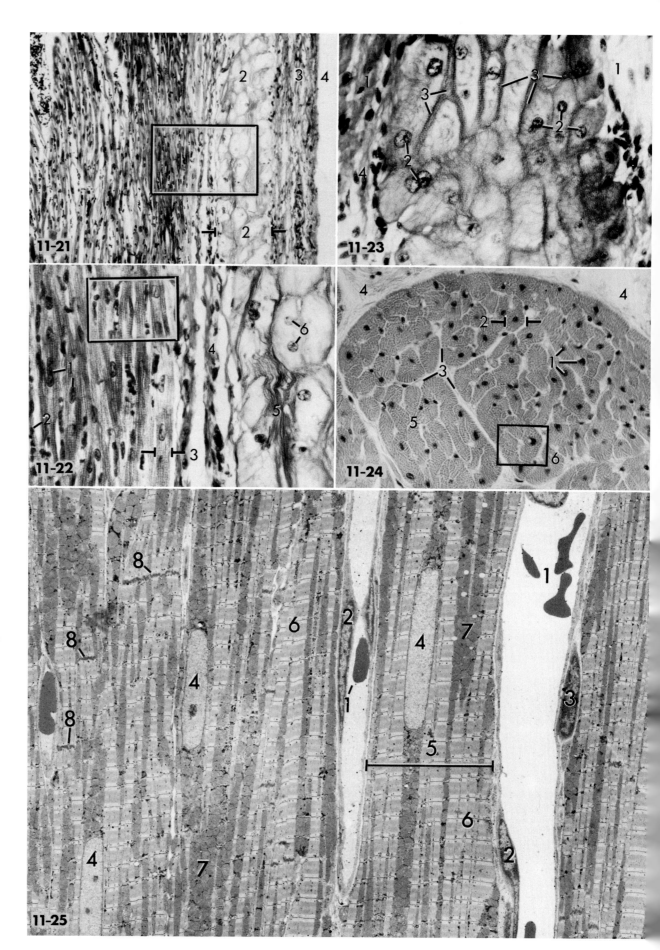

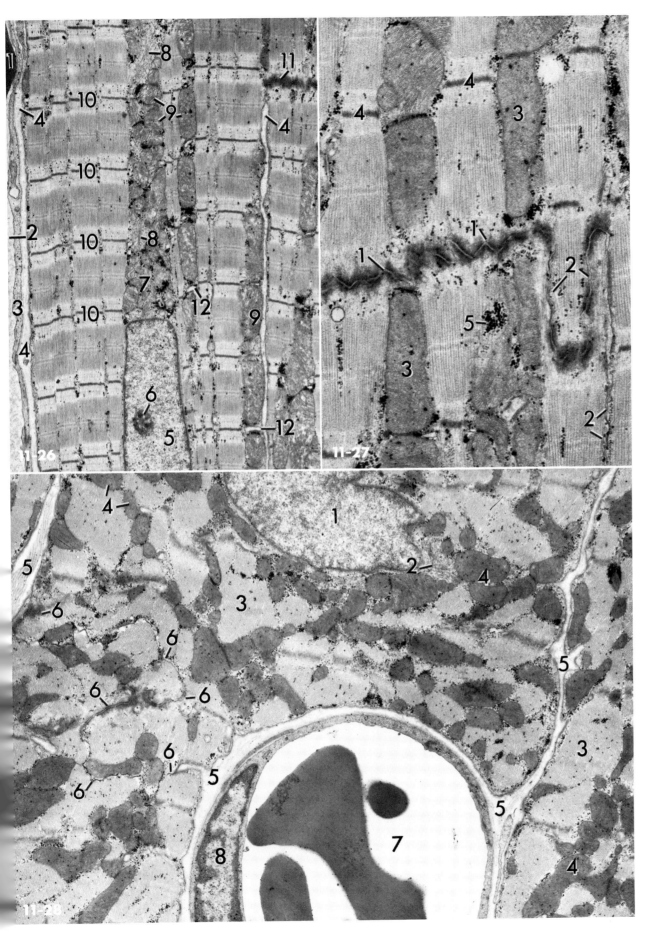

Fig. 11-26. Cardiac muscle cells. Longitudinal section. Heart. Rat. E.M. X 7500.
1. Erythrocyte. **2.** Lumen of longitudinally sectioned capillary. **3.** Endothelium.
4. Extracellular space with endomysium.
5. Nucleus of cardiac muscle cell.
6. Nucleolus. **7.** Extrafibrillar sarcoplasm in central conical space. **8.** Small Golgi zones. **9.** Mitochondria. **10.** Z-lines of myofibrils. **11.** Part of intercalated disk.

Fig. 11-27. Cardiac muscle cell. Longitudinal section. Heart. Rat. E.M. X 19,000.
1. Transverse part of intercalated disk.
2. Longitudinal part of intercalated disk.
3. Mitochondria. **4.** Z-lines of myofibrils.
5. Particulate glycogen.

Fig. 11-28. Cardiac muscle cells. Cross section. Enlargement of area similar to rectangle in Fig. 11-24. Heart. Rat. E.M. × 9000.
1. Nucleus of cardiac muscle cell. **2.** Small Golgi zone. **3.** Myofibrils. **4.** Mitochondria.
5. Endomysium of extracellular space.
6. Intercalated disk; lateral junction of two cells. **7.** Lumen of blood capillary with erythrocytes. **8.** Nucleus of endothelial cell.

Fig. 11-29. Detail of intercalated disk. Heart. Rat. E.M. × 99,000. **1.** Desmosomes (maculae adhaerentes). **2.** Intermediate junctions (fasciae adhaerentes). **3.** Rectangle: gap-junction (nexus). **4.** Web of fine cytoplasmic filaments. **5.** Myofilaments. **6.** Z-line. **7.** Glycogen particles. **8.** Outer mitochondrial membrane.

Fig. 11-30. Nexus (gap-junction). Enlargement of area similar to rectangle in Fig. 11-29. Intercalated disk. Heart. Rat. E.M. × 250,000. **1.** Apposing sarcolemmae. **2.** Intermembranous gap, about 20 Å wide. **3.** Glycogen particles.

Fig. 11-31. Periphery of cardiac muscle cell. Rat. E.M. × 64,000. **1.** Delicate collagenous fibrils. **2.** External (basal) lamina. **3.** Sarcolemma. **4.** Invagination of sarcolemma (T-tubule) with external lamina. **5.** Myofilaments. **6.** Mitochondria. **7.** Profiles of tubular sarcoplasmic reticulum. **8.** Glycogen particles.

Fig. 11-32. Longitudinal section of cardiac muscle cell. Rat. E.M. × 32,000. **1.** Z-lines. **2.** Mitochondria. **3.** Transverse tubule of T-system. **4.** Glycogen particles.

Fig. 11-33. Topography of Z-line in cardiac muscle cell. Rat. E.M. × 96,000. **1.** Z-lines. **2.** Thin filaments. **3.** Terminal portions of sarcoplasmic reticulum. **4.** Transverse tubule of T-system. **5.** Triad. **6.** Glycogen particles.

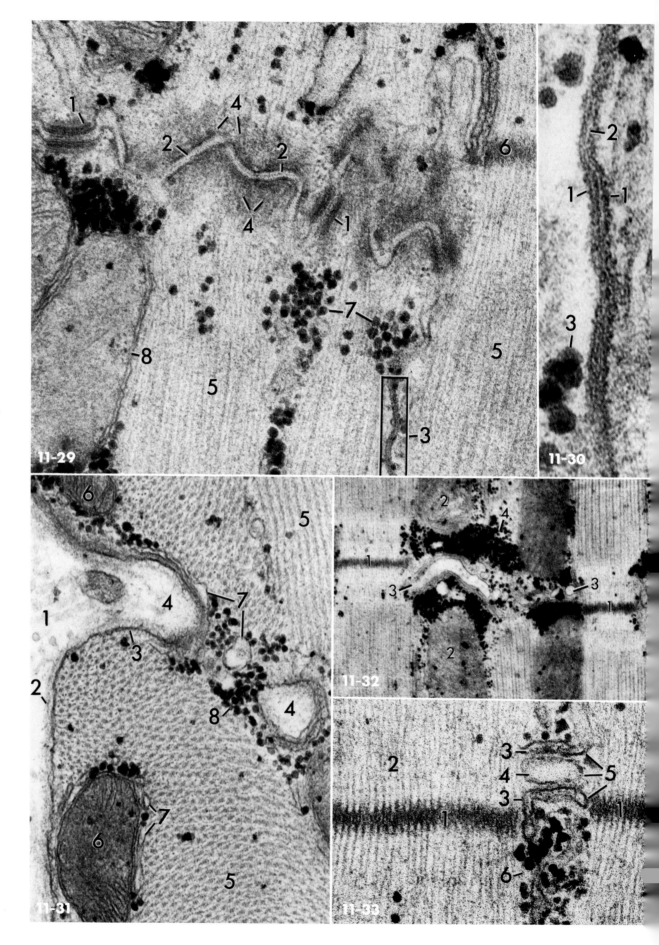

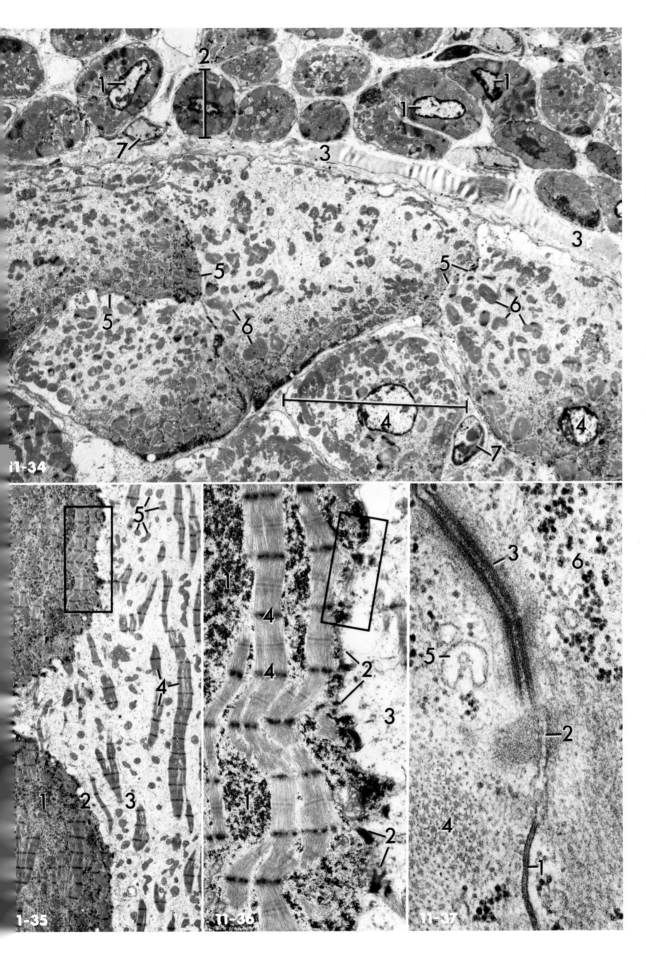

Fig. 11-34. Comparison between Purkinje fibers and ordinary cardiac muscle fibers. Interventricular septum. Steer heart. E.M. X 1800. **1.** Nuclei of ordinary cardiac muscle fibers. **2.** Width of fiber 10 μ. **3.** Bundles of collagenous fibrils. **4.** Nuclei of Purkinje fibers; width indicated 28 μ. **5.** Cell borders (sarcolemmae) of adjacent Purkinje fibers in close contact. Their course is easily seen because of differences in sarcoplasmic density of the Purkinje fibers. **6.** Cross-sectioned myofibrils. **7.** Blood capillaries.

Fig. 11-35. Longitudinal section of Purkinje fibers (cells). Steer heart. E.M. X 1800. **1.** Cells with dense sarcoplasm. **2.** Cell border. **3.** Cell with light sarcoplasm. **4.** Myofibrils. **5.** Mitochondria.

Fig. 11-36. Enlargement of area similar to rectangle in Fig. 11-35. Steer heart. E.M. X 9000. **1.** Density of sarcoplasm caused by large accumulations of particulate glycogen. **2.** Cell border. **3.** Glycogen particles present to limited extent in the sarcoplasm of this cell. **4.** Z-lines of myofibril.

Fig. 11-37. Detail of sarcolemmal specializations. Purkinje fibers. Steer heart. E.M. X 86,000. **1.** Gap-junction (nexus). **2.** Intermediate junction (fascia adhaerens). **3.** Desmosome (macula adhaerens). **4.** Myofilaments. **5.** Sarcoplasmic reticulum. **6.** Glycogen particles.

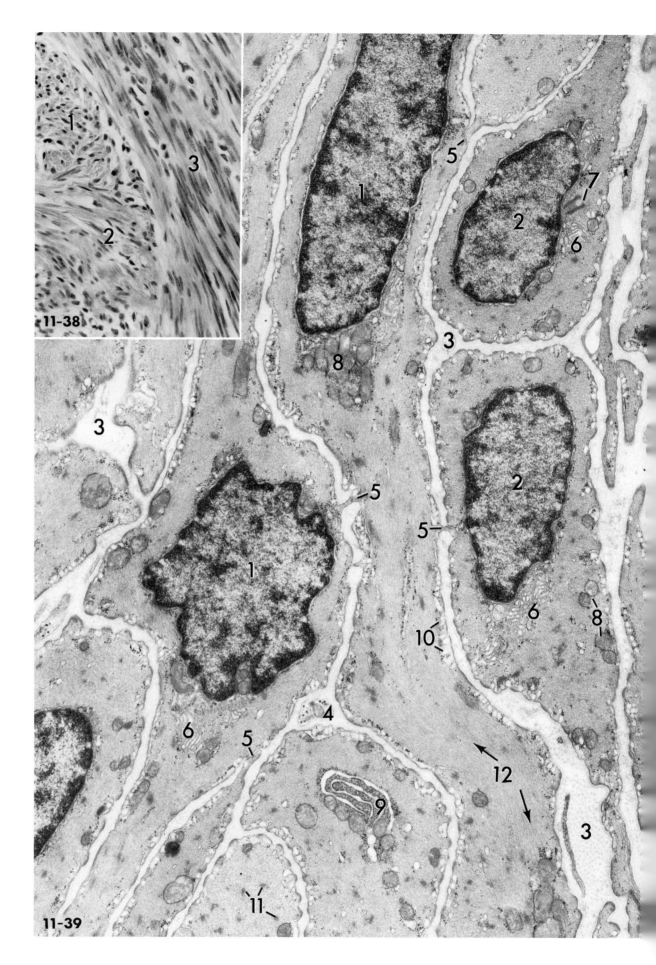

Fig. 11-38. Smooth muscle cells of myometrium. Uterus. Human. L.M. X 315.
  1. Cross-sectioned smooth muscle cells.
  2. Obliquely sectioned smooth muscle cells.
  3. Longitudinally sectioned smooth muscle cells.

Fig. 11-39. Smooth muscle cells. Ductus deferens. Rat. E.M. X 13,000. **1.** Nuclei of longitudinally sectioned smooth muscle cells. **2.** Nuclei of cross-sectioned smooth muscle cells. **3.** Narrow intercellular space with reticular and delicate collagenous fibrils. **4.** Denuded axon of nerve terminal. **5.** Narrow cell processes establishing intercellular contact. **6.** Golgi zones. **7.** Centriole. **8.** Mitochondria. **9.** Granular endoplasmic reticulum. **10.** Surface (micropinocytotic) vesicles. **11.** Fusiform densities. **12.** Longitudinal axis of myofilaments in sarcoplasm.

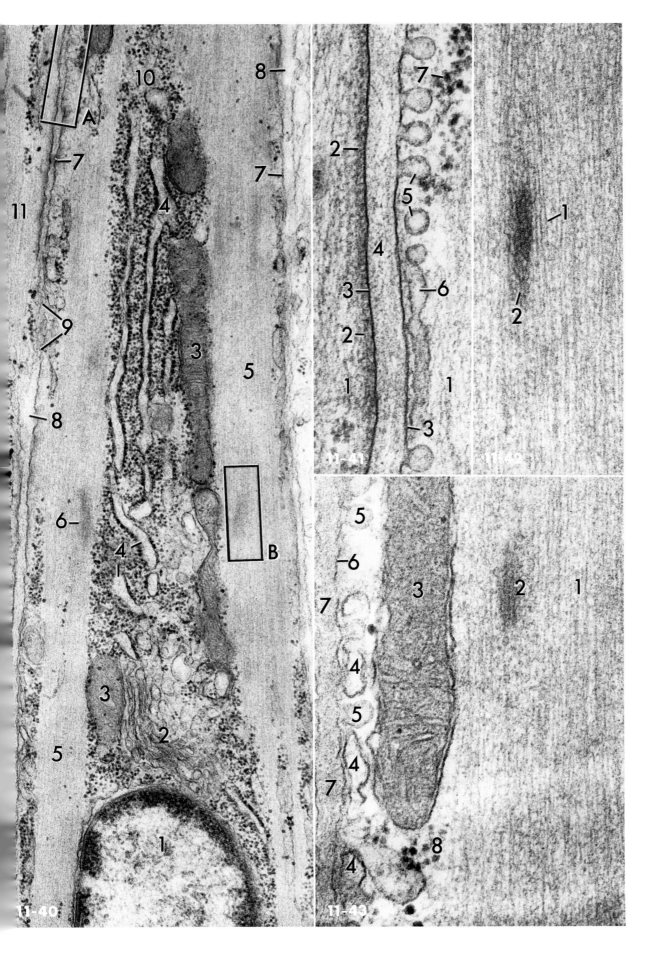

Fig. 11-40. Smooth muscle cell. Longitudinally sectioned. Prostate. E.M. × 32,000.
1. Nucleus. **2.** Golgi zone. **3.** Mitochondria.
4. Cisternae of granular endoplasmic reticulum. **5.** Myofilamentous part of sarcoplasm. **6.** Fusiform density (indistinct).
7. Sarcolemma. **8.** Intercellular space.
9. Membranous contact between two smooth muscle cells. Similar area enlarged in Fig. 11-49. **10.** Glycogen particles.
11. Adjacent smooth muscle cell.

Fig. 11-41. Detail of sarcolemmae of two apposing smooth muscle cells. Enlargement of area similar to rectangle (A) in Fig. 11-40. Ductus deferens. Mouse. E.M. × 90,000.
1. Sarcoplasm. **2.** Dense body (attachment plaque). **3.** Sarcolemma. **4.** Narrow intercellular space, about 900 Å wide, occupied only by thin external (basal) laminae. **5.** Surface (micropinocytotic) vesicles. **6.** Element of sarcoplasmic reticulum, in close proximity ("coupling") to sarcolemma. **7.** Glycogen particles.

Fig. 11-42. Myofilaments of smooth muscle cell, sectioned longitudinally. Enlargement of area similar to rectangle (B) in Fig. 11-40. Prostate. Rat. E.M. × 90,000. **1.** Only one kind of filaments present in this preparation, averaging 60 Å in width.
2. Fusiform density (dense oval body).

Fig. 11-43. Subsarcolemmal topography of smooth muscle cell. Prostate. Rat. E.M. × 90,000. **1.** Myofilaments. **2.** Fusiform density. **3.** Mitochondrion. **4.** Tubules of sarcoplasmic reticulum near sarcolemma ("coupling"). **5.** Surface vesicles.
6. Sarcolemma. **7.** External (basal) lamina.
8. Particulate glycogen.

Fig. 11-44. Cross-sectioned smooth muscle cells. Ureter. Rat. E.M. X 62,000.
1. Mitochondrion. **2.** Nucleus.
3. Myofilaments. **4.** Microtubules. **5.** Glycogen particles. **6.** Surface (micropinocytotic) vesicles. **7.** Dense bodies (attachment plaques). **8.** Narrow intercellular space with external (basal) laminae. **9.** Points of sarcolemmal contact.

Fig. 11-45. Cross-sectioned myofilaments. Smooth muscle. Ductus deferens. Mouse. E.M. X 32,000. See legend Fig. 11-47.

Fig. 11-46. Cross-sectioned myofilaments in lattice-like bundles. Smooth muscle. Muscularis externa. Large intestine. Rat. E.M. X 64,000. See legend Fig. 11-47.

Fig. 11-47 Cross-sectioned myofilaments. Smooth muscle. Ductus deferens. Mouse. E.M. X 96,000. **1.** Fusiform densities (dense oval bodies). **2.** Thick myofilaments (about 150 Å). **3.** Intermediate size myofilaments (about 100 Å). **4.** Thin myofilaments (about 50 Å).
5. Mitochondria. **6.** Tubules of sarcoplasmic reticulum.

Fig. 11-48. Myoneural junctions. Smooth muscle. Ductus deferens. Rat. E.M. X 9000.
1. Nucleus of smooth muscle cell.
2. Intercellular space. **3.** Sarcolemmal contacts between adjacent smooth muscle cells.
4. Fusiform densities. **5.** Denuded axons of autonomic nerve endings.

Fig. 11-49. Sarcolemmal point of contact. Enlargement of area similar to rectangle (A) in Fig. 11-48. E.M. X 90,000.
1. Sarcolemma. **2.** Gap-junction. **3.** Surface vesicles. **4.** Glycogen particles. **5.** Ribosomes.

Fig. 11-50. Myoneural junction. Smooth muscle. Enlargement of area similar to rectangle (B) in Fig. 11-48. E.M. X 63,000.
1. Sarcolemma. **2.** Intercellular space.
3. Axolemma of autonomic nerve ending.
4. Subneural sarcolemma. **5.** Granulated synaptic vesicles of nerve ending.
6. Sarcoplasmic reticulum. **7.** Glycogen particles. **8.** Mitochondrion.

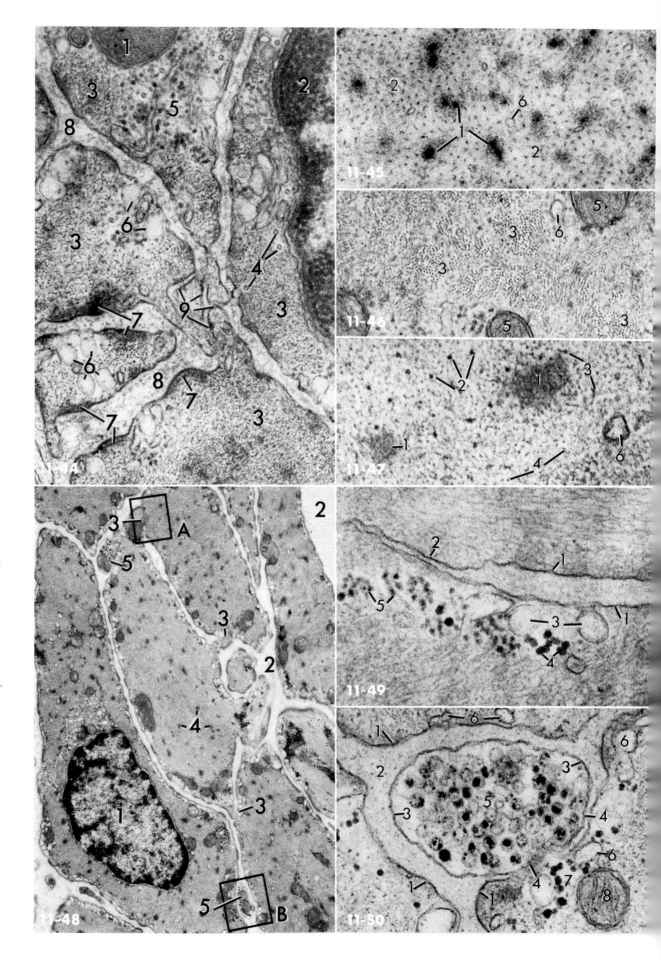

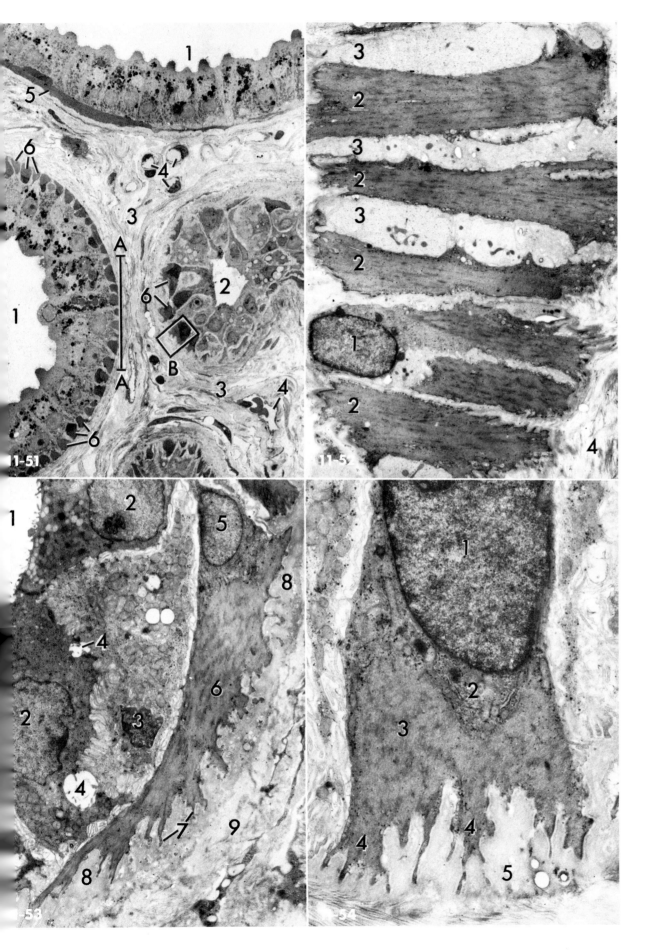

Fig. 11-51. Myoepithelial cells associated with sweat glands. Axilla. Human. E.M. X 600. **1.** Lumina of odoriferous sweat glands. **2.** Lumen of ordinary sweat gland. **3.** Connective tissue. **4.** Blood capillaries. **5.** Longitudinally sectioned myoepithelial cell. The gland is also sectioned longitudinally. **6.** Cross-sectioned myoepithelial cells.

Fig. 11-52. Myoepithelial cells. associated with odoriferous sweat gland, sectioned in the plane indicated by the bar A-A in Fig. 11-51. Axilla. Human. E.M. X 3600. **1.** Nucleus of myoepithelial cell. **2.** Cytoplasm of myoepithelial cells contains numerous fusiform densities. The myoepithelial cells of the odoriferous gland are all arranged quite regularly and in parallel with the long axis of the tubular gland. **3.** Secretory epithelial cells alternate with myoepithelial cells. **4.** Collagenous fibrils.

Fig. 11-53. Part of ordinary sweat gland. Axilla. Human. E.M. X 4000. **1.** Lumen of gland. **2.** Nuclei of dark (mucoid) cells. **3.** Nucleus of clear cell. **4.** Intercellular canaliculi. **5.** Nucleus of longitudinally sectioned myoepithelial cell. **6.** Filamentous part of sarcoplasm. **7.** Cell processes. **8.** Basal lamina (unusually thick). **9.** Connective tissue.

Fig. 11-54. Detail of myoepithelial cell of ordinary sweat gland. Enlargement of area similar to rectangle (B) in Fig. 11-51. Axilla. Human. E.M. X 9000. **1.** Nucleus **2.** Small perinuclear non-fibrillar part of sarcoplasm. **3.** Filamentous part of sarcoplasm. **4.** Cell processes. **5.** Basal lamina.

References

SKELETAL MUSCLE

Ashley, C. C. Calcium and the activation of skeletal muscle. Endeavour *30*: 18–25 (1971).

Bourne, G. H. (Ed.). The Structure and Function of Muscle Vol. I: Structure. Academic Press, New York, 1960.

Franzini-Armstrong, C. Studies on the triad. I. Structure of the junction in frog twitch fibers. J. Cell Biol. *47*: 488–499 (1970).

Franzini-Armstrong, C. Studies on the triad. II. Penetration of tracers into the junctional gap. J. Cell Biol. *49*: 196–203 (1971).

Franzini-Armstrong, C. and Porter, K. R. The Z disc of skeletal muscle fibrils. Z. Zellforsch. *61*: 661–672 (1964).

Hess, A. and Rosner, S. The satellite cell bud and myoblast in denervated mammalian muscle fibers. Am. J. Anat. *129*: 21–40 (1970).

Huxley, H. E. The mechanism of muscular contraction. Sci. Amer. *213*: 18–27 (1965).

Huxley, H. E. The mechanism of muscular contraction. Science *164*: 1356–1366 (1969).

Huxley, H. E. and Hanson, J. Molecular basis of contraction in cross-striated muscle. *In* Structure and Function of Muscle (Ed. G. H. Bourne), Vol. I, pp. 183–227. Academic Press, New York, 1960.

Kelly, D. E. Models of muscle Z-band fine structure based on a looping filament configuration. J. Cell Biol. *34*: 827–840 (1967).

Kelly, D. E. The fine structure of skeletal muscle triad junctions. J. Ultrastruct. Res. *29*: 37–49 (1969).

Kelly, D. E. and Cahill, M. A. Filamentous and matrix components of skeletal muscle Z-disks. Anat. Rec. *172*: 623–642 (1972).

Knappeis, G. G. and Carlsen, F. The ultrastructure of the Z-disc in skeletal muscle. J. Cell Biol. *13*: 323–331 (1962).

Mauro, A. Satellite cell of skeletal muscle fibers. J Biophys. Biochem. Cytol. *9*: 493–495 (1961).

Porter, K. R. The sarcoplasmic reticulum. Its recent history and present status. J. Biophys. Biochem. Cytol. *10*: (Suppl.) 219–226 (1961).

Rowe, R. W. Ultrastructure of the Z line of skeletal muscle fibers. J. Cell Biol. *51*: 674–685 (1971).

Schiaffino, S., Hanzlikova, V. and Pierobon, S. Relations between structure and function in rat skeletal muscle fibers. J. Cell Biol. *47*: 107–119 (1970).

Shafiq, S. A. Gorycki, M. Goldstone, L. and Milhorat, A. T. The fine structure of fiber types in normal human muscle. Anat. Rec. *156*: 283–302 (1966).

CARDIAC MUSCLE

Barr, L., Dewey, M. M. and Berger, W. Propagation of action potentials and the structure of the nexus in cardiac muscle. J. Gen. Physiol. *48*: 797–824 (1965).

Challice, C. E. Microstructure of specialized tissues in the mammalian heart. Ann. N.Y. Acad. Sci. *156*: 14–33 (1969).

DeFelice, L. J. and Challice, C. E. Anatomical and ultrastructural study of the electrophysiological atrioventricular node of the rabbit. Circulation Res. *24*: 457–474 (1969).

Fawcett, D. W. and McNutt, N. S. The ultrastructure of the cat myocardium. I. Ventricular papillary muscle. J. Cell Biol. *42*: 1–45 (1969).

Fishman, A. P. (Ed.) The Myocardium—Its Biochemistry and Biophysics. Circulation *24*: 323–548 (1961).

Hibbs, R. G. and Ferrans, V. J. An ultrastructural and histochemical study of rat atrial myocardium. Am. J. Anat. *124*: 251–280 (1969).

Jamieson, J. D. and Palade, G. E. Specific granules in atrial muscle cells. J. Cell Biol. *23*: 151–172 (1964).

Kawamura, K. and James, T. N. Comparative ultrastructure of cellular junctions in working myocardium and the conduction system under normal and pathological conditions. J. Molec. Cell Cardiol. *3*: 31–60 (1971).

Kim, S. and Baba, N. Atrioventricular node and Purkinje fibers in the guinea pig heart. Am. J. Anat. *132*: 339–354 (1971).

Leak, L. V. The ultrastructure of myofibers in a reptilian heart: the boa constrictor. Am. J. Anat. *120*: 553–582 (1967).

McNutt, N. S. and Fawcett, D. W. A comparison of the T system and sarcoplasmic reticulum in atrial and ventricular heart muscle. J. Cell Biol. *35*: 90A (1967).

McNutt, N. S. and Fawcett, D. W. The ultrastructure of the cat myocardium. II. Atrial muscle. J. Cell Biol. *42*: 46–67 (1969).

McNutt, N. S. and Weinstein, R. S. The ultrastructure of the nexus. A correlated thin-section and freeze-cleavage study. J. Cell Biol. *47*: 666–688 (1970).

Simpson, F. O. and Rayns, D. G. The relationship between the transverse tubular system and other tubules at the Z disc levels of myocardial cells in the ferret. Am. J. Anat. *122*: 193–208 (1968).

Simpson, F. O. and Oertelis, S. J. The fine structure of sheep myocardial cells: sarcolemmal invaginations and the transverse tubular system. J. Cell Biol. *12*: 91–100 (1962).

Sjöstrand, F. S., Andersson-Cedergren, E. and Dewey, M. M. The ultrastructure of the intercalated discs of frog, mouse and guinea pig cardiac muscle. J. Ultrastruct. Res. *1*: 271–287 (1958).

Sommer, J. R. and Johnson, E. A. A comparative study of Purkinje fibers and ventricular fibers. J. Cell Biol. *36*: 497–526 (1968).

Sonnenblick, E. H. Correlation of myocardial structure and function. Circulation *38*: 29–44 (1968).

Sperelakis, N., Rubio, R. and Radnick, J. Sharp discontinuity in sarcomere lengths across intercalated disks of fibrillating cat hearts. J. Ultrastruct. Res. *30*: 503–532 (1970).

Stenger, R. J. and Spiro, D. The ultrastructure of mammalian cardiac muscle. J. Biophys. Biochem. Cytol. *9*: 325–353 (1961).

Thaemert, J. C. Atrioventricular node innervation in ultrastructural three dimensions. Am. J. Anat. *128*: 239–264 (1970).

Thaemert, J. C. Fine structure of the atrioventricular node as viewed in serial sections. Am. J. Anat. *136*: 43–66 (1973).

SMOOTH MUSCLE

Bo, W. J., Odor, D. L. and Rothrock, M. L. Ultrastructure of uterine smooth muscle following progesterone or progesterone-estrogen treatment. Anat. Rec. *163*: 121–132 (1969).

Cobb, J. L. S. and Bennett, T. A study of nexuses in visceral smooth muscle. J. Cell Biol. *41*: 287–297 (1969).

Cooke, P. H. and Fay, F. S. Correlation between fiber length, ultrastructure, and the length-tension relationship of mammalian smooth muscle. J. Cell Biol. *52*: 105–116 (1971).

Dewey, M. M. and Barr, L. A study of the structure and distribution of the nexus. J. Cell Biol. *23*: 553–585 (1964).

Devine, C. E. and Somlyo, A. P. Thick filaments in vascular smooth muscle. J. Cell Biol. *49*: 636–649 (1971).

Devine, C. E., Somlyo, A. V. and Somlyo, A. P. Sarcoplasmic reticulum and excitation-contraction in mammalian smooth muscles. J. Cell Biol. *52*: 690–718 (1972).

Fay, F. S. and Cooke, P. H. Reversible disaggregation of myofilaments in vertebrate smooth muscle. J. Cell Biol. *56*: 399–411 (1973).

Goldstein, D. J. On the origin and morphology of myoepithelial cells of apocrine sweat glands. J. Investig. Dermatol. *37*: 301–309 (1961).

Kelly, R. E. and Arnold, J. W. Myofilaments of the muscles of the pupillary muscles of the iris fixed in situ. J. Ultrastruct. Res. *40*: 532–545 (1972).

Kelly, R. E. and Rice, R. V. Localization of myosin filaments in smooth muscle. J. Cell Biol. *37*: 105–116 (1968).

Kelly, R. E. and Rice, R. V. Ultrastructural studies on the contractile mechanism of smooth muscle. J. Cell Biol. *42*: 683–694 (1969).

Leeson, C. R. The electron microscopy of the myoepithelium in the rat exorbital lacrimal gland. Anat. Rec. *137*: 45–56 (1960).

Merrillees, N. C. R. The nervous environment of individual smooth muscle cells of the guinea pig vas deferens. J. Cell Biol. *37*: 794–317 (1968).

Nonomura, Y. Myofilaments in smooth muscle of guinea pig taenia coli. J. Cell Biol. *39*: 741–745 (1968).

Panner, B. J. and Honig, C. R. Filament ultrastructure and organization in vertebrate smooth muscle. Contraction hypothesis based on localization of actin and myosin. J. Cell Biol. *35*: 303–321 (1967).

Panner, B. J. and Honig, C. R. Locus and state of aggregation of myosin in tissue sections of vertebrate smooth muscle. J. Cell Biol. *44*: 52–61 (1970).

Rice, R. V., Moses, J. A., McManus, G. M., Brady, A. C. and Blasik, L. M. The organization of contractile filaments in mammalian smooth muscle. J. Cell Biol. *47*: 183–196 (1970).

Richardson, K. C. The fine structure of autonomic nerve endings in smooth muscle of the rat vas deferens. J. Anat. Lond. *96*: 427–442 (1962).

Rhodin, J. A. G. Fine structure of vascular walls in mammals with special reference to smooth muscle component. Physiol. Rev. *42* (Suppl.): 48–81 (1962).

Somlyo, A. P. and Somlyo, A. V. Vascular smooth muscle. I. Normal structure, pathology, biochemistry and biophysics. Pharmacol. Rev. *20*: 197–272 (1968).

Somlyo, A. P., Devine, C. E., Somlyo, A. V. and North, S. R. Sarcoplasmic reticulum and the temperature-dependent contraction of smooth muscle in calcium-free solutions. J. Cell Biol. *51*: 722–741 (1971).

Tandler, B. Ultrastructure of the human submaxillary gland. III. Myoepithelium. Z. Zellforsch. *68*: 852–863 (1965).

Uehara, Y. and Burnstock, G. Postsynaptic specialization of smooth muscle at close neuromuscular junctions in the guinea pig sphincter pupillae. J. Cell Biol. *53*: 849–853 (1972).

Uehara, Y., Campbell, G. R. and Burnstock, G. Cytoplasmic filaments in developing and adult vertebrate smooth muscle. J. Cell Biol. *50*: 484–497 (1971).

12 Nervous system—organization

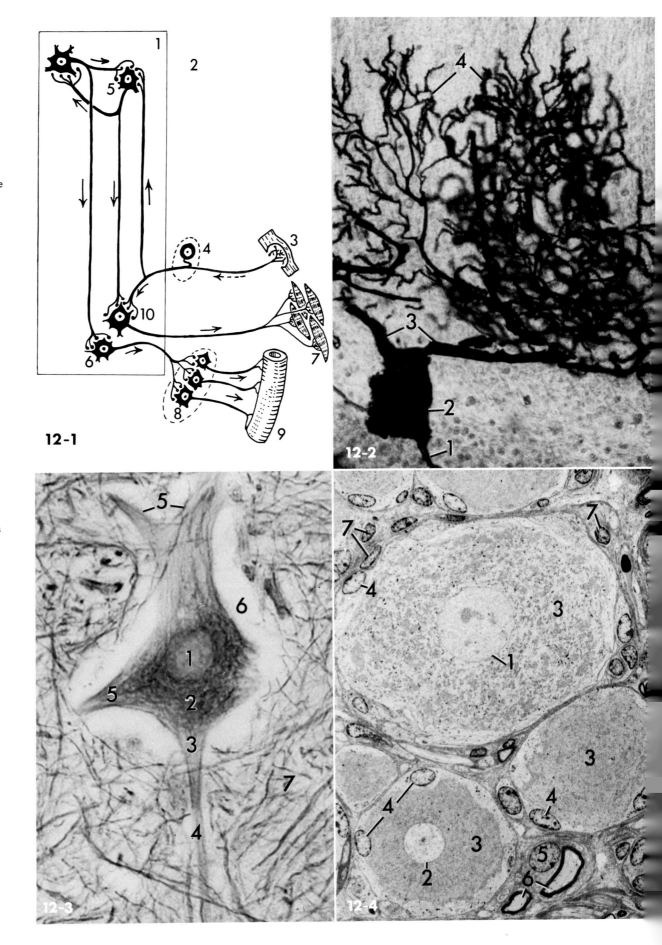

Fig. 12-1. Principal disposition of neurons in the central and peripheral nervous system. Arrows indicate direction of nerve impulses. **1.** Rectangle: central nervous system (brain and spinal cord). **2.** Peripheral nervous system (outside rectangle). **3.** Sense organ. **4.** Pseudo-unipolar nerve cell in sensory ganglion. **5.** Nerve cells in spinal cord and brain. **6.** Motor nerve cells. **7.** Skeletal muscle. **8.** Multipolar nerve cells in autonomic ganglion. **9.** Viscera (non-skeletal muscle and glands). **10.** Synapses.

Fig. 12-2. Purkinje nerve cell, made visible by gold impregnation technique. Cerebellum. Cat. L.M. X 450. **1.** Axon. **2.** Perikaryon (nucleus obliterated by impregnation technique). **3.** Dendrites. **4.** Dendritic arborization.

Fig. 12-3. Motor neuron. Anterior horn. Spinal cord. Gold chloride. Cat. L.M. X 800. **1.** Nucleus. **2.** Perikaryon with neurofilamentous network. **3.** Axon hillock. **4.** Axon. **5.** Dendrites. **6.** Artificial perineuronal shrinkage space. **7.** Neuropil with network of axons and dendrites.

Fig. 12-4. Pseudo-unipolar nerve cells. Spinal (sensory) ganglion. Cat. E.M. X 880. **1.** Nucleus of large nerve cell. **2.** Nucleus of small nerve cell. **3.** Perikaryon. **4.** Nuclei of satellite cells. **5.** Nucleus of Schwann cell. **6.** Myelinated nerve processes. **7.** Capsule cells.

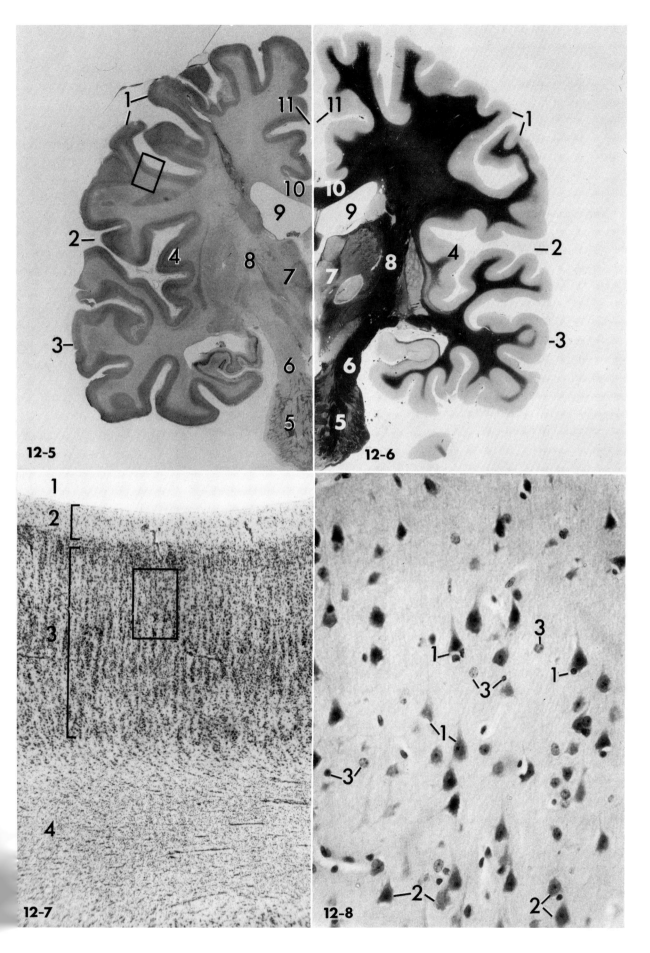

12-5

12-6

12-7

12-8

Figs. 12-5 & 12-6. *Frontal section through the cerebral hemispheres, thalami, and ventral pons.*

Fig. 12-5 is stained with cresyl-violet, showing nerve cells dark, and nerve processes light.

Fig. 12-6 is stained with the Weigert method, showing nerve cells light and myelinated nerve processes black. Human. X 1.4. **1.** Parietal lobe. **2.** Lateral fissure. **3.** Temporal lobe. **4.** Insula. **5.** Pons. **6.** Cerebral peduncle. **7.** Thalamus. **8.** Internal capsule. **9.** Lateral ventricle. **10.** Corpus callosum. **11.** Longitudinal cerebral fissure.

Fig. 12-7. Cerebral (temporal) cortex. Enlargement of area similar to rectangle in Fig. 12-5. Human. L.M. × 40. **1.** Surface of brain. **2.** Molecular layer of cortex (layer I). **3.** Cortex (nerve cell layers II–VI). **4.** Medulla (white matter).

Fig. 12-8. Detail of cerebral cortex (gray matter). Enlargement of area similar to rectangle in Fig. 12-7, corresponding to approximately nerve cell layers III–IV. Human. L.M. × 385. **1.** Pyramidal nerve cells of layer III. **2.** Stellate-shaped (granule) cells of layer IV. **3.** Neuroglial cells.

Fig. 12-9. Horizontal section of the cerebellum. Section stained with the Weigert method; myelinated nerve processes black. Human. L.M. X 1.1. **1.** Vermis of cerebellum. **2.** Cerebellar hemispheres.

Fig. 12-10. Cerebellar folia. Enlargement of area similar to rectangle in Fig. 12-9. Weigert staining method. Human. L.M. X 7.3. **1.** Folia. **2.** Sulci. **3.** Cerebellar cortex (gray matter). **4.** Cerebellar medulla (white matter).

Fig. 12-11. Cerebellar folium. Enlargement of area similar to rectangle in Fig. 12-10. Weigert staining method. Human. L.M. X 69. **1.** Interfoliary sulcus. **2.** Molecular layer of cerebellar cortex. **3.** Purkinje cell layer. **4.** Granule cell layer. **5.** White matter of folium (myelinated nerve processes).

Fig. 12-12. Detail of cerebellar cortex. Enlargement of area similar to rectangle in Fig. 12-11. Human. L.M. X 770. **1.** Nerve cells (basket cells). **2.** Purkinje nerve cells. **3.** Nuclei of granule cells. **4.** Golgi type II nerve cell. **5.** Nuclei of neuroglial cell.

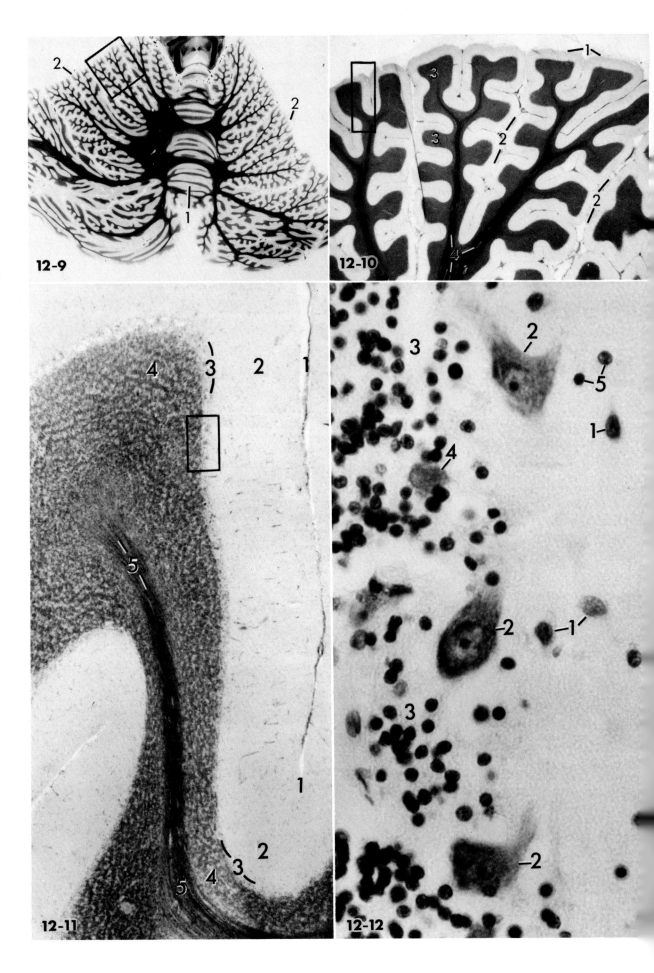

148

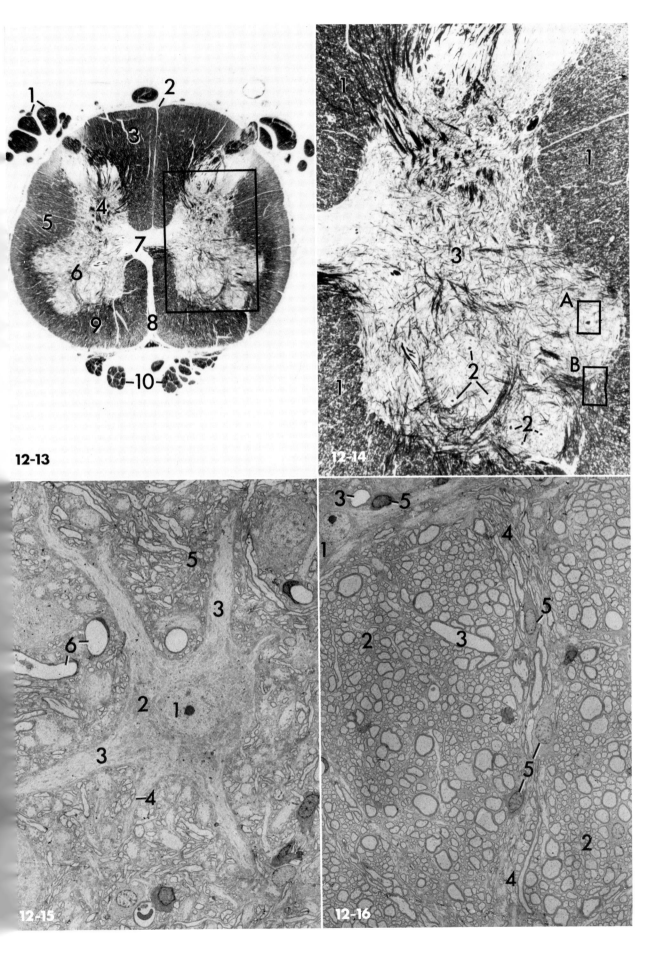

12-13

12-14

12-15

12-16

Fig. 12-13. Cross section through the spinal cord. Lumbar segment (L5). Weigert staining method; myelinated nerve processes black. Human. L.M. X 8.8. **1.** Dorsal root. **2.** Dorsal median septum. **3.** Dorsal funiculus (white matter). **4.** Posterior horn (gray matter). **5.** Lateral funiculus. **6.** Anterior horn. **7.** Gray commissure. **8.** Ventral median fissure. **9.** Anterior funiculus. **10.** Ventral roots.

Fig. 12-14. Enlargement of rectangle in Fig. 12-13. L.M. X 26. **1.** Columns of white matter (myelinated nerve processes). **2.** Motor neurons in anterior horn of gray matter. **3.** Myelinated and non-myelinated nerve processes form an irregular loose network in the gray matter of the spinal cord.

Fig. 12-15. Motor neuron. Anterior horn. Spinal cord. Thoracic segment. Enlargement of area similar to rectangle (A) in Fig. 12-14. Rat. E.M. X 780. **1.** Nucleus of motor neuron. **2.** Perikaryon. **3.** Dendrites. **4.** Axon. **5.** Network of myelinated and non-myelinated nerve processes. **6.** Lumen of capillary. This neuron is enlarged further in Fig. 13-1.

Fig. 12-16. Cross section of anterior funiculus. Spinal cord. Thoracic segment. Enlargement of area similar to rectangle (B) in Fig. 12-14. Rat. E.M. X 640. **1.** Motor neuron in anterior horn of gray matter. **2.** Myelinated nerve processes of varied diameters; arranged in parallel, make up the columns of white matter of the spinal cord. **3.** Lumen of capillary. **4.** Myelinated nerve processes (axons) traversing the white column on their way to the ventral root of the spinal nerve. **5.** Nuclei of neuroglial cells. Further enlargements of this area are seen in Figs. 13-9 and 13-10.

149

Fig. 12-17. Peripheral nerve. Cross section. Sciatic nerve. Human. L.M. × 27. **1.** Bundles of nerve fibers (nerve fascicles). **2.** Loose connective tissue (epineurium). **3.** Perineurium. **4.** Blood vessels.

Fig. 12-18. Bundle of nerve fibers. Cross section. Enlargement of area similar to rectangle in Fig. 12-17. Specimen fixed by osmium tetroxide. Monkey. L.M. × 220. **1.** Perineurium. **2.** Myelin sheaths show up as black rings. **3.** Nerve processes, largely unstained.

Fig. 12-19. Bundle of nerve fibers. Cross section. Enlargement of area similar to rectangle in Fig. 12-18. Rat. E.M. × 640. **1.** Perineurium. **2.** Myelin sheaths. **3.** Nerve processes. **4.** Schwann cells (neurolemma). **5.** Lumen of blood vessels. **6.** Endoneurium. Further enlargement of this area is seen in Fig. 13-18.

Fig. 12-20. Peripheral nerves. Longitudinal section. Sciatic nerve. Human. L.M. × 28. **1.** Bundles of nerve fibers. There is a great resemblance to tendons at this magnification. **2.** Epineurium. **3.** Perineurium.

Fig. 12-21. Bundle of nerve fibers. Longitudinal section. Specimen fixed by osmium tetroxide. Enlargement of area similar to rectangle in Fig. 12-20. Monkey. L.M. × 400. **1.** Myelin sheaths. **2.** Nodes of Ranvier. **3.** Schmidt-Lanterman's incisure.

Fig. 12-22. Bundle of nerve fibers. Longitudinal section. Enlargement of area similar to rectangle in Fig. 12-21. Rat. E.M. × 580. **1.** Myelin sheaths. **2.** Nerve processes. **3.** Node of Ranvier. **4.** Schmidt-Lanterman's incisure. **5.** Schwann cell (neurolemma). **6.** Blood vessel. Further enlargements of this area are seen in Figs. 13-20 to 13-24.

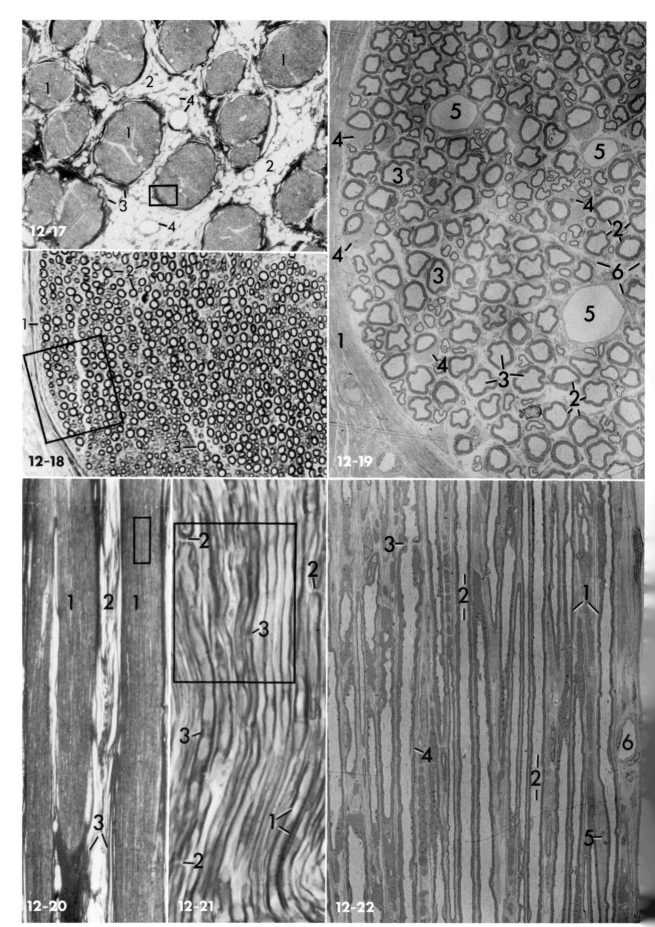

150

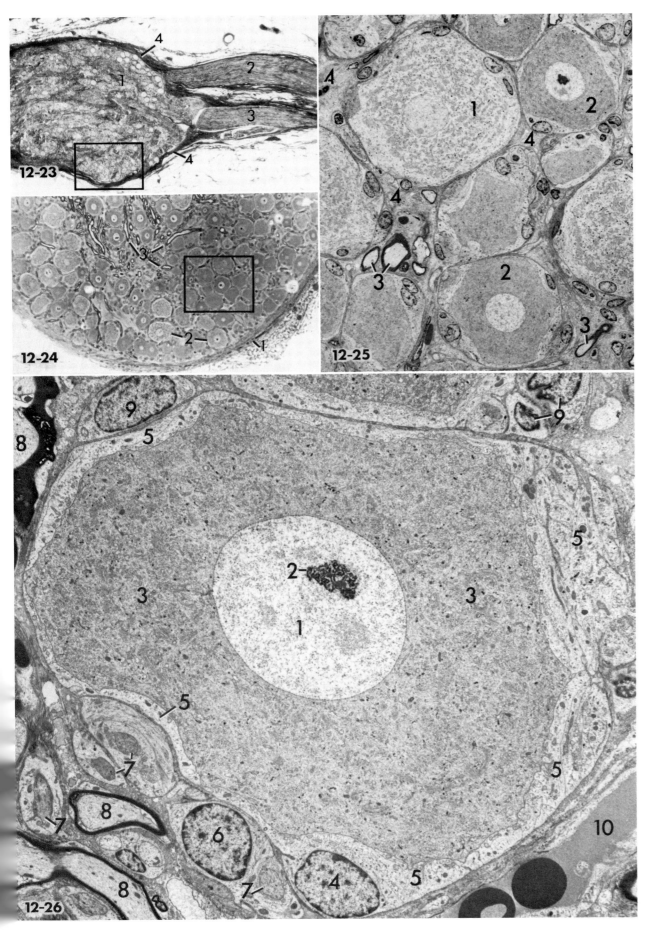

Fig. 12-23. Spinal (dorsal) root ganglion. Human. L.M. X 17. **1.** Spinal (sensory) ganglion. **2.** and **3.** Dorsal nerve root. **4.** Connective tissue capsule.

Fig. 12-24. Spinal root ganglion. Enlargement of area similar to rectangle in Fig. 12-23. Cat. L.M. X 110. **1.** Connective tissue capsule. **2.** Nerve cells. **3.** Myelinated nerve processes.

Fig. 12-25. Pseudo-unipolar nerve cells. Spinal ganglion. Enlargement of area similar to rectangle in Fig. 12-24. Cat. E.M. X 600. **1.** Large spinal ganglion cell. **2.** Small spinal ganglion cell. **3.** Myelinated nerve processes. **4.** Connective tissue elements.

Fig. 12-26. Pseudo-unipolar (sensory) ganglion cell. Spinal root ganglion. Cat. E.M. X 2400. **1.** Nucleus of ganglion cell. **2.** Nucleolus. **3.** Perikaryon. Note: origin of single nerve process of this pseudo-unipolar cell is not in the plane of section. **4.** Nucleus of satellite cell. **5.** Cytoplasm of satellite cells. **6.** Nucleus of Schwann cell. **7.** Nerve processes surrounded by cytoplasm of Schwann cell. **8.** Myelinated nerve processes. **9.** Nuclei of capsule cells. **10.** Lumen of capillary with erythrocytes.

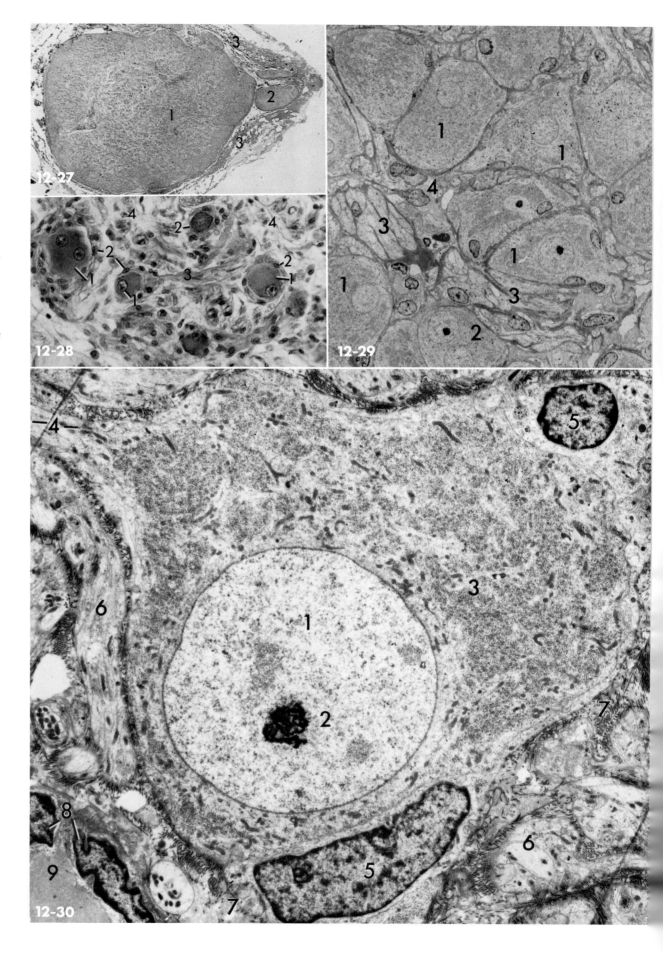

Fig. 12-27. Sympathetic ganglion. Thorax. Human. L.M. X 15.5. **1.** Sympathetic (motor) ganglion. **2.** Bundle of visceral nerve fibers. **3.** Connective tissue capsule.

Fig. 12-28. Sympathetic ganglion. Human. L.M. X 290. **1.** Nerve cells. **2.** Satellite cells. **3.** Non-myelinated nerve fibers. **4.** Loose connective tissue.

Fig. 12-29. Multipolar nerve cells. Sympathetic ganglion. Abdomen. Cat. E.M. X 600. **1.** Ganglion cells. **2.** Binucleate ganglion cell. **3.** Non-myelinated nerve fibers. **4.** Connective tissue elements.

Fig. 12-30. Multipolar sympathetic (motor) ganglion cell. Sympathetic ganglion. Abdomen. Cat. E.M. X 4600. **1.** Nucleus of ganglion cell. **2.** Nucleolus. **3.** Perikaryon. **4.** Cell process, presumably axon. **5.** Nucleus of satellite cells. **6.** Non-myelinated nerve fibers. **7.** Connective tissue fibers. **8.** Nuclei of endothelial cells. **9.** Lumen of capillary.

References

Babel, J. Ultrastructure of the Peripheral Nervous System. C. V. Mosby, St. Louis, 1970.

Barr, M. L. The Human Nervous System. Harper & Row, New York, 1972.

Bourne, G. H. (Ed.). The Structure and Function of Nervous Tissue. Vol. 1: Structure I. Academic Press, New York, 1968.

Everett, N. B. Functional Neuroanatomy. Lea & Febiger, Philadelphia, 1971.

Ford, D. H. and Schade, J. P. Atlas of Human Brain. Elsevier, Amsterdam, 1966.

Klüver, H. and Barrera, E. A method for the combined staining of cells and fibers in the nervous system. J. Neuropath. & Exper. Neurol. *12*: 400–403 (1953).

Noback, C. The Human Nervous System. McGraw-Hill, New York, 1967.

Rexed, B. A cytoarchitectonic atlas of the spinal cord in the cat. J. Comp. Neurol. *100*: 297–380 (1954).

Rodahl, K. and Issekutz, D. (Eds.). Nerve as a Tissue. Harper & Row, New York, 1966.

Truex, R. C. and Carpenter, M. B. Strong and Elwyn's Human Neuroanatomy. Williams & Wilkins, Baltimore, 1969.

Willis, W. D., Jr. and Grossman, R. G. Medical Neurobiology. Neuroanatomical and neurophysiological principles basic to clinical neuroscience. C. V. Mosby, St. Louis, 1973.

13 Nervous tissue— the neuron

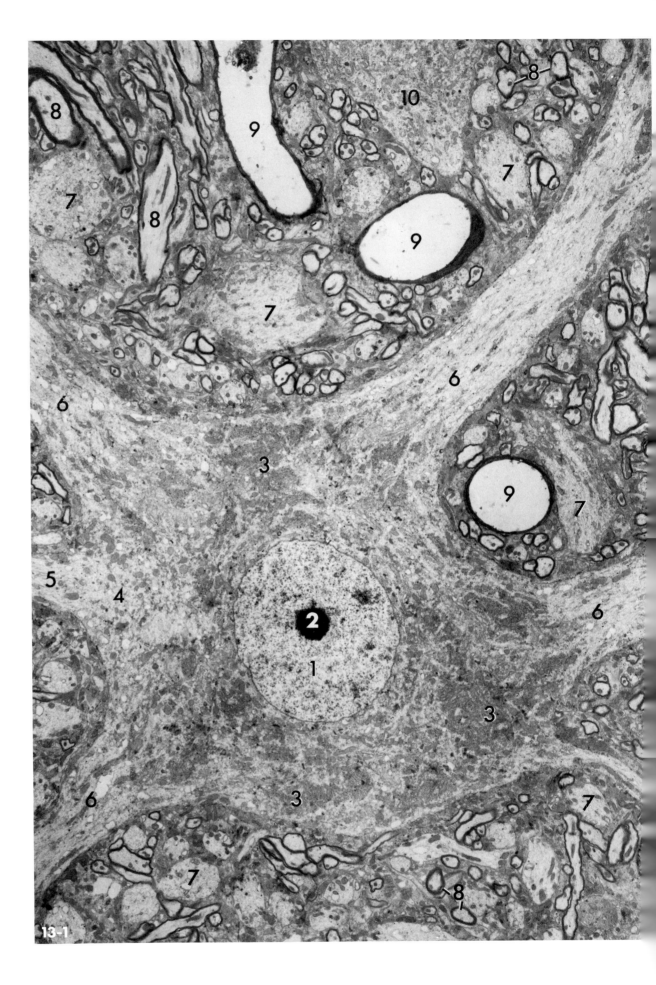

Fig. 13-1. Multipolar motor neuron. Anterior horn. Spinal cord. Thoracic segment. Rat. E.M. X 1920. **1.** Nucleus. **2.** Nucleolus. **3.** Nissl substance (granular endoplasmic reticulum). **4.** Axon hillock. **5.** Axon. **6.** Dendrites. **7.** Cross-sectioned dendrites. **8.** Myelinated nerve processes of the spinal cord gray matter. **9.** Lumen of capillary. **10.** Part of neighboring motor neuron.

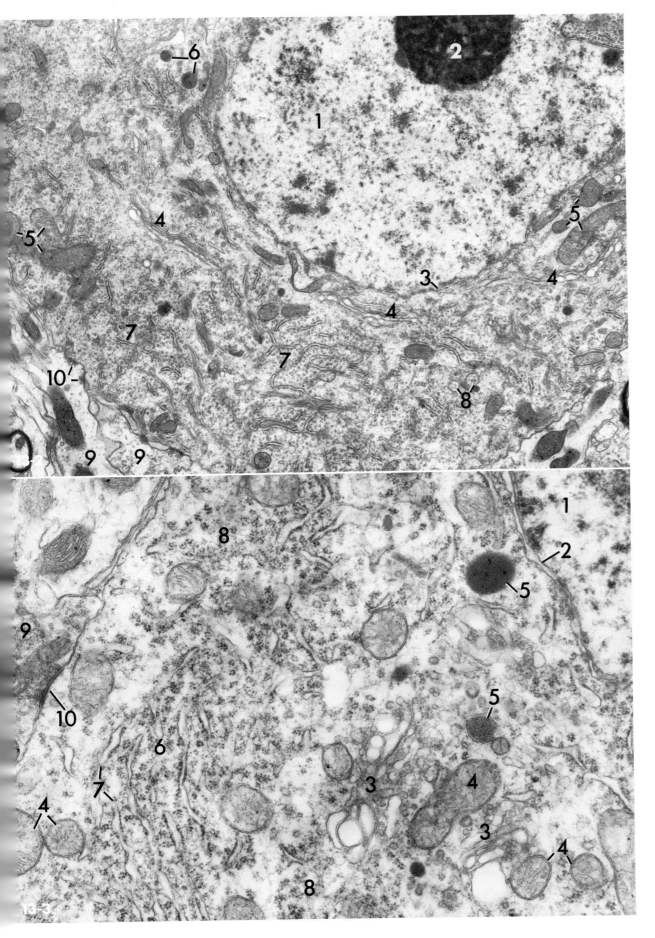

Fig. 13-2. Purkinje nerve cell. Cerebellar cortex. Rat. E.M. X 9000. **1.** Nucleus. **2.** Nucleolus. **3.** Nuclear membrane. **4.** Golgi zone. **5.** Mitochondria. **6.** Lysosomes. **7.** Granular endoplasmic reticulum (Nissl substance). **8.** Multivesicular bodies. **9.** Axon terminals. **10** Axo-somatic synapses.

Fig. 13-3. Detail of motor neuron. Anterior horn. Spinal cord. Thoracic segment. Rat. E.M. X 37,000. **1.** Nucleus. **2.** Nuclear membrane. **3.** Golgi zone. **4.** Mitochondria. **5.** Lysosome. **6.** Granular endoplasmic reticulum (Nissl substance). **7.** Cisternae of granular endoplasmic reticulum. **8.** Polyribosomes. **9.** Axon terminal (bouton terminal). **10.** Axo-somatic synapse.

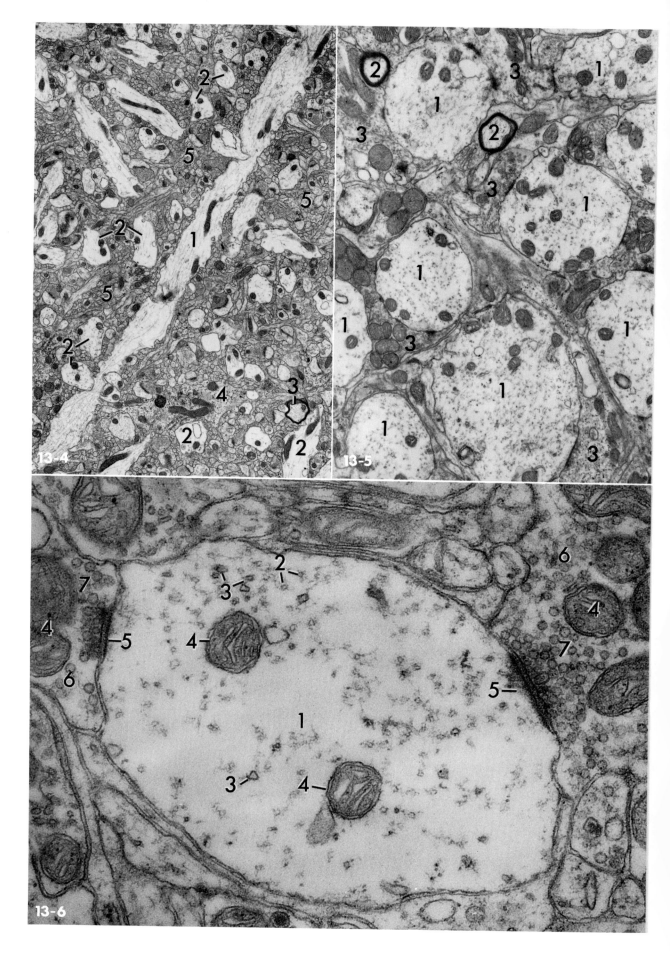

Fig. 13-4. Irregularly arranged dendrites. Molecular layer. Cerebral cortex. Rat. E.M. X 4800. **1.** Large dendrite: longitudinal section. **2.** Cross-sectioned large dendrites. **3.** Myelinated nerve process. **4.** Part of neuroglial cell. **5.** Neuropil: a mixture of abundant, delicate branching axon terminals (telodendria); small dendrites; and neuroglial cell processes.

Fig. 13-5. Cross-sectioned dendrites, arranged in parallel. Gray matter. Spinal cord. Rat. E.M. X 9000. **1.** Dendrites. **2.** Myelinated nerve processes. **3.** Axon terminals.

Fig. 13-6. Enlargement of cross-sectioned dendrite. Gray matter. Spinal cord. E.M. X 60,000. **1.** Dendritic cytoplasm. **2.** Microtubules. **3.** Profiles of tubular, agranular endoplasmic reticulum. **4.** Mitochondria. **5.** Axo-dendritic synapses. **6.** Axon terminals. **7.** Synaptic vesicles.

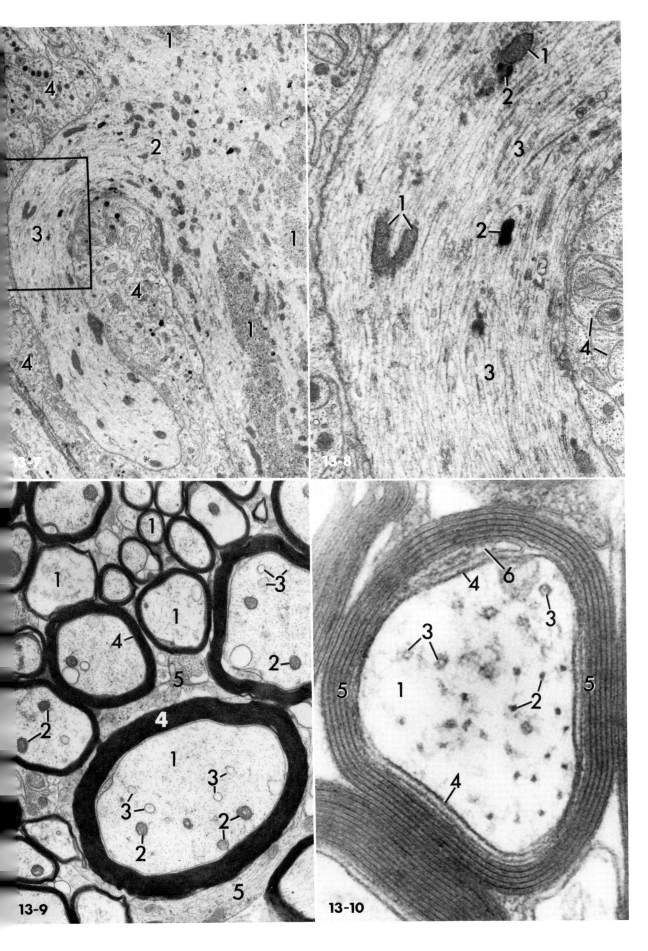

Fig. 13-7. Pseudo-unipolar neuron. Spinal root ganglion. Cat. E.M. X 4800. **1.** Nissl substance (granular endoplasmic reticulum) of spinal ganglion cell. **2.** Hillock. **3.** Initial segment of single nerve process of pseudo-unipolar neuron. **4.** Cell processes of satellite cells ensheath the nerve process. Axon terminals and synapses are not present in association with spinal (sensory) ganglion cells.

Fig. 13-8. Initial segment of single nerve process of pseudo-unipolar ganglion cell. Enlargement of rectangle in Fig. 13-7. Spinal root ganglion. Cat. E.M. X 18,000.
1. Mitochondria. **2.** Lysosomes.
3. Microtubules and neurofilaments. **4.** Cell processes of satellite cells with numerous glial filaments.

Fig. 13-9. Myelinated nerve processes of varied diameters. White matter. Spinal cord. Cross section. Rat. E.M. X 9000. **1.** Axon cytoplasm. **2.** Mitochondria. **3.** Profiles of agranular endoplasmic reticulum. **4.** Myelin sheaths. **5.** Cytoplasm of neuroglial cells.

Fig. 13-10. Detail of myelinated nerve process. White matter. Spinal cord. Rat. E.M. X 124,000. **1.** Axon cytoplasm.
2. Neurofilaments. **3.** Microtubules.
4. Axolemma. **5.** Myelin sheath. **6.** Ad-axonal oligodendroglial cytoplasm.

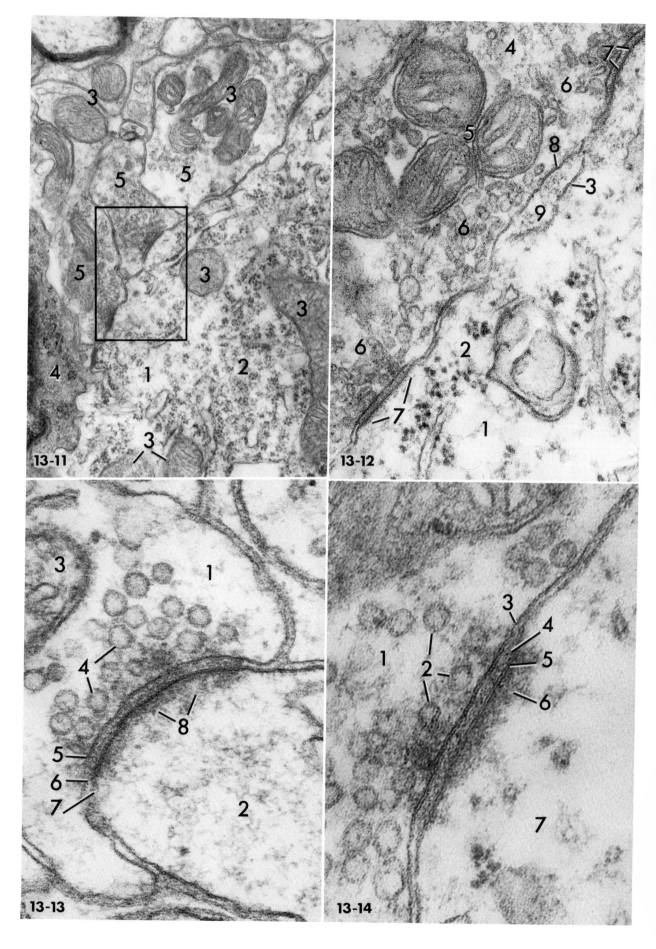

Fig. 13-11. Axo-somatic synapses. Motor neuron. Anterior horn. Spinal cord. Rat. E.M. X 37,000. **1.** Cytoplasm of motor neuron. **2.** Polysomes. **3.** Mitochondria. **4.** Cytoplasm and part of nucleus of perineuronal neuroglial cell (oligodendrocyte). **5.** Axon terminals with axo-somatic synapses.

Fig. 13-12. Axo-somatic synapses. Enlargement of area similar to rectangle in Fig. 13-11. Motor neuron. Anterior horn. Spinal cord. Rat. E.M. X 93,000. **1.** Cytoplasm of motor neuron. **2.** Ribosomes. **3.** Cell membrane of motor neuron. **4.** Axoplasm of bouton terminal (axon terminal). **5.** Mitochondria. **6.** Oval or flat synaptic vesicles. **7.** Synaptic region. **8.** Axolemma. **9.** Enlarged intercellular space.

Fig. 13-13. Axo-dendritic synapse. Molecular layer. Cerebellar cortex. Rat. E.M. X 172,000. **1.** Axon terminal. **2.** Dendrite. **3.** Mitochondrion. **4.** Round synaptic vesicles. **5.** Presynaptic membrane. **6.** Synaptic cleft. **7.** Postsynaptic membrane. **8.** Subsynaptic web.

Fig. 13-14. Detail of synaptic region. Axo-dendritic synapse. Gray matter. Spinal cord. Rat. E.M. X 172,000. **1.** Cytoplasm of axon terminal. **2.** Synaptic vesicles. **3.** Presynaptic membrane. **4.** Synaptic cleft. **5.** Postsynaptic membrane. **6.** Subsynaptic web. **7.** Cytoplasm of dendrite.

160

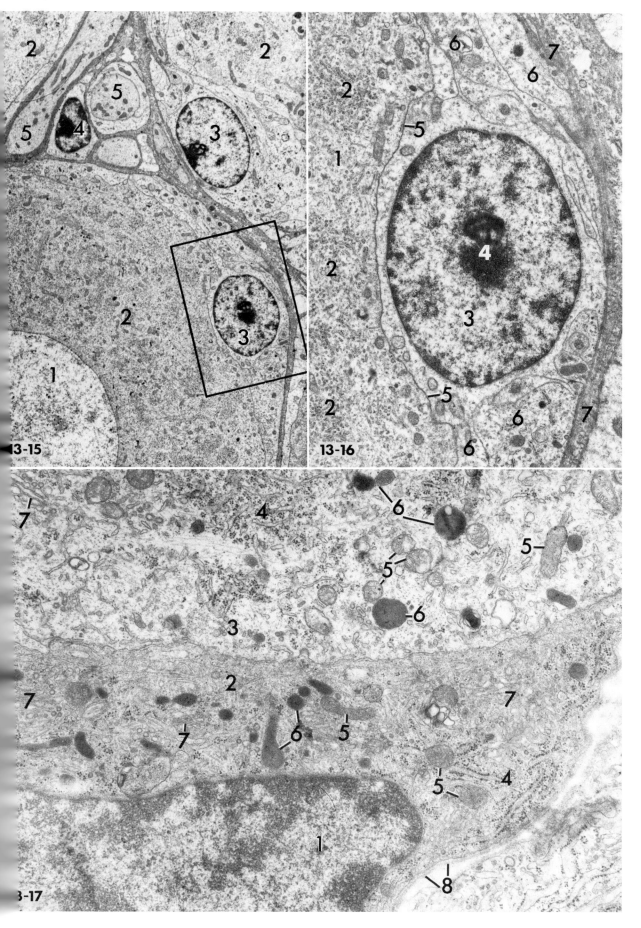

Fig. 13-15. Sheath surrounding spinal root ganglion cell. Cat. E.M. × 2500. **1.** Nucleus of pseudo-unipolar neuron. **2.** Perikaryon. **3.** Nucleus of satellite cell. **4.** Nucleus of capsule cell or Schwann cell. **5.** Nerve cell processes surrounded by cytoplasmic sheath of satellite or Schwann cells.

Fig. 13-16. Satellite cell. Enlargement of rectangle in Fig. 13-15. Spinal root ganglion. Cat. E.M. × 9000. **1.** Cytoplasm of spinal ganglion cell. **2.** Nissl substance (granular endoplasmic reticulum). **3.** Nucleus of satellite cell. **4.** Nucleolus. **5.** Cell membrane of satellite cell borders directly on cell membrane of ganglion cell. **6.** Cytoplasmic processes ensheathing the ganglion cell. **7.** Pericellular connective tissue fibrils.

Fig. 13-17. Detail of ganglion cell and satellite cell. Trigeminal (sensory) ganglion (Gasserian). Cat. E.M. × 28,000. **1.** Nucleus of satellite cell. **2.** Electron-dense cytoplasm of satellite cell. **3.** Electron-lucent cytoplasm of ganglion cell. **4.** Profiles of granular endoplasmic reticulum. **5.** Mitochondria. **6.** Lysosomes. **7.** Golgi zone. **8.** External (basal) lamina.

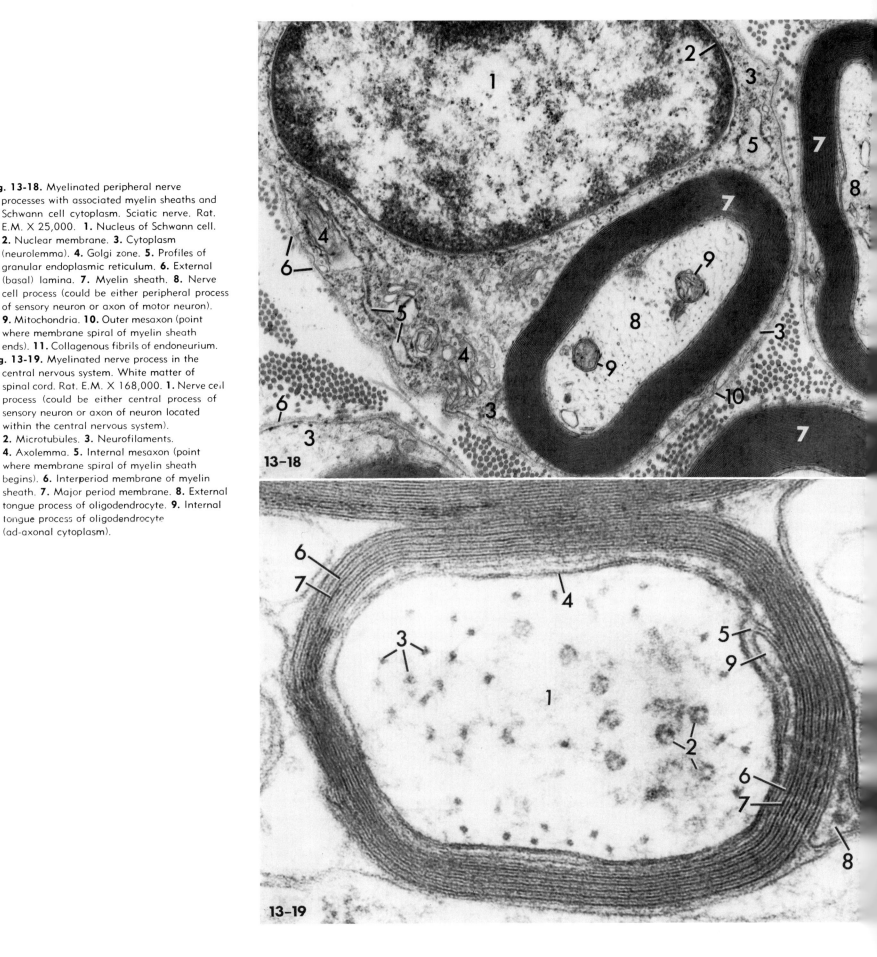

Fig. 13-18. Myelinated peripheral nerve processes with associated myelin sheaths and Schwann cell cytoplasm. Sciatic nerve. Rat. E.M. X 25,000. **1.** Nucleus of Schwann cell. **2.** Nuclear membrane. **3.** Cytoplasm (neurolemma). **4.** Golgi zone. **5.** Profiles of granular endoplasmic reticulum. **6.** External (basal) lamina. **7.** Myelin sheath. **8.** Nerve cell process (could be either peripheral process of sensory neuron or axon of motor neuron). **9.** Mitochondria. **10.** Outer mesaxon (point where membrane spiral of myelin sheath ends). **11.** Collagenous fibrils of endoneurium.

Fig. 13-19. Myelinated nerve process in the central nervous system. White matter of spinal cord. Rat. E.M. X 168,000. **1.** Nerve cell process (could be either central process of sensory neuron or axon of neuron located within the central nervous system). **2.** Microtubules. **3.** Neurofilaments. **4.** Axolemma. **5.** Internal mesaxon (point where membrane spiral of myelin sheath begins). **6.** Interperiod membrane of myelin sheath. **7.** Major period membrane. **8.** External tongue process of oligodendrocyte. **9.** Internal tongue process of oligodendrocyte (ad-axonal cytoplasm).

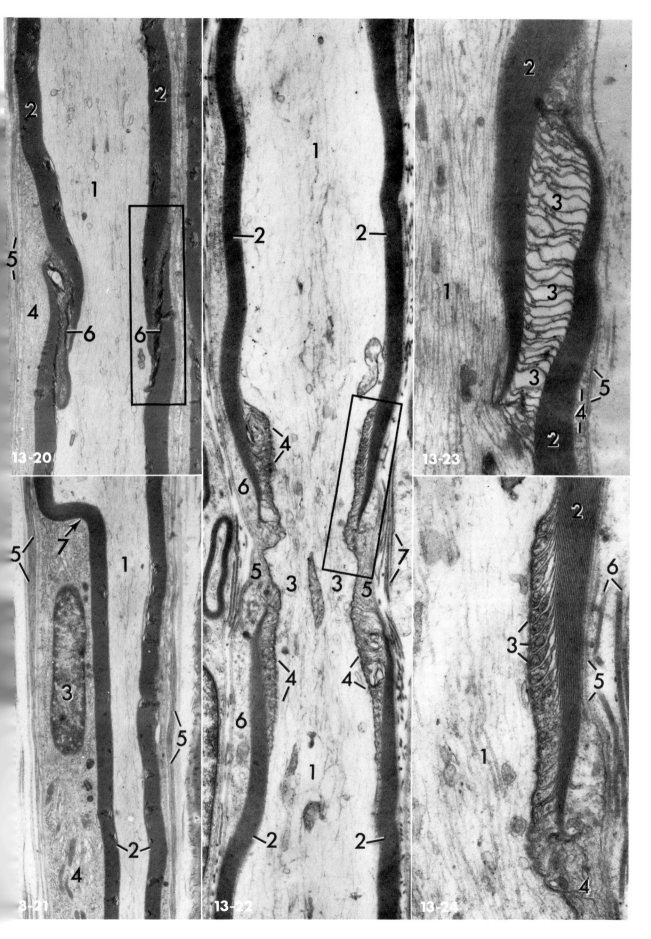

Fig. 13-20 & 13-21. Peripheral myelinated nerve process. Longitudinal section. Sciatic nerve. Rat. E.M. X 4500. **1.** Nerve process ("axon"). **2.** Myelin sheath. **3.** Nucleus of Schwann cell. **4.** Cytoplasm of Schwann cell (neurolemma). **5.** Collagenous fibrils of endoneurium. **6.** Incisure of Schmidt-Lantermann. **7.** Nuclear region of cytoplasm indents locally the myelin sheath.

Fig. 13-22. Node of Ranvier. Peripheral myelinated nerve process. Longitudinal section. Sciatic nerve. Rat. E.M. X 9000. **1.** Nerve process ("axon"). **2.** Myelin sheath. **3.** Nodal area of nerve process. **4.** Schwann cell processes. **5.** Outer collar of Schwann cell processes. **6.** Schwann cell cytoplasm (neurolemma). **7.** Collagenous fibrils of endoneurium.

Fig. 13-23. Detail of incisure of Schmidt-Lantermann. Enlargement of area similar to rectangle in Fig. 13-20. Sciatic nerve. E.M. X 18,000. **1.** Axoplasm with microtubules and neurofilaments. **2.** Myelin sheath. **3.** Schwann cell cytoplasm is retained in the region of the incisure, since the fusion of the inner leaflets of the cell membrane is locally opened up at these points. **4.** Schwann cell cytoplasm (neurolemma). **5.** External lamina.

Fig. 13-24. Detail of node of Ranvier. Enlargement of rectangle in Fig. 13-22. E.M. X 39,000. **1.** Nodal axoplasm with microtubules and neurofilaments. **2.** Myelin sheath. **3.** Successive laminae of the myelin sheath terminate as paranodal cytoplasmic swellings. **4.** Outer collar of Schwann cell processes. **5.** External (basal) lamina. **6.** Collagenous fibrils of endoneurium.

Fig. 13-25. Detail of myelin sheath. Longitudinal section. Sciatic nerve. E.M. X 130,000.
1. Collagenous fibrils of endoneurium. **2.** External (basal) lamina. **3.** Cell membrane of Schwann cell. **4.** Thin rim of Schwann cell cytoplasm (neurolemma). **5.** Myelin sheath: major period membranes are clearly resolved; interperiod membranes indistinct. **6.** Thin rim of ad-axonal Schwann cell cytoplasm. **7.** Axolemma. **8.** Cytoplasm of nerve cell process (axon).

Figs. 13-26 & 13-27. Detail of myelinated peripheral nerve process. Longitudinal section. Sciatic nerve. Rat. E.M. Fig. 13-26: X 102,000. Fig. 13-27: X 96,000.
1. Microtubules; average width 225 Å. **2.** Neurofilaments; average width 85 Å. **3.** Tubular profile of agranular endoplasmic reticulum; average width 400 Å.

Fig. 13-28. Autonomic nerve, consisting largely of non-myelinated nerve fibers. Cross section. Kidney. Rat. E.M. X 1700. **1.** Epineurium (in this case also perineurium). **2.** Nuclei of Schwann cells. **3.** Small circular profiles are non-myelinated nerve processes. **4.** Myelinated nerve processes. **5.** Lumen of capillary. **6.** Area similar to rectangle is enlarged in Fig. 13-29.

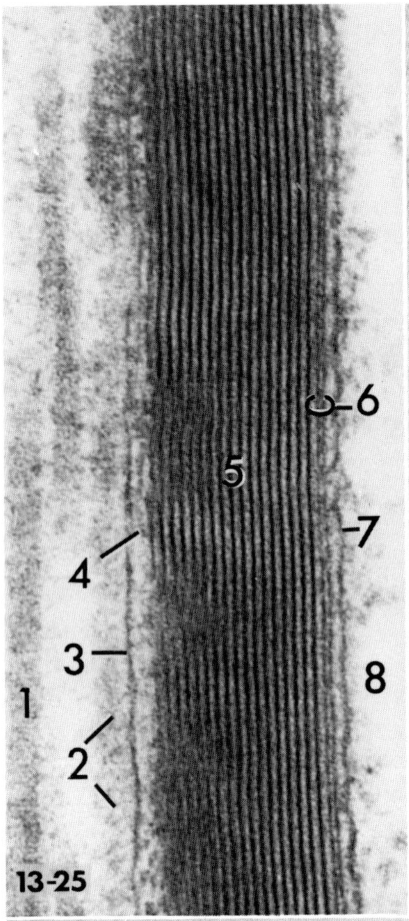

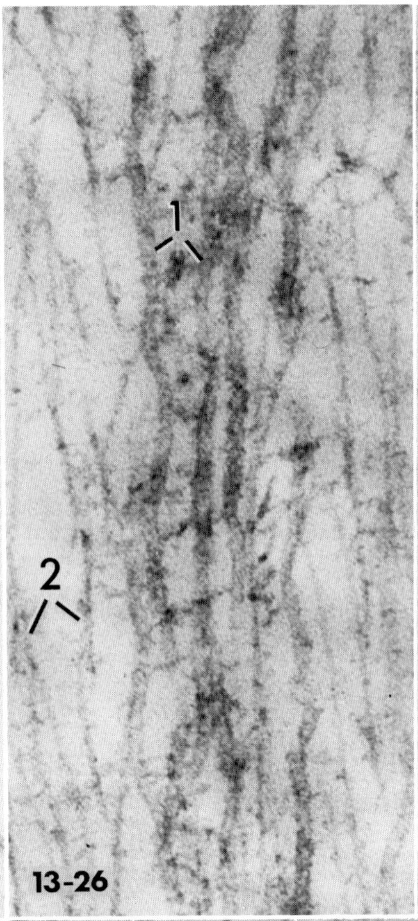

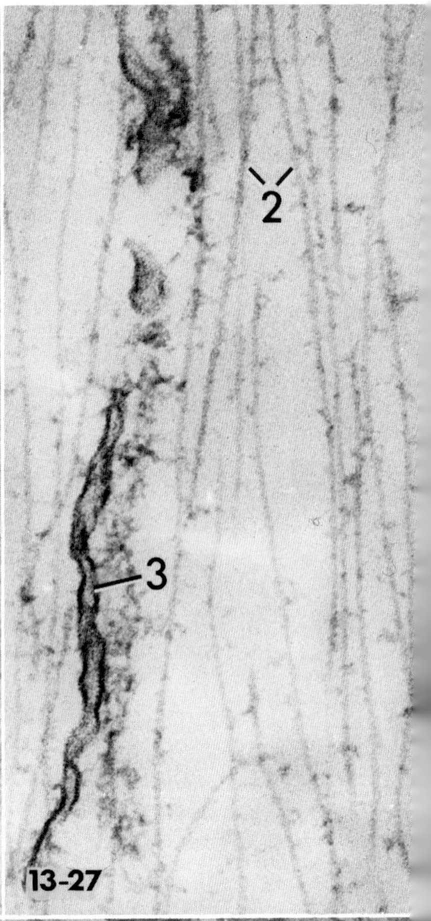

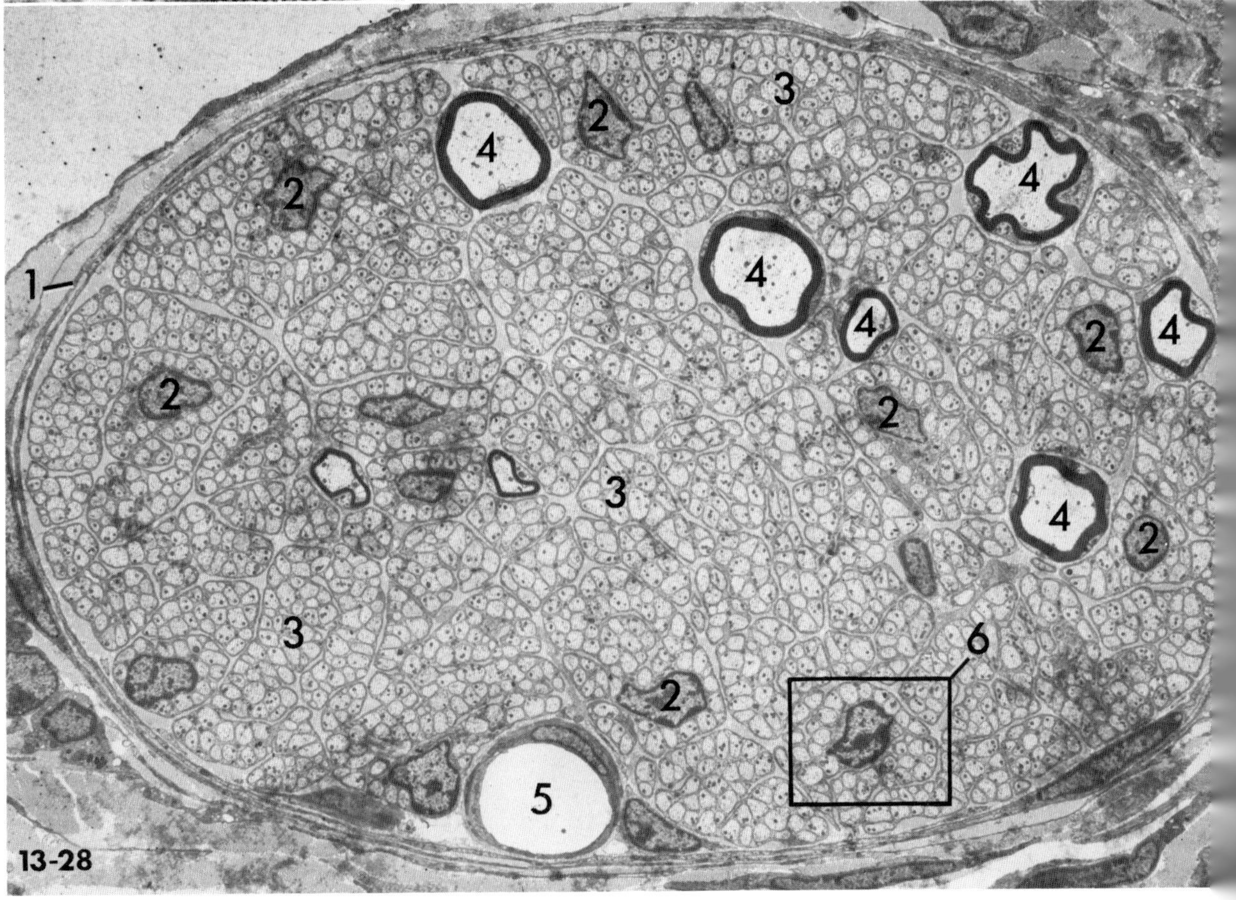

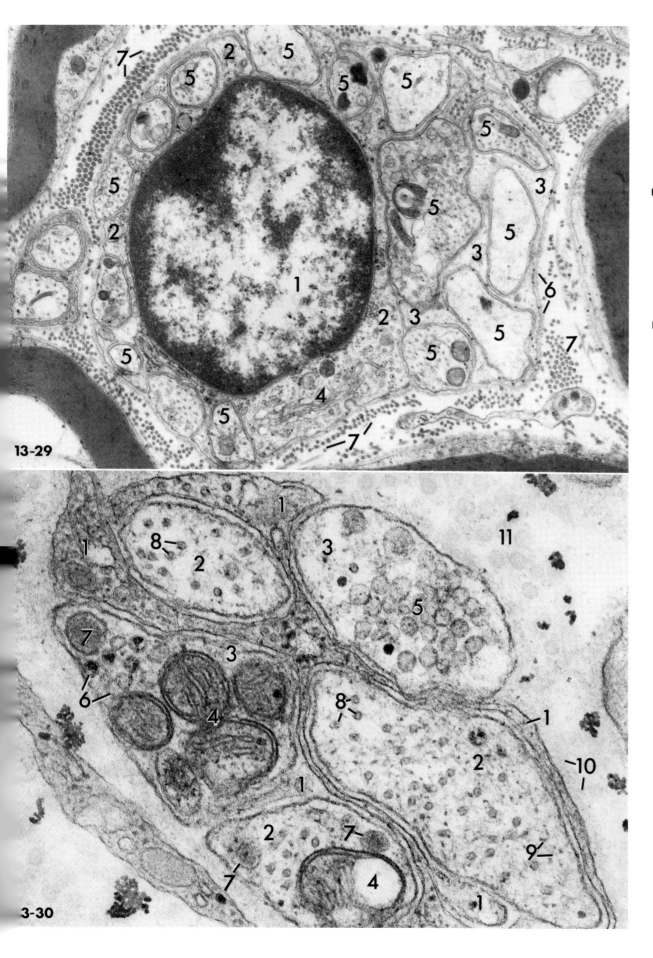

Fig. 13-29. Non-myelinated nerve processes. Cross section. Enlargement of area similar to rectangle in Fig. 13-28. Sciatic nerve. Rat. E.M. X 21,000. **1.** Nucleus of Schwann cell. **2.** Schwann cell cytoplasm. **3.** Cytoplasm of adjoining Schwann cell, interdigitating with neighboring cell. **4.** Golgi zone. **5.** Nerve cell processes partly or completely surrounded by Schwann cell cytoplasm. **6.** External (basal) lamina. **7.** Collagenous fibrils of endoneurium.

Fig. 13-30. Small non-myelinated nerve processes. Cross section. Smooth muscle layer. Ureter. Rat. E.M. X 90,000. **1.** Schwann cell cytoplasm. **2.** Delicate nerve processes. **3.** Bead-like swellings of nerve processes (boutons en passant). One is seen in longitudinal section in Fig. 16-58. **4.** Mitochondria. **5.** Clear synaptic vesicles. **6.** Granulated (dense-core) synaptic vesicles. **7.** Large granulated vesicles. **8.** Microtubules. **9.** Neurofilaments. **10.** Extremely delicate external (basal) lamina. **11.** Cross-sectioned collagenous fibrils.

References

Bischoff, A. and Moor, H. Ultrastructural differences between the myelin sheaths of peripheral nerve fibers and CNS white matter. Z. Zellforsch. *81*: 303–310 (1967).

Bodian, D. The generalized vertebrate neuron. Science *137*: 323–326 (1962).

Brunk, U. and Ericsson, J. L. E. Electron microscopical studies on rat brain neurons. Localization of acid phosphatase and mode of formation of lipofuscin bodies. J. Ultrastruct. Res. *38*: 1–15 (1972).

Burkel, W. E. The histological fine structure of perineurium. Anat. Rec. *158*: 177–190 (1967).

de Robertis, E. Submicroscopic morphology of the synapse. Int. Rev. Cytol. *8*: 61–96 (1959).

de Robertis, E. Ultrastructure and cytochemistry of the synaptic region. Science *156*: 907–914 (1967).

Eccles, J. C. The Physiology of Synapses. Academic Press, New York, 1964.

Elfvin, L. G. The ultrastructure of the superior cervical sympathetic ganglion of the cat. 1. The structure of the ganglion processes as studied by serial sections. J. Ultrastruct. Res. *8*: 403–440 (1963).

Friede, R. L. and Samorajski, T. The clefts of Schmidt-Lanterman: a quantative electron microscopic study of their structure in developing and adult sciatic nerves of the rat. Anat. Rec. *165*: 89–102 (1969).

Geren, B. B. The formation from the Schwann cell surface of myelin in the peripheral nerves of chick embryos. Exper. Cell Res. *7*: 558–562 (1954).

Gobel, S. Electron microscopical studies of the cerebellar molecular layer. J. Ultrastruct. Res. *21*: 430–458 (1968).

Gray, E. G. and Guillery, R. W. Synaptic morphology in the normal and degenerating nervous system. Int. Rev. Cytol. *19*: 111–182 (1966).

Herndon, R. M. The fine structure of the Purkinje cell. J. Cell Biol. *18*: 167–180 (1963).

Hirano, A. and Dembitzer, H. M. A structural analysis of the myelin sheath in the central nervous system. J. Cell Biol. *34*: 555–567 (1967).

Hydén, H. (Ed.). The Neuron. Elsevier, Amsterdam, 1967.

Karlsson, U. Three-dimensional studies of neurons in the lateral geniculate nucleus of the rat. II. Environment of perikarya and proximal part of their branches. J. Ultrastruct. Res. *16*: 482–504 (1966).

Metuzals, J. Ultrastructure of the nodes of Ranvier and their surrounding structures in the central nervous system. Z. Zellforsch. *65*: 719–759 (1965).

Palay, S. L. The morphology of synapses in the central nervous system. Exper. Cell Res. Suppl. *5*, 275–293 (1958).

Palay, S. L. and Palade, G. E. The fine structure of neurons. J. Biophys. Biochem. Cytol. *1*: 69–88 (1955).

Peters, A. and Kaiserman-Abramof, I. T. The small pyramidal neuron of the rat cerebral cortex. The perikaryon, dendrites and spines. Am. J. Anat. *127*: 321–356 (1970).

Peters, A. Stellate cells of the rat parietal cortex. J. Comp. Neurol. *141*: 345–373 (1971).

Peters, A., Palay, S. L. and Webster, H. de F. The Fine Structure of the Nervous System. The cells and their processes. Harper & Row, New York, 1970.

Pick, J., de Lemos, C. and Gerdin, C. The fine structure of sympathetic neurons in man. J. Comp. Neurol. *122*: 19–67 (1964).

Revel, J.-P. and Hamilton, D. W. The double nature of the intermediate dense line in peripheral nerve myelin. Anat. Rec. *163*: 7–16 (1969).

Siegesmund, K. A. The fine structure of subsurface cisterns. Anat. Rec. *162*: 187–196 (1968).

Sjöstrand, F. S. The lamellated structure of the nerve myelin sheath as revealed by high resolution electron microscopy. Experientia *9*: 68–69 (1953).

Sotelo, C. The fine structural localization of norepinephrine-³H in the substantia nigra and area postrema of the rat. An autoradiographic study. J. Ultrastruct. Res. *36*: 824–841 (1971).

Steer, J. M. Some observations on the fine structure of rat dorsal spinal nerve roots. J. Anat. *109*: 467–485 (1971).

Uga, S. and Ikui, H. Membrane modification occurring between neurons and Schwann cells. J. Electron Micr. *17*: 155 (1968).

Uzman, B. G. The spiral configuration of myelin lamellae. J. Ultrastruct. Res. *2*: 208–212 (1964).

van der Loos, H. Fine structure of synapses in the cerebral cortex. Z. Zellforsch. *60*: 815–825 (1963).

Wuerker, R. B. and Kirkpatrick, J. B. Neuronal microtubules, neurofilaments, and microtubules. Int. Rev. Cytol. *33*: 45–75 (1972).

14 Nervous tissue— nerve endings

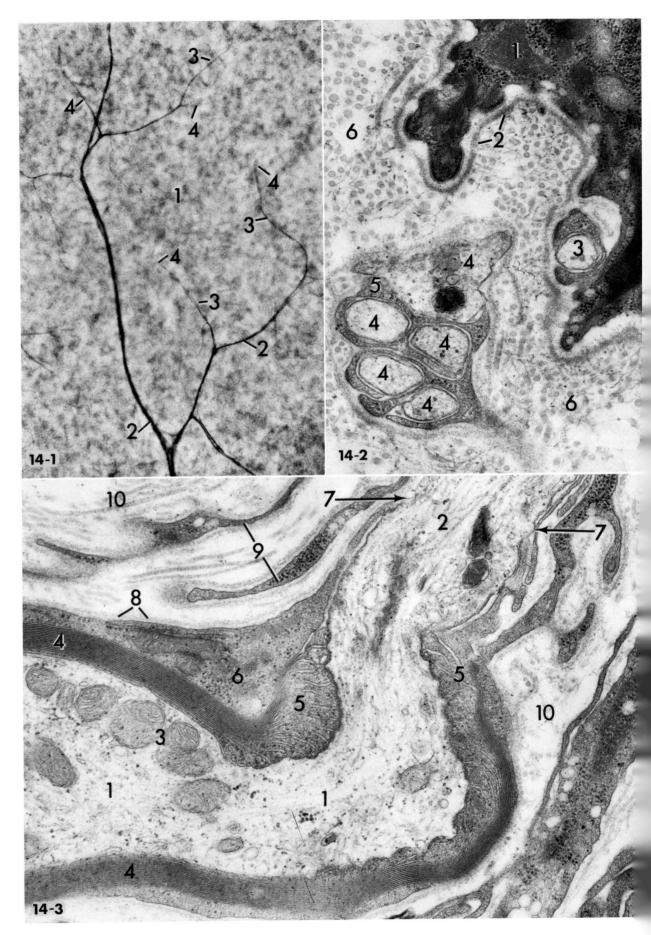

Fig. 14-1. Free nerve endings (sensory). Silver impregnation method. Cornea. Flat mount. Mouse (4 days old). L.M. X 225. **1.** Irregularly patterned background represents corneal epithelial cells and their nuclei. **2.** Myelinated nerves located in corneal connective tissue stroma. **3.** Points where myelin sheath is shed. **4.** Denuded nerve endings among corneal epithelial cells.

Fig. 14-2. Free nerve endings (sensory). Skin. Rat. E.M. X 31,000. **1.** Base of epidermis. **2.** Basal lamina. **3.** Nerve process within epithelium. **4.** Nerve processes in subepithelial connective tissue. **5.** Schwann cell cytoplasm. **6.** Network of reticulum and delicate collagenous fibrils.

Fig. 14-3. Termination of myelinated nerve process. Papillary layer of dermis. Rat. E.M. X 31,000. **1.** Peripheral nerve process of sensory neuron. **2.** Microtubules. **3.** Mitochondria. **4.** Myelin sheath. **5.** Successive laminae of the myelin sheath terminate as cytoplasmic swellings. **6.** Schwann cell cytoplasm (neurolemma). **7.** Level at which the nerve process becomes denuded. **8.** External (basal) lamina. **9.** A limited number of delicate cytoplasmic processes of the Schwann cell surround loosely the denuded nerve process. **10.** Connective tissue fibrils.

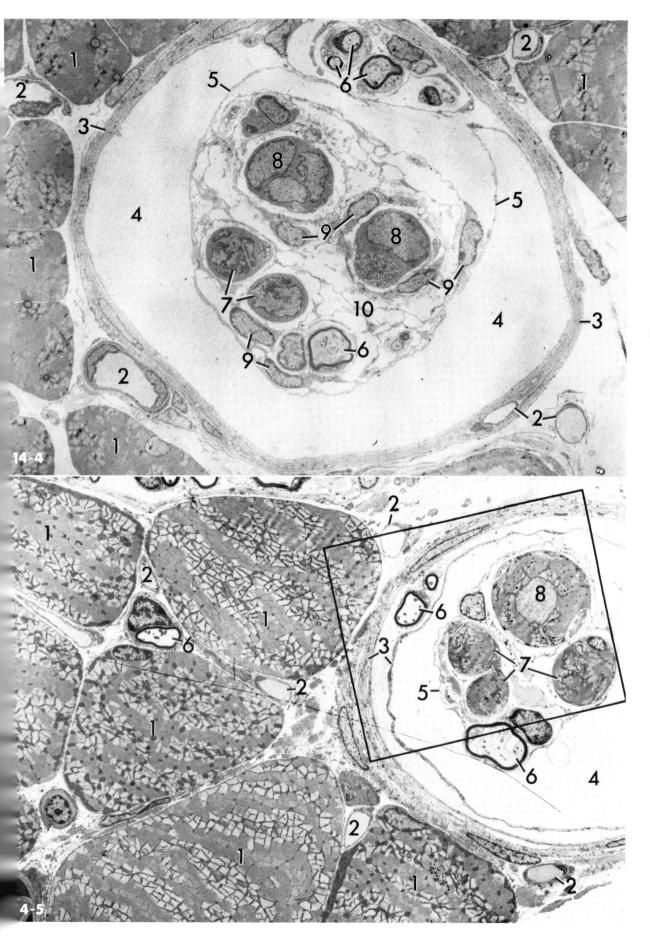

Fig. 14-4. Neuromuscular spindle. Cross section. Equatorial region. Triceps surae muscle. Rat. Embryo, 2 days before birth. E.M. × 1200. (From: Jacqueline H. Levy, 1972). **1.** Extrafusal skeletal muscle fibers. **2.** Lumen of blood capillary. **3.** Outer capsule. **4.** Periaxial space. **5.** Inner capsule. **6.** Myelinated nerve fibers. **7.** Intrafusal nuclear chain muscle fibers. **8.** Nuclear bag muscle fibers. **9.** Fibroblasts. **10.** Loose connective tissue.

Fig. 14-5. Neuromuscular spindle. Cross section. Juxta-equatorial region. Front leg muscle. Newborn rat. E.M. X 1900. **1.** Extrafusal skeletal muscle fibers. **2.** Lumen of capillary. **3.** Outer capsule. **4.** Periaxial space. **5.** Inner capsule. **6.** Myelinated nerve fibers. **7.** Nuclear chain muscle fibers. **8.** Nuclear bag muscle fibers. Rectangle enlarged in Fig. 14-6.

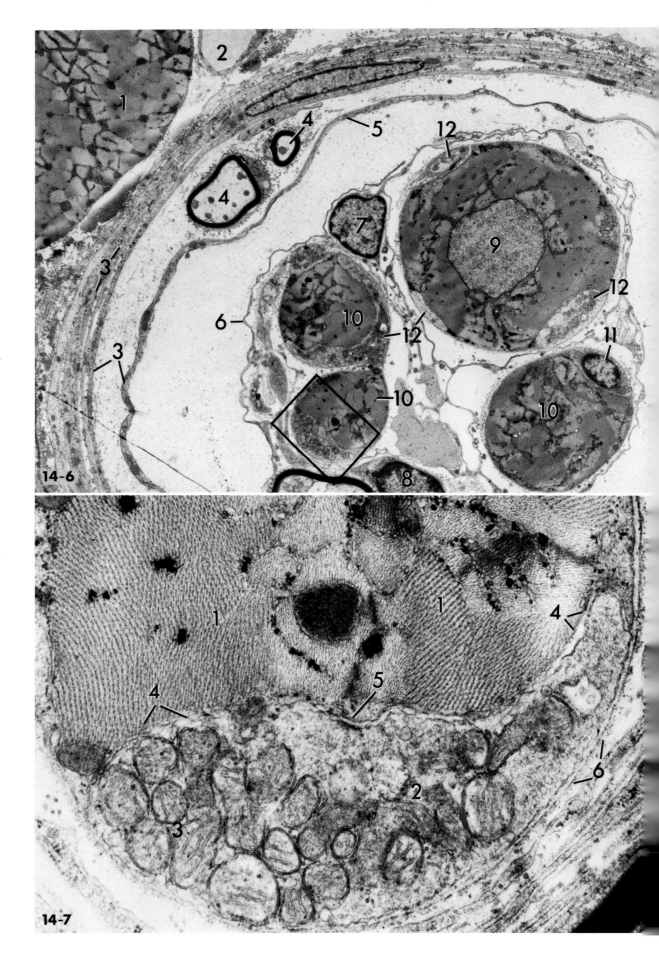

Fig. 14-6. Neuromuscular spindle. Cross section. Juxta-equatorial region. Enlargement of rectangle in Fig. 14-5. E.M. X 4500. **1.** Part of extrafusal muscle fiber. **2.** Lumen of capillary. **3.** Sheet-like cells of outer capsule. **4.** Myelinated nerve fibers. **5.** Periaxial space. **6.** Inner capsule. **7.** Nucleus of fibroblast. **8.** Nucleus of Schwann cell. **9.** Nucleus of nuclear bag fiber. **10.** Polar ends of nuclear chain fibers. **11.** Satellite muscle cell. **12.** Sensory nerve endings.

Fig. 14-7. Sensory nerve ending. Neuromuscular spindle. Enlargement of rectangle in Fig. 14-6. E.M. X 60,000. **1.** Myofilaments of intrafusal nuclear chain muscle fiber. **2.** Sensory nerve ending. **3.** Mitochondria. **4.** Membranous contact between sarcolemma and cell membrane of nerve ending. **5.** Zonula adhaerens junction. **6.** External (basal) lamina.

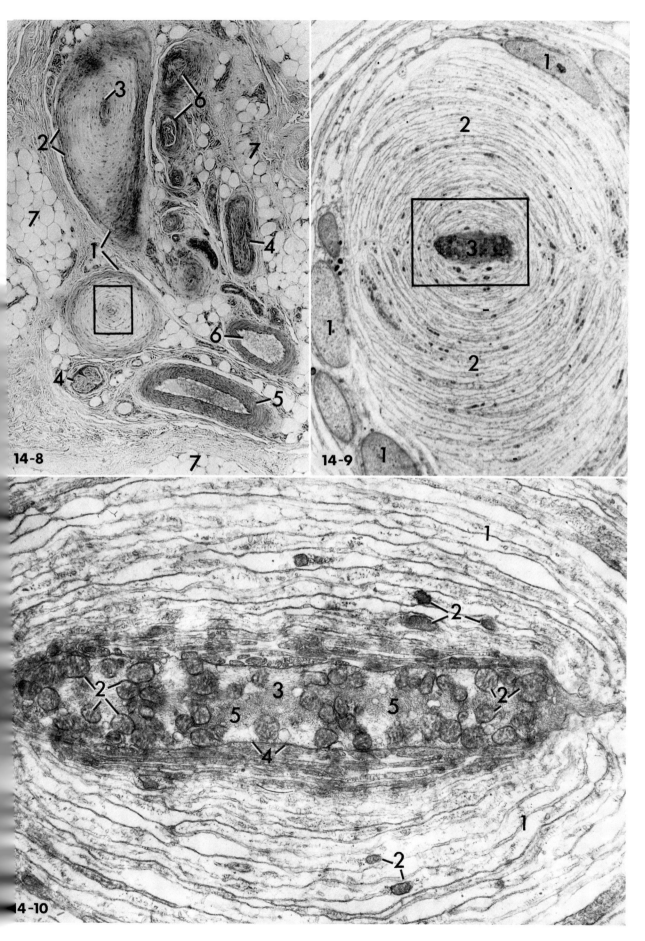

Fig. 14-8. Hypodermal region. Skin of palm of hand. Human. L.M. X 56. **1.** Pacinian corpuscles. **2.** Outer part. **3.** Central core. **4.** Bundle of nerve fibers. **5.** Artery. **6.** Veins. **7.** Adipose tissue.

Fig. 14-9. Pacini's corpuscle. Cross section. Central core. Enlargement of area similar to rectangle in Fig. 14-8. Pancreas. Cat. E.M. X 1800. **1.** Nuclei of flattened fibroblasts in outer part of corpuscle. **2.** Cytoplasmic lamellae of central core. **3.** Nerve fiber.

Fig. 14-10. Pacini's corpuscle. Cross section. Central core and nerve ending. Enlargement of area similar to rectangle in Fig. 14-9. Pancreas. Cat. E.M. X 16,000. **1.** Interdigitating lamellar cell processes of inner core. **2.** Mitochondria. **3.** Nerve ending. **4.** Cell membrane of nerve process. **5.** Neurofilaments.

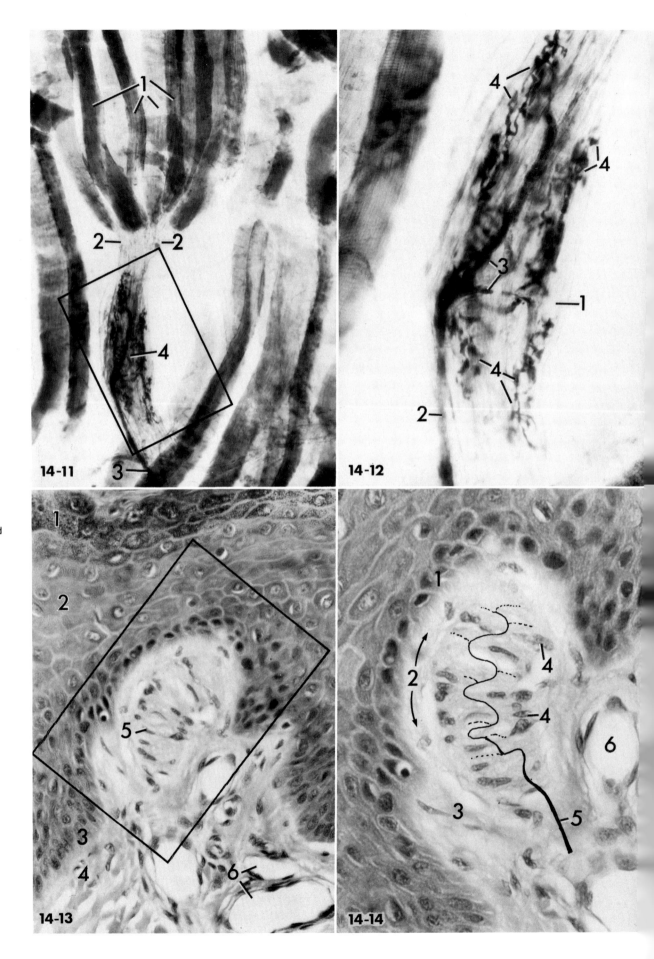

Fig. 14-11. Golgi tendon organ. Teased skeletal muscle. Impregnation method. Rat. L.M. X 154. **1.** Striated skeletal muscle fibers (cells). **2.** Muscle-tendon junction. **3.** Peripheral (sensory) nerve fiber. **4.** Arborization of nerve termination (tendon organ).

Fig. 14-12. Golgi tendon organ. Enlargement of rectangle in Fig. 14-11. L.M. X 418. **1.** Tendon. **2.** Peripheral (sensory) nerve fiber. **3.** Branching of nerve fiber. **4.** Terminal arborization of nerve fiber with club-shaped endings.

Fig. 14-13. Meissner's corpuscle. Skin. Human. L.M. X 385. **1.** Stratum granulosum of epidermis. **2.** Stratum spinosum. **3.** Stratum basale of epidermis. **4.** Papillary layer of dermis. **5.** Meissner's corpuscle. **6.** Dermal capillaries and venules.

Fig. 14-14. Meissner's corpuscle. Enlargement of rectangle in Fig. 14-13. L.M. X 600. **1.** Stratum basale of epidermis. **2.** Level of basal lamina. **3.** Connective tissue of dermal papillary layer. **4.** Nuclei of flat, transversely stacked fibroblasts. **5.** Distribution of terminal arborization of nerve fiber indicated by solid and dotted lines. **6.** Capillary.

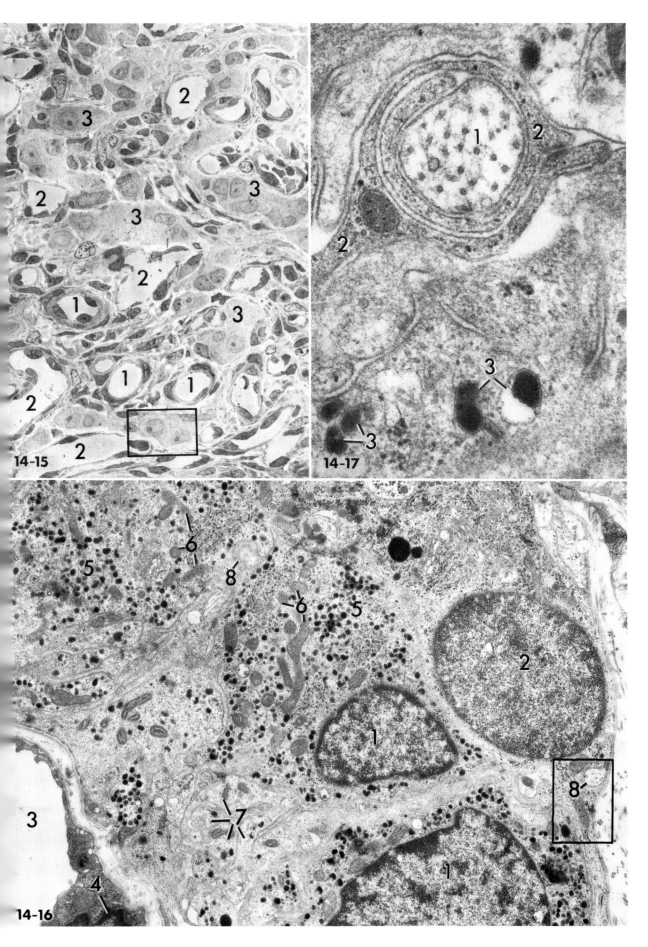

Fig. 14-15. Carotid body. Rat. E.M. X 640.
1. Lumen of small arteriole. **2.** Lumen of capillary. **3.** Glomus cells.

Fig. 14-16. Carotid body. Glomus cells. Enlargement of area similar to rectangle in Fig. 14-15. Rat. E.M. × 9000. **1.** Nucleus of type I glomus cell (chief cell). **2.** Nucleus of type II glomus cell (supporting cell.) **3.** Lumen of capillary. **4.** Nucleus of endothelial cell. **5.** Dense-core granules. **6.** Mitochondria. **7.** Effector type (motor) nerve processes with dense-core vesicles. **8.** Sensory type nerve process.

Fig. 14-17. Detail of glomus cells. Carotid body. Enlargement of area similar to rectangle in Fig. 14-16. Rat. E.M. X 58,000. **1.** Sensory type nerve fiber with microtubules. **2.** Cytoplasmic processes of type II glomus cell, encircling nerve fiber. **3.** Dense-core granules of type I glomus cell.

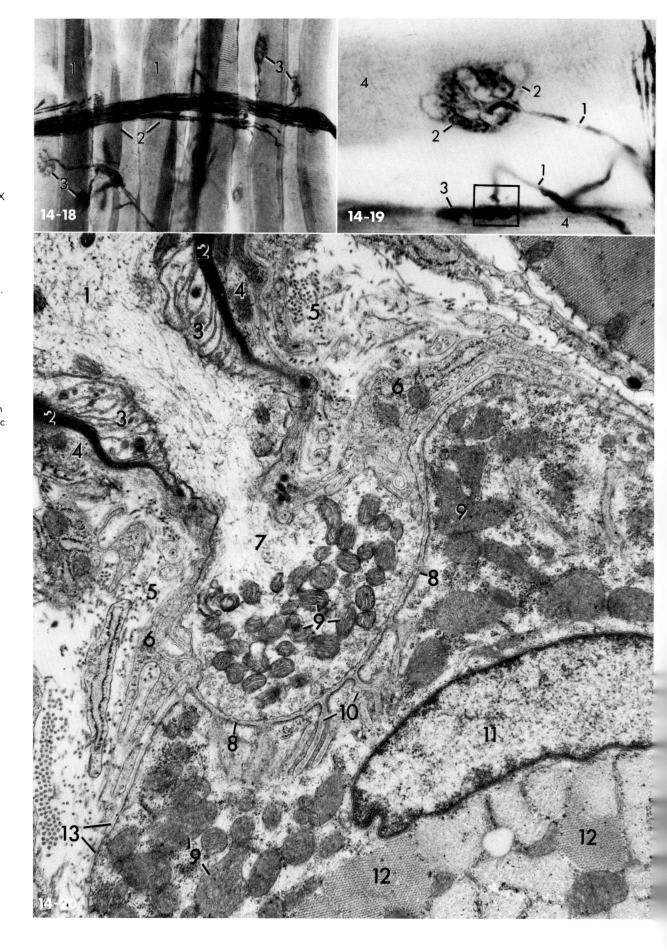

Fig. 14-18. Motor nerve endings. Skeletal muscle. Gold chloride method. Human. L.M. X 200. **1.** Striated muscle fibers. **2.** Bundle of myelinated nerve fibers. **3.** Motor end plates.

Fig. 14-19. Motor end plates. Gold chloride method. Skeletal muscle. Human. L.M. X 600. **1.** Efferent nerve fibers. **2.** Motor end plate in surface view. **3.** Motor end plate in side view. **4.** Striated skeletal muscle fibers.

Fig. 14-20. Motor end plate. Skeletal muscle. Enlargement of area approximately similar to rectangle in Fig. 14-19. Rat. E.M. X 30,000. **1.** Efferent nerve process (axon). **2.** Myelin sheath. **3.** Successive laminae of the myelin sheath terminate as cytoplasmic swellings. **4.** Cytoplasm of Schwann cell (neurolemma). **5.** Endoneurial connective tissue. **6.** Cytoplasm of teloglial cell (Schwann cell). **7.** Axon terminal (end knob). **8.** Synaptic trough (recess). **9.** Mitochondria. **10.** Subneural, synaptic clefts. **11.** Nucleus of skeletal muscle cell. **12.** Myofibrils. **13.** External (basal) lamina.

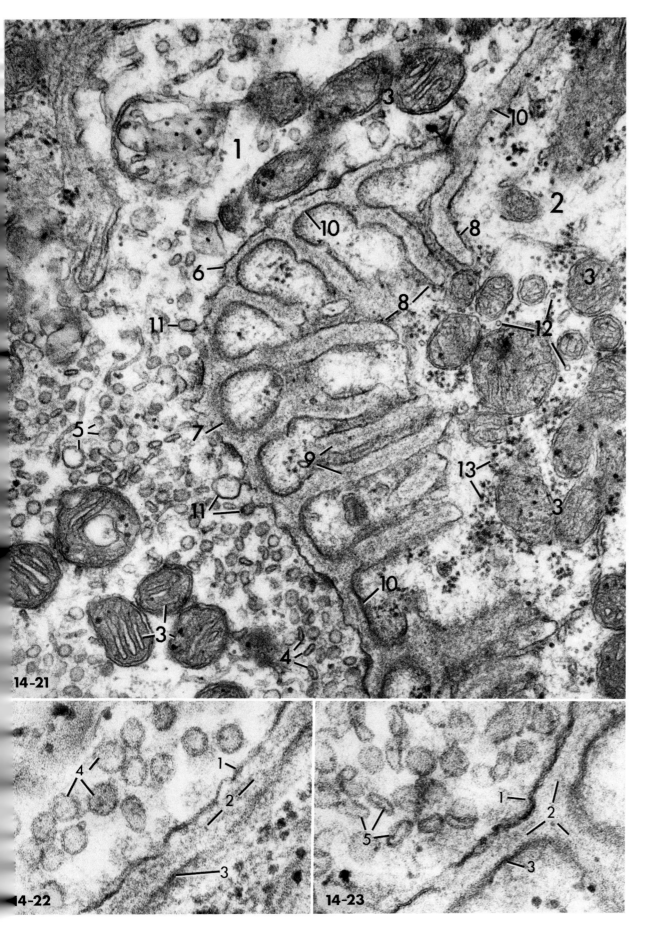

Fig. 14-21. Detail of motor end plate. Skeletal muscle. Rat. E.M. X 60,000. **1.** Axon terminal. **2.** Cytoplasm of muscle cell (sole plate). **3.** Mitochondria. **4.** Flat synaptic vesicles. **5.** Round synaptic vesicles. **6.** Presynaptic membrane. **7.** Synaptic cleft with glycoprotein material. **8.** Postsynaptic, junctional folds. **9.** Subneural primary and secondary clefts. **10.** Postsynaptic sarcolemma. **11.** Synaptic vesicles fusing with presynaptic membrane. **12.** Microtubules. **13.** Ribosomes.

Figs. 14-22 & 14-23. Detail of synaptic junctions of motor end plate. Skeletal muscle. Rat. E.M. X 124,000. **1.** Presynaptic cell membrane of axon terminal. **2.** Synaptic cleft. **3.** Postsynaptic sarcolemma. **4.** Round (excitatory?) electron-lucent, synaptic vesicles, bounded by a delicate, trilaminar membrane. **5.** Flat (inhibitory?) synaptic vesicles.

14-21

14-22

14-23

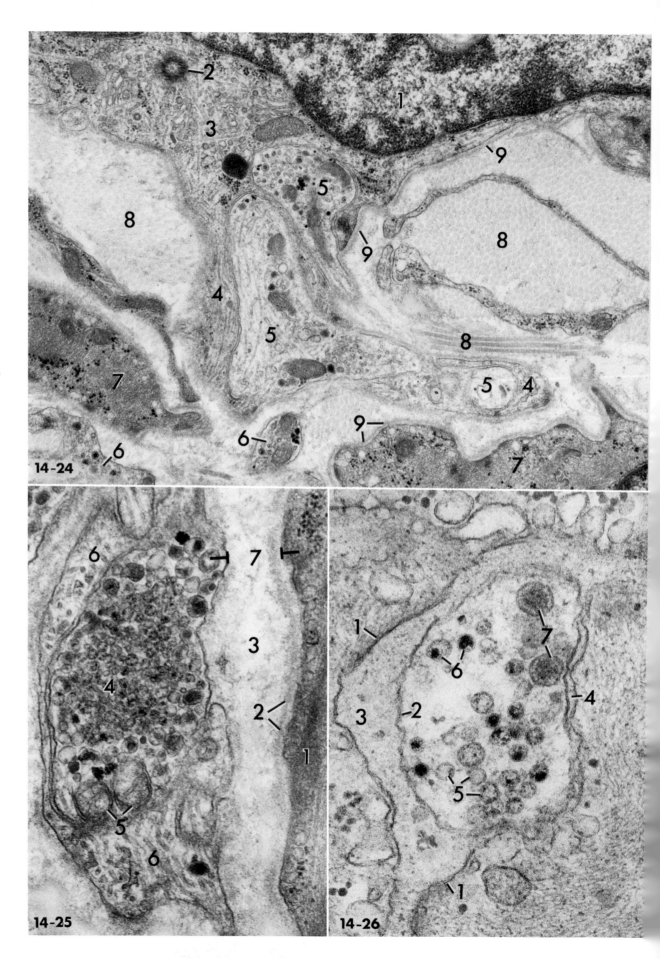

Fig. 14-24. Vasomotor nerve endings. Large helicine arteriole. Corpus cavernosum penis. Rat. E.M. X 31,000. **1.** Nucleus of Schwann cell. **2.** Centriole. **3.** Microtubules. **4.** Schwann cell cytoplasm. **5.** Sympathetic (adrenergic) nerve endings. **6.** Denuded adrenergic nerve endings. **7.** Cytoplasm of vascular smooth muscle cells. **8.** Collagenous fibrils. **9.** External (basal) lamina.

Fig. 14-25. Sympathetic (adrenergic) vasomotor nerve ending. Helicine arteriole. Corpus cavernosum penis. Rat. E.M. X 60,000. **1.** Vascular smooth muscle cell. **2.** External lamina. **3.** Perivascular connective tissue space. **4.** Adrenergic axon terminal with numerous small, granulated (dense-core) vesicles and some large granulated (dense-core) vesicles. **5.** Mitochondria. **6.** Schwann cell cytoplasm with microtubules. **7.** Minimum diffusion gap between axolemma and sarcolemma (indicated by T-bars) is 0.27 μ in this section.

Fig. 14-26. Myoneural junction. Smooth muscle. Ductus deferens. Rat. E.M. X 90,000. **1.** Sarcolemma of smooth muscle cells. **2.** Axolemma of sympathetic nerve ending. **3.** Intercellular space. **4.** Myoneural junction; intercellular space 175 Å. **5.** Clear vesicles. **6.** Small granulated vesicles. **7.** Large granulated vesicles.

References

Adal, M. N. The fine structure of the sensory region of cat muscle spindles. J. Ultrastruct. Res. 26: 332–354 (1969).

Abbott, C. P. and Howe, A. Ultrastructure of aortic body tissue in the cat. Acta Anat. 81: 609–619 (1972).

Andersson-Cedergren, E. Ultrastructure of motor endplate and sarcoplasmic components of mouse skeletal muscle fiber. J. Ultrastruct. Res. Suppl. 1, 1959.

Banker, B. Q. and Girvin, J. P. The ultrastructural features of the mammalian muscle spindle. J. Neuropath. Exp. Neurol. 30: 155–195 (1971).

Biscoe, T. J. and Stehbens, W. E. Ultrastructure of the carotid body. J. Cell Biol. 30: 563–578 (1966).

Böck, P., Stockinger, L. and Vyslonzil, E. Die Feinstruktur des Glomus caroticum beim Menschen. Z. Zellforsch. 105: 543–568 (1970).

Bridgman, C. F. The structure of tendon organs in the cat: a proposed mechanism for responding to muscle tension. Anat. Rec. 162: 209–220 (1968).

Cauna, N. and Ross, L. L. The fine structure of Meissner's touch corpuscles of human fingers. J. Biophys. Biochem. Cytol. 8: 467–482 (1960).

Cauna, N. Structure of digital touch corpuscles. Acta Anat. 32: 1–23 (1958).

Cauna, N. The mode of termination of the sensory nerves and its significance. J. Comp. Neurol. 113: 169–210 (1959).

Chiba, T. and Yamauchi, A. On the fine structure of the nerve terminals in the human myocardium. Z. Zellforsch. 108: 324–338 (1970).

Coërs, C. Structure and organization of the myoneural junction. Int. Rev. Cytol. 22: 239–268 (1967).

Coleridge, H. M., Coleridge, J. C. G. and Howe, A. Thoracic chemoreceptors in the dog. A histological and electrophysiological study of the location, innervation and blood supply of the aortic bodies. Circ. Res. 26: 235–247 (1970).

Devine, C. E. and Simpson, F. O. The fine structure of vascular sympathetic neuromuscular contacts in the rat. Am. J. Anat. 121: 153–174 (1967).

Edwards, C., Heath, D. and Harris, P. Ultrastructure of the carotid body in high-altitude guinea-pigs. J. Path. 107: 131–136 (1971).

Geffin, L. B., Livett, B. G. and Rush, R. A. Transmitter economy of sympathetic neurons. Circ. Res. 26: Suppl. II, 33–39 (1970).

Hökfelt, T. Distribution of noradrenaline storing particles in peripheral adrenergic neurons as revealed by electron microscopy. Acta Physiol. Scand. 76: 427–440 (1969).

Iggo, A. and Muir, A. R. The structure and function of a slowly adapting touch corpuscle in hairy skin. J. Physiol. 200: 763–796 (1969).

Levy, J. H. Development of the neuromuscular spindle in the rat: light and electron microscopy. Ph.D. Thesis 1972. Graduate School of Basic Medical Science. New York Medical College, Valhalla, N.Y. 10595.

Morita, E., Chiocchio, S. R. and Tramezzani, J. H. Four types of main cells in the carotid body of the cat. J. Ultrastruct. Res. 28: 399–410 (1969).

Niedorf, H. R., Rode, J. and Blümcke, S. Feinstruktur und Catecholamingehalt des Glomus caroticum der Ratte nach einmaliger Reserpin-injektion. Virchows Arch., Part B, Zellpath. 5: 113–123 (1970).

Ovalle, W. K., Jr. Fine structure of rat intrafusal muscle fibers. The polar region. J. Cell Biol. 51: 83–103 (1971).

Ovalle, W. K., Jr. Motor nerve terminals on rat intrafusal muscle fibers, a correlated light and electron microscopic study. J. Anat. 111: 239–252 (1972).

Ovalle, W. K., Jr. Fine structure of rat intrafusal muscle fibers. The equatorial region. J. Cell Biol. 52: 382–396 (1972).

Padykula, H. A. and Gauthier, G. F. The ultrastructure of the neuromuscular junctions of mammalian red, white and intermediate skeletal muscle fibers. J. Cell Biol. 46: 27–41 (1970).

Pick, J. Fine structure of nerve terminals in the human gut. Anat. Rec. 159: 131–145 (1967).

Quilliam, T. A. and Armstrong, J. Mechanoreceptors. Endeavour, 22: 55–60 (1963).

Rees, P. M. The distribution of biogenic amines in the carotid bifurcation region. J. Physiol. 193: 245–253 (1967).

Rees, P. M. Observations on the fine structure and distribution of presumptive baroreceptor nerves at the carotid sinus. J. Comp. Neurol. 131: 517–548 (1967).

Richardson, K. C. The fine structure of autonomic nerve endings in smooth muscle of the rat vas deferens. J. Anat. 96: 427–442 (1962).

Rumpelt, H.-J. and Schmalbruch, H. Zur Morphologie der Bauelements von Muskelspindeln bei Mensch und Ratte. Z. Zellforsch. 102: 601–630 (1969).

Scalzi, H. A. and Price, H. M. The arrangement and sensory innervation of the intrafusal fibers in the feline muscle spindle. J. Ultrastruct. Res. 36: 375–390 (1971).

Shuangshoti, S. and Netsky, M. G. Human choroid plexus: morphologic and histochemical alterations with age. Am. J. Anat. 128: 73–96 (1970).

Yates, R. D., Chen, I. and Duncan, D. Effects of sinus nerve stimulation on carotid body glomus cells. J. Cell Biol. 46: 544–552 (1970).

15 Nervous tissue— non-neural structures

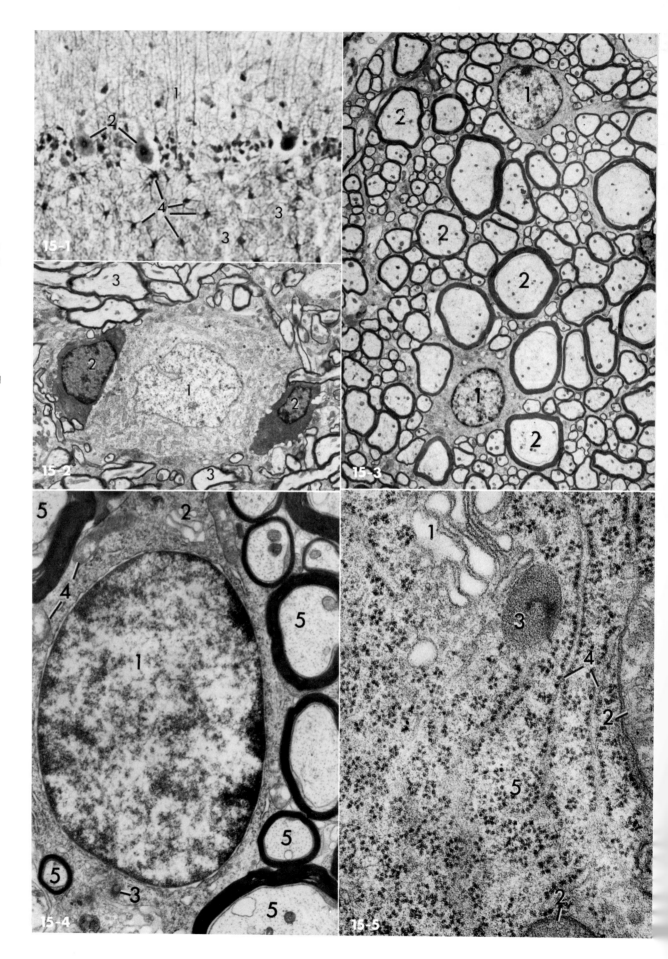

Fig. 15-1. Neuroglial cells. Cerebellar cortex. Impregnation method. Cat. L.M. X 242. **1.** Molecular layer. **2.** Purkinje nerve cells. **3.** Granule cell layer. **4.** Neuroglial cells.

Fig. 15-2. Oligodendrocytes. Gray matter. Spinal cord. Rat. E.M. X 1800. **1.** Nucleus of neuron in anterior horn. **2.** Nuclei of perineuronal (satellite) oligodendrocytes. **3.** Myelinated nerves.

Fig. 15-3. Oligodendroycytes. White matter. Spinal cord. Cross section. Rat. E.M. X 1800. **1.** Nuclei of interfascicular oligodendrocytes. **2.** Myelinated nerve processes of varied diameters.

Fig. 15-4. Oligodendrocyte. White matter. Spinal cord. Cross section. Rat. E.M. X 9000. **1.** Nucleus of oligodendrocyte. **2.** Golgi zone. **3.** Centriole. **4.** Mitochondria. **5.** Myelinated nerve processes. Sheet-like processes of the oligodendrocytes form the myelin sheaths of the central nervous system.

Fig. 15-5. Detail of oligodendrocyte. Gray matter. Spinal cord. Rat. E.M. X 62,000. **1.** Golgi zone. **2.** Mitochondria. **3.** Lysosome. **4.** Cisternae of granular endoplasmic reticulum. **5.** Polyribosomes and monoribosomes in electron-dense cytoplasm.

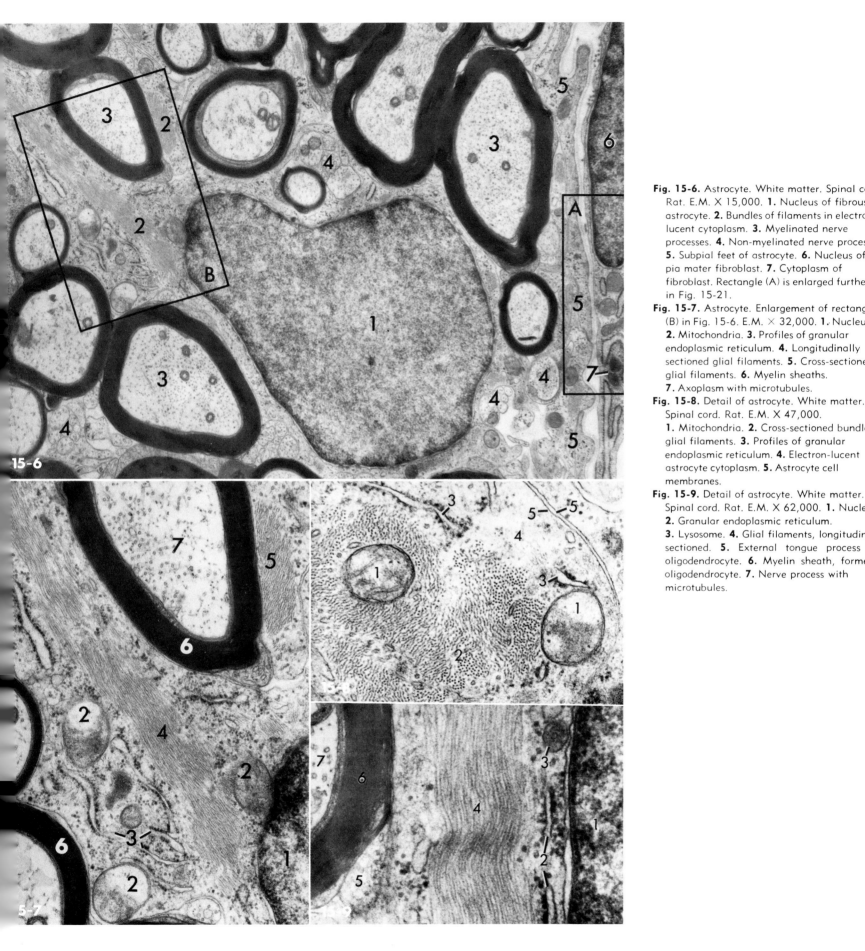

Fig. 15-6. Astrocyte. White matter. Spinal cord. Rat. E.M. X 15,000. **1.** Nucleus of fibrous astrocyte. **2.** Bundles of filaments in electron-lucent cytoplasm. **3.** Myelinated nerve processes. **4.** Non-myelinated nerve processes. **5.** Subpial feet of astrocyte. **6.** Nucleus of pia mater fibroblast. **7.** Cytoplasm of fibroblast. Rectangle (A) is enlarged further in Fig. 15-21.

Fig. 15-7. Astrocyte. Enlargement of rectangle (B) in Fig. 15-6. E.M. X 32,000. **1.** Nucleus. **2.** Mitochondria. **3.** Profiles of granular endoplasmic reticulum. **4.** Longitudinally sectioned glial filaments. **5.** Cross-sectioned glial filaments. **6.** Myelin sheaths. **7.** Axoplasm with microtubules.

Fig. 15-8. Detail of astrocyte. White matter. Spinal cord. Rat. E.M. X 47,000. **1.** Mitochondria. **2.** Cross-sectioned bundles of glial filaments. **3.** Profiles of granular endoplasmic reticulum. **4.** Electron-lucent astrocyte cytoplasm. **5.** Astrocyte cell membranes.

Fig. 15-9. Detail of astrocyte. White matter. Spinal cord. Rat. E.M. X 62,000. **1.** Nucleus. **2.** Granular endoplasmic reticulum. **3.** Lysosome. **4.** Glial filaments, longitudinally sectioned. **5.** External tongue process of oligodendrocyte. **6.** Myelin sheath, formed by oligodendrocyte. **7.** Nerve process with microtubules.

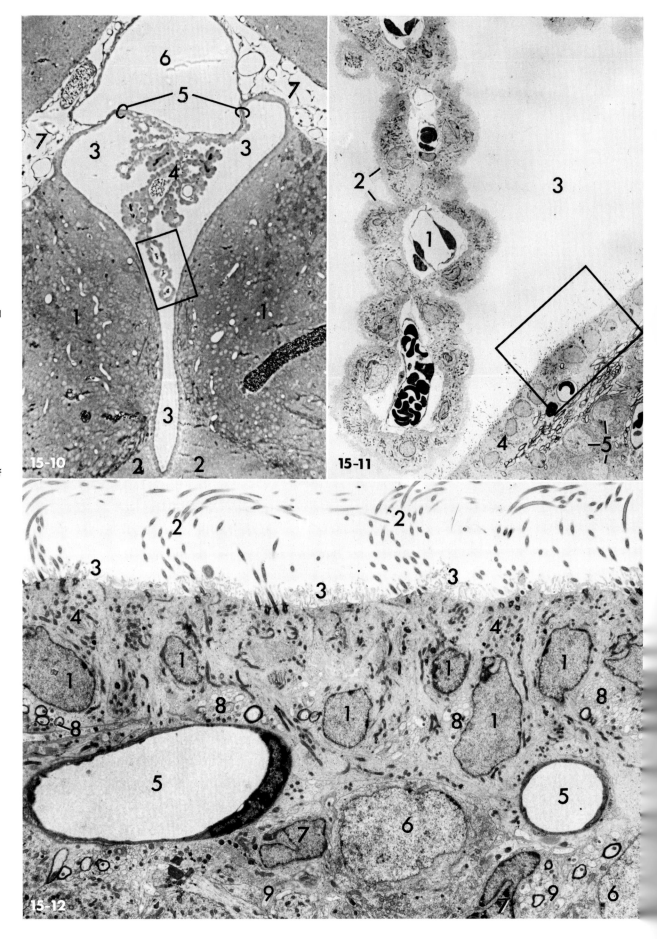

Fig. 15-10. Diencephalon. Frontal section. Rat. L.M. X 134. **1.** Thalamus. **2.** Hypothalamus. **3.** Third ventricle. **4.** Choroid plexus. **5.** Roof of third ventricle (tela choroidea: pia mater + ependyma). **6.** Venous sinus. **7.** Arachnoid.

Fig. 15-11. Choroid plexus. Enlargement of area indicated by rectangle in Fig. 15-10. E.M. X 640. **1.** Capillaries of choroid plexus with erythrocytes. **2.** Single layer of modified, non-ciliated ependymal cells. **3.** Third ventricle. **4.** Single layer of ciliated ependymal cells lining the third ventricle. **5.** Neurons of thalamus.

Fig. 15-12. Ependyma. Third ventricle. Enlargement of area similar to rectangle in Fig. 15-11. Rat. E.M. X 2100. **1.** Nuclei of ependymal cells. **2.** Cilia. **3.** Microvilli. **4.** Mitochondria. **5.** Lumen of capillary. **6.** Nuclei of neurons in thalamus. **7.** Nuclei of neuroglial cells. **8.** Myelinated and non-myelinated nerve processes border directly on the basal cell membrane of the ependymal cells. No basal lamina present. **9.** Neuropil of the thalamus.

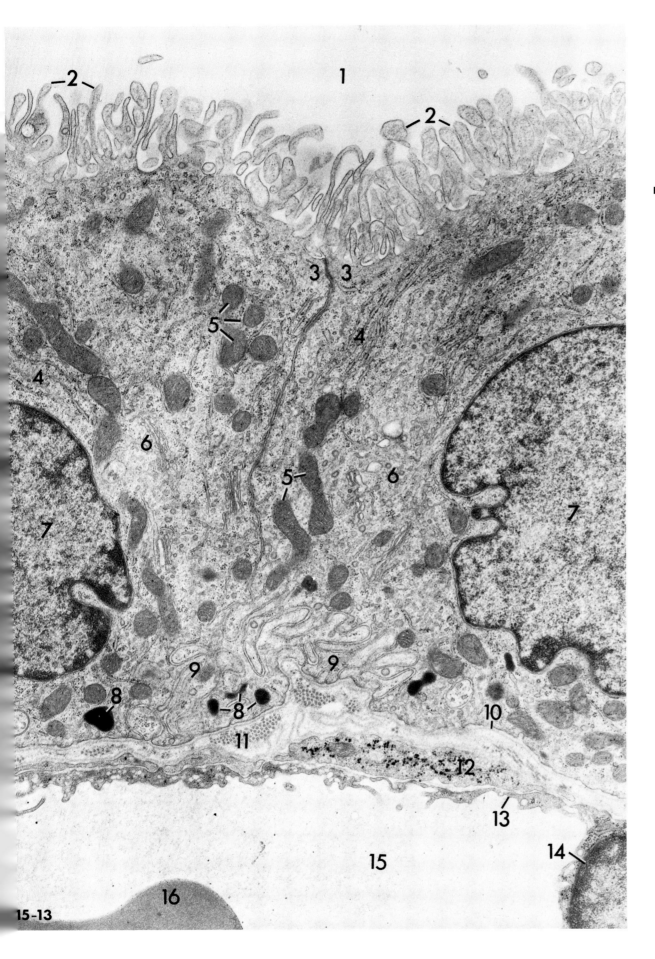

Fig. 15-13. Details of choroid plexus. Ependymal cells of the modified type that covers the vascular tufts of the choroid plexus. Diencephalon. Third ventricle. Rat. E.M. X 13,000. **1.** Third ventricle. **2.** Bulbous microvilli. **3.** Junctional specialization of apposing cell membranes. **4.** Profiles of granular endoplasmic reticulum. **5.** Mitochondria. **6.** Golgi zone. **7.** Nuclei. **8.** Lysosomes. **9.** Infolded and interdigitated basal cell membranes. **10.** Basal lamina. **11.** Pial connective tissue fibrils. **12.** Pericyte. **13.** Fenestrated thin endothelium. **14.** Nucleus of endothelial cell. **15.** Lumen of capillary. **16.** Erythrocyte.

15-13

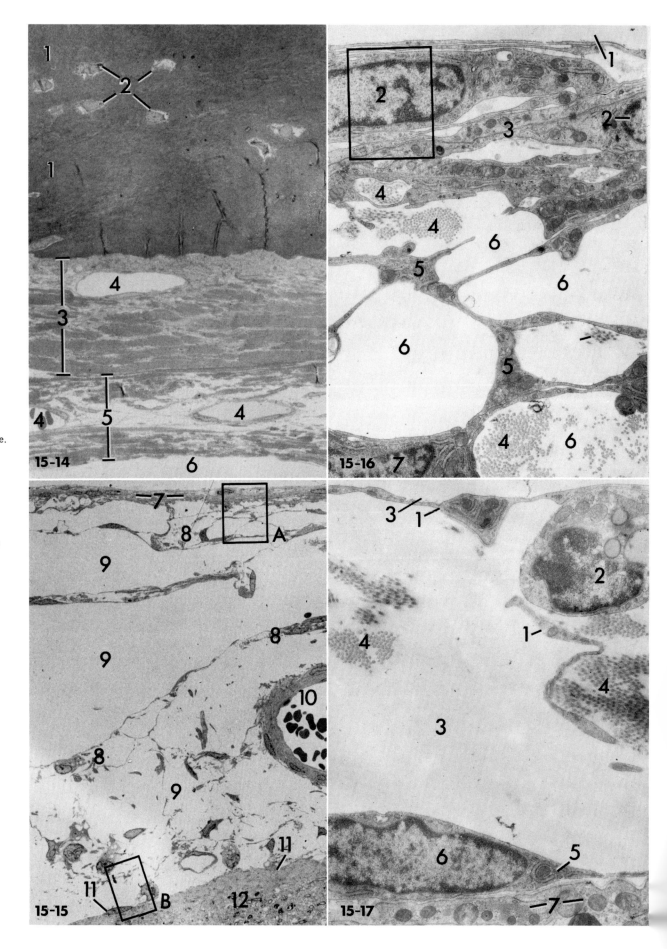

Figs. 15-14 & 15-15. Architecture of meninges. Survey. Parietal region. Frontal section. Kitten. E.M. X 640. **1.** Matrix of parietal bone. **2.** Osteocytes in bone lacunae. **3.** Outer layer of dura mater (= inner periosteum). **4.** Blood vessels. **5.** Inner layer of dura mater. **6.** Subdural space filled with lymph. **7.** Cellular membrane of arachnoid. **8.** Arachnoid trabeculae. **9.** Arachnoid space filled with cerebrospinal fluid. **10.** Small artery ("pial" blood vessel). **11.** Pia mater. **12.** Cortical nervous tissue of cerebral hemisphere.

Fig. 15-16. Arachnoid. Enlargement of area similar to rectangle (A) in Fig. 15-15. Parietal region. Kitten. E.M. X 9000. **1.** Subdural space. **2.** Nuclei of fibroblasts. **3.** Flat processes of cells forming the arachnoid cellular membrane. **4.** Bundles of collagenous fibrils. **5.** Arachnoid trabeculae. **6.** Arachnoid space. **7.** Nucleus of trabecular fibroblast.

Fig. 15-17. Pia-arachnoid membrane. Enlargement of area similar to rectangle (B) in Fig. 15-15. Parietal region. Kitten. E.M. X 9000. **1.** Arachnoid trabeculae. **2.** Nucleus of macrophage. **3.** Arachnoid space. **4.** Collagenous fibrils. **5.** Fibroblast of pial membrane. **6.** Nucleus. **7.** Subpial astroglial feet.

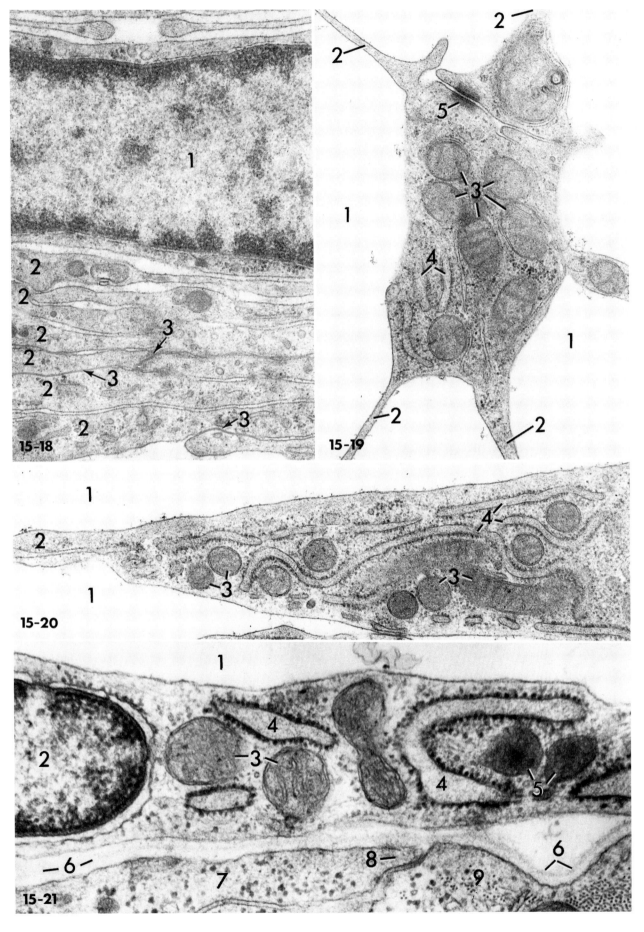

Fig. 15-18. Detail of arachnoid cellular membrane. Enlargement of area similar to rectangle in Fig. 15-16. Parietal region. Kitten. E.M. X 31,000. **1.** Nucleus of fibroblast. **2.** Many closely apposed, delicate, squamous fibroblasts make up the arachnoid membrane. **3.** Gap-junctions.

Fig. 15-19 & 15-20. Arachnoid trabecular fibroblasts. Parietal region. Kitten. E.M. X 31,000. **1.** Arachnoid space. **2.** Slender cell processes. **3.** Mitochondria. **4.** Cisternae of granular endoplasmic reticulum. **5.** Desmosome.

Fig. 15-21. Pia-glial membrane. Enlargement of rectangle (A) in Fig. 15-6. Spinal cord. Rat. E.M. X 62,000. **1.** Arachnoid space. **2.** Nucleus of pial fibroblast. **3.** Mitochondria. **4.** Cisternae of granular endoplasmic reticulum. **5.** Lysosomes. **6.** External (basal) lamina of the brain tissue of the central nervous system. **7.** Astrocytic cytoplasm of subpial feet. **8.** Gap-junction. **9.** Astrocytic filaments.

Fig. 15-22. Pia-arachnoid blood vessels. Cerebral cortex. Rat. E.M. X 600. **1.** Arachnoid space. **2.** Pial membrane. **3.** Small pial artery; lumen 70 μ. **4.** Arteriole entering the molecular layer of the cerebral cortex; lumen 25 μ. **5.** Small pial venule; lumen 40 μ. **6.** Brain capillary; lumen 5 μ. **7.** Molecular layer of cerebral cortex.

Fig. 15-23. Pia-arachnoid blood vessels. Enlargement of rectangle in Fig. 15-22. E.M. X 1500. **1.** Arachnoid space. **2.** Arachnoid macrophage. **3.** Nuclei of pial fibroblasts. **4.** Wall of arteriole; thickness 5 μ. **5.** Smooth muscle cell. **6.** Elastic membrane. **7.** Endothelium. **8.** Nucleus of astrocyte. **9.** Molecular layer of cerebral cortex. **10.** Small arteriole; lumen 25 μ.

Fig. 15-24. Topography of perivascular space in the brain tissue. Enlargement of area similar to rectangle in Fig. 15-23. Cerebral cortex. Rat. E.M. X 60,000. **1.** Lumen of arteriole; 25 μ. **2.** Endothelial cytoplasm. **3.** Tight junction. **4.** Basal lamina. **5.** Smooth muscle cells. **6.** External lamina of smooth muscle cells. **7.** Pial fibroblast. **8.** Subpial collagenous fibrils. **9.** Subpial astrocytic feet. **10.** Junctional specializations of apposed cell membranes of the glial feet.

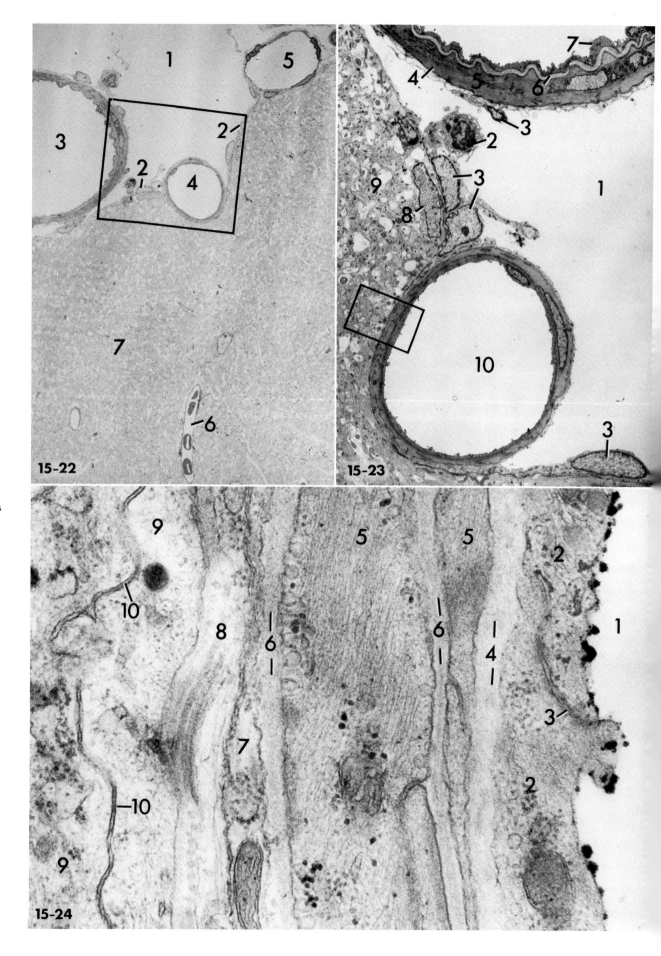

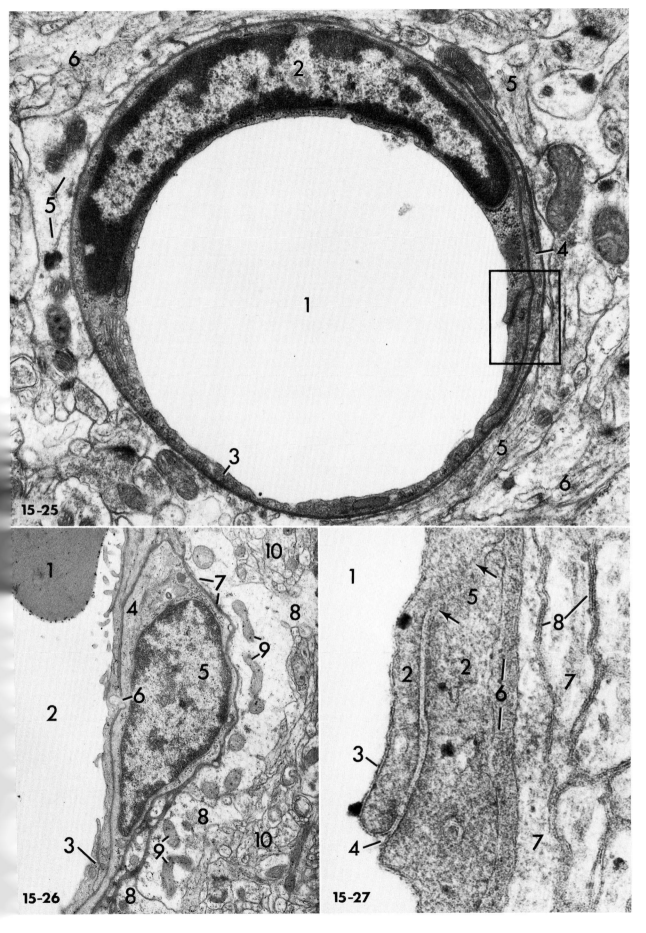

Fig. 15-25. Brain capillary. Molecular layer. Cerebral cortex. Rat. E.M. × 21,500.
1. Lumen; 5 μ. **2.** Nucleus of endothelial cell. **3.** Non-fenestrated, continuous endothelium. **4.** Pericytic process. **5.** Perivascular feet of astrocytes. **6.** Neuropil.

Fig. 15-26. Brain capillary. Molecular layer. Cerebral cortex. Rat. E.M. X 8400.
1. Erythrocyte. **2.** Capillary lumen; 8 μ. **3.** Endothelium. **4.** Cytoplasm of pericyte. **5.** Nucleus. **6.** Endothelial-pericytic junction. **7.** Basal lamina. **8.** Glial perivascular feet of astrocytes. **9.** Mitochondria. **10.** Neuropil of molecular layer of cerebral cortex.

Fig. 15-27. Blood-brain barrier. Brain capillary. Enlargement of area similar to rectangle in Fig. 15-25. Molecular layer. Cerebral cortex. Rat. E.M. X 120,000.
1. Capillary lumen. **2.** Overlapping endothelial processes. **3.** Trilaminar endothelial cell membrane. **4.** Tight junction (= fusion of outer leaflets of apposing cell membranes). **5.** Cell membranes sectioned obliquely between arrows. **6.** Basal lamina. **7.** Perivascular astroglial end-feet. **8.** Junctional specialization: gap-junctions.

References

Baron, M. and Gallego, A. The relation of the microglia with the pericytes in the cat cerebral cortex. Z. Zellforsch. *128*: 42–57 (1972).

Blakemore, W. F. The ultrastructure of the subependymal plate in the rat. J. Anat. *104*: 423–433 (1969).

Bondareff, W. and McLone, D. G. The external glial limiting membrane in Macaca: ultrastructure of a laminated glioepithelium. Am. J. Anat. *136*: 277–296 (1973).

Brightman, M. W. and Paley, S. L. The fine structure of ependyma in the brain of the rat. J. Cell Biol. *19*: 415–439 (1963).

Brightman, M. W. and Reese, T. S. Junctions between intimately apposed cell membranes in the vertebrate brain. J. Cell Biol. *40*: 648–677 (1969).

Bunge, R. Glial cells and the central myelin sheath. Physiol. Rev. *48*: 197–251 (1968).

Cammermeyer, J. Morphologic distinctions between oligodendrocytes and microglia cells in the rabbit cerebral cortex. Am. J. Anat. *118*: 227–248 (1966).

Cancilla, P. A., Baker, R. N., Pollock, P. S. and Frommes, S. P. The reaction of pericytes of the central nervous system to exogenous protein. Lab. Investig. *26*: 376–383 (1972).

Cserr, H. F. Physiology of the choroid plexus. Physiol. Rev. *51*: 273–311 (1971).

Davson, H. Physiology of the Cerebrospinal Fluid. Little, Brown, Boston, 1967.

Frederickson, R. G. and Low, F. N. Blood vessels and tissue space associated with the brain of the rat. Am. J. Anat. *125*: 123–146 (1969).

Himango, W. A. and Low, F. N. The fine structure of a lateral recess of the subarachnoid space in rat. Anat. Rec. *171*: 1–20 (1971).

Hirano, A. and Zimmerman, H. M. Some new cytological observations of the normal rat ependymal cell. Anat. Rec. *158*: 293–302 (1967).

Hydén, H. and Pigon, A. A cytophysiological study of the functional relationship between oligodendroglial cells of Deiters' nucleus. J. Neurochem. *6*: 57–72 (1960).

Jones, E. G. On the mode of entry of blood vessels into the cerebral cortex. J. Anat. *106*: 507–520 (1970).

Kruger, L. and Maxwell, D. S. Electron microscopy of oligodendrocytes in normal rat cerebrum. Am. J. Anat. *118*: 411–436 (1966).

Kuffler, S. W. and Nicholls, J. G. The physiology of neuroglial cells. Ergebn. Physiol. *57*: 1–90 (1966).

McCabe, J. S. and Low, F. N. The subarachnoid angle: an area of transition in peripheral nerve. Anat. Rec. *164*: 15–34 (1969).

Morse, D. E. and Low, F. N. The fine structure of the pia mater of the rat. Am. J. Anat. *133*: 349–368 (1972).

Millhouse, O. E. Light and electron microscopic studies of the ventricular wall. Z. Zellforsch. *127*: 149–174 (1972).

Nakai, J. Morphology of Neuroglia. C. C. Thomas, Springfield, Ill., 1963.

Peters, A. Anatomical considerations of the site of the blood-brain barrier. J. Anat. *95* (suppl): 20–22 (1961).

Pease, D. C. and Schultz, R. L. Electron microscopy of rat cranial meninges. Am. J. Anat. *102*: 301–313 (1958).

Vaughn, J. E. and Peters, A. Electron microscopy of the early postnatal development of fibrous astrocytes. Am. J. Anat. *121*: 131–152 (1967).

16 Cardiovascular system

Fig. 16-1. Schematic drawing of human heart. For simplicity, aorta and arteria pulmonalis are not shown. **1.** Right atrium. **2.** Left atrium. **3.** Right ventricle. **4.** Left ventricle. **5.** Venae cavae. **6.** Pulmonary veins. **7.** Right artioventricular valve (tricuspid). **8.** Left atrioventricular valve (bicuspid). **9.** Interatrial septum. **10.** Interventricular septum. **11.** SA-node. **12.** AV-node. **13.** AV-bundle. **14.** Right and left branches of impulse-conducting system. **15.** Terminal ramifications.

Fig. 16-2. Part of atrial and ventricular wall. Corresponds to area indicated by rectangle (A) in Fig. 16-1. Heart. Monkey. L.M. X 7. **1.** Wall of atrium, 1 mm thick. **2.** Wall of ventricle, 10 mm thick. **3.** Cusp of atrioventricular valve. **4.** Papillary muscles. **5.** Chordae tendineae (indicated by dashed lines). **6.** Delicate trabeculae carneae. **7.** Adipose tissue in coronary sulcus. **8.** Coronary artery.

Fig. 16-3. Ventricular wall. Human heart. Enlargement of area similar to rectangle (B) in Fig. 16-1. L.M. X 11. **1.** Ventricle. **2.** Cross-sectioned papillary muscles. **3.** Myocardium: bundles and layers of cardiac muscle cells with markedly alternating fiber directions. **4.** Connective tissue septa (perimysium). **5.** Blood vessel. **6.** Surface of heart (thin epicardium).

Fig. 16-4. Atrial wall. Monkey heart. Enlargement of rectangle (A) in Fig. 16-2. L.M. X 128. **1.** Endocardium, several times thicker than in ventricle. **2.** Myocardium: bundles and layers of cardiac muscle fibers. **3.** Coronary sulcus.

Fig. 16-5. Juncture of atrium and ventricle. Monkey heart. Enlargement of rectangle (B) in Fig. 16-2. L.M. X 30. **1.** Atrial wall. **2.** Annulus fibrosus. **3.** Ventricular wall. **4.** Base of cusp in atrioventricular valve. **5.** Adipose tissue in coronary sulcus.

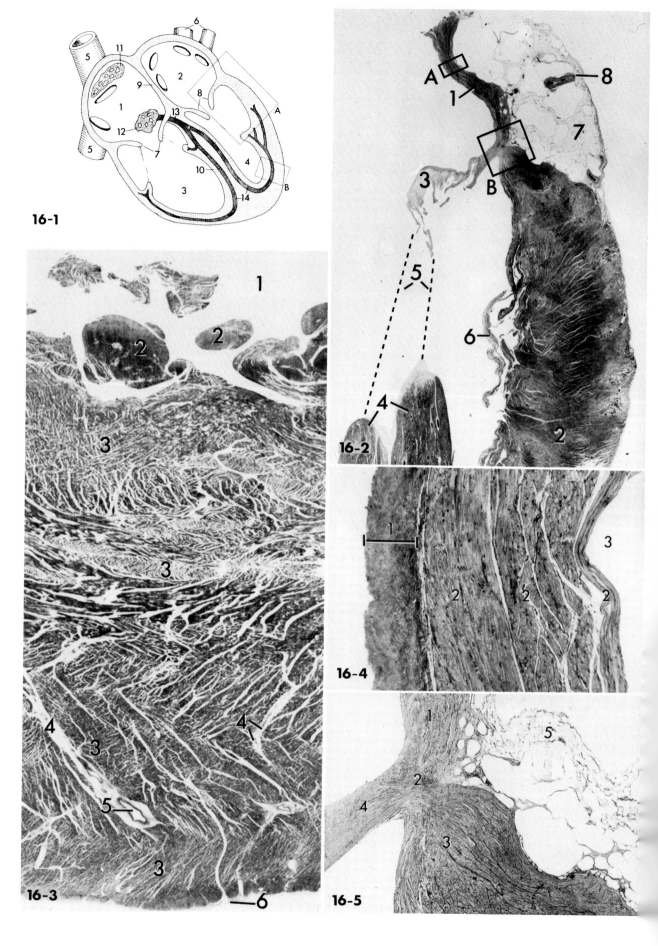

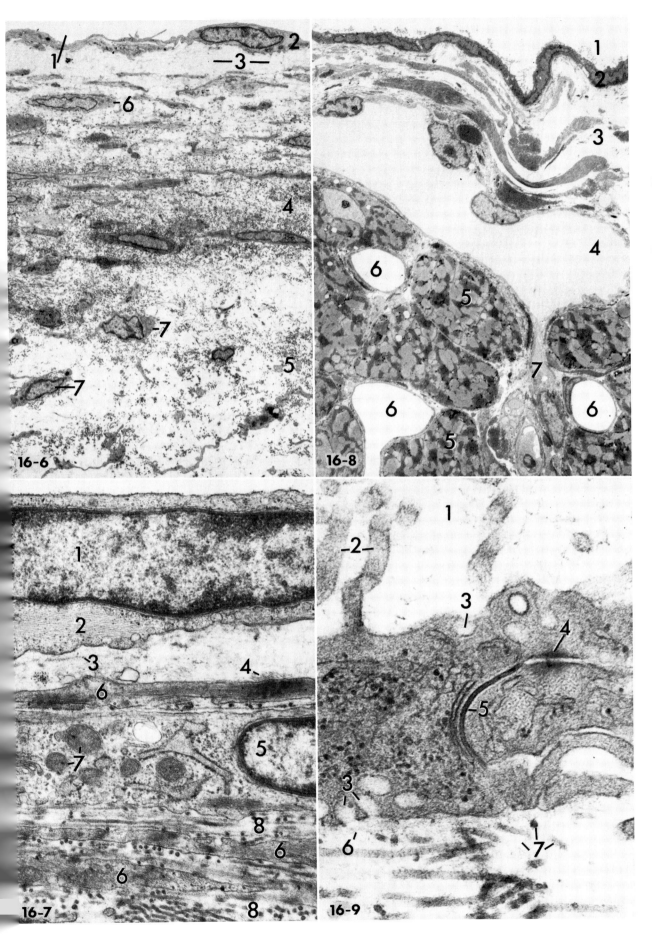

Fig. 16-6. Endocardium. Left atrium. Rat. E.M.
X 1800. **1.** Atrial cavity. **2.** Endothelial cells.
3. Basement membrane. **4.** Fibroelastic layer.
5. Subendocardial layer. **6.** Smooth muscle
cell. **7.** Fibroblasts.

Fig. 16-7. Detail of endocardium. Left ventricle.
Rat. E.M. X 29,000. **1.** Nucleus of endothelial
cell. **2.** Cytoplasmic filaments. **3.** Delicate and
incomplete basal lamina. **4.** Reticular and
elastic microfibrils. **5.** Nucleus of smooth
muscle cell. **6.** Cytoplasmic processes of
smooth muscle cells containing delicate
bundles of myofilaments. **7.** Mitochondria.
8. Collagenous fibrils.

Fig. 16-8. Epicardium. Right atrium. Rat. E.M.
X 1800. **1.** Cavity of pericardial sac.
2. Mesothelial cells. **3.** Loose connective tissue
with bundles of collagenous fibrils.
4. Pericardial lymphatic vessel. **5.** Cardiac
muscle fibers of atrial myocardium. **6.** Blood
capillaries. **7.** Connective tissue septum.

Fig. 16-9. Detail of epicardial mesothelial cells.
Right atrium. Rat. E.M. X 62,000.
1. Pericardial cavity. **2.** Microvilli. **3.** Surface
(micropinocytotic) vesicles. **4.** Desmosome.
5. Gap-junction. **6.** Thin basal lamina.
7. Delicate collagenous (or reticular)
fibrils 350 Å thick.

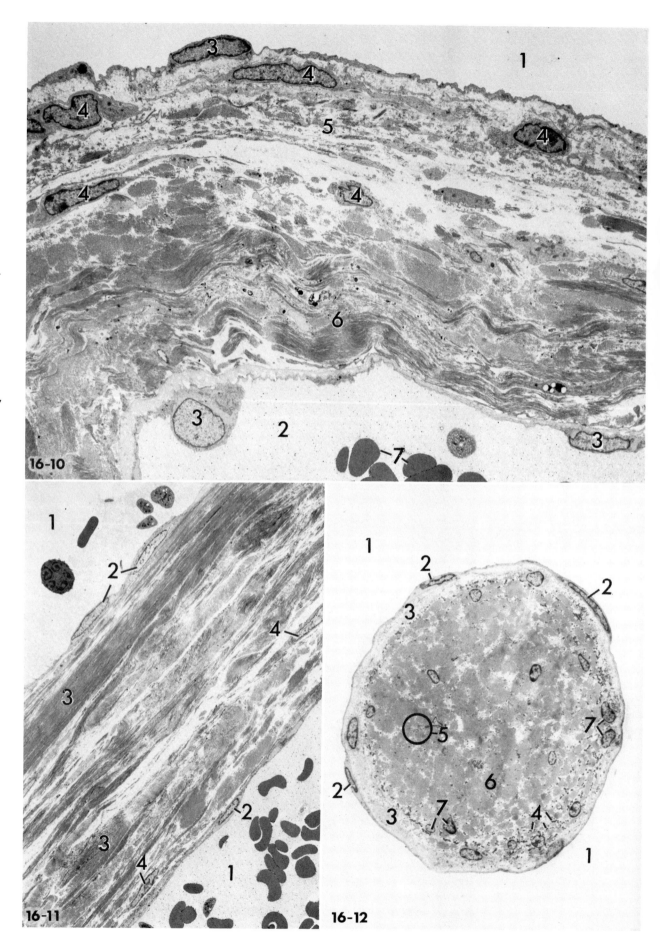

Fig. 16-10. Cusp of left atrioventricular valve. Rat. E.M. X 1900. **1.** Left atrium. **2.** Left ventricle. **3.** Nuclei of endothelial cells. **4.** Nuclei of fibroblasts. **5.** Loose connective tissue. **6.** Dense connective tissue. **7.** Erythrocytes.

Fig. 16-11. Chorda tendinea. Longitudinal section. Left ventricle. Heart. Rat. E.M. X 1100. **1.** Ventricular cavity. **2.** Nuclei of endothelial cells of thin endocardium. **3.** Collagenous fiber bundles. **4.** Nuclei of fibroblasts.

Fig. 16-12. Chorda tendinea. Cross section. Left ventricle. Heart. Rat. E.M. X 1500. **1.** Ventricular cavity. **2.** Nuclei of endothelial cells. **3.** Subendothelial loose connective tissue. **4.** Elastic fibers (dark dots). **5.** Circle: enlargement of this area is found in Fig. 7-7 (p. 83). **6.** Collagenous fibers. **7.** Fibroblasts.

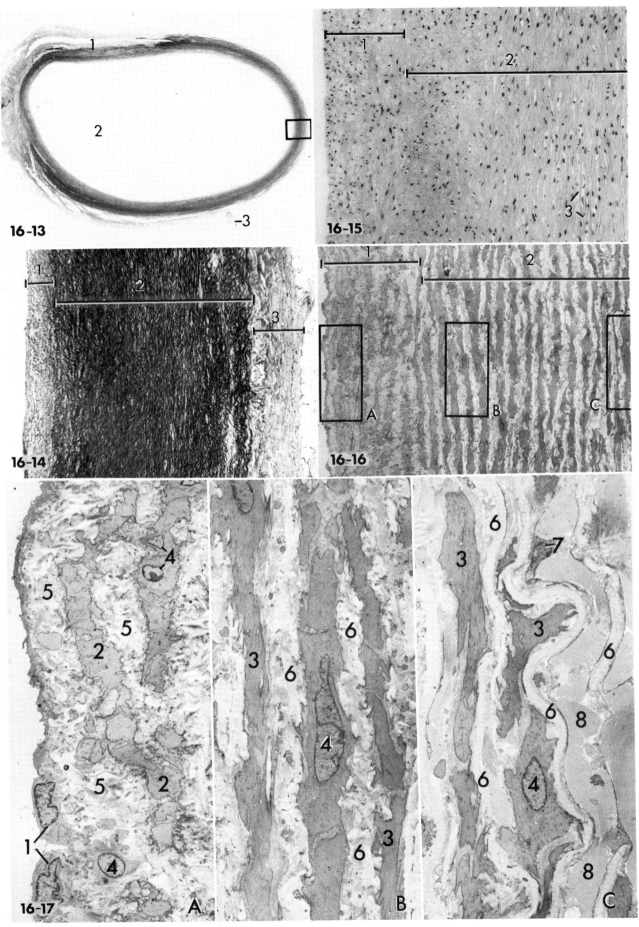

Fig. 16-13. Aorta. Cross section. Human. L.M. × 5. **1.** Wall thickness averages 1.5 mm. **2.** Diameter of lumen: max. distance 14 mm; min. distance 7 mm. **3.** Small artery in tunica adventitia.

Fig. 16-14. Aorta. Cross section. Human. Elastic stain. Enlargement of area similar to rectangle in Fig. 16-13. L.M. × 65. **1.** Intima (108 μ). **2.** Media. (820 μ). Elastic membranes of media stained black. No distinct inner or outer elastic membrane. **3.** Adventitia (215 μ) with peripheral adipose tissue.

Fig. 16-15. Aorta. Cross. section. Human. Hematoxylin and eosin stain. Area similar to Fig. 16-14. L.M. × 89. **1.** Intima. **2.** Media. Nuclei of smooth muscle cells appear as dark dots. **3.** Elastic membranes appear as faintly stained, slightly refractive, wavy lines.

Fig. 16-16. Aorta. Cross section. Squirrel monkey. E.M. × 380. **1.** Intima. **2.** Media.

Fig. 16-17. Aorta. Cross section. Enlargements of areas similar to rectangles in Fig. 16-16. A (intima), B (media), C (media-adventitia). Squirrel monkey. E.M. × 1800. **1.** Nuclei of endothelial cells. **2.** Longitudinally arranged smooth muscle cells. **3.** Circularly arranged smooth-muscle cells. **4.** Nuclei of smooth muscle cells. **5.** Irregularly arranged collagenous and elastic fibers. **6.** Elastic membranes. **7.** Nucleus of fibroblast in adventitia. **8.** Coarse bundles of collagenous fibrils in adventitia.

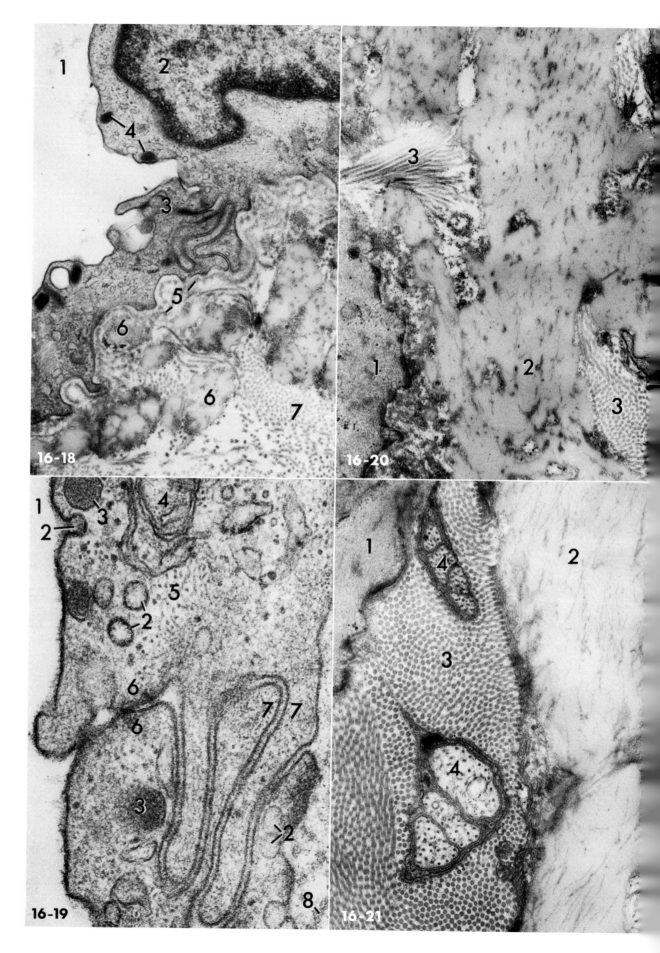

Fig. 16-18. Endothelium. Aorta. Cross section. Squirrel monkey. E.M. X 24,000. **1.** Lumen of aorta. **2.** Nucleus of endothelial cell. **3.** Junction of endothelial cells. **4.** Specific endothelial granules. **5.** Basal lamina. **6.** Elastic fibers with both amorphous substance and elastic microfibrils. **7.** Collagenous fibrils.

Fig. 16-19. Detail of aortic endothelial cells. Squirrel monkey. E.M. X 87,000. **1.** Lumen of aorta. **2.** Surface (micropinocytotic) vesicles. **3.** Specific endothelial granules without apparent inner microtubules. **4.** Mitochondrion. **5.** Cytoplasmic filaments. **6.** Gap-junction. **7.** Non-specialized junction of cell membranes. **8.** Indistinct basal lamina.

Fig. 16-20. Detail of aortic media. Squirrel monkey. E.M. X 24,000. **1.** Part of smooth muscle cell. **2.** Elastic membrane, consisting mostly of amorphous substance. **3.** Delicate bundles of collagenous fibrils.

Fig. 16-21. Detail of media-adventitia transitional zone. Squirrel monkey. E.M. X 24,000. **1.** Part of smooth muscle cell. **2.** Elastic membrane, consisting almost entirely of amorphous substance. **3.** Large accumulation of collagenous fibrils. **4.** Non-myelinated nerve fibers.

194

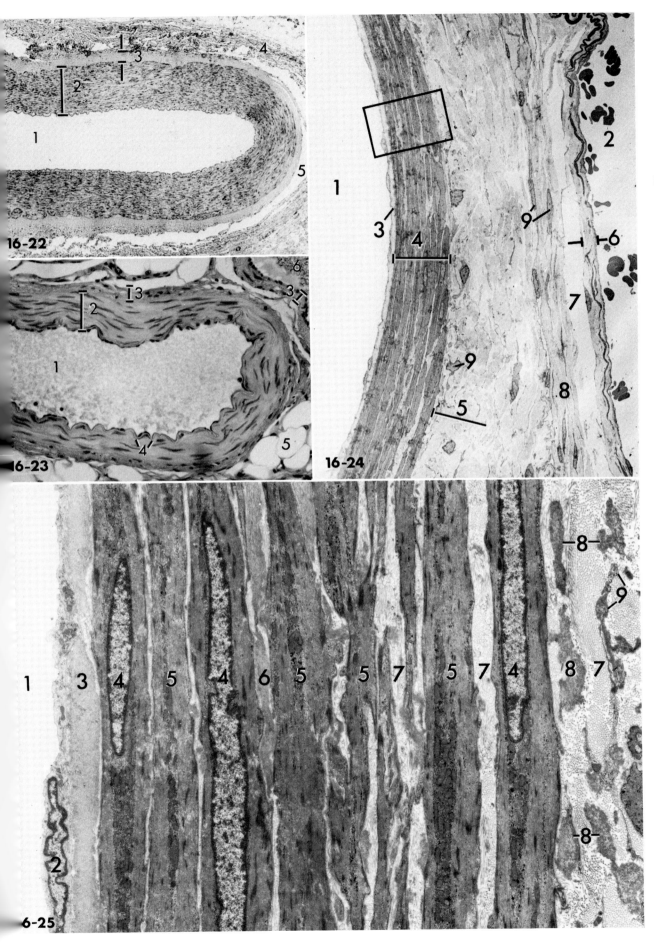

Fig. 16-22. Muscular artery. Finger. Human. L.M. × 27. **1.** Lumen; max. width 3 mm (3000 μ). **2.** Intima and media; width 250 μ. **3.** Adventitia; width 80 μ. **4.** Perivascular connective tissue. **5.** Tear (preparation artifact).

Fig. 16-23. Small muscular artery. Mesentery. Rabbit. L.M. × 135. **1.** Lumen; max. width 0.5 mm (500 μ). **2.** Intima and media; width 75 μ. **3.** Adventitia; width 22 μ. **4.** Internal elastic membrane (scalloped line). **5.** Perivascular adipose tissue. **6.** Lumen of small vein (entire vein seen in Fig. 16-48). **7.** Wall of vein; width 20 μ.

Fig. 16-24. Renal artery and vein. Cross section. Fixed by intra-arterial perfusion. Rat. E.M. × 660. **1.** Lumen of artery preserved in non-collapsed condition; width 650 μ. **2.** Lumen of vein; width 2600 μ. **3.** Endothelium and internal elastic membrane. **4.** Media; width 25 μ. **5.** Adventitia blending with perivascular connective tissue; width approx. 20 μ. **6.** Intima and media of vein; width averages 5 μ. **7.** Tear (preparation artifact). **8.** Adventitia. **9.** Fibroblasts.

Fig. 16-25. Wall of small muscular artery. Enlargement of area similar to rectangle in Fig. 16-24. Renal artery. Cross section. Rat. E.M. × 5000. **1.** Lumen. **2.** Nucleus of endothelial cell. **3.** Internal elastic lamina. **4.** Nuclei of smooth muscle cells. **5.** Circularly arranged smooth muscle cells. **6.** Elastic fibers. **7.** Collagenous fibrils. **8.** Profiles of incomplete external elastic membrane. **9.** Non-myelinated nerve axons.

Fig. 16-26. Detail of tunica intima of cross-sectioned muscular artery. Renal artery. Rat. E.M. X 17,000. **1.** Lumen. **2.** Nuclei of endothelial cells. **3.** Junctional area of adjacent endothelial cells. **4.** Internal elastic membrane, 1.6 μ thick. Note absence of subendothelial basal lamina. **5.** Mitochondria of smooth muscle cell. **6.** Slender cytoplasmic processes of smooth muscle cell reach toward the endothelial cell across an interruption (fenestra) of the elastic membrane. **7.** External lamina of smooth muscle cell. **8.** Small bundles of delicate collagenous fibrils.

Fig. 16-27. Detail of border zone between tunica media and tunica adventitia of cross-sectioned muscular artery. Renal artery. Rat. E.M. X 17,000. **1.** Fusiform densities of smooth muscle cell myofilaments. **2.** Delicate cytoplasmic processes, some of which establish membranous contacts with neighboring cell. **3.** External lamina of smooth muscle cell. **4.** Collagenous fibrils. **5.** Elastic fibers forming an incomplete external elastic membrane. **6.** Attachment plaque (dense body).

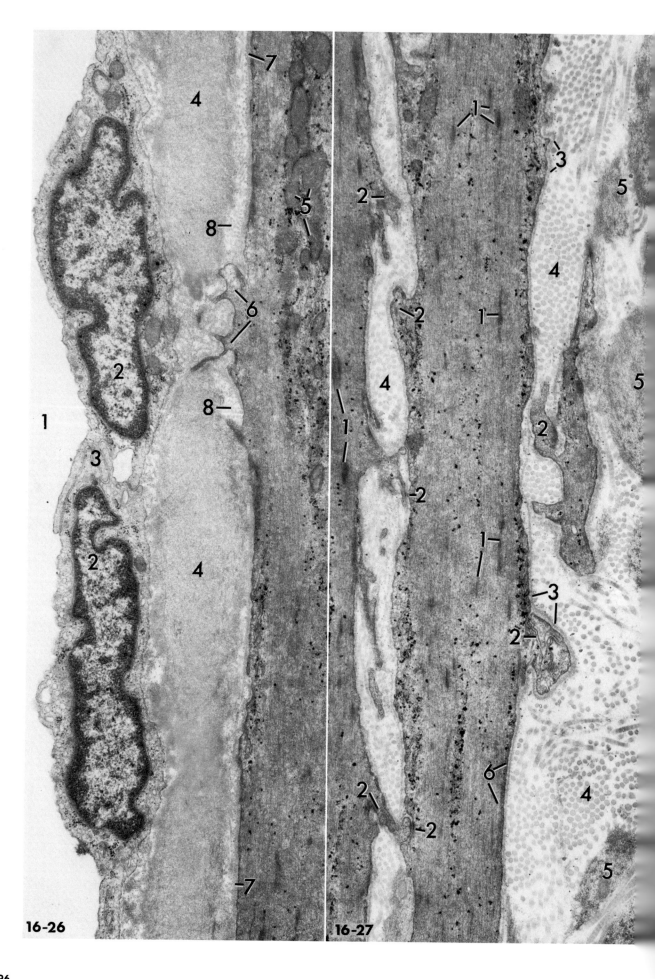

16-26

16-27

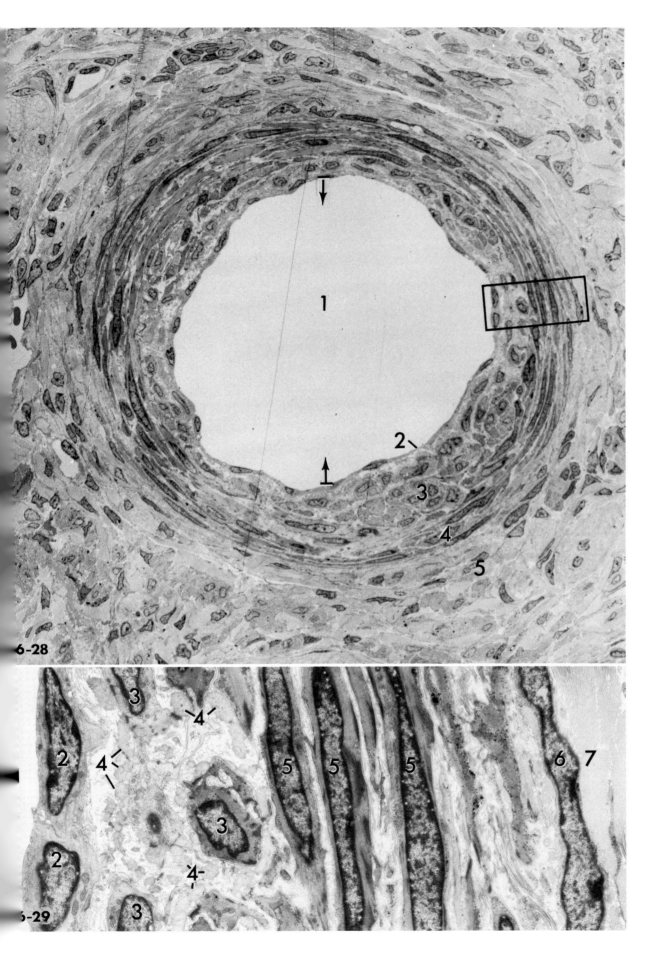

Fig. 16-28. Small helicine artery. Cross section. Fixed by intra-arterial perfusion. Cavernous tissue. Penis. Rat. E.M. X 800. **1.** Lumen; width between arrows 110 μ. **2.** Endothelium. **3.** Longitudinally arranged smooth muscle cells of intima. Aggregations of these cells form intima cushions. **4.** Circularly arranged smooth muscle cells of media. **5.** Adventitia.

Fig. 16-29. Wall of small helicine artery. Enlargement of rectangle in Fig. 16-28. E.M. X 4500. **1.** Lumen. **2.** Nuclei of endothelial cells. **3.** Nuclei of longitudinally arranged smooth muscle cells. **4.** Elastic fibers and scattered collagenous fibrils. **5.** Nuclei of circularly arranged smooth muscle cells. **6.** Nucleus of fibroblast. **7.** Bundles of collagenous fibrils.

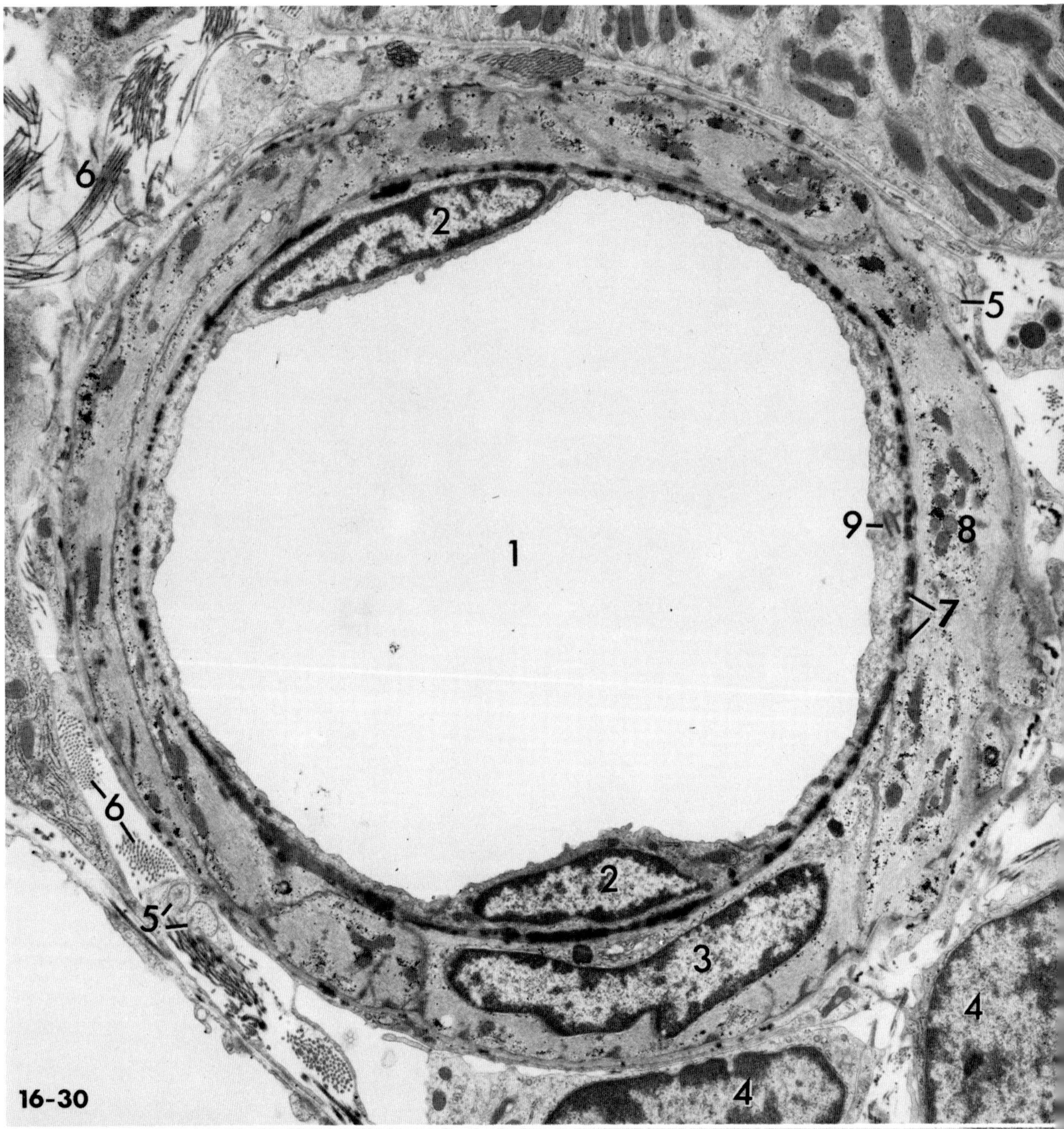

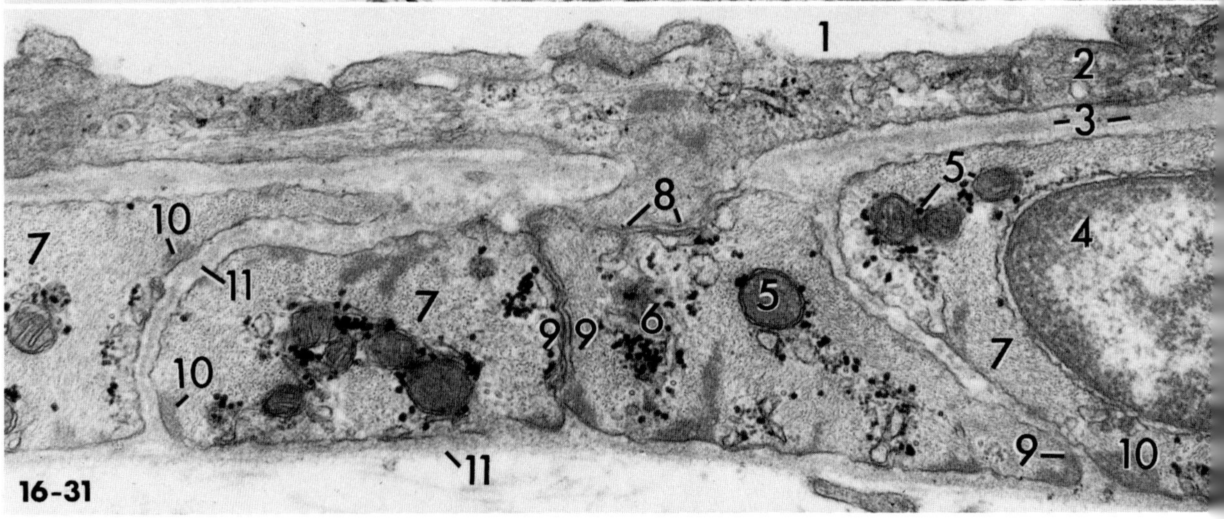

Fig. 16-30. Afferent arteriole. Cross section. Kidney. Rat. E.M. X 7000. **1.** Lumen; width 18 μ. **2.** Nuclei of endothelial cells. **3.** Nucleus of spirally arranged smooth muscle cell. **4.** Nuclei of perivascular connective tissue cells. **5.** Non-myelinated nerve axons. **6.** Collagenous fibrils. **7.** Profiles of incomplete internal elastic membrane. **8.** Mitochondria. **9.** Centriole.

Fig. 16-31. Afferent arteriole. Longitudinal section. Kidney. Rat. E.M. X 31,000. **1.** Lumen. **2.** Endothelial cytoplasm. **3.** Basal lamina. **4.** Nucleus of smooth muscle cell. **5.** Mitochondria. **6.** Glycogen particles. **7.** Myofilaments. **8.** Myoendothelial junction. **9.** Junctional area of smooth muscle cells. **10.** Attachment plaques (dense bodies). **11.** External (basal) lamina.

16-30

16-31

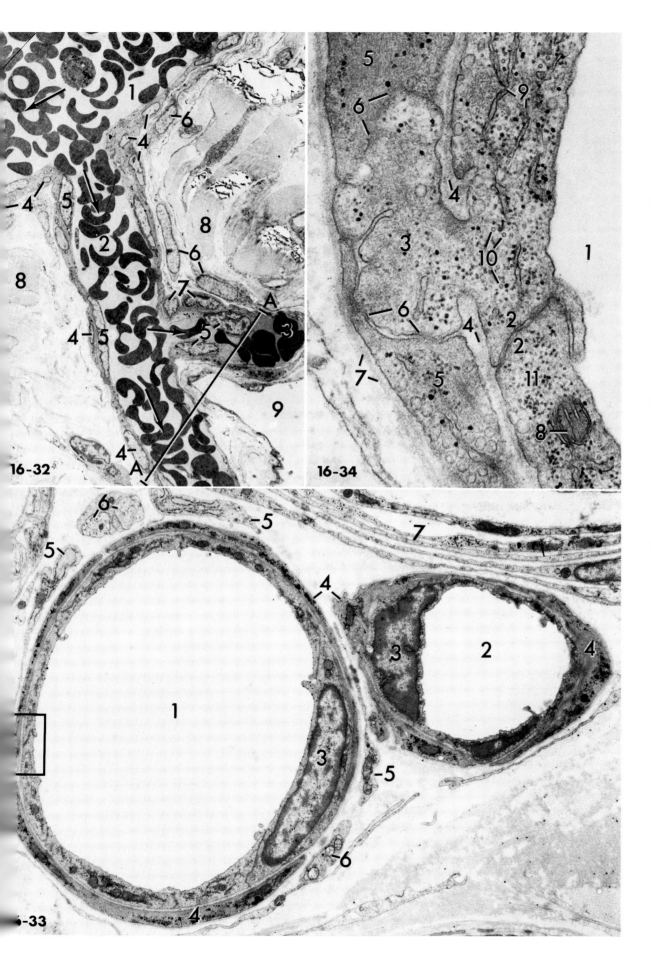

Fig. 16-32. Precapillary sphincter area. Longitudinal section. Dermis. Rabbit. E.M. X 1600. Arrows indicate direction of blood flow. **1.** Lumen of 30 μ arteriole. **2.** Lumen of 12 μ terminal arteriole. **3.** Beginning of arterial capillary; lumen 7.5 μ wide. **4.** Nuclei of smooth muscle cells. **5.** Nuclei of endothelial cells. **6.** Nuclei of fibroblasts. **7.** Nuclei of smooth muscle cells. In this position around the origin of an arterial capillary, these smooth muscle cells form a true precapillary sphincter. **8.** Bundles of collagenous fibrils. **9.** Lymphatic capillary (After Rhodin: J. Ultrastr. Res. *18*, 181, 1967).

Fig. 16-33. Precapillary sphincter area. Cross section in the plane indicated by line A-A in Fig. 16-32. Enlarged detail of Fig. 11-4 (p. 223). Skeletal muscle. Rat. E.M. X 9000. **1.** Lumen of terminal arteriole; width 10 μ. **2.** Lumen of beginning of arterial capillary; width 5 μ. **3.** Nuclei of endothelial cells. **4.** Cytoplasm of smooth muscle cells. **5.** Fibroblast cytoplasm. **6.** Non-myelinated nerve axons. **7.** Lamellated capsular cells of neuromuscular spindle.

Fig. 16-34. Myoendothelial junction in arteriole. Enlargement of area indicated by rectangle in Fig. 16-33, several sections deeper. Skeletal muscle. Rat. E.M. X 47,000. **1.** Lumen. **2.** Junctional area of endothelial cells. **3.** Foot-like process from base of endothelial cell. **4.** Basal lamina. **5.** Cytoplasm of smooth muscle cell. **6.** Junctional area of smooth muscle cell and endothelial cell (myoendothelial junction). **7.** External lamina. **8.** Mitochondrion. **9.** Profiles of granular endoplasmic reticulum. **10.** Microtubules. **11.** Ribosomes.

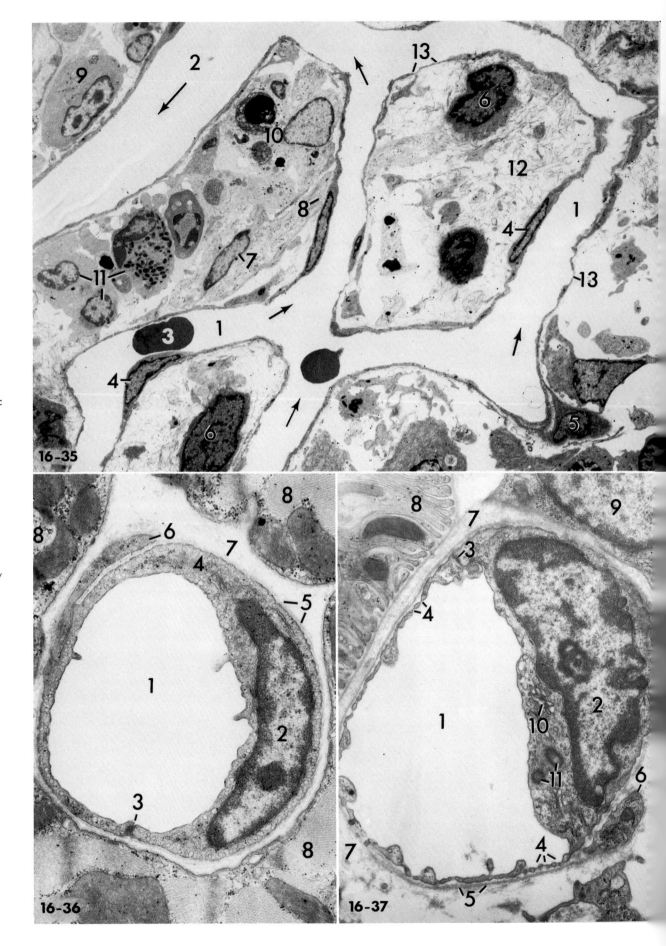

Fig. 16-35. Capillary network. Longitudinal section. Connective tissue core of intestinal villus. Rat. E.M. X 1900. Arrows indicate assumed direction of blood flow. **1.** True capillaries. Lumen averages 4 μ in width. **2.** Postcapillary venule; lumen 9 μ wide. **3.** Erythrocyte. **4.** Nuclei of endothelial cells. **5.** Pericyte. **6.** Fibroblast. **7.** Schwann cell nucleus. **8.** Non-myelinated nerve axons. **9.** Plasma cell. **10.** Macrophage. **11.** Leukocytes. **12.** Loose network of collagenous fibrils. **13.** Stretches of fenestrated endothelium near the venous end of the capillary network. (After Rhodin: Topics in the Study of Life; The Bio Source Book. Harper & Row, 1971.)

Fig. 16-36. True capillary. Cross section. Cardiac muscle. Rat. E.M. X 19,000. **1.** Lumen; width 3.5 μ. **2.** Nucleus of endothelial cell. **3.** Junction of cytoplasmic arms of same endothelial cell. **4.** Cytoplasm rich in micropinocytotic vesicles. **5.** Basal lamina. **6.** Cytoplasmic process of pericyte. **7.** Pericapillary connective tissue space. **8.** Part of cardiac muscle cells.

Fig. 16-37. Peritubular capillary. Kidney. Rat. E.M. X 16,000. **1.** Lumen; width 5 μ. **2.** Nucleus of endothelial cell. **3.** Junction of endothelial cytoplasmic arms. **4.** Highly fenestrated cytoplasm. Each fenestra closed by a thin membrane (diaphragm). **5.** Basal lamina. **6.** Part of pericyte. **7.** Pericapillary connective tissue space. **8.** Base of kidney tubule cell. **9.** Nucleus of fibroblast. **10.** Golgi zone. **11.** Centrioles.

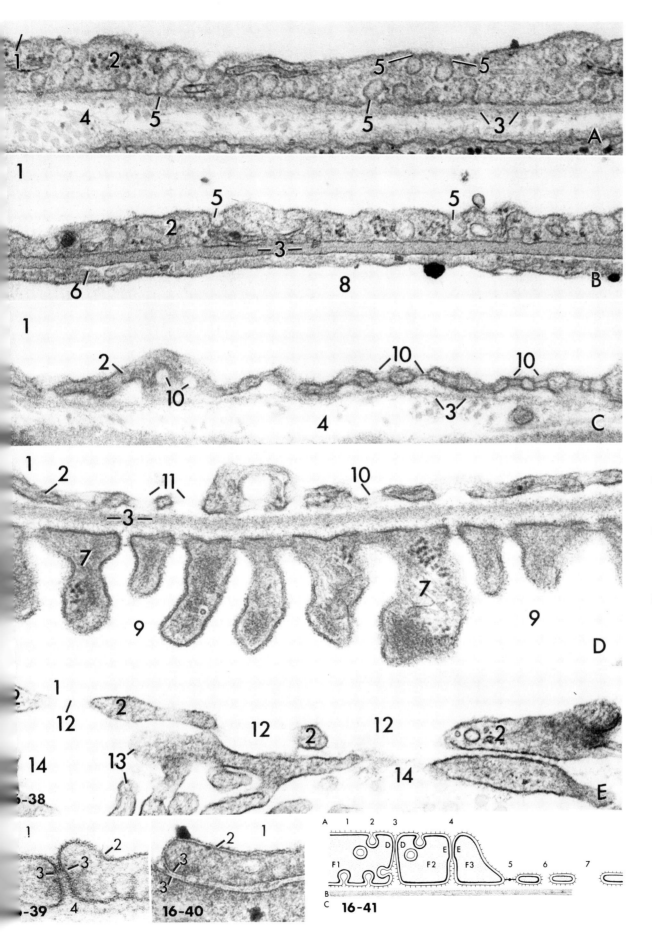

Fig. 16-38. A comparison of capillary walls in rat tissue. E.M. × 60,000. (A–E). **A.** Continuous thick endothelium. Cardiac muscle. **B.** Continuous thin endothelium. Lung. **C.** Fenestrated thin endothelium. Kidney. Peritubular capillary. **D.** Fenestrated thin endothelium. Kidney. Glomerular capillary. **E.** Discontinuous endothelium. Liver. Sinusoid. **1.** Lumen of capillary. **2.** Endothelial cytoplasm. **3.** Basal lamina. **4.** Pericapillary space. **5.** Surface (micropinocytotic) vesicles. **6.** Cytoplasm of alveolar epithelial cell. **7.** Cytoplasm of visceral epithelial cell of Bowman's capsule. **8.** Pulmonary alveolus (air sac). **9.** Urinary space. **10.** Fenestration bridged by a thin membrane (diaphragm). **11.** Open fenestrations. **12.** Cytoplasmic holes (gaps). **13.** Microvilli of hepatic parenchymal cell. **14.** Pericapillary space of Disse. (After Rhodin: Topics in the Study of Life: The Bio Source Book. Harper & Row, 1971.)

Fig. 16-39. Junctional area. Capillary. Skeletal muscle. Rat. E.M. × 120,000. **1.** Lumen. **2.** Trilaminar cell membrane. **3.** Gap-junction. **4.** Basal lamina.

Fig. 16-40. Junctional area. Capillary. Cerebral cortex. Rat. E.M. × 120,000. **1.** Lumen. **2.** Trilaminar cell membrane. **3.** True tight junction (fusion of outer leaflets of apposing trilaminar cell membranes).

Fig. 16-41. Routes of transport across capillary endothelial cells are schematized in this composite drawing. The transport may occur in either direction across the cell. F1, F2, and F3 are adjoining segments of endothelial cells. The cell membrane is composed of a superficial glycoprotein layer (illustrated as pegs) and three laminae (leaflets). **A.** Capillary lumen. **B.** Basal lamina. **C.** Pericapillary space. **D.** True tight junction. **E.** Gap-junction. *Transport routes:* **1.** Through plasma membrane. **2.** Surface (micropinocytotic) vesicles. **3.** True tight junction (impenetrable). **4.** Gap-junction (penetrable). **5.** Fenestrations (with closing membrane). **6.** Fenestrations (open). **7.** Holes (gaps). (After Rhodin: Topics in the Study of Life: The Bio Source Book. Harper & Row 1971.)

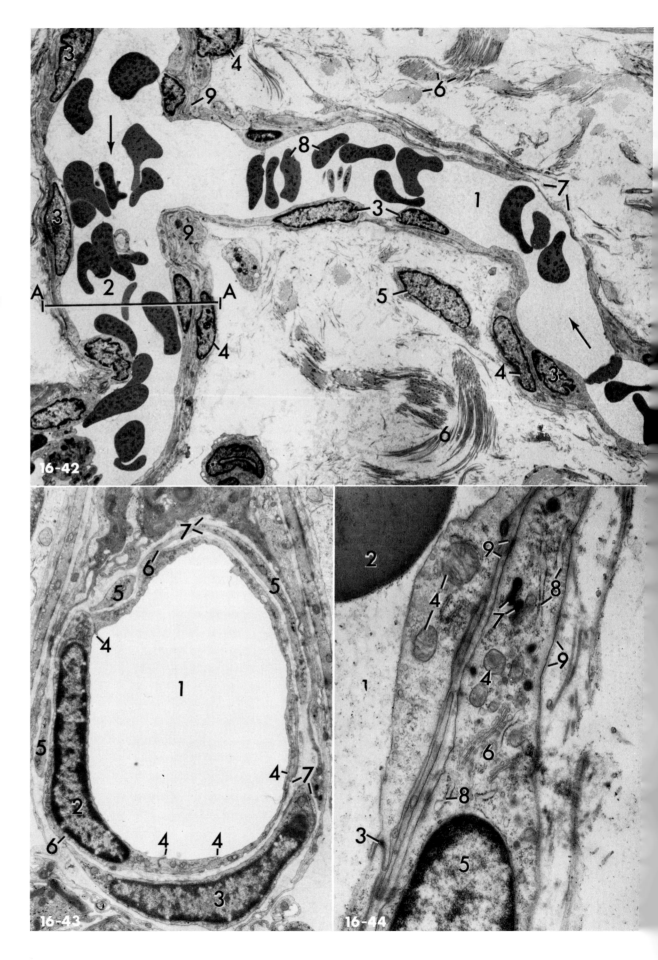

Fig. 16-42. Connection between venous capillary and postcapillary venule. Longitudinal section. Dermis. Rabbit. E.M. X 2300. Arrows indicate direction of blood flow. **1.** Lumen of venous capillary; width averages 8 μ. **2.** Lumen of postcapillary venule; lumen averages 12 μ. **3.** Nuclei of endothelial cells. **4.** Nuclei of pericytes. **5.** Fibroblast. **6.** Collagenous fibrils. **7.** Stretch of fenestrated endothelium. **8.** Erythrocytes. **9.** Processes of pericytic cytoplasm surround junction of capillary and postcapillary venule. Smooth muscle cells do not occur here.

Fig. 16-43. Cross section of postcapillary venule, corresponding approximately to level indicated by line A-A in Fig. 16-42. Interstitial tissue. Testis. Rat. E.M. X 7000. **1.** Lumen; width 10 μ. **2.** Nucleus of endothelial cell. **3.** Nucleus of pericyte. **4.** Junctions of endothelial cells. **5.** Strands of pericytic cytoplasm. **6.** Junctions of pericytes and endothelial cells. **7.** Basal lamina.

Fig. 16-44. Postcapillary venule. Longitudinal section. Dermis. Rat. E.M. X 20,000. **1.** Lumen. **2.** Erythrocyte. **3.** Junction of endothelial cells. **4.** Mitochondria. **5.** Nucleus of pericyte. **6.** Golgi zone. **7.** Lysosomes. **8.** Profiles of granular endoplasmic reticulum. **9.** Basal (external) lamina.

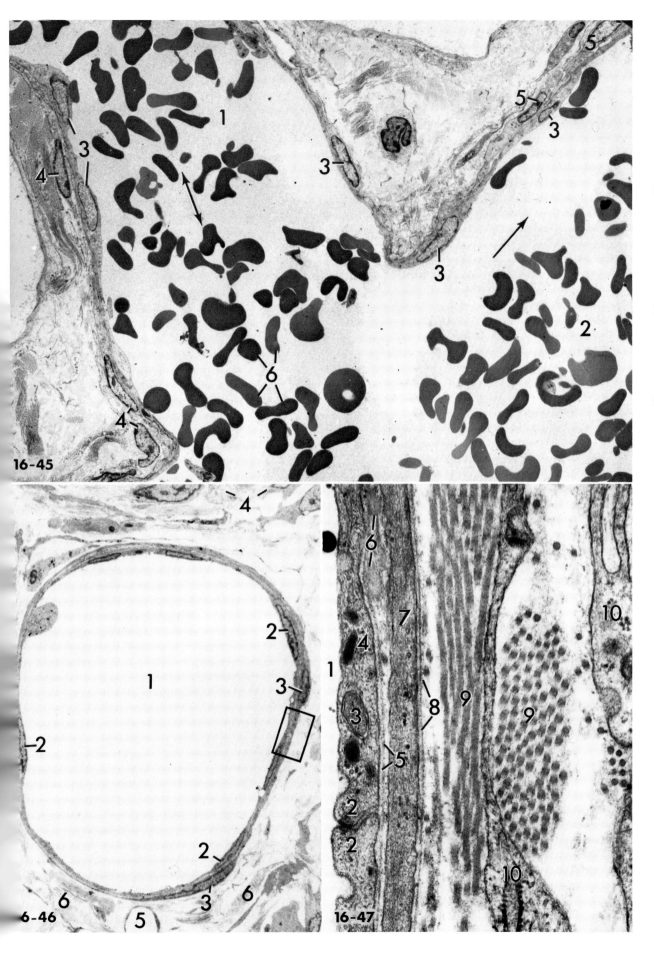

Fig. 16-45. Connection between collecting venule and muscular venule. Longitudinal section. Dermis. Rabbit. E.M. X 1800. Arrows indicate direction of blood flow. **1.** Lumen of collecting venule; width averages 50 μ. **2.** Lumen of muscular venule; width averages 90 μ. **3.** Nuclei of endothelial cells. **4.** Nuclei of pericytes. **5.** Smooth muscle cells. **6.** Erythrocytes.

Fig. 16-46. Muscular venule. Cross section. Submucosa. Small intestine. Rat. E.M. X 1200. **1.** Lumen; width 70 μ. **2.** Nuclei of endothelial cells. **3.** Nuclei of smooth muscle cells. **4.** Base of crypt of Lieberkühn. **5.** Lumen of capillary; width 7 μ. **6.** Loosely arranged collagenous fibrils.

Fig. 16-47. Wall of cross-sectioned muscular venule. Enlargement of area similar to rectangle in Fig. 16-46. Skeletal muscle. Rat. E.M. X 47,000. **1.** Lumen of venule; width 80 μ. **2.** Junction of endothelial cells. **3.** Mitochondrion. **4.** Specific endothelial granules. **5.** Basal lamina. **6.** Delicate elastic fibers. **7.** Smooth muscle cell. **8.** External lamina. **9.** Collagenous fibrils. **10.** Cytoplasm of fibroblast.

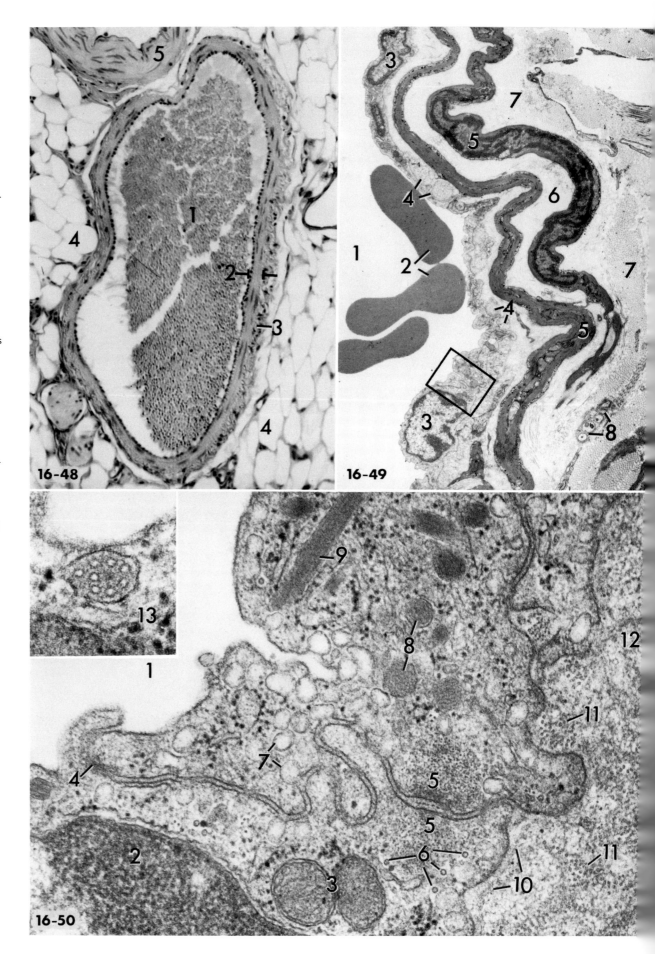

Fig. 16-48. Small vein. Mesentery. Rabbit. L.M. X 190. **1.** Lumen (max. width 570 μ) with coagulated blood. **2.** Intima and media; width 20 μ. **3.** Adventitia blending with perivascular connective tissue. **4.** Adipose tissue **5.** Wall of small artery (width 90 μ).

Fig. 16-49. Wall of cross-sectioned renal vein. Same preparation as in Fig. 16-24. Rat. E.M. X 4500. **1.** Lumen; width 2600 μ. **2.** Erythrocytes. **3.** Nuclei of endothelial cells. **4.** Elastic fibers, unevenly distributed immediately adjacent to the endothelial cells in the subendothelial connective tissue. **5.** Smooth muscle cells. **6.** Collagenous fibrils between smooth muscle cells. **7.** Bundles of collagenous fibrils in adventitia. **8.** Non-myelinated nerve axons.

Fig. 16-50. Junctional area of endothelial cells. Renal vein. Enlargement of rectangle in Fig. 16-49. Rat. E.M. X 64,000. **1.** Lumen. **2.** Nucleus. **3.** Mitochondria. **4.** Gap-junction. **5.** Intermediate-type junction with adjacent accumulation of cytoplasmic filaments. **6.** Microtubules. **7.** Surface (micropinocytotic) vesicles. **8.** Specific endothelial granules. **9.** Longitudinally sectioned specific endothelial granule. **10.** Indistinct basal lamina. **11.** Cross-sectioned microfibrils of elastic fiber. **12.** Amorphous substance of elastic fiber. **13.** Inset: Enlargement (X 128,000) of specific endothelial granule, showing its boundary membrane and component small tubules which are not present in all specific endothelial granules.

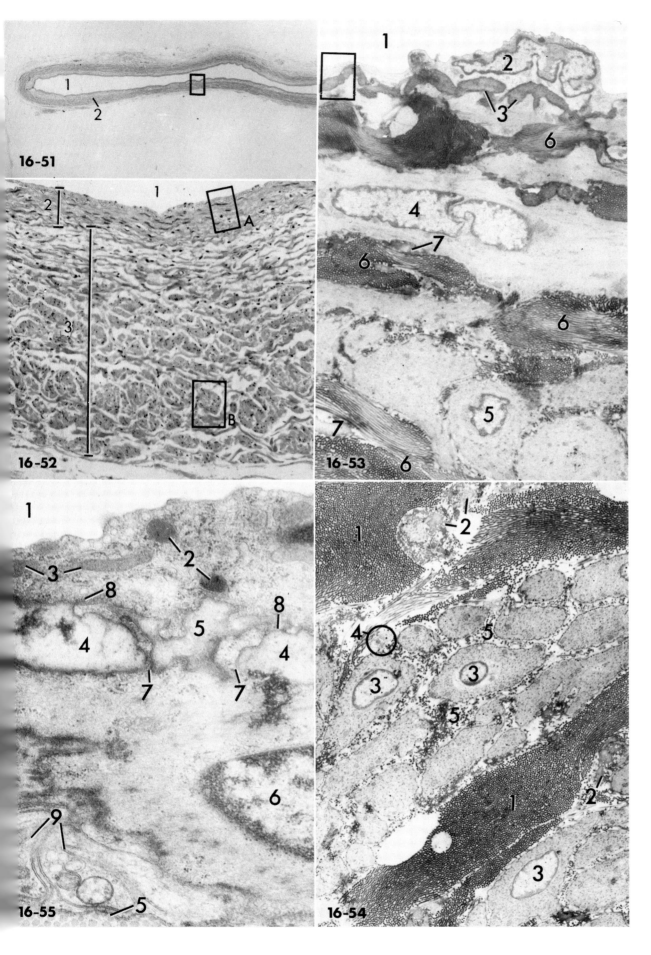

Fig. 16-51. Vena cava. Cross section. Human. L.M. × 5. **1.** Lumen, highly collapsed; width 21 mm. **2.** Wall thickness approximately 700 µ (0.7 mm).

Fig. 16-52. Wall of cross-sectioned vena cava. Enlargement of area similar to rectangle in Fig. 16-51. Human. L.M. × 100. **1.** Lumen **2.** Intima and media (100 µ) with circularly arranged smooth muscle cells. **3.** Adventitia (600 µ) with longitudinally arranged smooth muscle cells.

Fig. 16-53. Intima and media of cross-sectioned vena cava. Enlargement of area similar to rectangle (A) in Fig. 16-52. Squirrel monkey. E.M. × 5100. **1.** Lumen. **2.** Nucleus of endothelial cell. **3.** Subendothelial elastic fibers, forming an incomplete internal elastic membrane. **4.** Nucleus of circularly arranged smooth muscle cell. **5.** Nucleus of longitudinally arranged smooth muscle cell. **6.** Bundles of collagenous fibrils. **7.** Elastic fibers.

Fig. 16-54. Adventitia of cross-sectioned vena cava. Enlargement of area similar to rectangle (B) in Fig. 16-52. Squirrel monkey. E.M. × 5100. **1.** Coarse bundles of collagenous fibrils. **2.** Scattered elastic fibers. **3.** Nuclei of longitudinally arranged smooth muscle cells. **4.** Circle: non-myelinated nerve axons. **5.** Scattered collagenous fibrils.

Fig. 16-55. Detail of vena cava. Enlargement of area similar to rectangle in Fig. 16-53. Squirrel monkey. E.M. × 27,000. **1.** Lumen. **2.** Specific granules of endothelial cell. **3.** Mitochondria. **4.** Elastic fibers. **5.** Collagenous fibrils. **6.** Nucleus of circularly arranged smooth muscle cell. **7.** Slender cytoplasmic processes of smooth muscle cell establish contacts with endothelial cell. **8.** Myoendothelial junctions. **9.** Non-myelinated nerve axons.

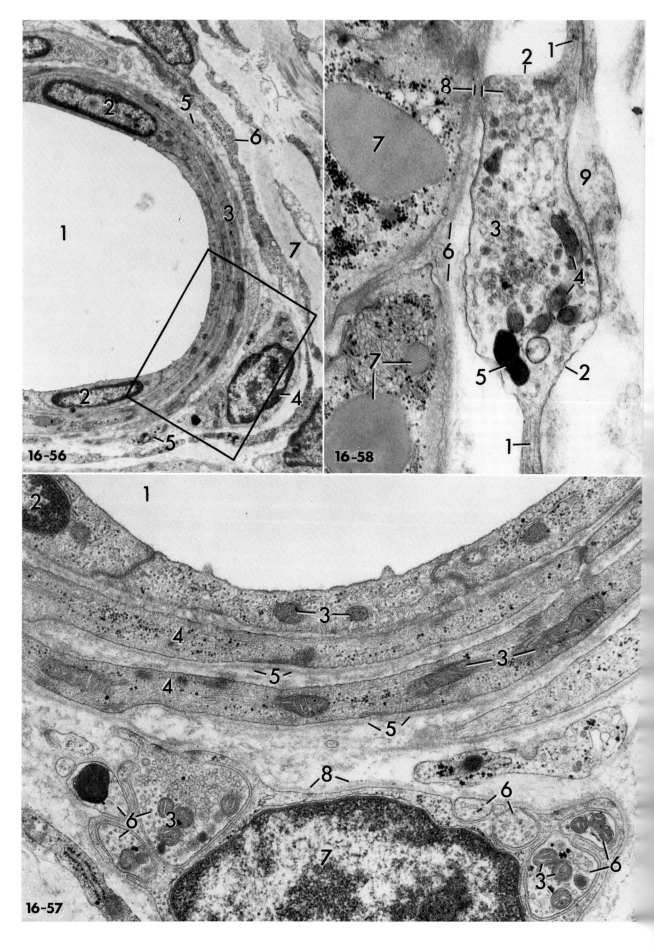

Fig. 16-56. Helicine arteriole. Cavernous tissue. Penis. Rat. E.M. × 9000. **1.** Lumen; width 15 μ. **2.** Nuclei of endothelial cells. **3.** Smooth muscle cells. **4.** Nucleus of Schwann cell. **5.** Non-myelinated nerve axons. **6.** Fibroblast. **7.** Collagenous fibrils.

Fig. 16-57. Helicine arteriole. Enlargement of rectangle in Fig. 16-56. Cavernous tissue. Penis. Rat. E.M. × 36,000. **1.** Lumen. **2.** Nucleus of endothelial cell. **3.** Mitochondria. **4.** Smooth muscle cells. **5.** External lamina. **6.** Non-myelinated nerve axons with synaptic vesicles and mitochondria. **7.** Nucleus of Schwann cell. **8.** External lamina.

Fig. 16-58. Sympathetic nerve axon terminal. Afferent arteriole at the level of the juxtaglomerular (JG) cells. Kidney. Rat. E.M. × 31,000. **1.** Denuded nerve axon terminal, cut longitudinally. **2.** Local swelling (widening) of terminal axon. **3.** Granulated (dense-core) vesicles. **4.** Mitochondria. **5.** Secondary lysosome. **6.** External lamina. **7.** Secretory granule of juxtaglomerular (JG) cells. **8.** Minimum diffusion gap between axolemma and sarcolemma is 670 Å. **9.** Schwann cell cytoplasm.

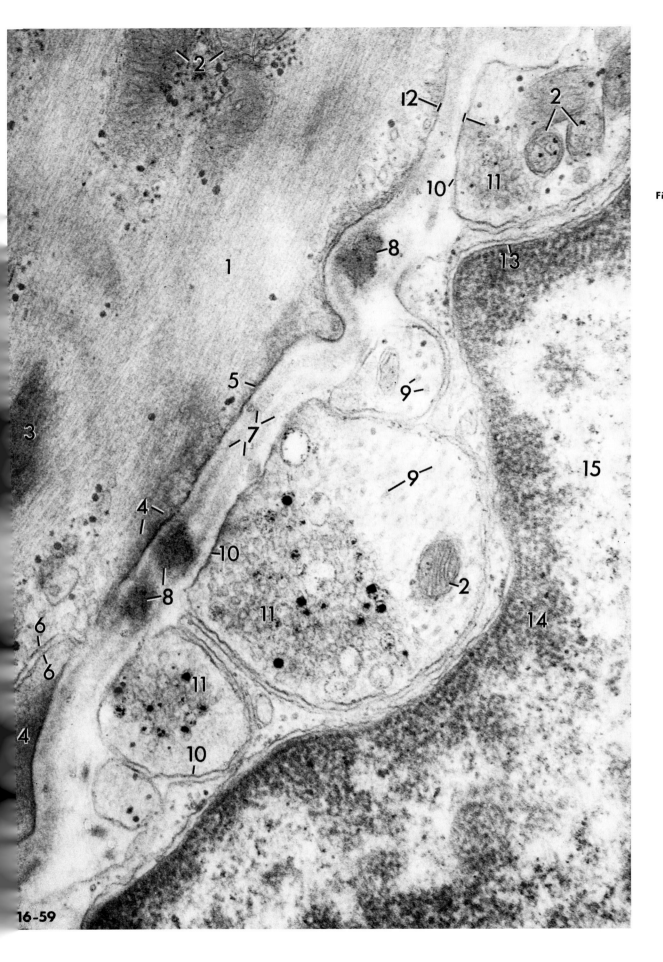

Fig. 16-59. Detail of vascular smooth muscle innervation. Afferent arteriole. Kidney. Rat. E.M. X 68,000. **1.** Myofilaments of smooth muscle cell. **2.** Mitochondria. **3.** Fusiform density. **4.** Attachment plaque (dense body). **5.** Cell membrane of smooth muscle cell. **6.** Junctional area of smooth muscle cell membranes. **7.** External laminae. **8.** Delicate elastic fibers. **9.** Microtubules of non-myelinated nerve axons. **10.** Axolemma. **11.** Mixture of granulated (dense-core) and non-granulated vesicles of non-myelinated nerve axon swellings. **12.** Minimum diffusion gap between axolemma and sarcolemma (for neurotransmitter substances) is 0.1 μ (indicated by T-bars). **13.** Nuclear membrane of Schwann cell nucleus. **14.** Dense heterochromatin. **15.** Light euchromatin.

References

HEART

Chiba, T. and Yamauchi, A. On the fine structure of the nerve terminals in the human myocardium. Z. Zellforsch. *108*: 324–338 (1970).

Forssmann, W. G. and Girardier, L. A study of the T-system in rat heart. J. Cell Biol. *44*: 1–19 (1970).

Hirano, H. and Ogawa, K. Ultrastructural localization of cholinesterase activity in the guinea pig heart. J. Electron Micr. *16*: 313–321 (1967).

Kolb, R., Pischinger, A. and Stockinger, L. Ultrastruktur der Pulmonalisklappe des Meerschweinchens. Zeitschr. mikr. anat. Forsch. *76*: 184–211 (1967).

Lannigan, R. A. and Zaki, S. A. Ultrastructure of the normal atrial endocardium. Brit. Heart J. *28*: 785–795 (1966).

Luisada, A. A. (Ed.). Development and Structure of the Cardiovascular System. McGraw-Hill, New York, 1961.

Mitomo, Y., Nakao, K. and Angrist, A. The fine structure of the heart valves in the chicken. I. Mitral valve. Am. J. Anat. *125*: 147–167 (1969).

Novi, A. M. An electron microscopic study of the innervation of papillary muscles in the rat. Anat. Rec. *160*: 123–142 (1968).

Rhodin, J. A. G., Del Missier, P. and Reid, L. C. The structure of the specialized impulse-conducting system of the steer heart. Circulation *24*: 349–367 (1969).

Stotler, W. A. and McMahon, R. A. The innervation and structure of the conductive system of the human heart. J. Comp. Neurol. *87*: 57–83 (1947).

Thaemert, J. C. Fine structure of neuromuscular relationships in mouse heart. Anat. Rec. *163*: 575–586 (1969).

ARTERIES AND VEINS

Abramson, D. I. (Ed.). Blood Vessels and Lymphatics. Academic Press, New York, 1962.

Albert, E. N. and Pease, D. C. An electron microscopic study of uterine arteries during pregnancy. Am. J. Anat. *123*: 165–194 (1968).

Bucciante, L. Microscopie optique de la paroi veineuse. Angiologica *2*: part II, 211–308 (1966).

Bunce, D. F. M. Structural differences between distended and collapsed arteries. Angiology *16*: 53–56 (1965).

Burri, P. H. and Weibel, E. R. Beeinflussung einer spezifischen cytoplasmatischen Organelle von Endothelzellen durch Adrenalin. Z. Zellforsch. *88*: 426–440 (1968).

Devine, C. E. and Simpson, F. O. The fine structure of vascular sympathetic neuromuscular contacts in the rat. Am. J. Anat. *121*: 153–173 (1967).

Fillenz, M. Innervation of pulmonary and bronchial blood vessels of the dog. J. Anat. *106*: 449–461 (1970).

Lang, J. Mikroskopische Anatomie der Arterien. Angiologica *2*: part I, 225–284 (1965).

Pease, D. C. and Paule, W. J. Electron microscopy of elastic arteries; the thoracic aorta of the rat. J. Ultrastruct. Res. *3*: 469–483 (1960).

Pease, D. C. and Molinari, S. Electron microscopy of muscular arteries: pial vessels of the cat and monkey. J. Ultrastruct. Res. *3*: 447–468 (1960).

Peters, T. J., Müller, M. and de Duve, C. Lysosomes of the arterial wall. I. Isolation and subcellular fractionation of cells from normal rabbit aorta. J. Exp. Med. *136*: 1117–1139 (1972).

Piezzi, R. S., Santolaya, R. S. and Bertini, F. The fine structure of endothelial cells of toad arteries. Anat. Rec. *165*: 229–236 (1969).

Ratschow, M. (Ed.). Angiologie. George Thieme, Stuttgart, 1959.

Reale, E. and Ruska, H. Die Feinstruktur der Gefässwände. Angiologica *2*: part I, 314–366 (1965).

Rhodin, J. A. G. Fine structure of vascular walls in mammals with special reference to smooth muscle component. Physiol. Rev. *42*: 48–87 (1962).

Sato, S. An electron microscopic study on the innervation of the intracranial artery of the rat. Am. J. Anat. *118*: 873–890 (1966).

Schwartz, S. M. and Benditt, E. P. Studies on aortic intima. I. Structure and permeability of rat thoracic aortic intima. Am. J. Path. *66*: 241–264 (1972).

Sengel, A. and Stoebner, P. Golgi origin of tubular inclusions in endothelial cells. J. Cell Biol. *44*: 223–226 (1970).

Silva, D. G. and Ikeda, M. Ultrastructural and acetylcholinesterase studies on the innervation of the ductus arteriosus, pulmonary trunk and aorta of the fetal lamb. J. Ultrastruct. Res. *34*: 358–374 (1971).

Takayanagi, T., Rennels, M. L. and Nelson, E. An electron microscopic study of intimal cushions in intracranial arteries of the cat. Am. J. Anat. *133*: 415–430 (1972).

Ts'ao, C., Glagov, S. and Kelsey, B. F. Structure of mammalian portal vein: postnatal establishment of two mutually perpendicular medial muscle zones in the rat. Anat. Rec. *171*: 457–470 (1971).

Weibel, E. R. and Palade, G. E. New cytoplasmic components in arterial endothelia. J. Cell Biol. *23*: 101–112 (1964).

Wissler, R. W. The arterial medial cell, smooth muscle or multifunctional mesenchyme? J. Atherosclerosis Res. *8*: 201–213 (1968).

Wood, E. The venous system. Sci. American *218*: 86–96 (1968).

MICROVASCULAR BED

Bennett, H. S., Luft, J. H. and Hampton, J. C. Morphological classification of vertebrate blood capillaries. Am. J. Physiol. *196*: 381–390 (1959).

Bensley, R. R. and Vintrup, B. On the nature of the Rouget cells of capillaries. Anat. Rec. *39*: 37–55 (1929).

Brightman, M. W. and Reese, T. S. Junctions between intimately apposed cell membranes in the vertebrate brain. J. Cell Biol. *40*: 648–677 (1969).

Bruns, R. R. and Palade, G. E. Studies on blood capillaries. I. General organization of blood capillaries in muscle. J. Cell Biol. *37*: 244–276 (1968).

Bruns, R. R. and Palade, G. E. Studies on blood capillaries. II. Transport of ferritin molecules across the wall of muscle capillaries. J. Cell Biol. *37*: 277–299 (1968).

Cecio, A. Ultrastructural features of cytofilaments within mammalian endothelial cells. Z. Zellforsch. *83*: 40–48 (1967).

Clementi, F. and Palade, G. E. Intestinal capillaries. I. Permeability to peroxidase and ferritin. J. Cell Biol. *41*: 33–58 (1969).

Clementi, F. and Palade, G. E. Intestinal capillaries. II. Structural effects of EDTA and histamine. J. Cell Biol. *42*: 706–714 (1969).

Crone, C. and Lassen, N. A. (Eds.). Capillary Permeability. Academic Press, New York, 1970.

Fernando, N. V. P. and Movat, H. Z. The fine structure of the terminal vascular bed. II. The smallest arterial vessels: terminal arterioles and metarterioles. Exp. Molec. Path. *3*: 1–9 (1964).

Fernando, N. V. P. and Movat, H. Z. Fine structure of the terminal vascular bed. III. Capillaries. Exp. Molec. Path. *3*: 87–97 (1964).

Karnovsky, M. J. The ultrastructural basis of capillary permeability studied with peroxidase as a tracer. J. Cell Biol. *35*: 213–236 (1967).

Lever, J. D., Spriggs, T. L. B. and Graham, J. D. P. A formol-fluorescence, fine-structural and autoradiographic study of the adrenergic innervation of the vascular tree in the intact and sympathectomized pancreas of the cat. J. Anat. *103*: 15–34 (1968).

Majno, G. Ultrastructure of the vascular membrane. *In* Handbook of Physiology, Section 2, Vol. III, Circulation, 1965, pp. 2293–2375.

Majno, G., Shea, S. M. and Leventhal, M. Endothelial contraction induced by histamine-type mediators. An electron microscopic study. J. Cell Biol. *42*: 647–672 (1969).

Marchesi, V. T. The role of pinocytic vesicles in the transport of material across the walls of small blood vessels. Investig. Ophthalmol. *4*: 1111–1121 (1965).

Maul, G. G. Structure and formation of pores in fenestrated capillaries. J. Ultrastruct. Res. *36*: 768–782 (1971).

Movat, H. Z. and Fernando, N. V. P. The fine structure of the terminal vascular bed. II. Small arteries with an internal elastic lamina. Exp. Molec. Path. *2*: 549–563 (1963).

Movat, H. Z. and Fernando, N. V. P. The fine structure of the terminal vascular bed. IV. The venules and their perivascular cells. Exp. Molec. Path. *3*: 98–114 (1963).

Pappenheimer, J. R. Passage of molecules through capillary walls. Physiol. Rev. *33*: 386–423 (1953).

Phelps, P. C. and Luft, J. H. Electron microscopical study of relaxation and constriction in frog arterioles. Am. J. Anat. *125*: 399–428 (1969).

Reese, T. S. and Karnovsky, M. J. Fine structural localization of a blood brain barrier to exogenous peroxidase. J. Cell Biol. *34*: 207–217 (1962).

Rhodin, J. A. G. The diaphragm of capillary endothelial fenestrations. J. Ultrastruct. Res. *6*: 171–185 (1962).

Rhodin, J. A. G. The ultrastructure of mammalian arterioles and precapillary sphincters. J. Ultrastruct. Res. *18*: 181–223 (1967).

Rhodin, J. A. G. Ultrastructure of mammalian venous capillaries, venules, and small collecting veins. J. Ultrastruct. Res. *25*: 452–500 (1968).

Rhodin, J. A. G. Fine structure of capillaries. *In* Topics in the Study of Life. The Bio Source Book (Ed. H. Ris), pp. 215–224. Harper & Row, New York, 1971.

Simon, G. Ultrastructure des capillaires. Angiologica *2*: part I, 370–434 (1965).

Venkatachalam, M. A. and Karnovsky, M. J. Extravascular protein in the kidney. An ultrastructural study of its relation to renal peritubular capillary permeability using protein tracers. Lab. Investig. *27*: 435–444 (1972).

Wolff, J. and Merker, H. J. Ultrastruktur und Bildung von Poren im Endothel von porösen und geschlossenen Kapillaren. Z. Zellforsch. *73*: 174–191 (1966).

17 Lymphatic system

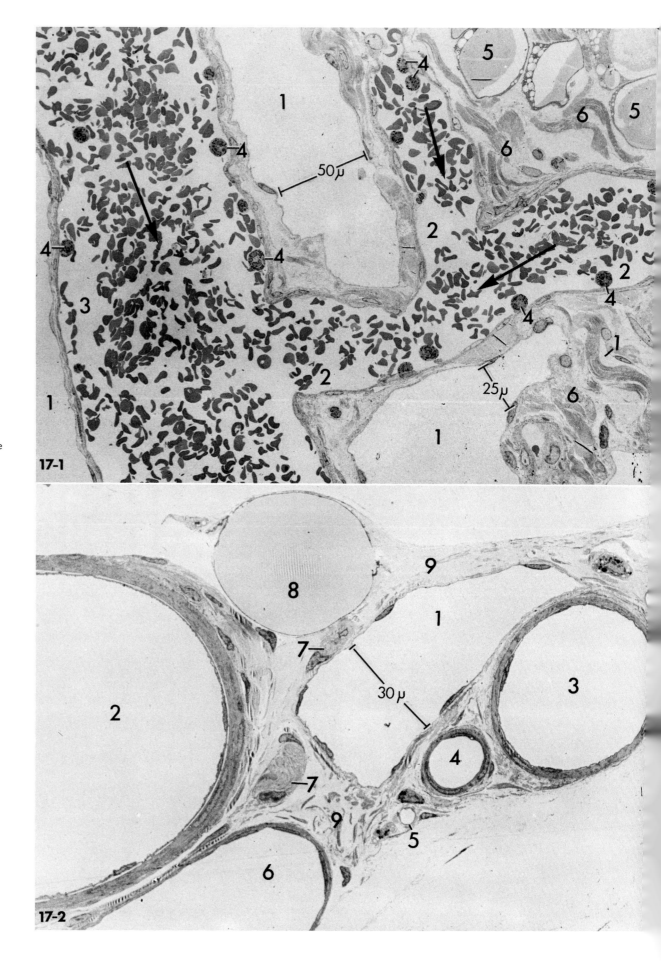

Fig. 17-1. Longitudinal section of lymphatic capillaries and venules in the dermal connective tissue. Skin. Rabbit. E.M. X 600. **1.** Lymphatic capillaries of varied cross-sectional diameters. These vessels drain the skin and are largely devoid of lymphocytes before reaching the first lymph node. **2.** Venules. **3.** Small vein (diameter about 90 μ). Arrows indicate direction of blood flow. **4.** Marginated granulocytes. **5.** Fat cells. **6.** Collagenous fibers.

Fig. 17-2. Microvascular dimensions. Cross section of vascular bundle. Mesentery. Rat. E.M. X 870. **1.** Lymphatic capillary: lumen 30 μ; wall 0.1 μ. **2.** Arteriole: lumen 85 μ; wall 5 μ. **3.** Arteriole: lumen 45 μ; wall 2.5 μ. **4.** Precapillary arteriole; lumen 14 μ; wall 2 μ. **5.** Capillary: lumen 5 μ; wall 0.2 μ. **6.** Venule: lumen 40 μ; wall 1 μ. **7.** Non-myelinated nerves. **8.** Fat cell. **9.** Loose connective tissue.

210

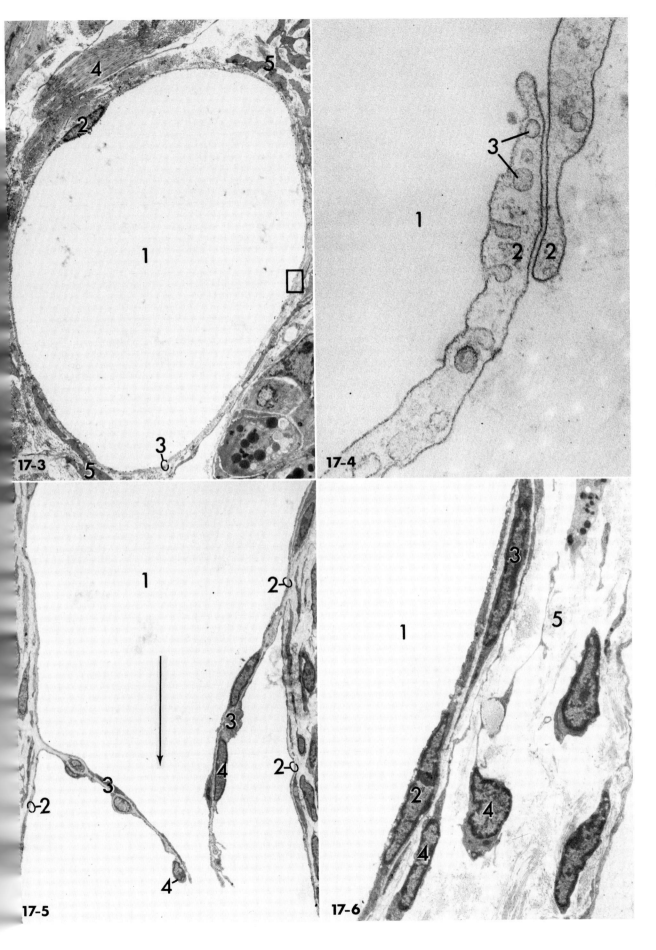

Fig. 17-3. Cross section of intestinal lymphatic capillary (lacteal). Small intestine. Rat. E.M. X 1400. **1.** Lumen (50 μ). **2.** Nucleus of endothelial cell. **3.** Endothelial cytoplasm. **4.** Bundles of collagenous fibrils. **5.** Smooth muscle cells of lamina muscularis mucosae (not part of the wall of the lacteal).

Fig. 17-4. Enlargement of area similar to rectangle in Fig. 17-3. Wall of lymphatic capillary. Mouse. E.M. X 64,000. **1.** Lumen. **2.** Overlapping edges of the endothelial cells. No special junctional arrangements. **3.** Pinocytotic vesicles. No basal lamina.

Fig. 17-5. Longitudinal section of collecting lymphatic vessel. Ovary. Rat. E.M. X 2800. **1.** Lumen. **2.** Endothelium. **3.** Valves. **4.** Nuclei of endothelial cells in the cusps. Arrow indicates direction of lymph flow.

Fig. 17-6. Cross section of part of afferent lymphatic vessel near entrance to lymph node. Rat. E.M. X 4000. **1.** Lumen. **2.** Nucleus of endothelial cell. **3.** Nucleus of smooth muscle cell. **4.** Nuclei of fibroblasts. **5.** Collagenous fibrils.

Fig. 17-7. Lingual tonsil. Monkey. L.M. X 100.
1. Stratified squamous, non-keratinized epithelium of upper surface of base of tongue.
2. Aggregation of lymphocytes, forming a lymphatic nodule without germinal center.
3. Ducts of salivary gland.

Fig. 17-8. Lingual tonsil. Detail. Monkey. L.M. X 260. **1.** Surface epithelium **2.** Subepithelial aggregation of lymphocytes. **3.** Extensive infiltration of surface epithelium by invading lymphocytes. **4.** Level of basement membrane. **5.** The most superficial layers of the squamous epithelium are not invaded by lymphocytes.

Fig. 17-9. Solitary lymphatic nodule. Appendix. Human. L.M. X 185. **1.** Germinal center of solitary lymphatic nodule. **2.** Peripheral aggregation of small lymphocytes. **3.** Diffuse infiltration of lamina propria by lymphocytes. **4.** Lumen of appendix. **5.** Crypts of Lieberkühn.

Fig. 17-10. Palatine tonsil. Human. L.M. X 14. **1.** Oropharyngeal cavity. **2.** Surface epithelium. **3.** Longitudinally sectioned crypt. **4.** Cross-sectioned crypt. **5.** Multiple lymphatic nodules with germinal centers. **6.** Capsule.

Fig. 17-11. Peyer's patch. Ileum. Monkey. L.M. X 39. **1.** Lumen of gut. **2.** Intestinal villi. **3.** Crypts of Lieberkühn. **4.** Multiple lymphatic nodules without germinal centers. **5.** Muscularis externa.

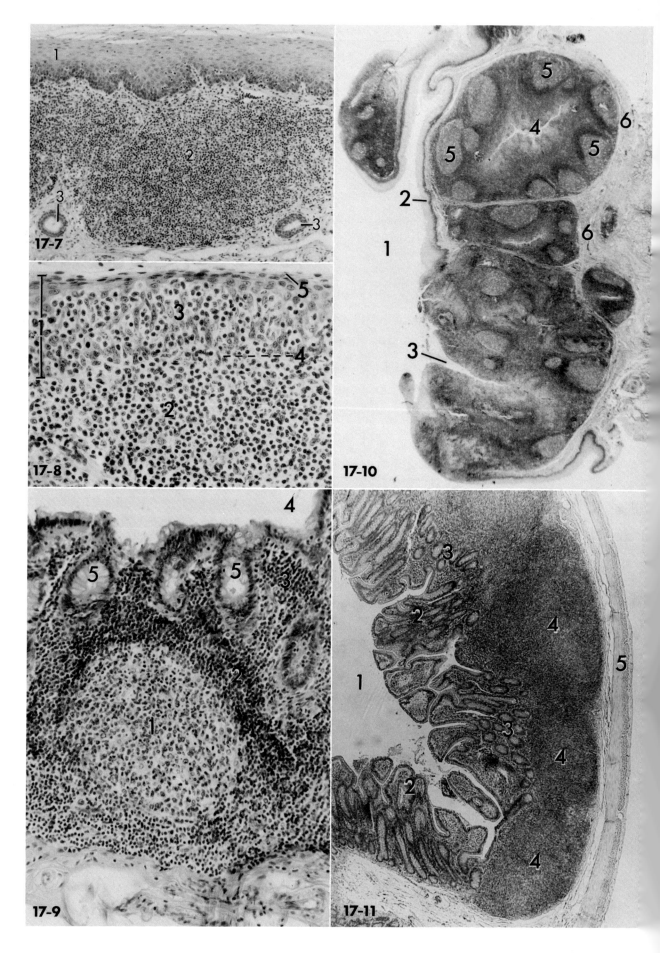

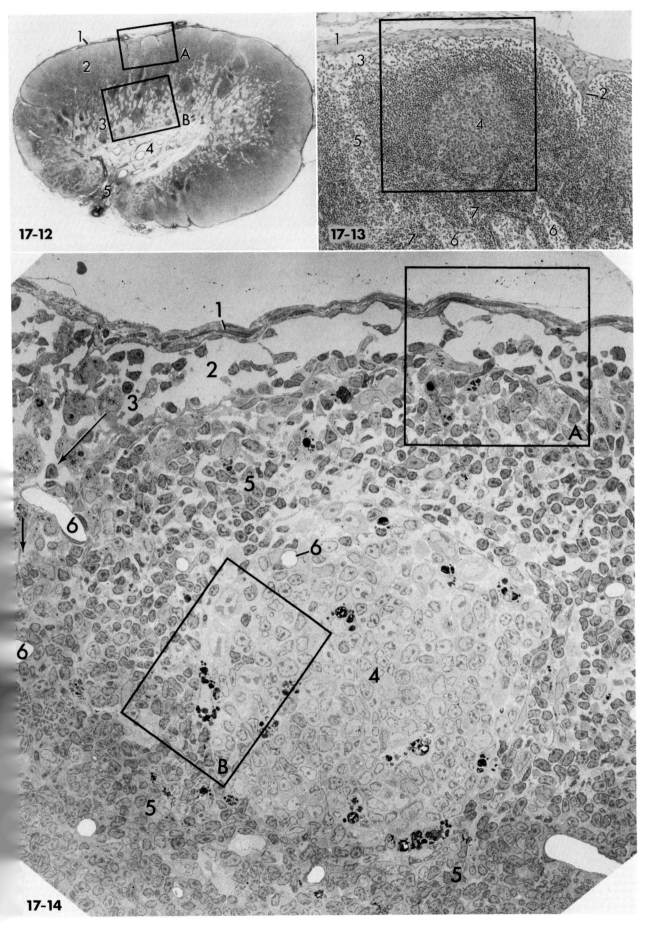

Fig. 17-12. Section of entire lymph node. Monkey. L.M. X 9. **1.** Capsule. **2.** Cortex. **3.** Medulla. **4.** Hilus. **5.** Blood vessels and efferent lymphatic vessel.

Fig. 17-13. Enlargement of area similar to rectangle (A) in Fig. 17-12. Lymph node. L.M. X 91. **1.** Capsule. **2.** Part of trabecula. **3.** Subcapsular sinus. **4.** Germinal center of lymphatic nodule. **5.** Penetrating sinus. **6.** Medullary sinuses. **7.** Medullary cords.

Fig. 17-14. Enlargement of area similar to square in Fig. 17-13. Lymph node. Rat. E.M. X 620. **1.** Capsule. **2.** Subcapsular sinus. **3.** Penetrating sinus. Arrows indicate direction of lymph flow. **4.** Germinal center of lymphatic nodule. Dominated by lymphoblasts and medium-sized lymphocytes. **5.** Peripheral aggregation of small lymphocytes (corona). **6.** Blood capillaries, fixed by intravascular perfusion. Rectangle (A) enlarged in Fig. 17-15; rectangle (B) in Fig. 17-16.

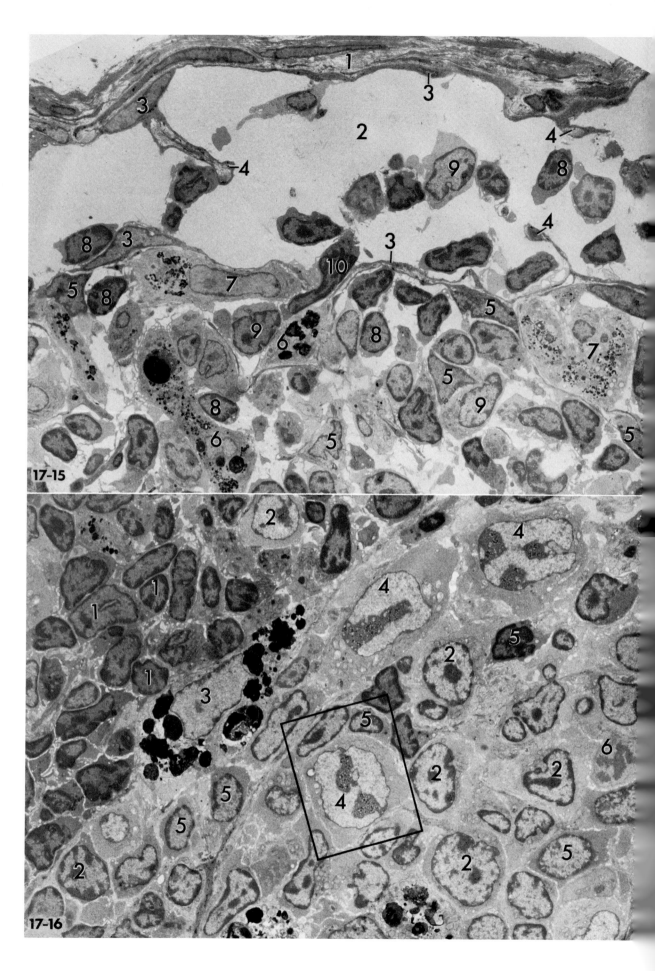

Fig. 17-15. Survey of subcapsular lymph sinus. Enlargement of rectangle (A) in Fig. 17-14. Lymph node. Rat. E.M. × 1800. **1.** Collagenous fibers of capsule. **2.** Lumen of subcapsular sinus. **3.** Littoral (lining) cell, endothelial in nature. **4.** Narrow bundles of collagenous fibrils, covered by thin cytoplasm of littoral cells, crossing sinus. **5.** Reticular cells. **6.** Macrophages. **7.** Monocytes (or macrophages). **8.** Small lymphocytes. **9.** Medium-sized lymphocytes. **10.** Small lymphocyte going through wall of lymph sinus.

Fig. 17-16. Survey of area between germinal center and peripheral corona of lymph nodule. Enlargement of rectangle (B) in Fig. 17-14. Lymph node. Rat. E.M. × 1800. **1.** Small lymphocytes of corona. **2.** Medium-sized lymphocytes. **3.** Macrophage at border between germinal center of corona. **4.** Large lymphocytes (lymphoblasts). Rectangle enlarged in Fig. 17-27. **5.** Small lymphocytes of germinal center. **6.** Lymphoid cell in mitosis.

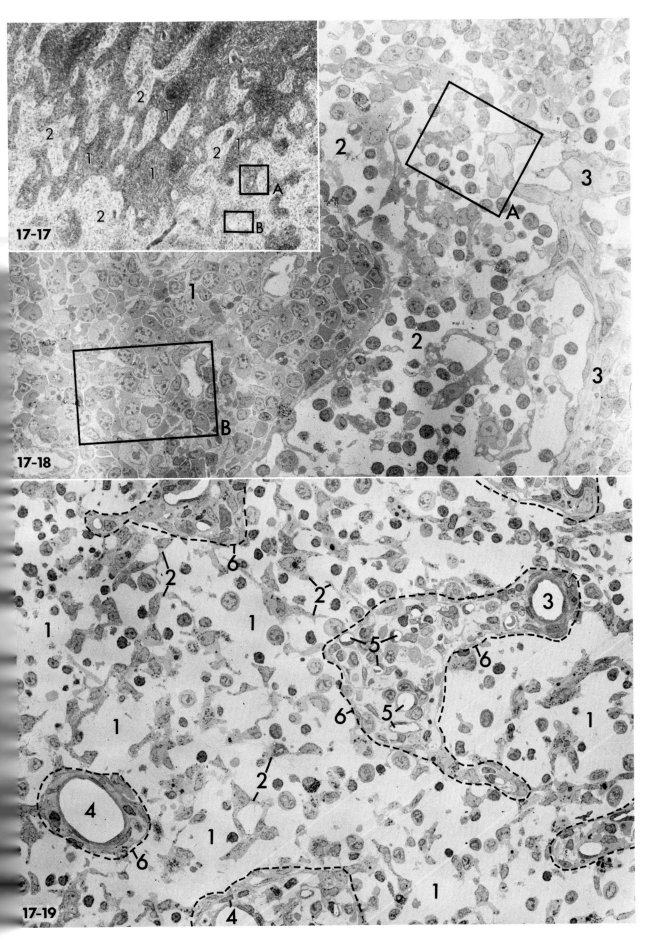

Fig. 17-17. Medulla of lymph node. Enlargement of rectangle (B) in Fig. 17-12. Lymph node. Monkey. L.M. X 40.
1. Medullary cords. **2.** Medullary sinuses.

Fig. 17-18. Survey of medullary cord and sinus. Enlargement of area similar to rectangle (A) in Fig. 17-17. Lymph node. Cat. E.M. X 640.
1. Medullary cord of densely packed plasma cells and lymphocytes. **2.** Medullary lymph sinus with a variety of circulating lymphoid cells. **3.** Trabeculae of dense connective tissue. Area similar to rectangle (A) is enlarged in Fig. 17-20 and area similar to rectangle (B) is enlarged in Fig. 17-30.

Fig. 17-19. Survey of medullary sinus near hilus. Enlargement of area similar to rectangle (B) in Fig. 17-17. Lymph node. Rat. E.M. × 570.
1. Lumen of sinus with circulating lymphoid cells. **2.** Cells forming a reticular network across sinus represent fixed macrophages. **3.** Small artery. **4.** Small veins. **5.** Capillaries. **6.** Dotted lines indicate trabeculae of loose connective tissue. Blood vessels of lymph nodes travel within the trabecular connective tissue compartment.

Fig. 17-20. Survey of medullary sinus. Enlargement of area similar to rectangle (A) in Fig. 17-18. Lymph node. Cat. E.M. X 1800. **1.** Lumen of sinus. **2.** Densely packed collagenous fibrils in trabeculae. **3.** Fibroblasts. **4.** Littoral cells cover the large dense connective tissue trabeculae. **5.** Fixed macrophages cover the narrow bundles of collagenous fibrils (*asterisks*). **6.** Small lymphocytes. **7.** Medium-sized lymphocytes. **8.** Unclassified lymphoid cells, similar to the cell enlarged in Fig. 17-29. These cells are probably intermediate between medium-sized and larger lymphocytes and/or plasma cells. **9.** Erythrocytes occasionally in the lymph sinus.

Fig. 17-21. Fixed macrophage in medullary lymph sinus. Lymph node. Cat. E.M. X 3300. **1.** Lumen of sinus. **2.** Nucleus of fixed macrophage. **3.** Golgi zone. **4.** Mitochondria. **5.** Lysosomes. **6.** Small numerous profiles most of which represent pinocytotic vesicles. **7.** Narrow bundles of fine and densely packed collagenous fibrils, surrounded by cytoplasmic processes of the macrophage.

Fig. 17-22. Enlargement of square in Fig. 17-21. Lymph node. Cat. E.M. X 25,000. **1.** Cross-sectioned narrow bundle of fine collagenous fibrils. **2.** Cytoplasmic arms of macrophage surround extracellular bundle of collagenous fibrils. **3.** Nucleus **4.** Filamentous layer of cell membrane (glycocalyx).

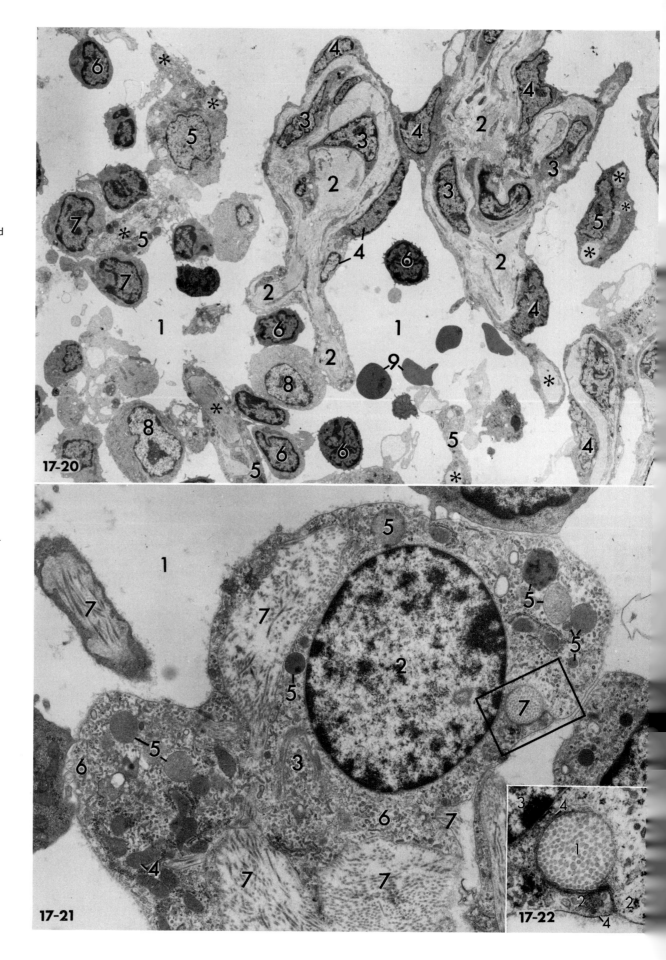

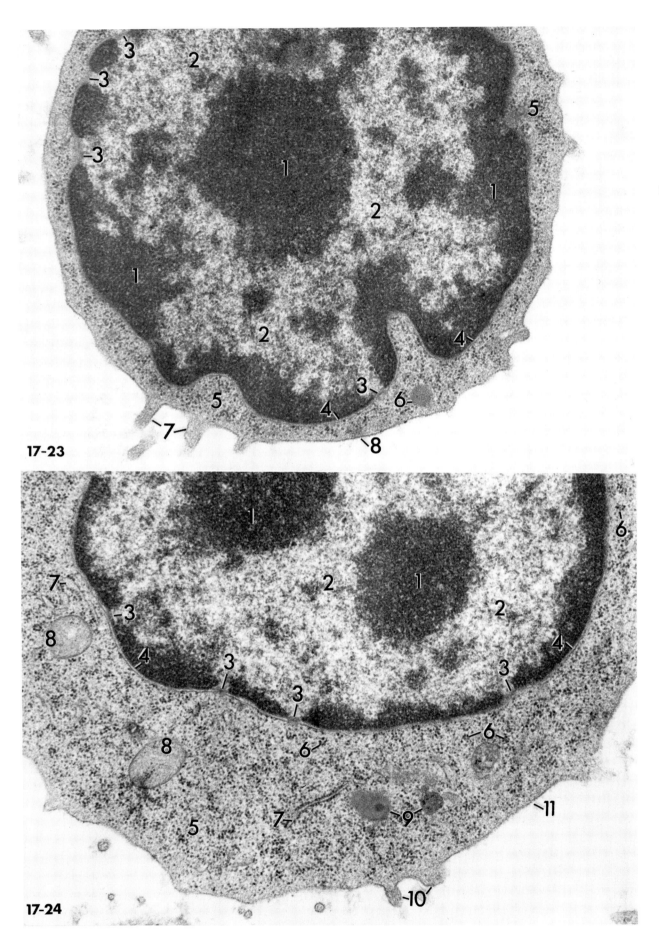

17-23

17-24

Fig. 17-23. Small lymphocyte (5 μ in diameter) in medullary sinus of lymph node. Cat. E.M. X 32,000. **1.** Heterochromatin of nucleus. **2.** Euchromatin of nucleus. **3.** Nuclear pore areas. **4.** Nuclear membrane. **5.** Free ribosomes in narrow zone of cytoplasm. **6.** Small granule. **7.** Microvilli. **8.** Surface membrane.

Fig. 17-24. Medium-sized lymphocyte (7 μ in diameter) in medullary sinus of lymph node. Cat. E.M. X 33,000. **1.** Heterochromatin of nucleus. **2.** Euchromatin of nucleus. **3.** Nuclear pore areas. **4.** Nuclear membrane. **5.** Numerous free ribosomes. Cytoplasmic zone is wider than in a small lymphocyte. **6.** Some free polysomes. **7.** Short profiles of granular endoplasmic reticulum. **8.** Mitochondria. **9.** Small granules. **10.** Microvilli. **11.** Surface membrane.

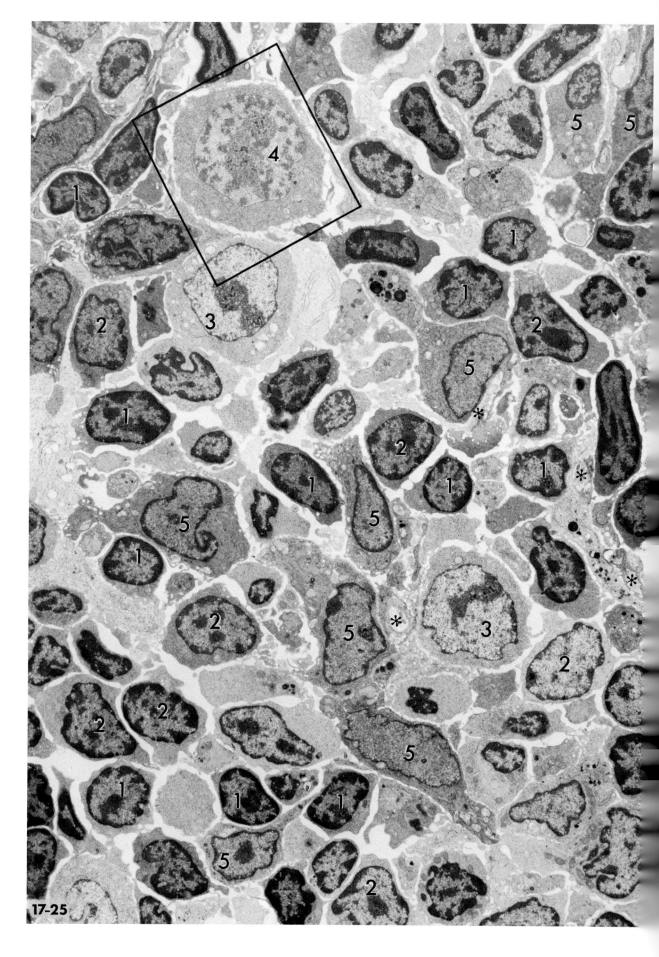

Fig. 17-25. Survey of germinal center in nodule of white pulp of spleen. Same preparation and area as seen in Fig. 18-6. Rat. E.M. × 2500. **1.** Small lymphocytes (average 5 μ in width). **2.** Medium-sized lymphocytes (average 8 μ in width). **3.** Large lymphocytes or lymphoblasts (average 12 μ in width). **4.** Large lymphocyte in prophase of mitotic division. Further enlarged in Fig. 17-26. **5.** Reticular cells. **6.** *Asterisks* indicate bundles of collagenous fibrils. Note that some of the lymphoid cells in this field of view cannot be categorized with certainty unless they are studied at higher magnifications.

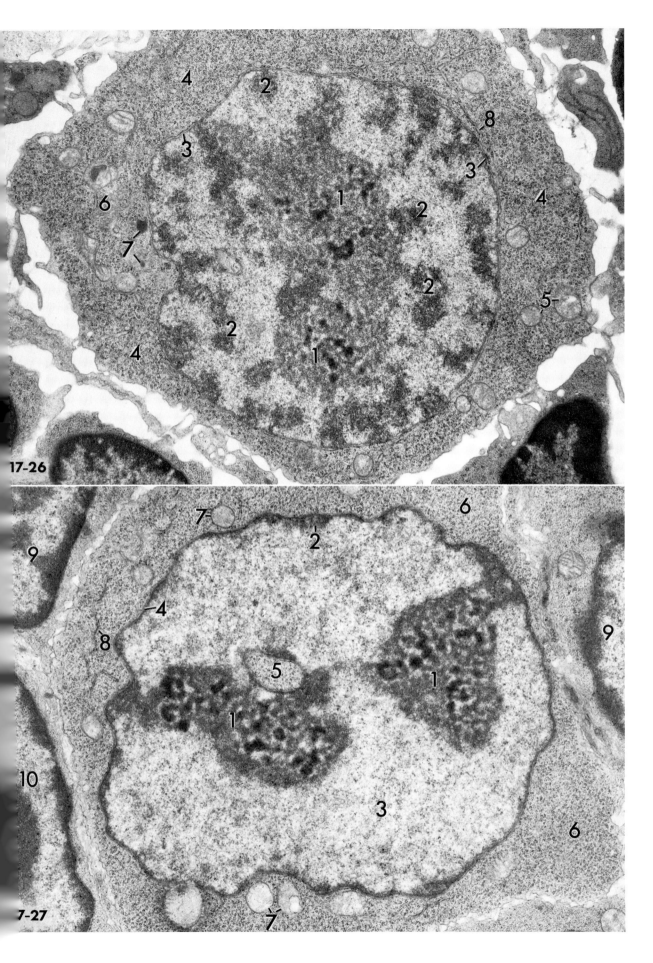

Fig. 17-26. Large lymphocyte (lymphoblast) in germinal center of splenic nodule. Cell width 14 μ. Nucleus in prophase of mitotic division. Enlargement of rectangle in Fig. 17-25. Spleen. Rat. E.M. X 12,000. **1.** Nucleoli. **2.** Chromosomes. **3.** Nuclear membrane. **4.** Cytoplasm filled with polyribosomes. **5.** Mitochondria. **6.** Small Golgi zone. **7.** Small granules. **8.** Short profiles of granular endoplasmic reticulum.

Fig. 17-27. Large lymphocyte (lymphoblast) in germinal center of lymphatic nodule. Cell width 12 μ. Nucleus in interphase. Enlargement of rectangle in Fig. 17-16. Lymph node. Rat. E.M. × 12,000. **1.** Nucleoli. **2.** Narrow zone of heterochromatin. **3.** Euchromatin. **4.** Nuclear membrane. **5.** Finger-like cytoplasmic indentation of nuclear surface cut across. **6.** Cytoplasm overcrowded with polyribosomes. **7.** Mitochondria. **8.** Short profiles of granular endoplasmic reticulum. Note the great similarity in cytoplasmic ultrastructure of lymphoblasts from spleen and lymph node. **9.** Nuclei of small lymphocytes. **10.** Nucleus of reticular cell.

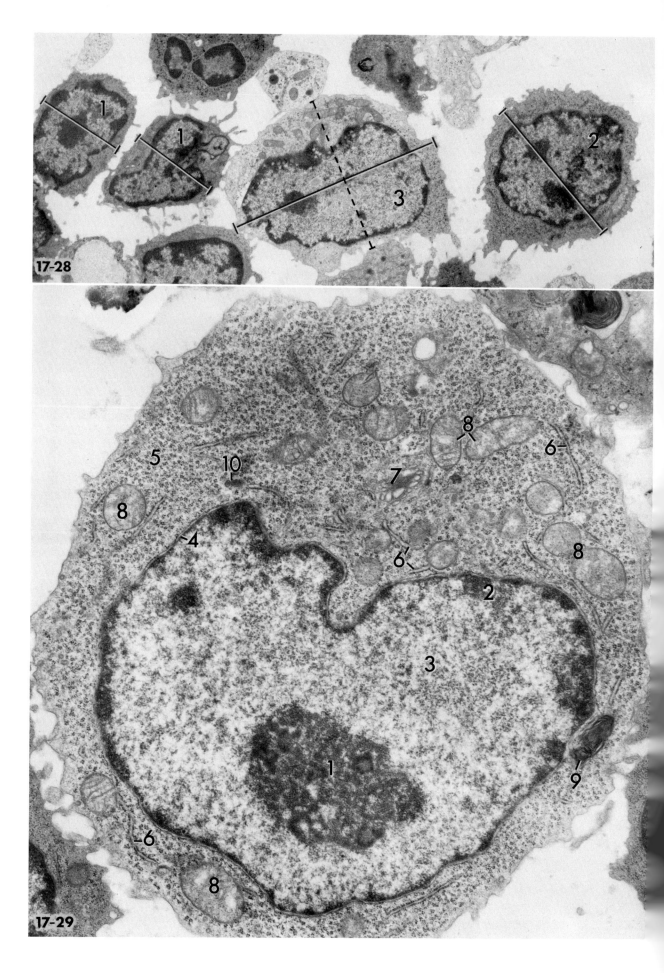

Fig. 17-28. Lymphocytes in medullary sinus. Lymph node. Cat. E.M. × 5500. This demonstrates the difficulty one encounters in trying to categorize lymphocytes solely on morphological grounds. **1.** Small lymphocytes, width indicated by line is 4.4 μ. **2.** Medium-sized lymphocyte, width indicated by line is 7.8 μ. **3.** Large lymphocyte. Width indicated by solid line is 11 μ; by dotted line 7.8 μ.

Fig. 17-29. Intermediate lymphoid cell from medullary sinus of lymph node. Cell width 10–11 μ. This is an example of the great heterogeneity among lymphoid cells. This cell could represent: a lymphoblast, a plasmablast, a monoblast, or the stem cell of the unitarian hemopoietic theory—a hemocytoblast. Lymph node. Cat. E.M. × 17,000. **1.** Nucleolus. **2.** Marginated heterochromatin. **3.** Euchromatin. **4.** Nuclear membrane. **5.** Polyribosomes. **6.** Short profiles of granular endoplasmic reticulum. **7.** Golgi zone. **8.** Mitochondria. **9.** Inclusion body (secondary lysosome). **10.** Small granules. *Conclusion.* If this cell is encountered in the circulating blood, it would be classified as a monocyte and not a lymphoblast, since the latter normally does not enter the peripheral circulation. Since this cell is found in a medullary lymph sinus, it probably represents a *large lymphocyte* (lymphoblast), possibly undergoing differentiation toward a plasma cell, particularly considering the abundant cytoplasm, the eccentric nucleus, and the relatively large number of profiles of granular endoplasmic reticulum.

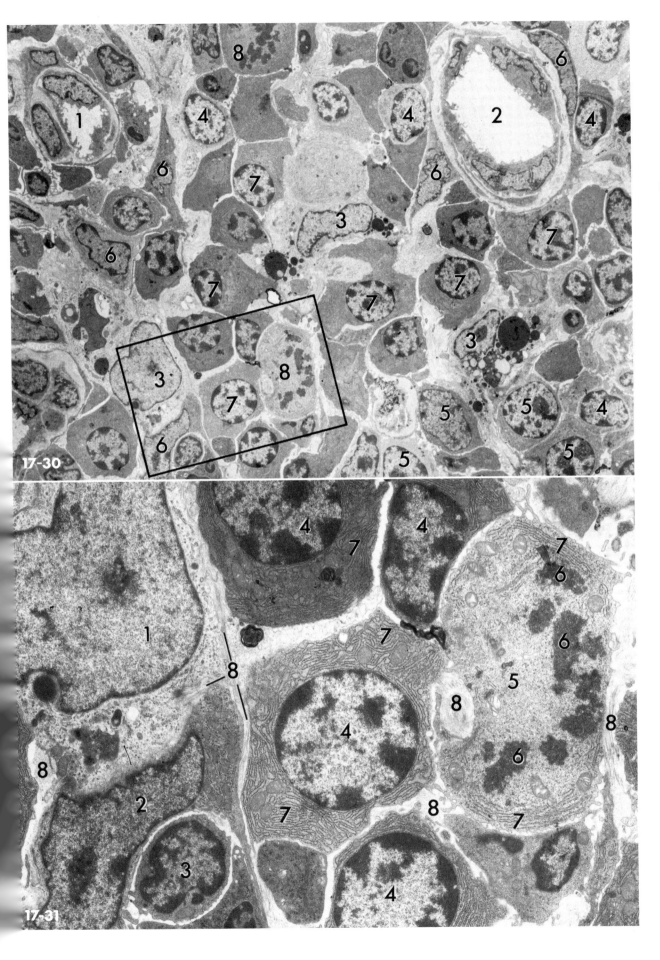

Fig. 17-30. Survey of medullary cord. Enlargement of area similar to rectangle (B) in Fig. 17-18. Lymph node. Cat. E.M. X 1900. **1.** Lumen of blood capillary. **2.** Lumen of venule. **3.** Macrophages. **4.** Small lymphocytes. **5.** Medium-sized lymphocytes. **6.** Reticular cells. **7.** Plasma cells. **8.** Dividing plasma cells.

Fig. 17-31. Detail of medullary cord. Enlargement of rectangle in Fig. 17-30. Lymph node. Cat. E.M. X 6900. **1.** Nucleus of macrophage. **2.** Nucleus of reticular cell. **3.** Nucleus of small lymphocyte. **4.** Nuclei of plasma cells. **5.** Dividing plasma cell. **6.** Chromosomes. **7.** Granular endoplasmic reticulum. **8.** Bundles of extracellular fine collagenous and reticular fibrils. Note that they are not only associated with reticular cells but occur freely in between the plasma cells.

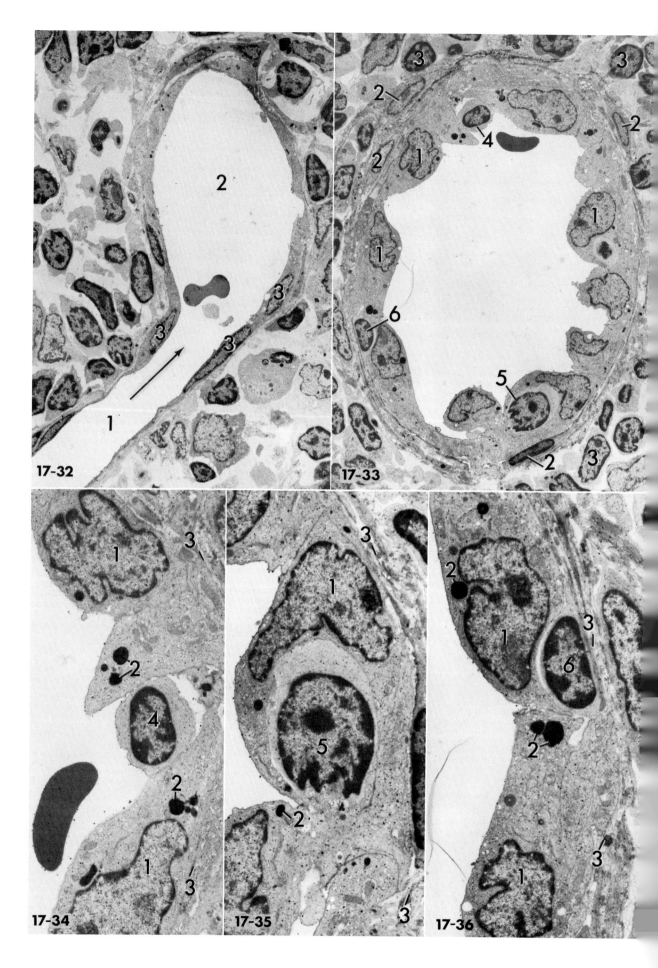

Fig. 17-32. Blood vessels of lymph node. Rat. E.M. X 1700. **1.** Venous capillary. Width of lumen 5 μ. Arrow indicates direction of blood flow. **2.** Postcapillary venule. Width of lumen 22 μ. **3.** Nuclei of endothelial cells.

Fig. 17-33. Cross section of lymph node postcapillary venule. Width of lumen approximately 30 μ. High endothelial cells characterize this kind of venule. Rat. E.M. X 960. **1.** Nuclei of endothelial cells. **2.** Nuclei of pericytes. **3.** Perivascular lymphocytes. **4.** Lymphocyte leaving lumen of venule (enlarged in Fig. 17-34). **5.** Lymphocyte partly surrounded by endothelial cell cytoplasm (enlarged in Fig. 17-35). **6.** Lymphocyte located between endothelium and pericytic sheath of venule (enlarged in Fig. 17-36).

Figs. 17-34, 17-35 & 17-36. Mechanism of lymphocyte recirculation. Enlargements of parts of venule in Fig. 17-33. Rat. E.M. X 4500. **1.** Nuclei of endothelial cells. **2.** Lysosomes. **3.** Basal lamina. **4.** This lymphocyte is leaving the venule by route between endothelial cells. **5.** This lymphocyte is engulfed by endothelial cell. **6.** This lymphocyte is temporarily lodged outside of endothelium.

222

References

Ackerman, G. A. The lymphocyte: its morphology and embryological origin. *In* The Lymphocyte in Immunology and Haematopoiesis. (Ed. J. M. Yoffey), pp. 11–30. Edward Arnold, London, 1967.

Ackerman, G. A. Structural studies of the lymphocyte and lymphocyte development. *In* Regulation of Hematopoiesis. (Ed. A. S. Gordon), Vol. 2: 1297–1338. Appleton-Century-Crofts, New York, 1970.

Bernhard, W. and Leplus, R. Fine Structure of the Normal and Malignant Human Lymph Node. Macmillan, New York, 1964.

Brooks, R. E. and Siegel, B. V. Normal human lymph node cells: an electron microscopic study. Blood *27*: 687–705 (1966).

Casley-Smith, J. R. and Clark, E. L. The structure of normal small lymphatics. Q. J. Exp. Physiol. *46*: 101–106 (1961).

Cliff, W. J. and Nicoll, P. A. Structure and function of lymphatic vessels of the bat's wing. Q. J. Exp. Physiol. *55*: 112–121 (1970).

de Petris, S., Karslbad, G. and Pernis, B. Localization of antibodies in plasma cells by electron microscopy. J. Exp. Med. *117*: 849–862 (1963).

Everett, N. B. and Tyler, R. W. Lymphopoiesis in the thymus and other tissues: functional implications. Int. Rev. Cytol. *21*: 205–237 (1967).

Feldman, J. D. and Nordquist, R. E. Immunologic competence of thoracic duct cells. II. Ultrastructure. Lab. Investig. *16*: 564–579 (1967).

Gowans, J. L. Life-span, recirculation and transformation of lymphocytes. Int. Rev. Exp. Path. *5*: 1–24 (1966).

Hostetler, J. R. and Ackerman, G. A. Lymphopoiesis and lymph node histogenesis in the embryonic and neonatal rabbit. Am. J. Anat. *124*: 57–76 (1969).

Leak, L. V. Studies on the permeability of lymphatic capillaries. J. Cell Biol. *50*: 300–323 (1971).

Leak, L. V. and Burke, J. F. Fine structure of the lymphatic capillary and the adjoining connective tissue area. Am. J. Anat. *118*: 785–810 (1966).

Marchesi, V. T. and Gowans, J. L. Migration of lymphocytes through the endothelium of venules in lymph nodes. An electron microscopic study. Proc. R. Soc. B. *159*: 283–290 (1964).

Mayerson, H. S. The Lymphatic System. Sci. American *208*: 80–90 (1963).

Mikata, A. and Niki, R. Permeability of postcapillary venules of the lymph node. An electron microscopic study. Exp. & Molec. Pathol. *14*: 289–305 (1971).

Miller, J. A. F. P., Basten, A., Sprent, J. and Cheers, C. Interaction between lymphocytes in immune responses. (Review). Cellular Immunology *2*: 469–495 (1971).

Movat, H. Z. and Fernando, N. V. P. The fine structure of lymphoid tissue. Exp. & Molec. Pathol. *3*: 546–568 (1964).

Movat, H. Z. and Fernando, N. V. P. The fine structure of lymphoid tissue during antibody formation. Exp. & Molec. Pathol. *4*: 155–188 (1965).

Nopajaroonsri, C., Luk, S. and Simon, G. T. Ultrastructure of the normal lymph node. Am. J. Path. *65*: 1–24 (1971).

Nossal, G. J. V. How cells make antibodies. Sci. American *211*: 106–115 (1964).

Nossal, G. J. V. The cellular basis of immunity. Harvey Lect. Series *63*: 179–211 (1968).

Nowell, P. C. and Wilson, D. B. Lymphocytes and hemic stem cells. Am. J. Path. *65*: 641–652 (1971).

Sainte-Marie, G. and Sin, Y. M. Structures of the lymph node and their possible function during the immune response. Rev. Can. Biol. *27*: 191–207 (1968).

Schipp, R. Der Feinstruktur filamentärer Strukturen im Endothel peripherer Lymphgefässe. Acta Anat *71*: 341–351 (1968).

Schwarz, M. R. Transformation of rat small lymphocytes with allogeneic lymphoid cells. Am. J. Anat. *121*: 559–570 (1967).

Smith, J. B., McIntosh, G. H. and Morris, B. The traffic of cells through tissues: a study of peripheral lymph in sheep. J. Anat. *107*: 87–100 (1970).

Takada, M. The ultrastructure of lymphatic valves in rabbits and mice. Am. J. Anat. *132*: 207–217 (1971).

Turner, D. R. The vascular tree of the haemal node in the rat. J. Anat. *104*: 481–493 (1969).

Wenk, E. J., Orlic, D., Reith, E. J. and Rhodin, J. A. G. The ultrastructure of mouse lymph node venules and the passage of lymphocytes across their walls. J. Ultrastruct. Res. *47* (1974).

Willingham, M. C., Spicer, S. S. and Graber, C. D. Immunological labeling of calf and human lymphocyte surface antigens. Lab. Investig. *25*: 211–219 (1971).

Zucker-Franklin, D. The ultrastructure of lymphocytes. Seminars in Hematology *6*: 4–27 (1969).

18 Spleen

Fig. 18-1. Spleen. Human. L.M. X 10.
1. Capsule. **2.** Trabeculae. **3.** Trabeculae with vein. **4.** Red pulp. **5.** White pulp with splenic nodules.

Fig. 18-2. Spleen fixed by intra-arterial perfusion. Rat. L.M. X 50. **1.** Capsule (thin). **2.** Red pulp. **3.** White pulp. **4.** Splenic nodule. **5.** Central artery. **6.** Trabecula.

Fig. 18-3. Enlargement of rectangle (A) in Fig. 18-2. Spleen. Rat. L.M. X 240. **1.** Red pulp. **2.** Venous sinuses. **3.** Germinal center of splenic nodule. **4.** Central artery. **5.** Marginal zone. **6.** Dilated funnel-shaped terminations of arterial capillaries. **7.** Trabecula.

Fig. 18-4. Spleen. Same preparation as in Fig. 18-2. Rat. L.M. X 230. **1.** Red pulp. **2.** Trabecula. **3.** Penicilli with sleeves of lymphoid tissue (sheathed arterioles). **4.** Cross-sectioned arterial capillary, luminal diameter about 5 μ. **5.** Venous sinus.

Fig. 18-5. Enlargement of rectangle (B) in Fig. 18-2. Spleen. Rat. L.M. X 230. **1.** Pulp arteriole (first segment of penicillus). **2.** Sheathed arteriole (second segment of penicillus). **3.** Venous sinuses. **4.** Red pulp.

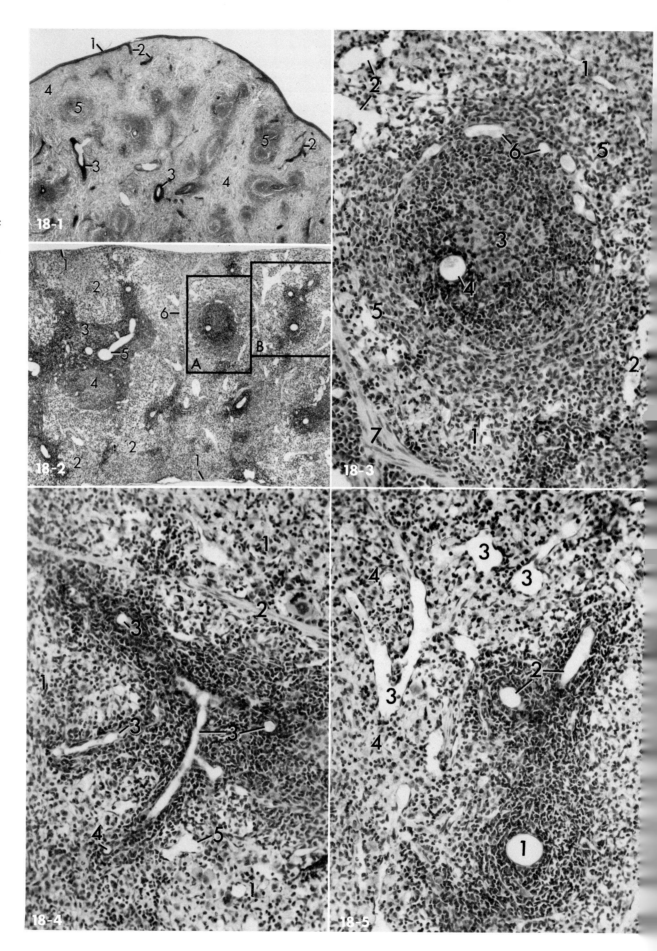

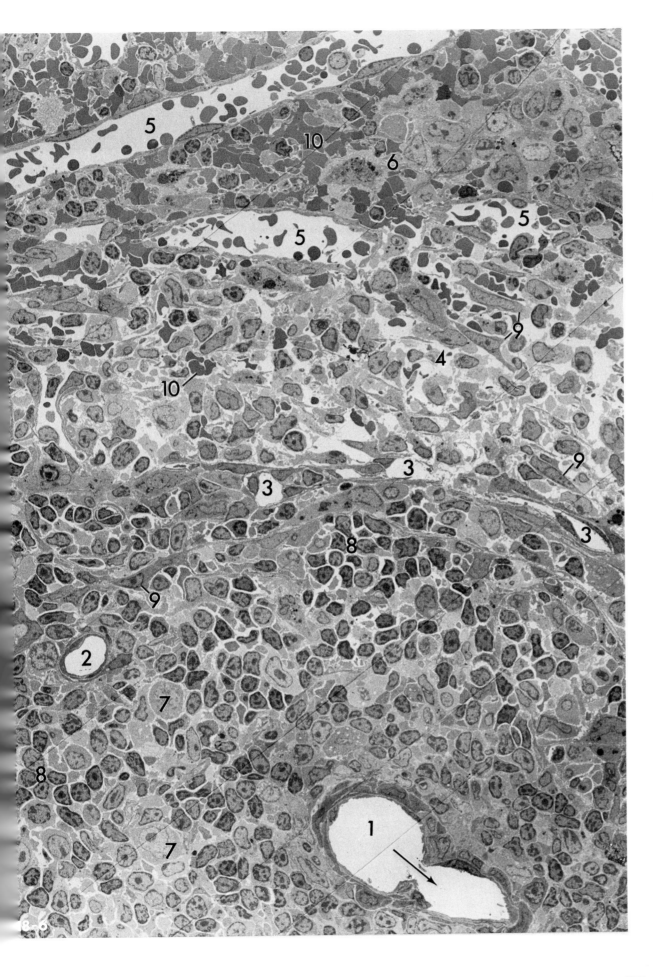

Fig. 18-6. Survey of white and red pulp of spleen. Fixation by intra-arterial perfusion. Rat. E.M. X 800. **1.** Central artery (lumen 30 μ) with branch (arrow) surrounded by a thick sleeve of white pulp. Details of the lymphoid tissue of the white pulp is seen in Fig. 17-25. **2.** Arteriole (lumen 11 μ) in white pulp. This is a branch of the central artery. **3.** Funnel-shaped open terminations of arterial capillaries. **4.** Marginal zone with large interstitial spaces. **5.** Venous sinuses. **6.** Red pulp. **7.** Large lymphocytes (lymphoblasts). **8.** Small lymphocytes. **9.** Reticular cells. **10.** Erythrocytes.

Fig. 18-7. Cross-sectioned central artery (arteriole) of white pulp. Spleen. Rat. E.M. X 1900. **1.** Lumen, 30 μ wide. **2.** Squamous endothelium. **3.** Media consists of 2–3 layers of smooth muscle cells. **4.** Periarteriolar sheath of lymphoid cells. Note that adventitial connective tissue cells are missing.

Fig. 18-8. Wall of central arteriole (artery) of spleen. Enlargement of rectangle in Fig. 18-7. Rat. E.M. X 14,000. **1.** Lumen. **2.** Endothelium. **3.** Basal lamina (elastica interna is missing). **4.** Smooth muscle cells. **5.** Small bundles of reticular and collagenous fibrils. **6.** Lymphocytes.

Fig. 18-9. Marginal zone of white pulp. Spleen. Rat. E.M. X 960. **1.** Edge of white pulp. **2.** Funnel-shaped open termination of arterial capillary. Arrow indicates direction of blood flow. **3.** Erythrocytes. **4.** Interstitial space, communicating with lumen of arterial capillary. **5.** Lymphocytes (mostly medium-sized). **6.** Macrophages. **7.** Reticular cells.

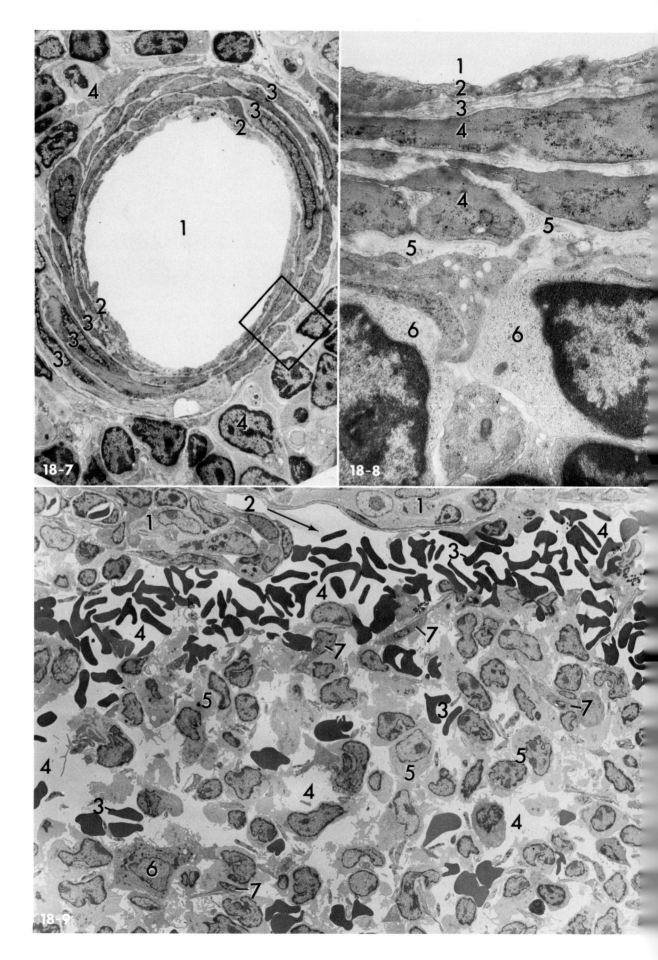

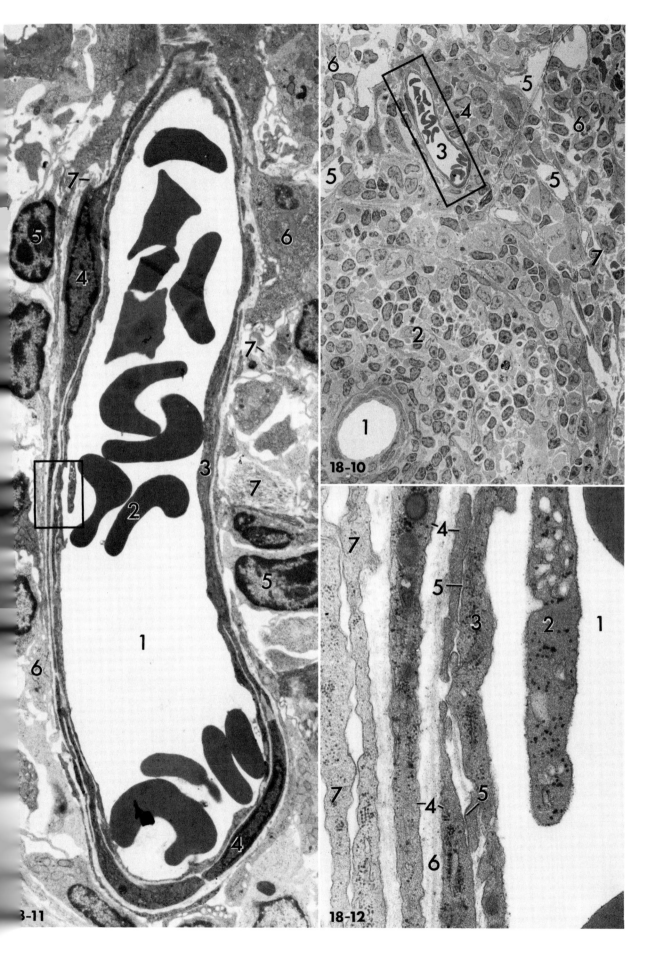

Fig. 18-10. Survey of spleen. Rat. E.M. X 580. **1.** Central artery (arteriole). Width of lumen 30 μ. **2.** White pulp. **3.** Sheathed arteriole (lumen 10 μ) originating from the central artery. **4.** Thin sleeve of lymphoid tissue. **5.** Funnel-shaped open terminations of arterial capillaries. **6.** Red pulp. **7.** Marginal zone.

Fig. 18-11. Sheathed arteriole. Enlargement of rectangle in Fig. 18-10. Rat. E.M. X 3700. **1.** Lumen. **2.** Erythrocytes. **3.** Endothelium. **4.** Nuclei of smooth muscle cells. **5.** Lymphocytes. **6.** Reticular cells. **7.** Bundles of collagenous fibrils.

Fig. 18-12. Wall of sheathed arteriole. Enlargement of rectangle in Fig. 18-11. Spleen. Rat. E.M. X 29,000. **1.** Lumen. **2.** Platelet. **3.** Endothelium. **4.** Smooth muscle cells. **5.** Myoendothelial junctions. **6.** Basal lamina. **7.** Thin cytoplasmic strands of reticular cells.

Fig. 18-13. Survey of red pulp preserved by intra-arterial perfusion and serial-sectioned. This is section No. 328 in a series of 500 sections. Spleen. Rat. E.M. X 2500. **1.** Smooth muscle cells of trabecula. **2.** Elastic fibers. **3.** Bundles of collagenous fibrils. **4.** Longitudinal section of open termination of arterial capillary (end of penicillus). Arrow indicates direction of blood flow. **5.** Endothelial cells. **6.** Reticular cells. **7.** Interstitial space. **8.** Cross-sectioned venous sinuses. **9.** Littoral cells (lining cells). **10.** Macrophages. **11.** Erythrocytes. **12.** Small lymphocytes. **13.** Proerythroblasts in mitotic prophase. This is a clonal formation of erythrocytes near phagocytes. Erythropoiesis is common in the spleen of young rats. **14.** Medium-sized lymphocyte. This could possibly also represent a hemocytoblast, a precursor of the proerythroblasts. **15.** Erythrocytes passing through stomata between littoral cells. **16.** Thrombocytes (platelets).

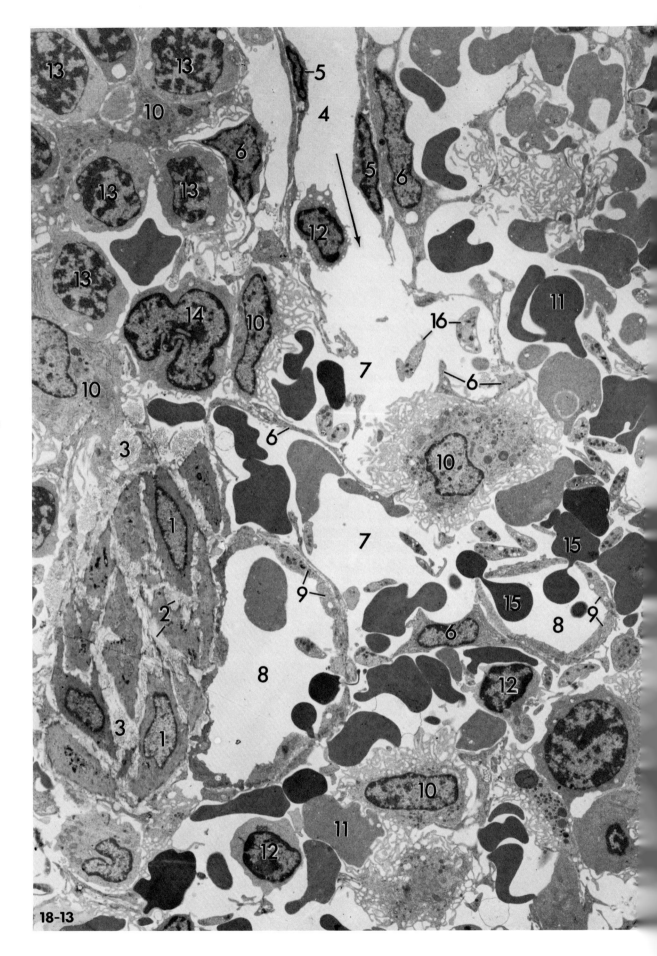

18-13

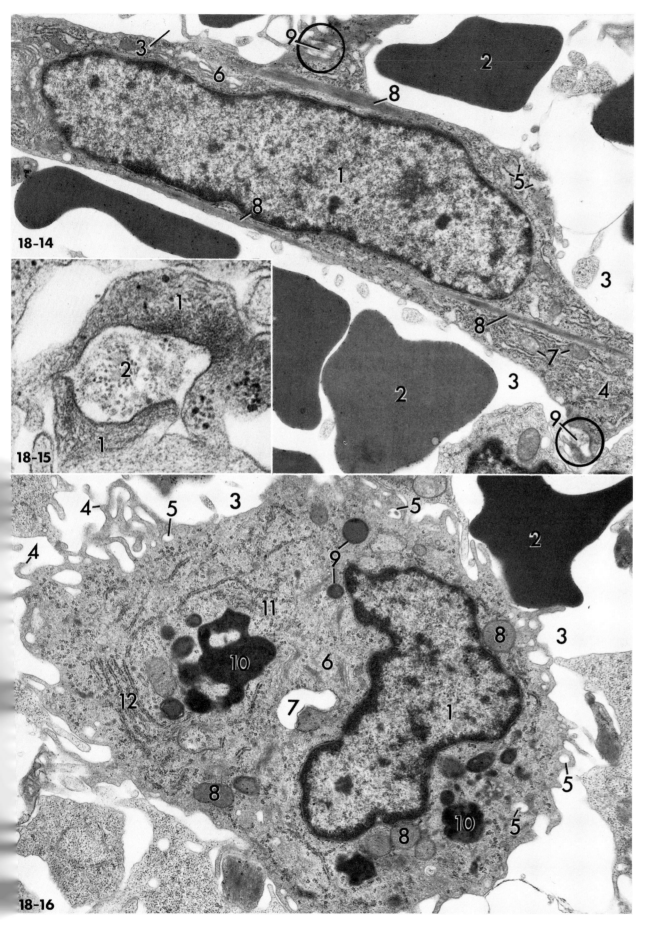

Fig. 18-14. Detail of reticular cell in red pulp of spleen. Rat. E.M. X 9500. **1.** Nucleus of reticular cell. **2.** Erythrocytes. **3.** Interstitial space of red pulp. **4.** Free ribosomes. **5.** Profiles of granular endoplasmic reticulum. **6.** Golgi zone. **7.** Mitochondria. **8.** Bundles of filaments. **9.** Reticular (extracellular) fibrils.

Fig. 18-15. Enlargement of areas similar to circles in Fig. 18-14. Spleen. Rat. E.M. X 74,000. **1.** Cytoplasmic processes of reticular cells containing densely packed filaments. **2.** Bundle of reticular fibrils with some elastic microfibrils.

Fig. 18-16. Detail of macrophage in the red pulp of spleen. Rat. E.M. X 18,000. **1.** Nucleus of macrophage. **2.** Erythrocyte. **3.** Interstitial space of red pulp. **4.** Microvilli. **5.** Micropinocytotic vesicles and vacuoles. **6.** Golgi zone. **7.** Dilated Golgi cisterna. **8.** Mitochondria. **9.** Primary lysosomes. **10.** Secondary lysosomes. **11.** Free polysomes. **12.** Profiles of granular endoplasmic reticulum.

Fig. 18-17 & 18-18. Survey of venous sinuses traversing the red pulp. Spleen. Rat. E.M. X 1600. **1.** Cross section of venous sinus (lumen 22 μ). **2.** Longitudinally sectioned venous sinuses. **3.** Nuclei of littoral (lining) cells. **4.** Nuclei of reticular cells. **5.** Erythrocytes. **6.** Thrombocytes. **7.** Macrophages. **8.** Small lymphocytes. **9.** Medium-sized lymphocytes. **10.** Monocyte. **11.** Erythrocytes passing through stomata in wall of venous sinus. **12.** Point of confluence of two venous sinuses. **13.** Interstitial space of red pulp. **14.** Tangential section through microvillous excrescences of macrophage. **15.** Plasma cell.

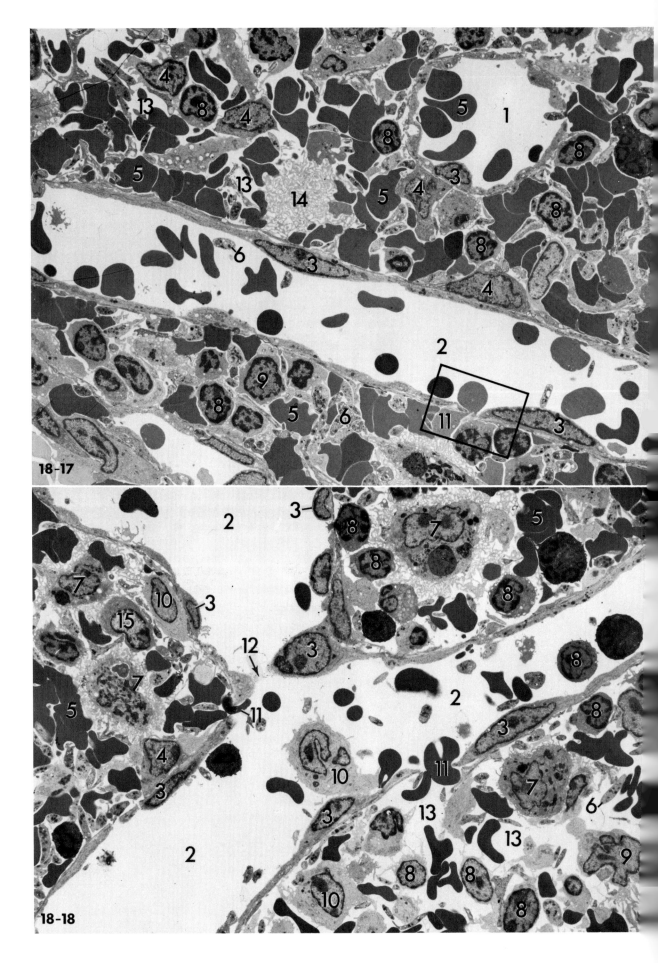

232

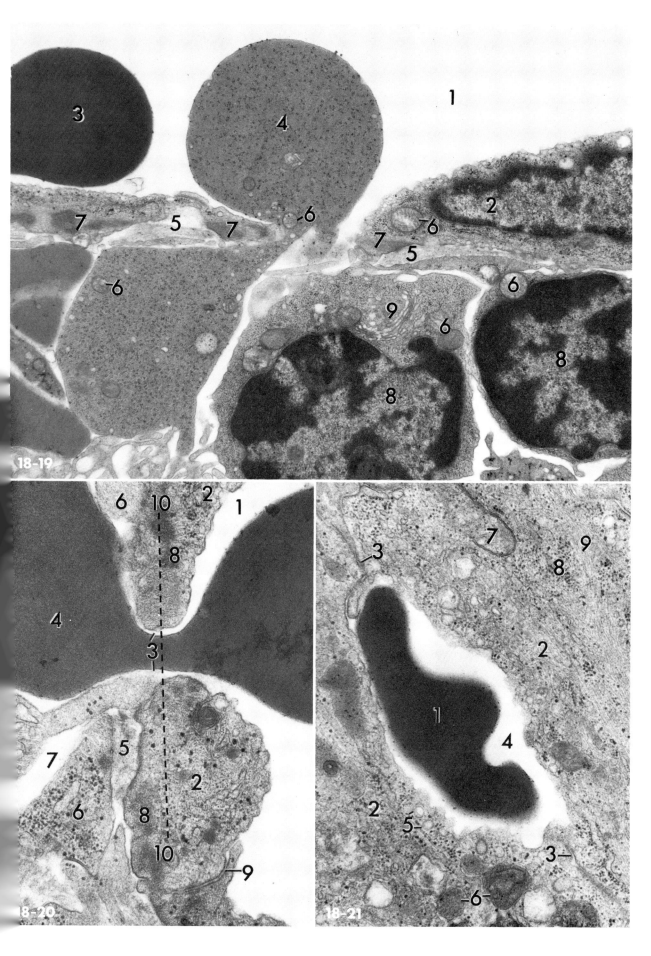

Fig. 18-19. Detail of venous sinus. Longitudinal section of wall. Enlargement of rectangle in Fig. 18-17. Spleen. Rat. E.M. X 15,000. **1.** Lumen of venous sinus. **2.** Nucleus of littoral (lining) cell. **3.** Erythrocyte. **4.** Young erythrocyte (reticulocyte) passing through a stoma in the wall of the venous sinus from the interstitial space of the red pulp to the lumen of the sinus. **5.** Bundles of delicate reticular fibrils. **6.** Mitochondria. **7.** Bundles of cytoplasmic filaments. **8.** Nuclei of small lymphocytes. **9.** Golgi zone.

Fig. 18-20. Detail of wall of cross-sectioned venous sinus. Spleen. Rat. E.M. X 15,000. **1.** Lumen of sinus. **2.** Littoral cells. **3.** Stoma (opening) between two littoral (lining) cells. **4.** Erythrocyte passing through stoma. **5.** Narrow strand of basal lamina. **6.** Parts of reticular cell. **7.** Interstitial space of red pulp. **8.** Cross-sectioned cytoplasmic filaments. **9.** Junction of two littoral cells. **10.** Plane of section in Fig. 18-21.

Fig. 18-21. Stoma in the wall of venous sinus. Tangential section of littoral cells through plane indicated by dotted line between 10 and 10 in Fig. 18-20. Section No. 139 in a series of 500 sections. Spleen. Rat. E.M. X 29,000. **1.** Erythrocyte. **2.** Cytoplasm of littoral cells. **3.** Cell membranes of adjoining littoral cells. **4.** Stoma represents a true, probably permanent slit-like opening between two littoral cells. **5.** Pinocytotic vesicles. **6.** Lysosomes. **7.** Mitochondrion. **8.** Free ribosomes. **9.** Cytoplasmic filaments.

References

Björkman, S. E. The splenic circulation. With special reference to the function of the spleen sinus wall. Acta Med. Scand. *128*, Suppl. 191, 1–89 (1947).

Burke, J. S. and Simon, G. T. Electron microscopy of the spleen. I. Anatomy and microcirculation. Am. J. Path. *58*: 127–155 (1970).

Burke, J. S. and Simon, G. T. Electron microscopy of the spleen. II. Phagocytosis of colloid carbon. Am. J. Path. *58*: 157–181 (1970).

Edwards, V. D. and Simon, G. T. Ultrastructural aspects of red cell destruction in the normal rat spleen. J. Ultrastruct. Res. *33*: 187–201 (1970).

Hirasawa, Y. and Tokuhiro, H. Electron microscopic studies on the normal human spleen: especially on the red pulp and the reticulo-endothelial cells. Blood *35*: 201–212 (1970).

Knisely, M. H. Spleen studies. I. Microscopic observations of the circulatory system of living unstimulated mammalian spleen. Anat. Rec. *65*: 23–50 (1936).

Lewis, O. J. The blood vessels of the adult mammalian spleen. J. Anat. *91*: 245–250 (1957).

MacKenzie, D., Whipple, W. A. O. and Wintersteiner, M. P. Studies on the microscopic anatomy and physiology of living and transilluminated mammalian spleens. Am. J. Anat. *68*: 397–456 (1941).

MacNeal, W. J. The circulation of blood through the spleen pulp. Arch. Path. 7: 215–227 (1929).

Moore, R. D., Mumaw, V. R. and Schoenberg, M. D. The structure of the spleen and its functional implications. Exp. & Molec. Pathol. *3*: 31–50 (1964).

Parpart, A. K., Whipple, A. O. and Chang, J. J. The microcirculation of the spleen of the mouse. Angiology *6*: 350–362 (1955).

Peck, H. M. and Hoerr, N. L. The intermediary circulation in the red pulp of the mouse spleen. Anat. Rec. *109*: 447–477 (1951).

Pictet, R., Orci, L., Forssmann, W. G. and Girardier, L. An electron microscope study of the perfusion-fixed spleen. I. The splenic circulation and the RES concept. Z. Zellforsch. *96*: 372–399 (1969).

Pictet, R., Orci, L., Forssmann, W. G. and Girardier, L. An electron microscope study of the perfusion-fixed spleen. II. Nurse cells and erythrophagocytosis. Z. Zellforsch. *96*: 400–417 (1969).

Roberts, D. K. and Latta, J. S. Electron microscopic studies on the red pulp of the rabbit spleen. Anat. Rec. *148*: 81–101 (1964).

Robinson, W. L. The vascular mechanism of the spleen. Am. J. Path. 2: 341–355 (1926).

Simon, G. T. and Burke, J. S. Electron microscopy of the spleen. III. Erythro-leukophagocytosis. Am. J. Path. *58*: 451–469 (1970).

Simon, G. and Pictet, R. Étude au microscope électronique des sinus spléniques et des cordons de Billroth chez le rat. Acta Anat. *57*: 163–171 (1964).

Snook, T. A comparative study of the vascular arrangements in mammalian spleens. Am. J. Anat. *87*: 31–77 (1950).

Snook, T. The histology of the vascular terminations in the rabbit spleen. Anat. Rec. *130*: 711–729 (1958).

Snook, T. Studies of the perifollicular region of the rat's spleen. Anat. Rec. *148*: 149–160 (1964).

Stutte, H. J. Nature of human spleen red pulp cells with special reference to sinus lining cells. Z. Zellforsch. *91*: 300–314 (1968).

Thomas, C. E. An electron- and light-microscope study of sinus structure in perfused rabbit and dog spleens. Am. J. Anat. *120*: 527–552 (1967).

Weiss, L. The structure of the intermediate vascular pathways in the spleen of rabbits. Am. J. Anat. *113*: 51–92 (1963).

Weiss, L. The white pulp of the spleen. Bull. Johns Hopkins Hosp. *115*: 99–173 (1964).

Zwillenberg, L. O. and Zwillenberg, H. H. Zur Struktur und Funktion der Hülsenkapillaren in der Milz. Z. Zellforsch. *59*: 908–921 (1963).

19 Thymus

Fig. 19-1. Thymus. Kitten. L.M. X 22.
1. Capsule at surface of gland. **2.** Connective tissue septa. **3.** Blood vessels. **4.** Lobules.

Fig. 19-2. Part of thymic lobule. Enlargement of area similar to rectangle in Fig. 19-1. Thymus. Kitten. L.M. X 215. **1.** Capsule at surface of lobule. **2.** Cortex. **3.** Medulla. **4.** Hassall's (thymic) corpuscles.

Fig. 19-3. Survey of thymic lobule. Enlargement of area similar to rectangle in Fig. 19-2. Thymus. Kitten. E.M. X 630. **1.** Capsule. **2.** Cortex. **3.** Medulla. **4.** Hassall's corpuscles. **5.** Blood capillaries.

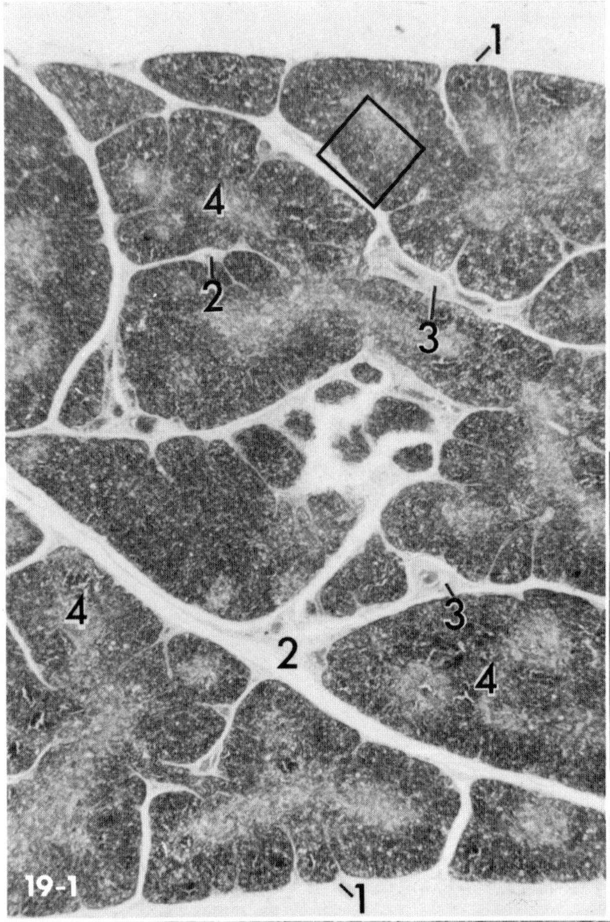

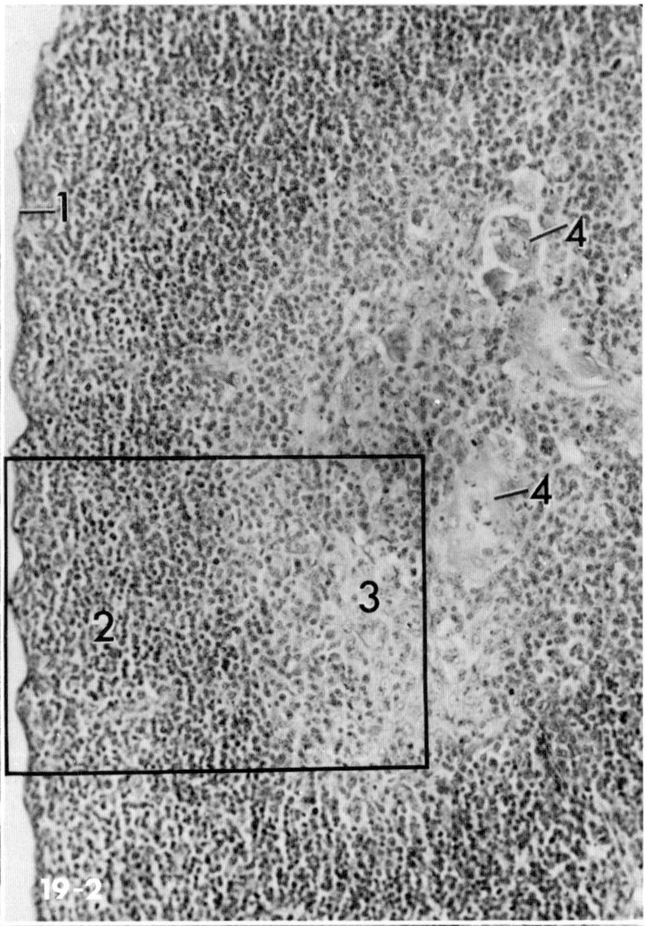

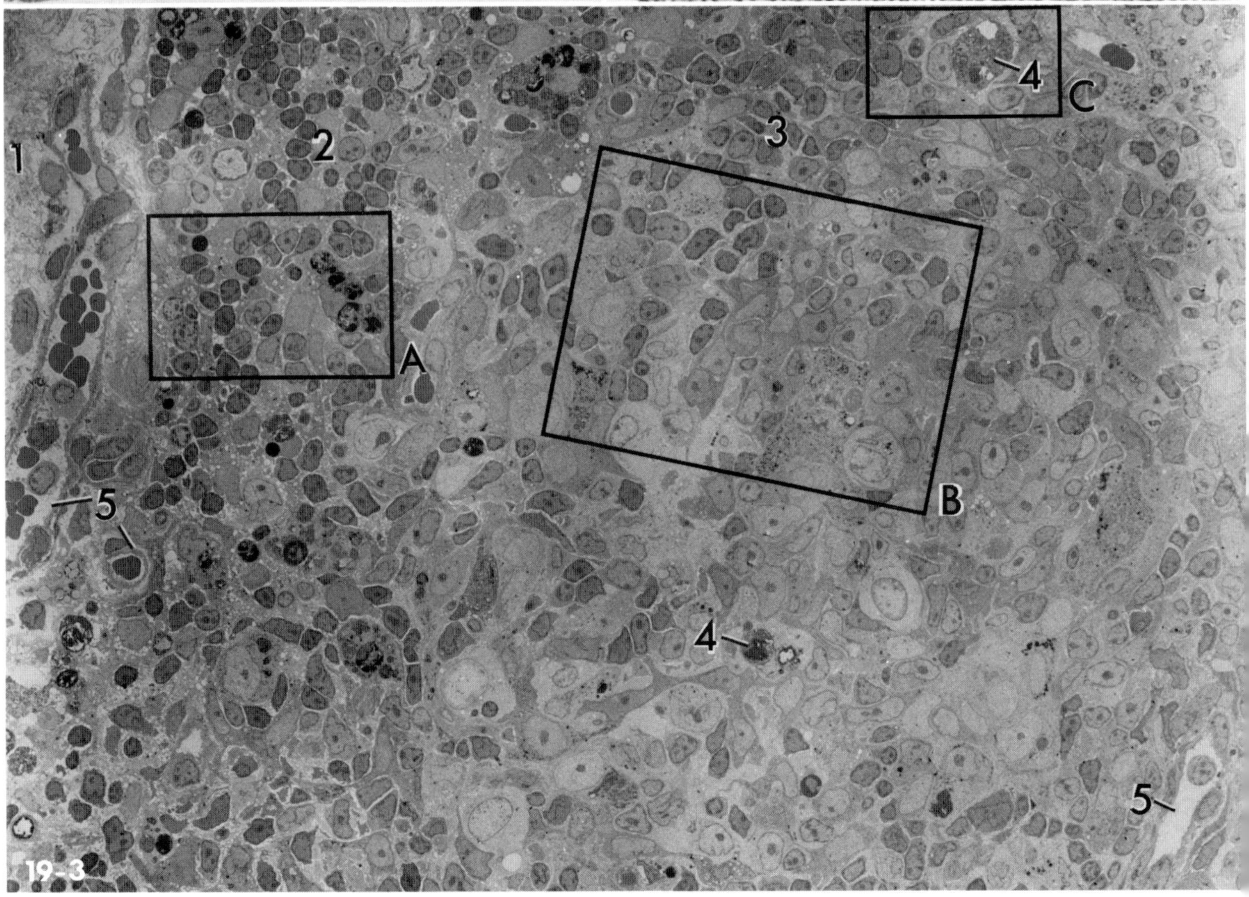

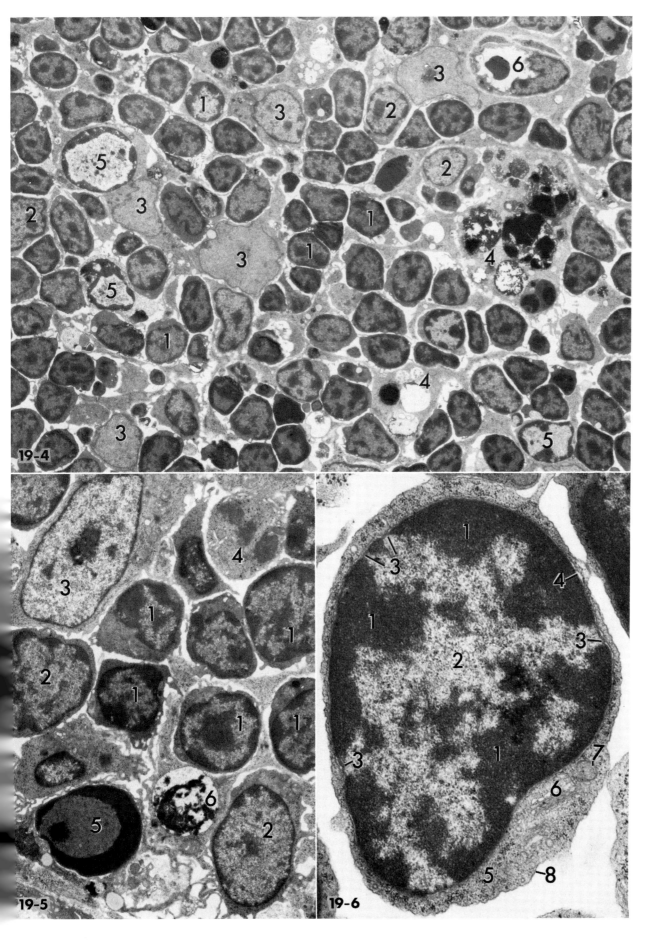

Fig. 19-4. Survey of thymic cortex. Enlargement of area similar to rectangle (A) in Fig. 19-3. Thymus. Kitten. E.M. X 1800. **1.** Small thymic lymphocytes. **2.** Medium-sized thymic lymphocytes. **3.** Nuclei of epithelial reticular cells. **4.** Macrophage. **5.** Thymic lymphocytes with dense marginated nuclear chromatin. **6.** Lumen of blood capillary.

Fig. 19-5. Detail of thymic cortex. Kitten. E.M. X 4500. **1.** Nuclei of small thymic lymphocytes. **2.** Nuclei of medium-sized thymic lymphocytes. **3.** Nucleus of epithelial reticular cell. **4.** Thymic lymphocyte in mitosis. **5.** Nucleus of small thymic lymphocyte with marginated nucleoplasm, indicating imminent cell death. **6.** Digestive vacuole or secondary lysosome in cytoplasm of macrophage.

Fig. 19-6. Small thymic lymphocyte (T cell) from cortex of thymus. Cell width 5 μ. Thymus. Kitten. E.M. X 18,000.
1. Heterochromatin. **2.** Euchromatin.
3. Nuclear pores. **4.** Nuclear membrane.
5. Ribosomes. **6.** Golgi zone. **7.** Mitochondria.
8. Surface (cell) membrane.

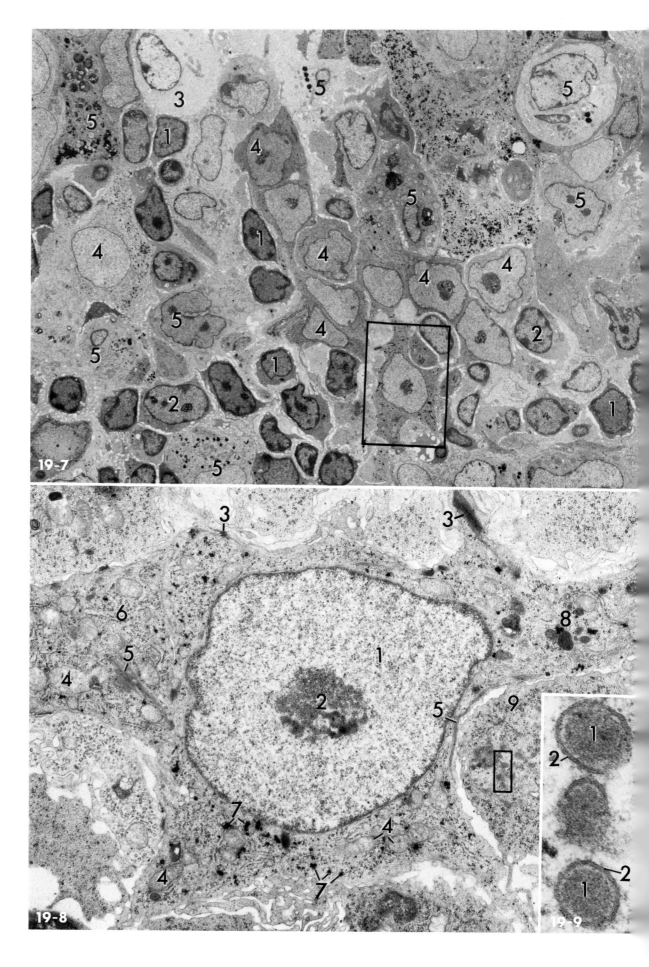

Fig. 19-7. Survey of thymic medulla. Enlargement of area similar to rectangle (B) in Fig. 19-3. Thymus. Kitten. E.M. X 1800. **1.** Small thymic lymphocytes. **2.** Medium-sized thymic lymphocytes. **3.** Large thymic lymphocyte. **4.** Epithelial reticular cells. **5.** Macrophages. Note that the identification of these cells is based on an analysis of each cell at higher magnifications.

Fig. 19-8. Epithelial reticular cell. Enlargement of rectangle in Fig. 19-7. Thymus. Kitten. E.M. X 13,000. **1.** Nucleus of epithelial reticular cell. **2.** Nucleolus. **3.** Desmosomes. **4.** Mitochondria. **5.** Cytoplasmic filaments. **6.** Ribosomes. **7.** Particulate glycogen. **8.** Small granules, most of which represent primary lysosomes. **9.** Adjacent epithelial reticular cell. Note that the reticular cell of the thymus is not necessarily in contact with reticular and collagenous fibrils in contrast to the reticular cells in lymph nodes and spleen.

Fig. 19-9. Small dense spherical granules in epithelial reticular cell. Enlargement of area similar to rectangle in Fig. 19-8. Thymus. Kitten. E.M. X 96,000. **1.** Core of granule. **2.** Trilaminar boundary membrane.

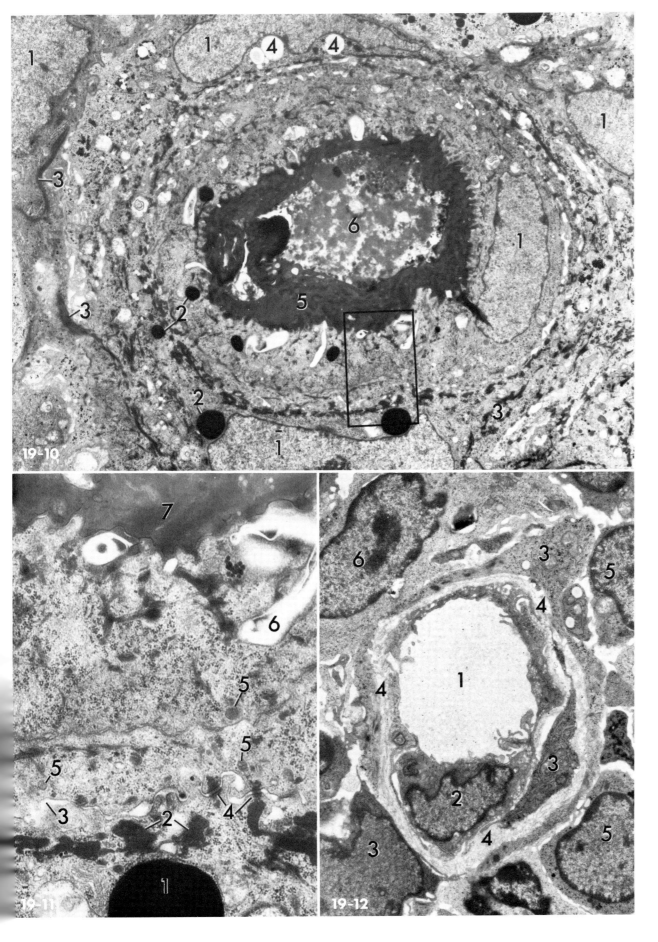

Fig. 19-10. Survey of Hassall's corpuscle. Enlargement of area similar to rectangle (C) in Fig. 19-3. Thymus. Kitten. E.M. X 4500. **1.** Nuclei of concentrically arranged epithelial reticular cells. **2.** Keratohyalin granules. **3.** Bundles of cytoplasmic filaments (tonofilaments). **4.** Lipid droplets. **5.** Fully keratinized epithelial reticular cell. **6.** Slightly cystic center of Hassall's corpuscle.

Fig. 19-11. Enlargement of rectangle in Fig. 19-10. Thymus. Kitten. E.M. X 18,000. **1.** Keratohyalin granule. **2.** Cross-sectioned bundles of tonofilaments. **3.** Intercellular space. **4.** Desmosomes. **5.** Membrane-coating granules. **6.** Cholesterol crystal space. **7.** Keratinized cell.

Fig. 19-12. Cross section of capillary in the medulla of the thymus. Kitten. E.M. X 4800. **1.** Lumen. **2.** Nucleus of endothelial cell. **3.** Pericytes. **4.** Basement membrane consisting of fine collagenous fibrils. **5.** Nuclei of thymic lymphocytes. **6.** Epithelial reticular cells.

239

References

Ackerman, G. A. and Hostetler, J. R. Morphological studies of the embryonic rabbit thymus: the in situ epithelial versus the extrathymic derivation of the initial population of lymphocytes in the embryonic thymus. Anat. Rec. *166*: 27–46 (1970).

Burnet, M. The thymus gland. Sci. American *207*: 50–57 (1962).

Chapman, W. L. and Allen, J. R. The fine structure of the thymus of the fetal and neonatal monkey (Macaca mulatta). Z. Zellforsch. *114*: 220–233 (1971).

Clark, S. L., Jr. The thymus in mice of strain 129/J, studied with the electron microscope. Am. J. Anat. *112*: 1–34 (1963).

Everett, N. B. and Tyler (Caffrey), R. W. Lymphopoiesis in the thymus and other tissues: functional implications. Int. Rev. Cytol. *22*: 205–286 (1967).

Gad, P. and Clark, S. L., Jr. Involution and regeneration of the thymus in mice, induced by bacterial endotoxin and studied by quantitative histology and electron microscopy. Am. J. Anat. *122*: 573–606 (1968).

Goldstein, G. and Mackay, I. R. The Thymus, pp. 1–352. Warren H. Green, St. Louis, 1969.

Haelst, U. G. J. van. Light and electron microscopic study of the normal and pathological thymus of the rat. I. The normal thymus. Z. Zellforsch. *77*: 534–553 (1967).

Haelst, U. G. J. van. Light and electron microscopic study of the normal and pathological thymus of the rat. III. A mesenchymal histiocytic type of cell. Z. Zellforsch. *99*: 198–209 (1969).

Hoshino, T. Electron microscopic studies of the epithelial reticular cells of the mouse thymus. Z. Zellforsch. *59*: 513–529 (1963).

Ito, T. and Hoshino, T. Fine structure of the epithelial reticular cells of the medulla of the thymus in the golden hamster. Z. Zellforsch. *69*: 311–318 (1966).

Izard, J. Ultrastructure of the thymic reticulum in guinea pig. Cytological aspects of the problem of the thymic secretion. Anat. Rec. *155*: 117–132 (1966).

Kohnen, P. and Weiss, L. An electron microscopic study of thymic corpuscles in the guinea pig and the mouse. Anat. Rec. *148*: 29–57 (1964).

20 Hypophysis

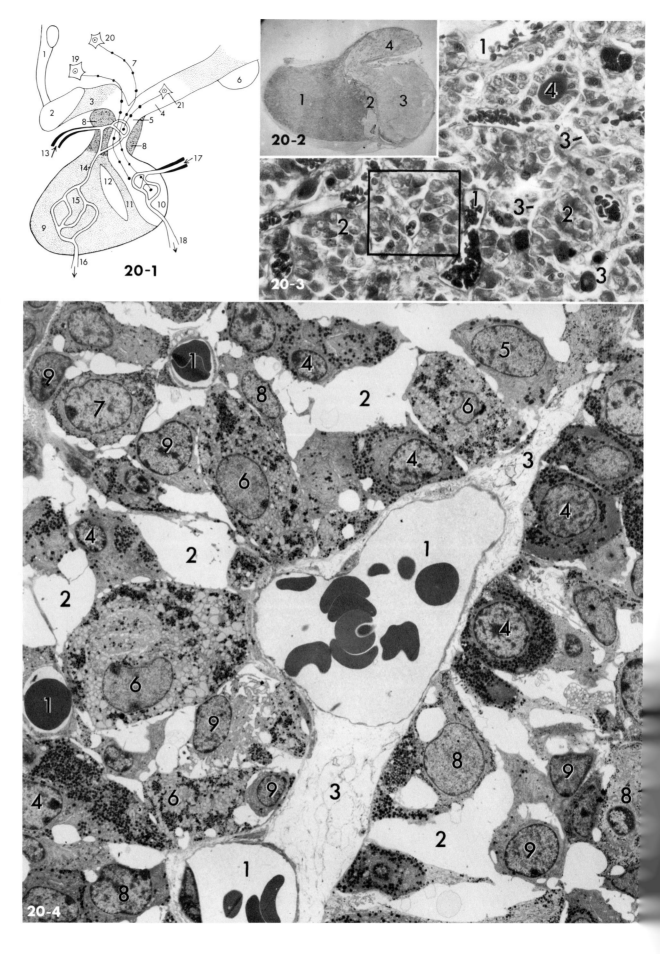

Fig. 20-1. Schematic drawing of the pituitary and the hypothalamo-hypophysial tract.
1. Anterior commissure and lamina terminalis.
2. Optic chiasm. **3.** Tuber cinereum. **4.** Median eminence. **5.** Infundibular stalk. **6.** Mamillary body. **7.** Third ventricle. **8.** Pars tuberalis.
9. Anterior lobe. **10.** Posterior lobe. **11.** Pars intermedia. **12.** Cleft. **13.** Superior hypophysial arteries. **14.** Portal vessels.
15. Sinusoids of adenohypophysis. **16.** Veins to cavernous sinuses. **17.** Inferior hypophysial arteries. **18.** Veins to cavernous sinuses.
19. Nerve cells in supraoptic nuclei. **20.** Nerve cells in paraventricular nuclei. **21.** Nerve cells in median eminence.

Fig. 20-2. Midsagittal section of pituitary. Human. L.M. X 4. **1.** Anterior lobe. **2.** Pars intermedia. **3.** Posterior lobe. **4.** Infundibular stalk.

Fig. 20-3. Survey of adenohypophysis. Human. L.M. X 340. **1.** Sinusoids (capillaries). **2.** Cords of endocrine secretory cells. **3.** Intercordal spaces. **4.** Follicle.

Fig. 20-4. Enlargement of area similar to rectangle in Fig. 20-3. Rat. E.M. X 1700.
1. Capillaries (sinusoids). **2.** Intercellular space.
3. Intercordal space with some collagenous fibrils. **4.** Somatotroph. **5.** Mammotroph.
6. Gonadotroph. **7.** Thyrotroph.
8. Adrenocorticotroph. **9.** Precursor (chromophobe) cell. The identification of these cells cannot be made accurately at this magnification. It is based on the study of these cells at higher magnifications.

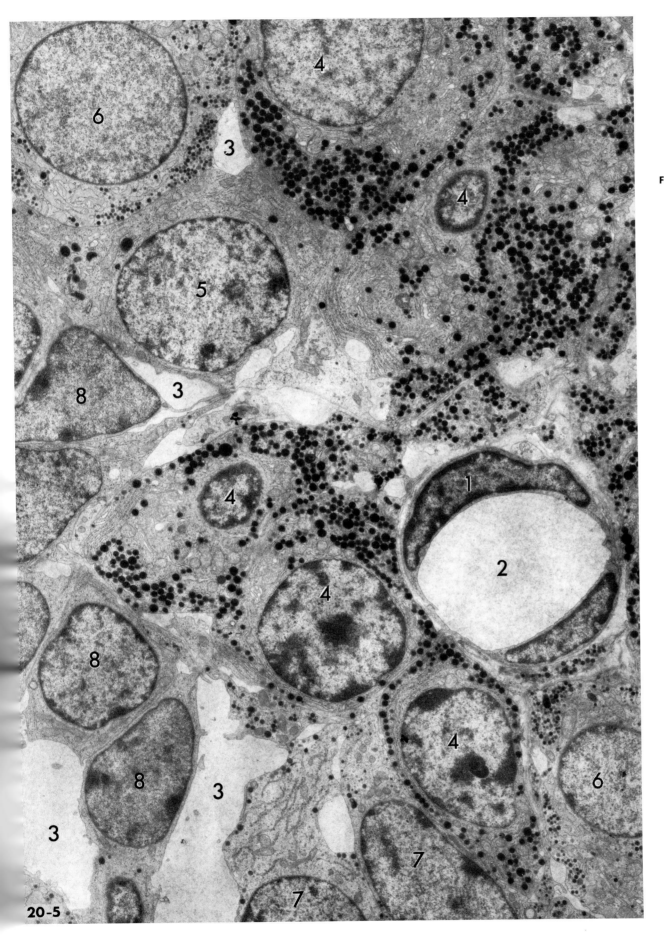

Fig. 20-5. Survey of several types of epithelial cells in the adenohypophysis. Rat. E.M. X 5300. At this magnification, cell types can be recognized more readily than in Fig. 20-4, based on the size, shape and number of secretory granules. **1.** Nucleus of capillary endothelial cell. **2.** Capillary lumen. **3.** Intercellular space. **4.** Nuclei of somatotrophs. **5.** Nucleus of mammotroph. **6.** Nuclei of thyrotrophs. **7.** Nuclei of adrenocorticotrophs. **8.** Nuclei of chromophobe precursor cells.

20-5

Fig. 20-6. Detail of somatotrophs. Adenohypophysis. Rat. E.M. X 9500. **1.** Nucleus. **2.** Cell membranes. **3.** Granular endoplasmic reticulum with narrow cisternae. **4.** Mitochondria. **5.** Secretory granules (3000 Å–3500 Å).

Fig. 20-7. Detail of mammotroph. Posterolateral lobe of adenohypophysis. Rat. E.M. X 9000. **1.** Nucleus. **2.** Cell membranes. **3.** Granular endoplasmic reticulum. **4.** Mitochondria. **5.** Golgi complex. **6.** Secretory granules (6000 Å–9000 Å).

Fig. 20-8. Detail of gonadotroph. Adenohypophysis. Rat. E.M. X 9000. **1.** Nucleus. **2.** Cell membranes. **3.** Granular endoplasmic reticulum with dilated cisternae. **4.** Mitochondria. **5.** Golgi complex. **6.** Presecretory granules. **7.** Secretory granules (1000 Å–3000 Å).

Fig. 20-9. Detail of thyrotrophs. Adenohypophysis. Rat. E.M. X 9000. **1.** Nuclei of thyrotrophs. **2.** Cell membranes. **3.** Granular endoplasmic reticulum. **4.** Mitochondria. **5.** Golgi complex. **6.** Secretory granules (1000 Å–1600 Å). **7.** Nucleus of precursor cell.

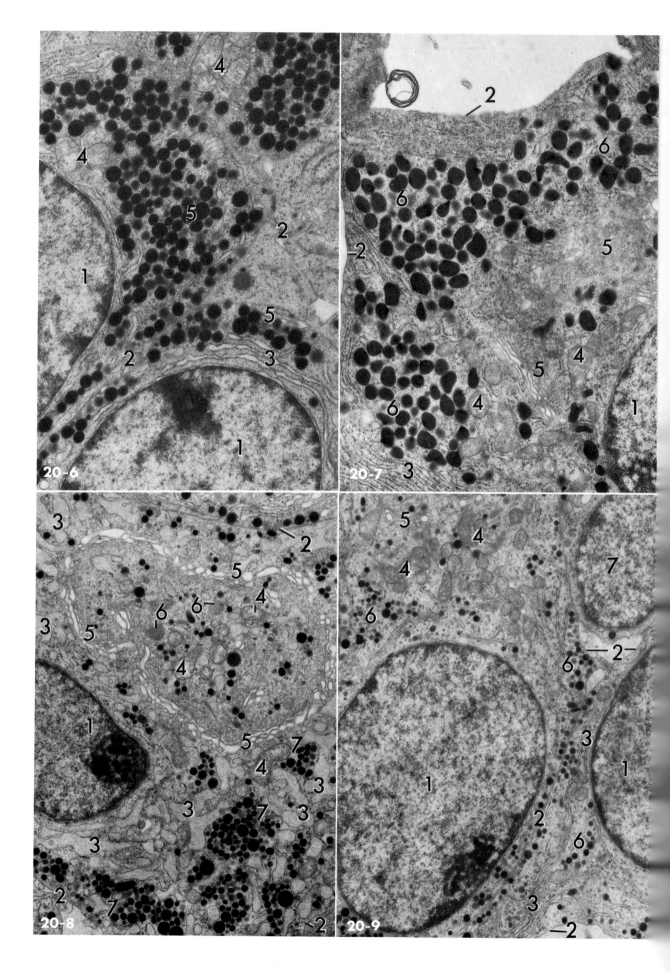

244

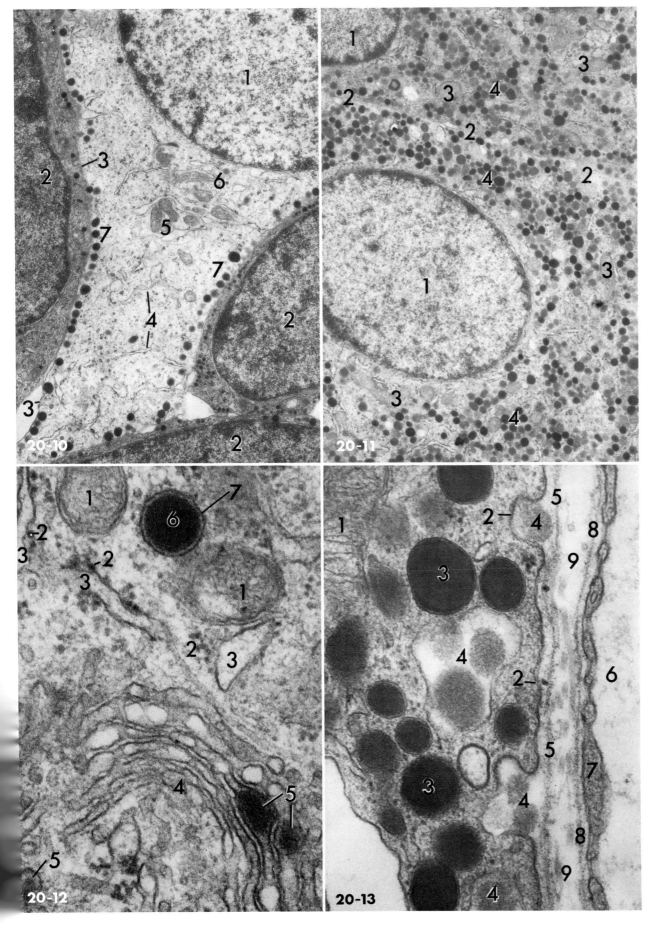

Fig. 20-10. Detail of corticotroph. Adenohypophysis. Rat. E.M. X 9000. **1.** Nucleus of corticotroph. **2.** Nuclei of precursor cells. **3.** Cell membranes. **4.** Granular endoplasmic reticulum. **5.** Mitochondria. **6.** Golgi complex. **7.** Marginated layer of secretory granules (2000 Å).

Fig. 20-11. Detail of cell in pars intermedia of the pituitary. Rat. E.M. X 9000. **1.** Nuclei. **2.** Cell membranes. **3.** Mitochondria. **4.** Secretory granules (2000 Å).

Fig. 20-12. Detail of gonadotroph. Adenohypophysis. Rat. E.M. X 87,000. **1.** Mitochondria. **2.** Ribosomes. **3.** Cisternae of granular endoplasmic reticulum. **4.** Golgi complex. **5.** Presecretory granules forming within the Golgi saccules. **6.** Mature secretory granule. **7.** Limiting membrane.

Fig. 20-13. Detail of gonadotroph at the moment of discharging secretory granules. Adenohypophysis. Rat. E.M. X 86,000. **1.** Mitochondrion. **2.** Cell membrane. **3.** Secretory granules. **4.** Discharging secretory granules. **5.** Basal lamina of cell cords. **6.** Capillary (sinusoidal) lumen. **7.** Fenestrated (closed) endothelium of capillary (sinusoid). **8.** Capillary basal lamina. **9.** Intercordal space with fine collagenous fibrils.

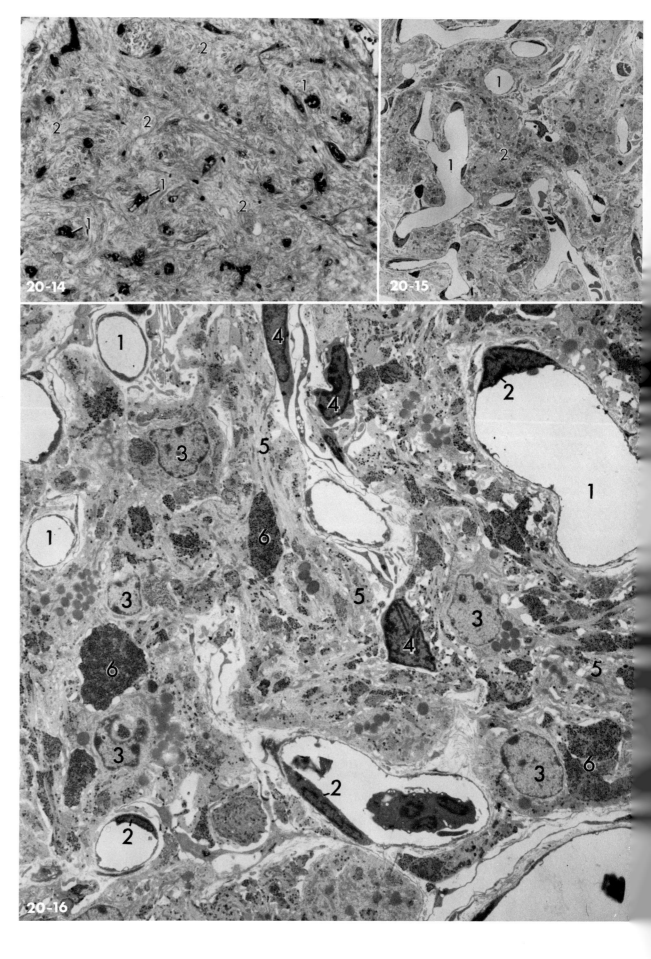

Fig. 20-14. Detail of the posterior lobe (pars nervosa) of the pituitary. Human. L.M. X 180. **1.** Capillaries (sinusoids). **2.** Meshwork of interweaving nerve processes, pituicytes and Herring bodies.

Fig. 20-15. Detail of the base of the neurohypophysis, fixed by intravascular perfusion. Rat. E.M. × 560. **1.** Capillary (sinusoids) with the lumen open. **2.** Meshwork of nerve fibers and pituicytes.

Fig. 20-16. Detail of the neurohypophysis. Same area and fixation as in Fig. 20-15. Rat. E.M. X 1900. **1.** Capillaries (sinusoids). **2.** Endothelial nuclei. **3.** Nuclei of pituicytes. **4.** Nuclei of fibroblasts. **5.** Nerve processes. **6.** Herring bodies.

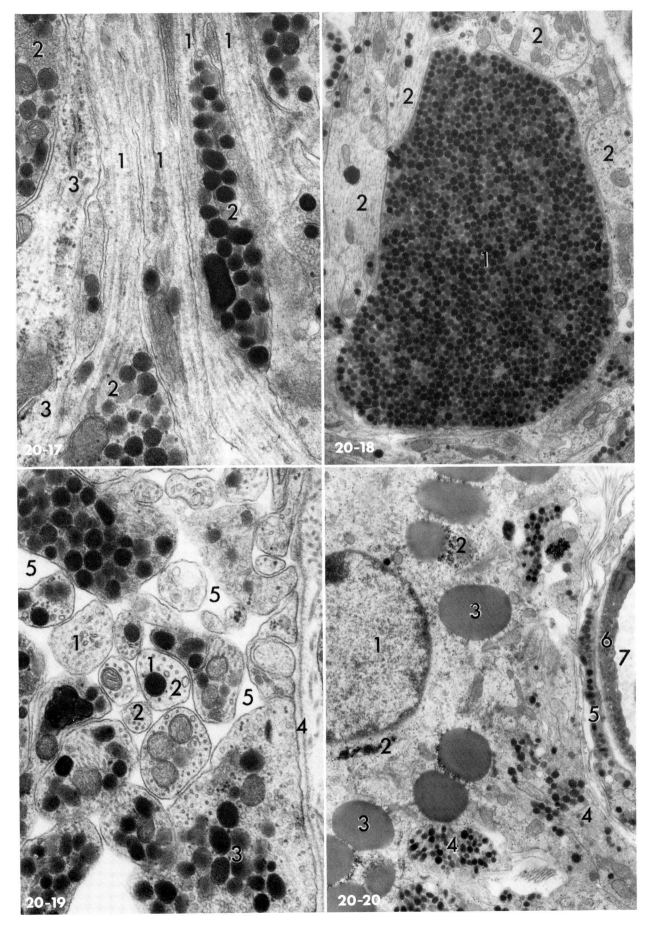

Fig. 20-17. Detail of neurohypophysis. Rat. E.M. X 37,000. **1.** Longitudinally sectioned nerve processes with microtubules. **2.** Neurosecretory granules being passed along the nerve processes. **3.** Part of pituicyte.

Fig. 20-18. Detail of neurohypophysis. Rat. E.M. X 9000. **1.** Local accumulation of numerous neurosecretory granules, referred to as Herring body. **2.** Nerve processes.

Fig. 20-19. Detail of neurohypophysis. Rat. E.M. X 36,000. **1.** Cross-sectioned nerve processes with few or no neurosecretory granules. **2.** Microtubules. **3.** Club-shaped nerve ending with neurosecretory granules and vesicles. **4.** Basal lamina. **5.** Intercellular (extracellular) space.

Fig. 20-20. Detail of neurohypophysis. Rat. E.M. X 9000. **1.** Nucleus of pituicyte. **2.** Particulate glycogen. **3.** Lipid droplets. **4.** Nerve processes. **5.** Nerve ending. **6.** Capillary endothelium. **7.** Capillary lumen.

References

ADENOHYPOPHYSIS

Coates, P. W., Ashby, E. A., Krulich, L., Dhariwal, A. P. S. and McCann, S. M. Morphologic alterations in somatotrophs of the rat adenohypophysis following administration of hypothalamic extracts. Am. J. Anat. *128*: 389–412 (1970).

Dekker, A. Electron microscopic study of somatotropic and lactotropic pituitary cells of the Syrian hamster. Anat. Rec. *162*: 132–136 (1968).

Heath, E. Cytology of the pars anterior of the bovine adenohypophysis. Am. J. Anat. *127*: 131–158 (1970).

Herlant, M. The cells of the adenohypophysis and their functional significance. Int. Rev. Cytol. *17*: 299–381 (1964).

Mikami, S. Light and electron microscopic investigations of six types of glandular cells of the bovine adenohypophysis. Z. Zellforsch. *105*: 457–482 (1970).

Paiz, C. and Hennigar, G. R. Electron microscopy and histochemical correlation of human anterior pituitary cells. Am. J. Path. *59*: 43–73 (1970).

Siperstein, E. R. and Miller, K. J. Further cytophysiologic evidence for the identity of the cells that produce adrenocorticotrophic hormone. Endocrinology *86*: 451–486 (1970).

Wislocki, G. B. The vascular supply of the hypophysis cerebri of the rhesus monkey and man. *In*: The Pituitary Gland, pp. 48–68. Williams & Wilkins, Baltimore, 1938.

NEUROHYPOPHYSIS

Barer, R. and Lederis, K. Ultrastructure of the rabbit neurohypophysis with special reference to the release of hormones. Z. Zellforsch. *75*: 201–239 (1966).

Bargmann, W. Neurosecretion. Int. Rev. Cytol. *19*: 183–201 (1966).

Bodian, D. Herring bodies and neuroapocrine secretion in the monkey. An electron microscopic study of the fate of the neurosecretory product. Bull. Johns Hopkins Hosp. *118*: 282–326 (1966).

Dellmann, H. D. and Rodriguez, E. M. Herring bodies; an electron microscopic study of local degeneration and regeneration of neurosecretory axons. Z. Zellforsch. *111*: 293–315 (1970).

Heller, H. (Ed.). The Neurohypophysis. Academic Press, New York, 1957.

Lederis, K. An electron microscopical study of the human neurohypophysis. Z. Zellforsch. *65*: 847–868 (1965).

Sawyer, C. H. Brain-endocrine interactions. A symposium presented at the 83rd session of the American Association of Anatomists. Am. J. Anat. *129*: 193–246 (1970).

Scharrer, E. Principles of Neuroendocrine Integration. Endocrines and the Central Nervous System, *43*: 1–35 (1966).

Scharrer, E. and Scharrer, B. Neurosekretion. *In*: Handbuch der mikroskopischen Anatomie des Menschen. (Eds. W. von Möllendorff and W. Bargmann), Vol. 6, part 5, pp. 953–1066. Springer, Berlin, 1954.

Scharrer, E. and Scharrer, B. Neuroendocrinology. Columbia Univ. Press, New York, 1963.

21 Thyroid gland

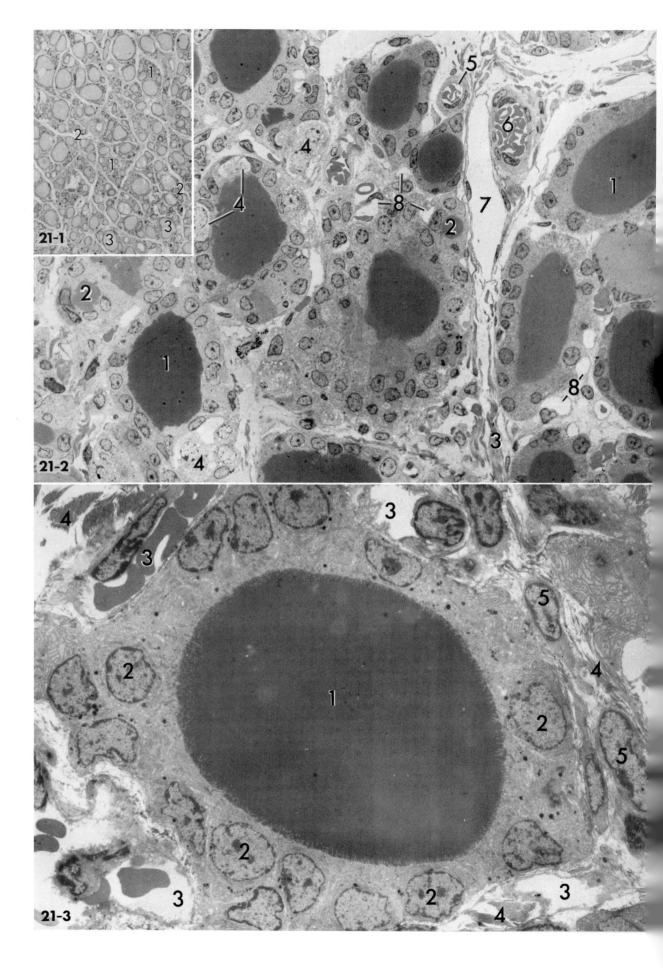

Fig. 21-1. Segment of thyroid gland. Human. L.M. X 23. **1.** Lobules. **2.** Septa. **3.** Follicles.

Fig. 21-2. Survey of thyroid gland. Rat. E.M. X 600. **1.** Large follicles. **2.** Small follicles. **3.** Connective tissue septa. **4.** Parafollicular cells. **5.** Arteriole. **6.** Venule. **7.** Lymphatic capillary. **8.** Blood capillaries.

Fig. 21-3. Detail of thyroid follicle. Rat. E.M. X 1800. **1.** Colloid in center of follicle. **2.** Nuclei of follicular epithelial cells. **3.** Perifollicular capillaries. **4.** Perifollicular bundles of collagenous fibrils. **5.** Nuclei of fibroblasts.

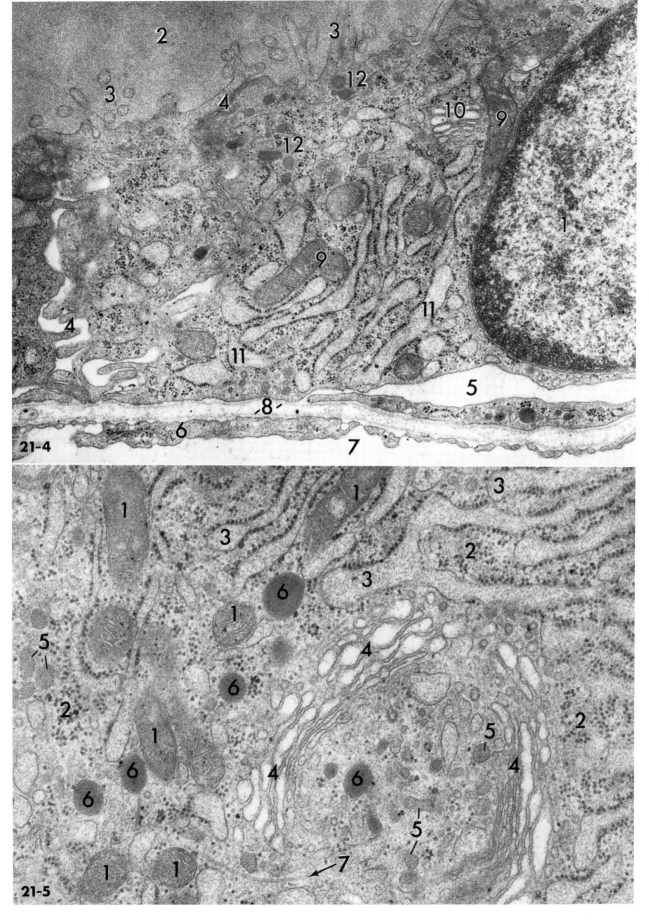

Fig. 21-4. Detail of epithelial cell of thyroid follicle. Rat. E.M. X 22,000. **1.** Nucleus. **2.** Colloid in center of follicle **3.** Microvilli. **4.** Cell membranes. **5.** Intercellular space. **6.** Endothelium of blood capillary. **7.** Capillary lumen. **8.** Basal laminae. **9.** Mitochondria. **10.** Golgi complex. **11.** Cisternae of granular endoplasmic reticulum. **12.** Secretory granules (colloid droplets).

Fig. 21-5. Enlargement of the central part of epithelial cell of thyroid follicle. Center of follicle to the left, base of epithelial cell to the right. Rat. E.M. X 47,000. **1.** Mitochondria. **2.** Ribosomes. **3.** Cisternae of granular endoplasmic reticulum. **4.** Vesicles, membranes, and flattened sacs of the Golgi complex. **5.** Secretory granules (colloid droplets). **6.** Primary lysosomes. **7.** Microtubule.

Fig. 21-6. Detail of the wall of thyroid follicle. Rat. E.M. × 10,000. **1.** Nucleus of parafollicular cell. **2.** Nucleus of principal follicular cell. **3.** Lumen of follicle. **4.** Lumen of perifollicular capillary. **5.** Fenestrated (closed) endothelium. **6.** Basal lamina of thyroid follicle. **7.** Close association of parafollicular cell and blood capillary. **8.** Golgi complexes. **9.** Dilated cisternae of the granular endoplasmic reticulum. **10.** Mitochondria. **11.** Secretory granules of parafollicular cell. **12.** Lysosomes. **13.** Collagenous fibrils of perifollicular connective tissue.

Fig. 21-7. Enlargement of area similar to rectangle in Fig. 21-6. Secretory granules of parafollicular cell. Thyroid. Rat. E.M. × 47,500. **1.** Mitochondria. **2.** Cisternae of granular endoplasmic reticulum. **3.** Ribosomes. **4.** Very dense-core secretory granule. **5.** Secretory granule with medium-dense core. **6.** Secretory granule with very light center. These granules are structurally rather similar to some of the cisternae of the nearby granular endoplasmic reticulum. The variation in core density represents intermediate stages of either hormone release or synthesis.

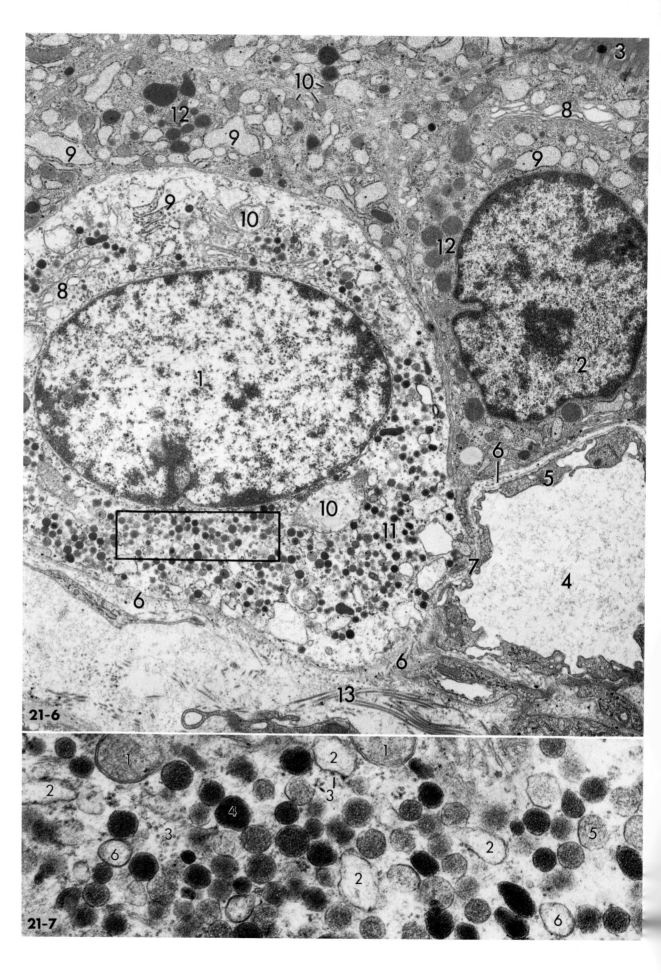

References

PRINCIPAL FOLLICULAR CELLS

Ekholm, R. Thyroid gland. *In* Electron Microscopic Anatomy (Ed. S. M. Kurtz), pp. 221–238. Academic Press, New York, 1964.

Ekholm, R. and Sjöstrand, F. S. The ultrastructural organization of the mouse thyroid gland. J. Ultrastruct. Res. *1*: 178–199 (1957).

Ekholm, R. and Strandberg, U. Thyroglobulin biosynthesis in the rat thyroid. J. Ultrastruct. Res. *20*: 103–110 (1967).

Heimann, P. Ultrastructure of human thyroid. Acta Endocrinologica *53*: Suppl. 110, 1–102 (1966).

Klinck, G. H. Structure of the thyroid. *In* The Thyroid (Eds. J. B. Hazard and D. E. Smith), pp. 1–31. Williams & Wilkins, Baltimore, 1964.

Klinck, G. H., Oertel, J. E. and Winship, T. Ultrastructure of normal human thyroid. Lab. Investig. *22*: 2–22 (1970).

Lupulescu, A. and Petrovici, A. Ultrastructure of the thyroid gland. Williams & Wilkins, Baltimore, 1968.

Nunez, E. A. and Becker, D. Secretory processes in follicular cells of the bat thyroid. Am. J. Anat. *129*: 369–398 (1970).

Seljelid, R. Endocytosis in thyroid follicle cells. I. Structure and significance of different types of single membrane-limited vacuoles and bodies. J. Ultrastruct. Res. *17*: 195–219 (1967).

Seljelid, R.: Endocytosis in thyroid follicles. II. A micro injection study of the origin of colloid droplets. J. Ultrastruct. Res. *17*: 401–420 (1967).

Seljelid, R. Endocytosis in thyroid follicle cells. III. An electron microscopic study of the cell surface and related structures. J. Ultrastruct. Res. *18*: 1–24 (1967).

Seljelid, R. Endocytosis in thyroid follicle cells. IV. On the acid phosphatase activity in thyroid follicle cells, with special reference to the quantitative aspects. J. Ultrastruct. Res. *18*: 237–256 (1967).

Seljelid, R. Endocytosis in thyroid follicle cells. V. On the redistribution of cytosomes following stimulation with thyrotropic hormone. J. Ultrastruct. Res. *18*: 479–488 (1967).

Whur, P., Herscovics, A. and Leblond, C. P. Radioautographic visualization of the incorporation of galactose-^{3}H and mannose-^{3}H by rat thyroids in vitro in relation to the stages of thyroglobulin synthesis. J. Cell Biol. *43*: 289–311 (1969).

Wissig, S. L. The anatomy of secretion in the follicular cells of the thyroid gland. I. The fine structure of the gland in the normal rat. J. Biophys. Biochem. Cytol. *7*: 419–432 (1960).

Wissig, S. L. The anatomy of secretion in the follicular cells of the thyroid gland. II. The effect of acute thyrotrophic hormone stimulation on the secretory apparatus. J. Cell Biol. *16*: 93–117 (1963).

PARAFOLLICULAR CELLS

Chan, A. S. and Conen, P. E. Ultrastructural observations on cytodifferentiation of parafollicular cells in the human fetal thyroid. Lab. Investig. *25*: 249–259 (1971).

Ekholm, R. and Ericson, L. E. The ultrastructure of the parafollicular cells of the thyroid gland in the rat. J. Ultrastruct. Res. *23*: 378–402 (1968).

Ericson, L. E. Subcellular localization of 5-hydroxytryptamine in the parafollicular cells of the mouse thyroid gland. An autoradiographic study. J. Ultrastruct. Res. *31*: 162–177 (1970).

Gershon, M. D., Belshaw, B. E. and Nunez, E. A. Biochemical, histochemical and ultrastructural studies of thyroid serotonin, parafollicular and follicular cells during development in the dog. Am. J. Anat. *132*: 5–20 (1971).

Nonidez, J. F. The origin of the parafollicular cell, a second epithelial component of the thyroid gland of the dog. Am. J. Anat. *49*: 479–505 (1932).

Strum, J. M. and Karnovsky, M. J. Cytochemical localization of endogenous peroxidase in thyroid follicular cells. J. Cell Biol. *44*: 655–666 (1970).

Teitelbaum, S. L., Moore, K. E. and Shiebler, W. C-Cell follicles in the dog thyroid: demonstration by in vivo perfusion. Anat. Rec. *168*: 69–78 (1970).

22 Parathyroid glands

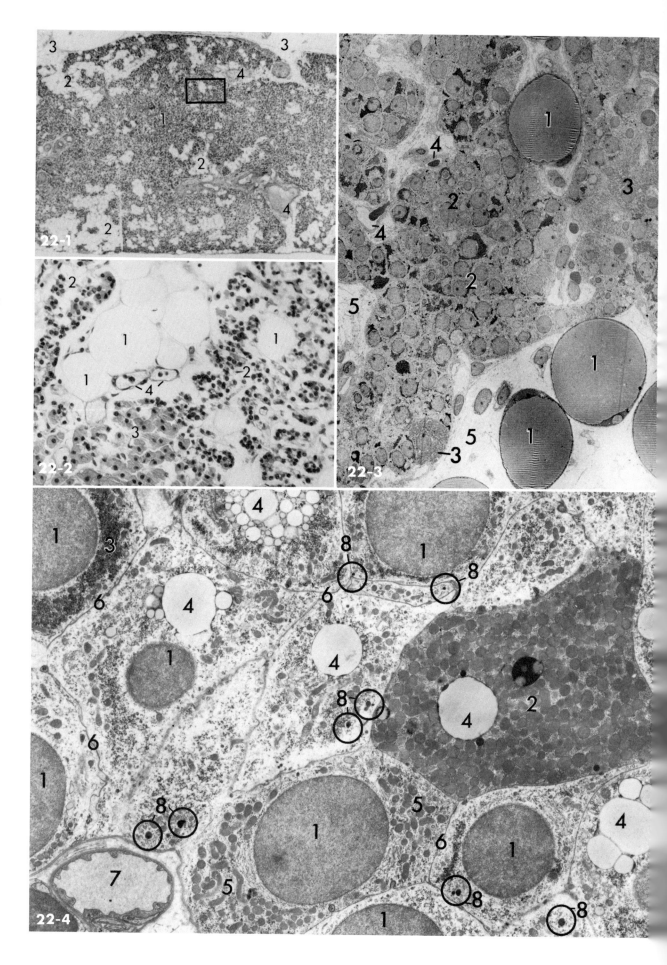

Fig. 22-1. Parathyroid gland. Human. L.M. X 24. **1.** Glandular tissue. **2.** Adipose tissue. **3.** Capsule. **4.** Connective tissue septa with blood vessels.

Fig. 22-2. Enlargement of area similar to rectangle in Fig. 22-1. Parathyroid gland. Human. L.M. X 260. **1.** Fat cells. **2.** Chief cells. **3.** Oxyphil cells. **4.** Blood capillaries.

Fig. 22-3. Survey of cords of cells in parathyroid gland. Human. E.M. X 570. **1.** Fat cells. **2.** Chief cells. **3.** Oxyphil cells. **4.** Blood capillaries. **5.** Connective tissue septa.

Fig. 22-4. Detail of parathyroid gland. Human. E.M. X 4500. **1.** Nuclei of chief cells. **2.** Oxyphil cell, crowded with mitochondria. **3.** Large accumulations of particulate glycogen. **4.** Lipid droplets. **5.** Mitochondria. **6.** Cell borders. **7.** Lumen of blood capillary. **8.** Circles indicate possible secretory granules.

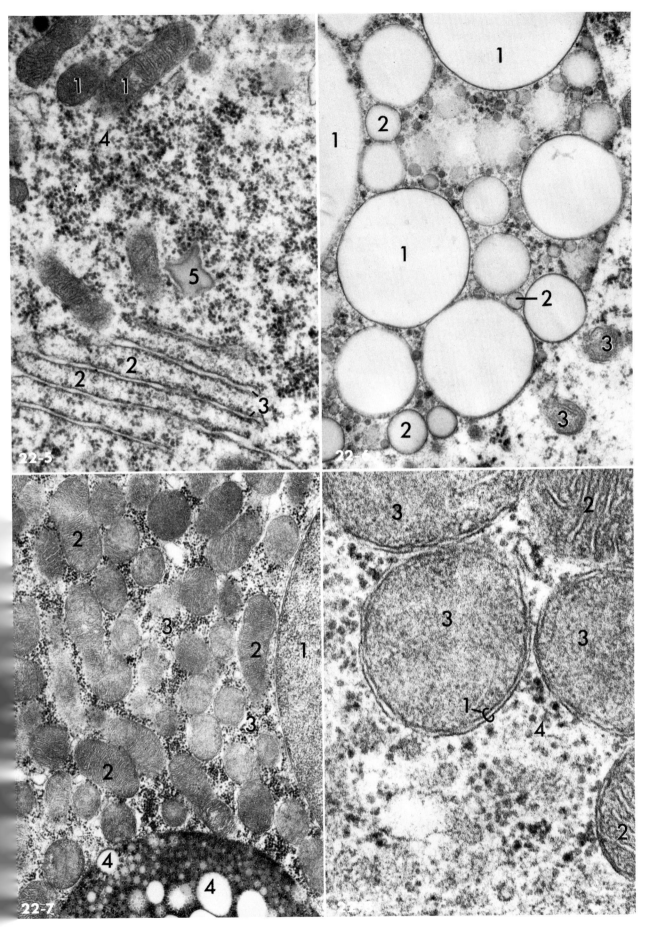

Fig. 22-5. Detail of chief cell. Parathyroid gland. Human. E.M. X 34,000. **1.** Mitochondria. **2.** Ribosomes. **3.** Flattened cisternae of granular endoplasmic reticulum. **4.** Accumulation of particulate glycogen. **5.** Partly collapsed small lipid droplet.

Fig. 22-6. Detail of chief cell. Parathyroid gland. Human. E.M. X 34,000. **1.** Large lipid droplets. **2.** Small lipid droplets. **3.** Mitochondria.

Fig. 22-7. Detail of oxyphil cell. Parathyroid gland. Human. E.M. X 17,000. **1.** Nucleus. **2.** Mitochondria. **3.** Particulate glycogen. **4.** Accumulation of lipid droplets of various sizes.

Fig. 22-8. Detail of mitochondria in oxyphil cell. Parathyroid gland. Human. E.M. X 87,000. **1.** Mitochondrial external envelope. **2.** Mitochondrial cristae. **3.** Mitochondrial matrix. **4.** Glycogen particles.

References

Capen, C. C. and Rowland, G. N. The ultrastructure of the parathyroid glands of young cats. Anat. Rec. *162*: 327–340 (1968).

Fetter, A. W. and Capen, C. C. The ultrastructure of the parathyroid glands of young pigs. Acta Anat. *75*: 359–372 (1970).

Munger, B. L. and Roth, S. I. The cytology of the normal parathyroid glands of man and Virginia deer. J. Cell Biol. *16*: 379–400 (1963).

Nakagima, K., Yamazaki, Y. and Isunoda, Y. An electron microscopic study of the human fetal parathyroid gland. Z. Zellforsch. *85*: 89–95 (1968).

Nunez, E. A., Whalen, J. P. and Krook, L. An ultrastructural study of the natural secretory cycle of the parathyroid gland of the bat. Am. J. Anat. *134*: 459–480 (1972).

23 Adrenal (suprarenal) glands

Fig. 23-1. Section of entire adrenal gland. Monkey. L.M. X 12. **1.** Capsule. **2.** Cortex. **3.** Medulla.

Fig. 23-2. Enlargement of rectangle in Fig. 23-1. Adrenal gland. Monkey. L.M. X 53. **1.** Capsule. **2.** Zona glomerulosa of cortex. **3.** Zona fasciculata of cortex. **4.** Zona reticularis of cortex. **5.** Adrenal medulla. **6.** Large medullary vein.

Fig. 23-3. Enlargement of area similar to rectangle (A) in Fig. 23-2. Adrenal gland. Rat. E.M. X 725. **1.** Capsule. **2.** Capsular arteriole. **3.** Capillaries of the zona glomerulosa. **4.** Capillaries of the zona fasciculata. Arrows indicate direction of blood flow. **5.** Approximate border between zona glomerulosa and zona fasciculata. **6.** Cords of glandular epithelial cells.

Fig. 23-4. Enlargement of area similar to rectangle (B) in Fig. 23-2. Adrenal gland. Rat. E.M. X 725. **1.** Capillaries of the zona fasciculata. **2.** Capillaries of the zona reticularis. **3.** Approximate border between fasciculata and reticularis. **4.** Adrenal medulla. **5.** Cell cords.

Fig. 23-5. Enlargement of area similar to rectangle in Fig. 23-3. Zona fasciculata. Adrenal cortex. Rat. E.M. X 5200. **1.** Lumina of capillaries. **2.** Nucleus of endothelial cell. **3.** Fenestrated (closed) endothelium. **4.** Subendothelial space. **5.** Nucleus of epithelial cell. **6.** Lipid droplets within the cell. **7.** Lipid droplets discharging at the cell surface. **8.** Mitochondria. **9.** Glycogen accumulations. **10.** Crystal.

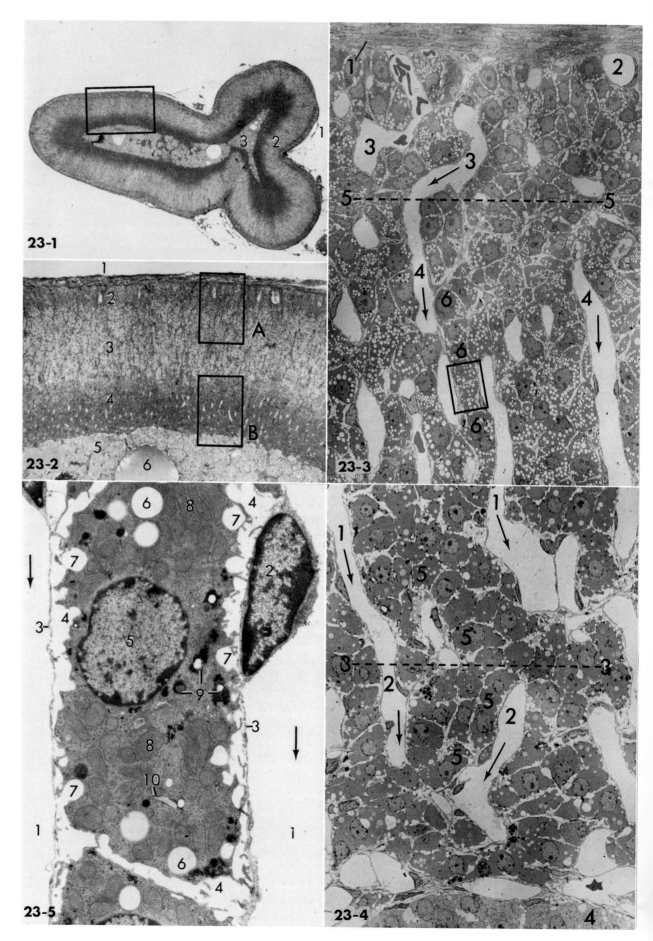

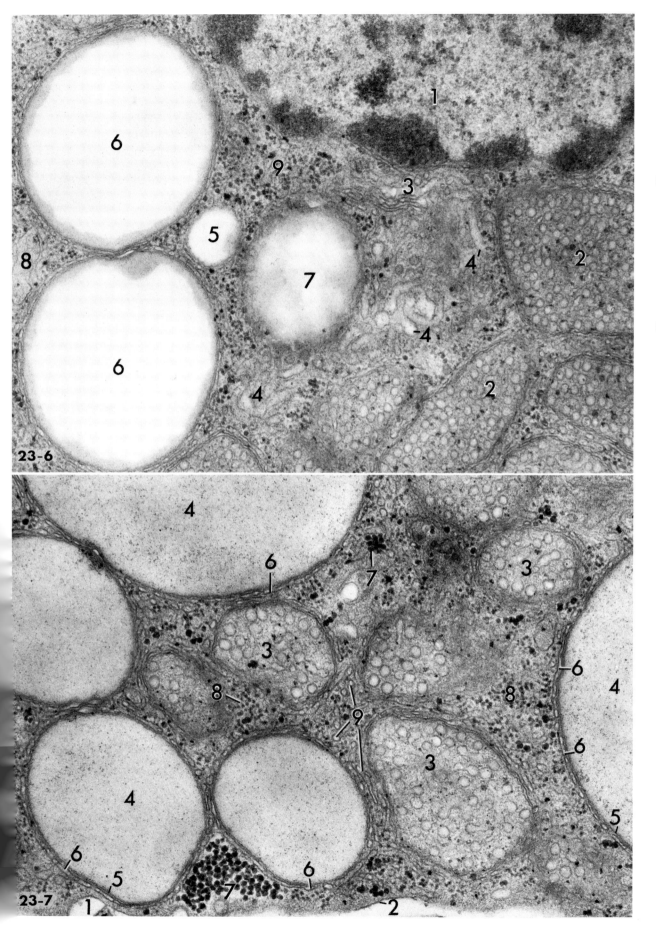

Fig. 23-6. Detail of cell from zona fasciculata. Adrenal cortex. Rat. E.M. X 60,000. **1.** Nucleus. **2.** Mitochondria with vesicular cristae. **3.** Golgi membranes. **4.** Tubular agranular endoplasmic reticulum, some profiles enlarging to form minute lipid droplets. **5.** Small lipid droplet. **6.** Large lipid droplets with center of lipid matrix slightly dissolved during preparation. **7.** Tangential section of large lipid droplet. **8.** Primary lysosome. **9.** Ribosomes.

Fig. 23-7. Detail of cell from zona fasciculata. Adrenal cortex. Rat. E.M. X 60,000. **1.** Intercellular space. **2.** Cell membrane. **3.** Mitochondria with vesicular cristae. **4.** Lipid droplets with matrix well preserved. **5.** Interface lipid droplet/cytoplasm. **6.** Profiles of agranular endoplasmic reticulum adhering to interface membrane of lipid droplet. **7.** Particulate glycogen. **8.** Free ribosomes. **9.** Profiles of agranular endoplasmic reticulum free in the cytoplasm.

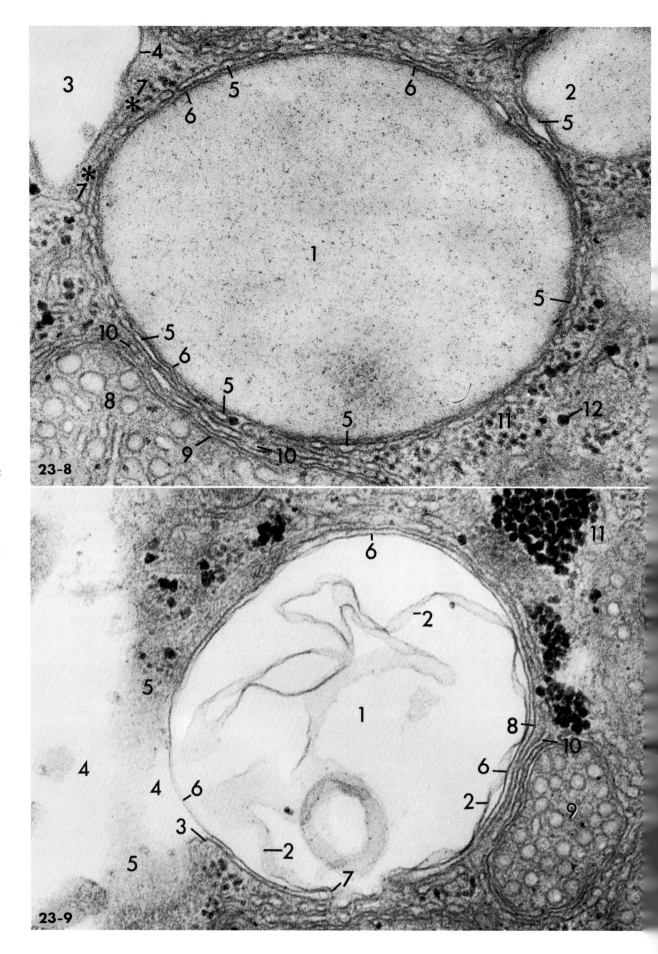

Fig. 23-8. Lipid droplet approaching the cell surface. Zona fasciculata. Adrenal cortex. Rat. E.M. × 116,000. From: Rhodin, J. Ultrastruct. Res. *34*: 23 (1971). **1.** Matrix of large lipid droplet. **2.** Small lipid droplet. **3.** Subendothelial space. **4.** Cell surface membrane. **5.** Bilaminar casing of merged profiles of agranular endoplasmic reticulum. **6.** Interface lipid droplet/cytoplasm appears as a thin, 40 Å boundary membrane. **7. Asterisks:** thin sheath of cytoplasm interposed between lipid droplet and extracellular space. **8.** Mitochondrion with vesicular cristae. **9.** Mitochondrial envelope. **10.** Bilaminar casing of merged profiles of agranular endoplasmic reticulum surrounds the mitochondrion. **11.** Ribosomes. **12.** Glycogen particle.

Fig. 23-9. Lipid droplet at the moment of presumed release of the droplet matrix. Zona fasciculata. Adrenal cortex. Rat. E.M. × 120,000. From: Rhodin, J. Ultrastruct. Res. *34*: 23 (1971). **1.** Center of droplet. **2.** Droplet boundary membrane, partly collapsed. **3.** Peripheral membrane of bilaminar endoplasmic casing has fused with surface cell membrane. **4.** Subendothelial space. **5.** Grazing section through edge of cytoplasmic opening. **6.** Intact central membrane of endoplasmic reticulum casing. **7.** Occasional continuity between peripheral and central membranes. **8.** Peripheral membrane of endoplasmic reticulum casing. **9.** Mitochondria. **10.** Agranular endoplasmic reticulum. **11.** Accumulation of glycogen particles.

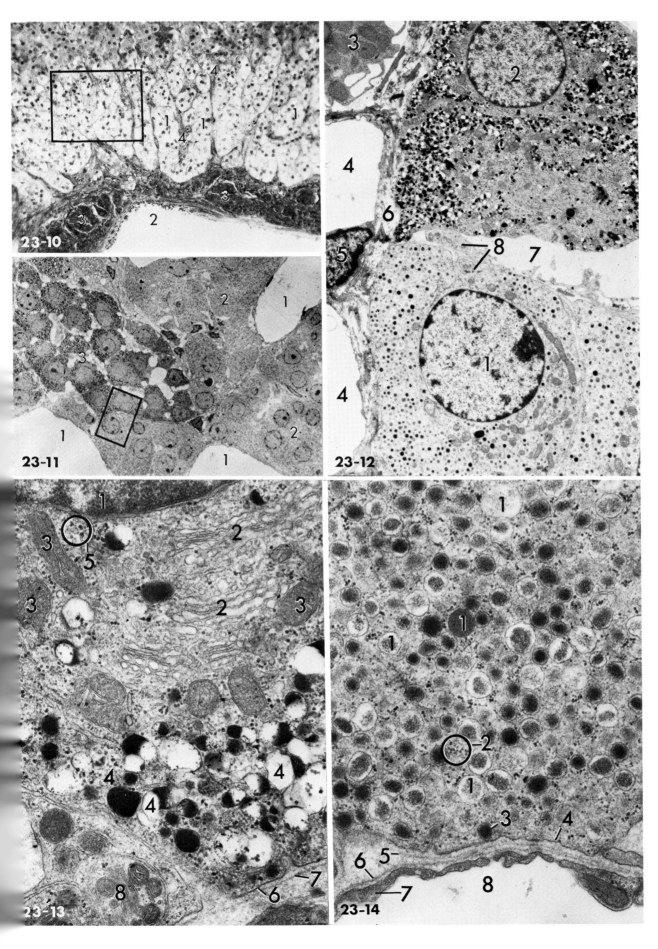

Fig. 23-10. Adrenal gland. Medulla. Human. L.M. X 133. **1.** Cords of medullary cells. **2.** Lumen of large medullary vein. **3.** Smooth muscle cells arranged longitudinally in the wall of the vein. **4.** Area of collapsed capillaries and venules.

Fig. 23-11. Enlargement of area similar to rectangle in Fig. 23-10. Adrenal medulla. Rat. E.M. X 650. **1.** Medullary capillaries and venules. **2.** Cords of epinephrine cells. **3.** Clusters of norepinephrine cells.

Fig. 23-12. Enlargement of area similar to rectangle in Fig. 23-11. Adrenal medulla. Rat. E.M. X 4500. **1.** Nucleus of epinephrine cell. **2.** Nucleus of norepinephrine cell. **3.** Corner of cell belonging to zona reticularis. **4.** Capillary lumen. **5.** Endothelial nucleus. **6.** Subendothelial space. **7.** Intercellular space. **8.** Nerve endings.

Fig. 23-13. Detail of norepinephrine cell. Adrenal medulla. Rat. E.M. X 32,500. **1.** Nucleus. **2.** Golgi complex. **3.** Mitochondria. **4.** Secretory granules (inadequately preserved). **5.** Circle: particulate glycogen. **6.** Cell membrane. **7.** Parenchymal external (basal) lamina. **8.** Mitochondria in nerve ending.

Fig. 23-14. Detail of epinephrine cell. Adrenal medulla. Rat. E.M. X 27,000. **1.** Secretory granules of varied size and density. **2.** Circle: particulate glycogen. **3.** Secretory granule on the verge of being extruded. **4.** Cell membrane. **5.** Parenchymal basal (external) lamina. **6.** Capillary basal lamina. **7.** Capillary endothelium. **8.** Capillary lumen.

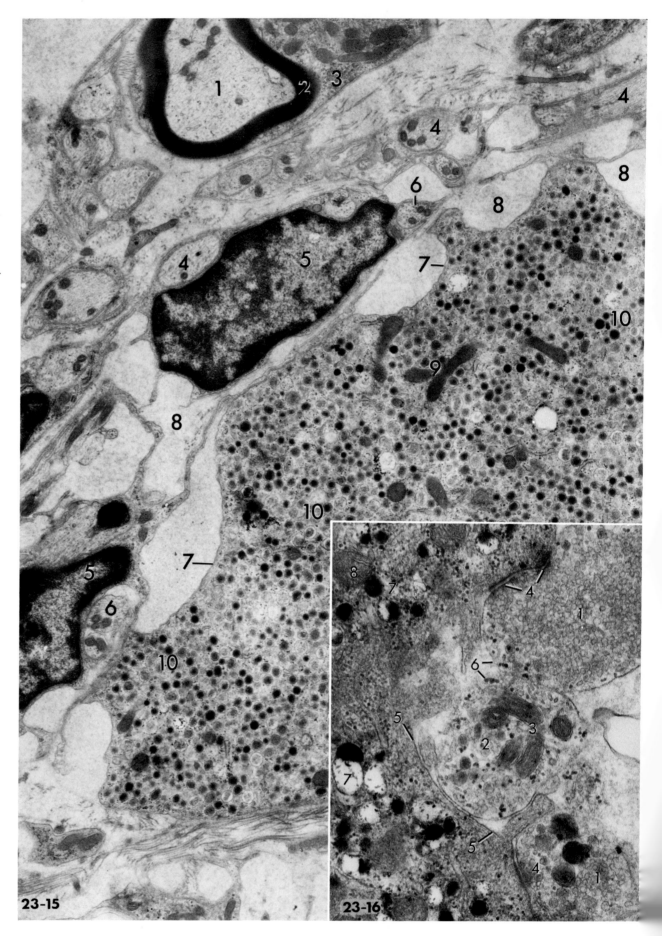

Fig. 23-15. Relationship between nerves and endocrine cells of the adrenal medulla. Rat. E.M. X 10,000. **1.** Axon of myelinated nerve. **2.** Myelin sheath. **3.** Schwann cell cytoplasm. **4.** Axons of non-myelinated nerves. **5.** Nuclei of Schwann cells. **6.** Nerve axons near cell membrane of endocrine cell. **7.** Cell membrane of epinephrine cell. **8.** Intercellular space. **9.** Mitochondria. **10.** Secretory granules.

Fig. 23-16. Terminal contacts of nerve endings. Adrenal medulla. Rat. E.M. X 36,000. **1.** Nerve endings with numerous clear vesicles. **2.** Dense-core vesicles in nerve ending. **3.** Mitochondria. **4.** Synaptic junctions. **5.** Cell membrane of norepinephrine cell. **6.** Particulate glycogen. **7.** Secretory granules. **8.** Mitochondrion.

References

ADRENAL CORTEX

Bennett, H. S. The life history and secretion of the cells of the adrenal cortex of the cat. Am. J. Anat. *67*: 151–228 (1940).

Bloodworth, J. M. B. and Powers, K. L. The ultrastructure of the normal dog adrenal. J. Anat. *102*: 457–476 (1968).

Brenner, R. M. Fine structure of adrenocortical cells in adult male rhesus monkeys. Am. J. Anat. *119*: 429–453 (1966).

Ford, J. K. and Young, R. W. Cell proliferation and displacement in the adrenal cortex of young rats injected with tritiated thymidine. Anat. Rec. *146*: 125–138 (1963).

Friend, D. S. and Brassil, G. E. Osmium staining of endoplasmic reticulum and mitochondria in the rat adrenal cortex. J. Cell Biol. *46*: 252–266 (1970).

Giacomelli, F., Wiener, J. and Spiro, D. Cytological alterations related to stimulation of the zona glomerulosa of the adrenal gland. J. Cell Biol. *26*: 499–522 (1965).

Idelman, S. Ultrastructure of the mammalian adrenal cortex. Int. Rev. Cytol. *27*: 181–281 (1970).

Long, J. A. and Jones, A. L. The fine structure of the zona glomerulosa and the zona fasciculata of the adrenal cortex of the opossum. Am. J. Anat. *120*: 463–488 (1967).

Long, J. A. and Jones, A. L. Observations on the fine structure of the adrenal cortex of man. Lab. Investig. *17*: 355–370 (1967).

Luse, S. Fine structure of adrenal cortex. *In*: The Adrenal Cortex (Ed. A. B. Eisenstein), pp. 1–60. Little, Brown, Boston, 1967.

Pauly, J. E. Morphological observations on the adrenal cortex of the laboratory rat. Endocrinology *60*: 247–264 (1957).

Penney, D. P. and Brown, G. M. The fine structural morphology of adrenal cortices of normal and stressed squirrel monkeys. J. Morph. *134*: 447–466 (1971).

Rhodin, J. A. G. The ultrastructure of the adrenal cortex of the rat under normal and experimental conditions. J. Ultrastruct. Res. *34*: 23–71 (1971).

Sheridan, M. N. and Belt, W. D. Fine structure of the guinea pig adrenal cortex. Anat. Rec. *149*: 73–98 (1964).

Zelander, T. The adrenal gland. *In*: Electron Microscopic Anatomy (Ed. S. M. Kurtz), pp. 199–220. Academic Press, New York, 1964.

Wood, J. G. Identification of and observation on epinephrine and norepinephrine containing cells in the adrenal medulla. Am. J. Anat. *112*: 285–303 (1963).

ADRENAL MEDULLA

Al-Lami, F. Light and electron microscopy of the adrenal medulla of macaca mulata monkey. Anat. Rec. *164*: 317–332 (1969).

Bennett, H. S. Cytological manifestations of secretion in the adrenal medulla of the cat. Am. J. Anat. *69*: 333–383 (1941).

Brown, W. J., Barajas, L. and Latta, H. The ultrastructure of the human adrenal medulla: with comparative studies of white rat. Anat. Rec. *169*: 173–184 (1971).

Coupland, R. E. Electron microscopic observations on the structure of the rat adrenal medulla. I. The ultrastructure and organization of chromaffin cells in the normal adrenal medulla. J. Anat. *99*: 231–254 (1965).

Coupland, R. E. Electron microscopic observations on the structure of the rat adrenal medulla. II. Normal innervation. J. Anat. *99*: 255–272 (1965).

Coupland, R. E. and Weakley, B. S. Electron microscopic observations on the adrenal medulla and extra-adrenal chromaffin tissue of the postnatal rabbit. J. Anat. *106*: 213–231 (1970).

D'Anzi, F. A. Morphological and biochemical observations on the catecholamine-storing vesicles of rat adrenomedullary cells during insulin-induced hypoglycemia. Am. J. Anat. *125*: 381–398 (1969).

Elfvin, L. G. The development of the secretory granules in the rat adrenal medulla. J. Ultrastruct. Res. *17*: 45–62 (1967).

PARAGANGLIA

Böck, P. Die Feinstruktur des paraganglionären Gewebes im Plexus suprarenalis des Meerschweinchens. Z. Zellforsch. *105*: 389–404 (1970).

Dawson, I. The endocrine cells of the gastrointestinal tract. Histochem. J. *2*: 527–549 (1970).

24 Pineal body

Fig. 24-1. Pineal body. Human. L.M. × 168.
1. Lobules of parenchyma. **2.** Connective tissue septa. **3.** Concretion.

Fig. 24-2. Pineal body concretion. Human. L.M. × 780. Concentric lamellae of hydroxy apatite, calcium carbonate apatite and organic matrix.

Fig. 24-3 & 24-4. Pineal body. Human. L.M. × 315. **1.** Connective tissue septa. **2.** Lumen of blood vessel. **3.** Parenchyma. Difference in cell types is not discernible. **4.** Cell shrinkage enhances the elongated shape of the cell processes and their allegedly club-shaped termination toward the connective tissue septa.

Fig. 24-5. Pineal body. Enlargement of area similar to rectangle in Fig. 24-4. Rat. E.M. × 2300. **1.** Nuclei of pinealocytes. **2.** Nuclei of pineal neuroglial cells (astrocytes). Note that differences in cell types have been verified at higher magnifications and are not discernible at this magnification. **3.** Dashed line indicates level of external (basal) lamina which surrounds the parenchymal lobule. **4.** Connective tissue septum. **5.** Lumen of capillary.

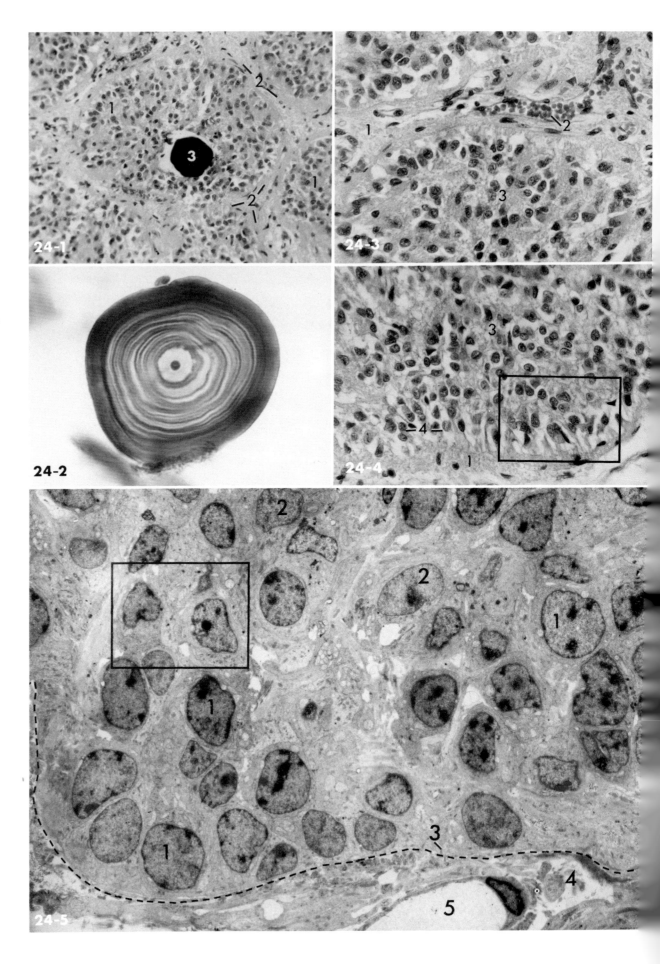

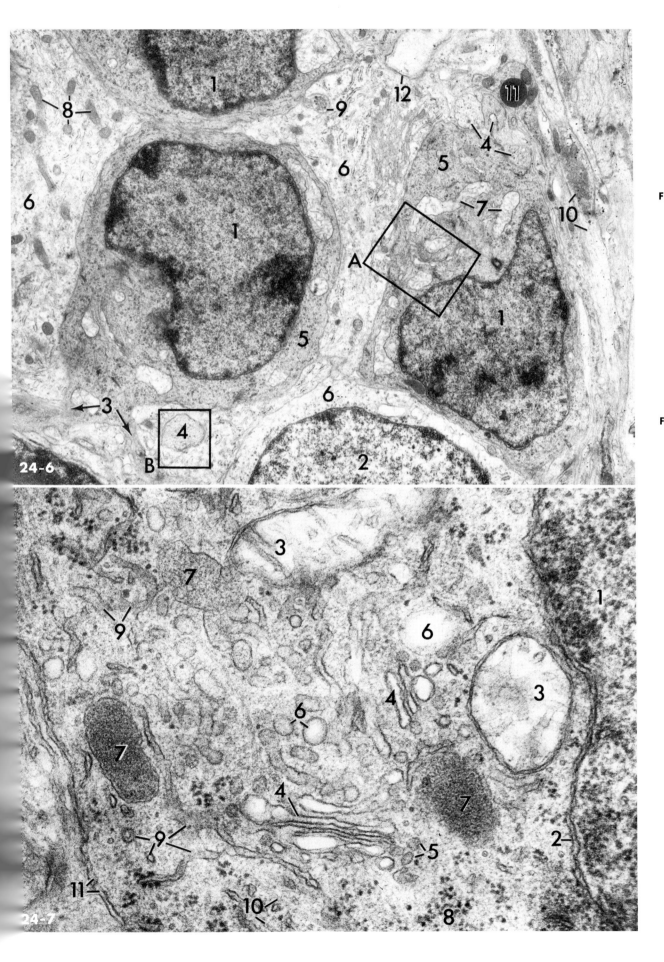

Fig. 24-6. Parenchymal cells. Pineal body. Enlargement of area similar to rectangle in Fig. 24-5. Rat. E.M. X 8400. **1.** Nuclei of pinealocytes. **2.** Nucleus of pineal neuroglial cell (astrocyte). **3.** Initial segment of two pinealocyte processes. **4.** Cross-sectioned pinealocyte processes. **5.** Electron-dense cytoplasm of pinealocyte. **6.** Electron-lucent cytoplasm of astrocyte. **7.** Large electron-lucent mitochondria. **8.** Small electron-dense mitochondria. **9.** Cross-sectioned sympathetic nerve process (enlarged further in Fig. 24-8, inset). **10.** Longitudinally sectioned sympathetic nerve processes. **11.** Large secondary lysosome. **12.** Glial cell membrane facing connective tissue space and external (basal) lamina.

Fig. 24-7. Detail of pinealocyte. Enlargement of area similar to rectangle (A) in Fig. 24-6. Pineal body. Rat. E.M. X 56,000. **1.** Nucleus. **2.** Nuclear membrane. **3.** Mitochondria with tubular cristae. **4.** Golgi saccules. **5.** Golgi vesicles. **6.** Condensing Golgi vacuoles. **7.** Primary lysosomes and/or grumose bodies. **8.** Ribosomes. **9.** Agranular endoplasmic reticulum. **10.** Microtubules. **11.** Cell membrane.

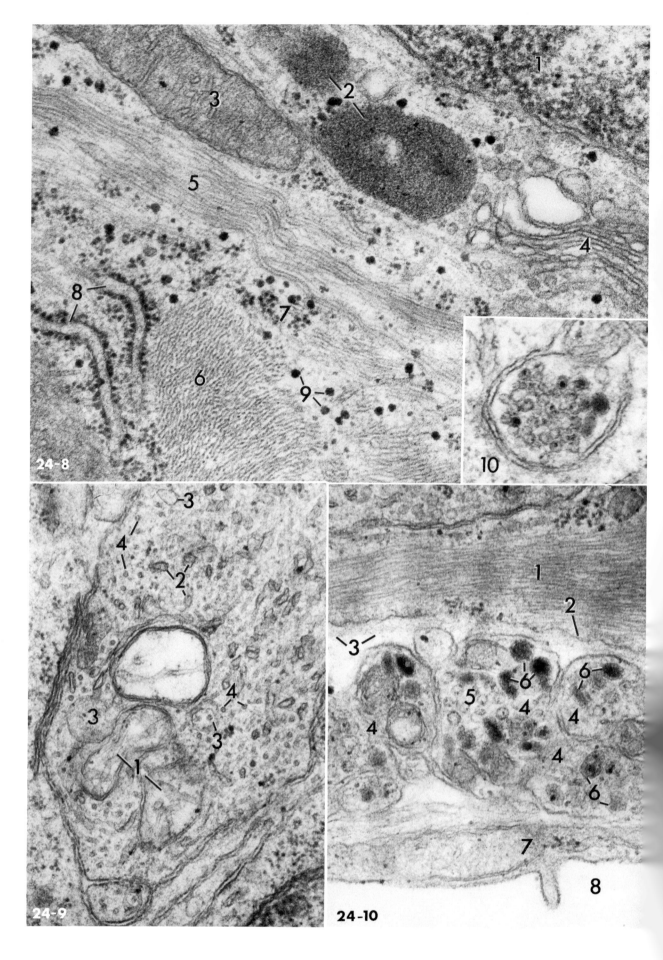

Fig. 24-8. Detail of pineal neuroglial cell (astrocyte). Pineal body. Rat. E.M. X 60,000. **1.** Nucleus. **2.** Lysosomes. **3.** Mitochondrion with membranous cristae. **4.** Golgi apparatus. **5.** Longitudinally sectioned bundle of cytoplasmic filaments. **6.** Cross-sectioned bundle of filaments. **7.** Ribosomes. **8.** Profiles of granular endoplasmic reticulum. **9.** Glycogen particles (beta type). **10.** Inset: cross-sectioned sympathetic nerve fiber, surrounded by astrocytic cytoplasm, containing clear vesicles, small and large dense-core vesicles.

Fig. 24-9. Cross-sectioned process of pinealocyte. Enlargement of area similar to rectangle (B) in Fig. 24-6. Pineal body. Rat. E.M. X 54,000. **1.** Mitochondria. **2.** Tubular elements of agranular endoplasmic reticulum. **3.** Clear vesicles. **4.** Microtubules.

Fig. 24-10. Detail of perivascular area. Pineal body. Rat. E.M. X 54,000. **1.** Cytoplasmic filaments in pineal neuroglial astrocyte. **2.** Cell membrane. **3.** External (basal) lamina of parenchymal lobule. **4.** Terminations of nerve endings. **5.** Small dense-cored vesicles. **6.** Large dense-core vesicles. **7.** Endothelium of postcapillary venule. **8.** Venular lumen.

References

Anderson, E. The anatomy of bovine and ovine pineals. Light and electron microscopic studies. J. Ultrastruct. Res. Suppl. 8 (1965).

Bertler, A., Falck, B. and Owman, Ch. Studies on 5-hydroxytryptamine stores in pineal gland of rat. Acta Physiol. Scand. *63*, Suppl. 239 (1964).

Clabough, J. W. Ultrastructural features of the pineal gland in normal and light deprived golden hamsters. Z. Zellforsch. *114*: 151–164 (1971).

Duffy, P. E. and Markesbery, W. R. Granulated vesicles in sympathetic nerve endings in the pineal gland: observations on the effect of the pharmacological agents by electron microscopy. Am. J. Anat. *128*: 97–116 (1970).

Duncan, D. and Micheletti, G. Notes on the fine structure of the pineal organ of cats. Texas Report Biol. Med. *24*: 576–587 (1966).

Hoffman, R. A. and Reiter, R. J. Pineal gland influence on gonads of male hamsters. Science *148*: 1609–1611 (1965).

Kappers, J. A. The mammalian pineal organ. J. Neuro-Visceral Relations. Suppl. 9, 140–184 (1969).

Kappers, J. A. and Schadé, J. P. (Eds.). Structure and function of the epiphysis cerebri. Progr. in Brain Res. *10*: 1–694 (1965).

Lederis, K. An electron microscopical study of the human neurohypophysis. Z. Zellforsch. *65*: 847–868 (1965).

Lues, G. Die Feinstruktur der Zirbeldrüse normaler, trächtiger und experimentell beeinflusster Meerschweinchen. Z. Zellforsch. *114*: 38–60 (1971).

Reiter, R. J. and Fraschini, F. Endocrine aspects of the mammalian pineal gland: a review. Neuroendocrinology *5*: 219–255 (1969).

Sano, Y. and Mashimo, T. Elektronenmikroskopische Untersuchungen an der Epiphysis Cerebri beim Hund. Z. Zellforsch. *69*: 129–139 (1966).

Sheridan, M. N. and Reiter, R. J. The fine structure of the hamster pineal gland. Am. J. Anat. *122*: 357–376 (1968).

Sheridan, M. N. and Reiter, R. J. Observations on the pineal system in the hamster. II. Fine structure of the deep pineal. J. Morph. *131*: 163–178 (1970).

Wartenberg, H. The mammalian pineal organ: electron microscopic studies on the fine structure of pinealocytes, glial cells, and on the perivascular compartment. Z. Zellforsch. *86*: 74–97 (1968).

Wolstenhome, G. E. and Knight, J. (Eds.). The Pineal Gland. Ciba Foundation Symposium, Churchill, London, 1971.

Wurtman, R. J. and Axelrod, J. The formation, metabolism and physiological effects of melatonin in mammals. Progr. Brain Res. *10*: 520–529 (1965).

25 Skin and appendages

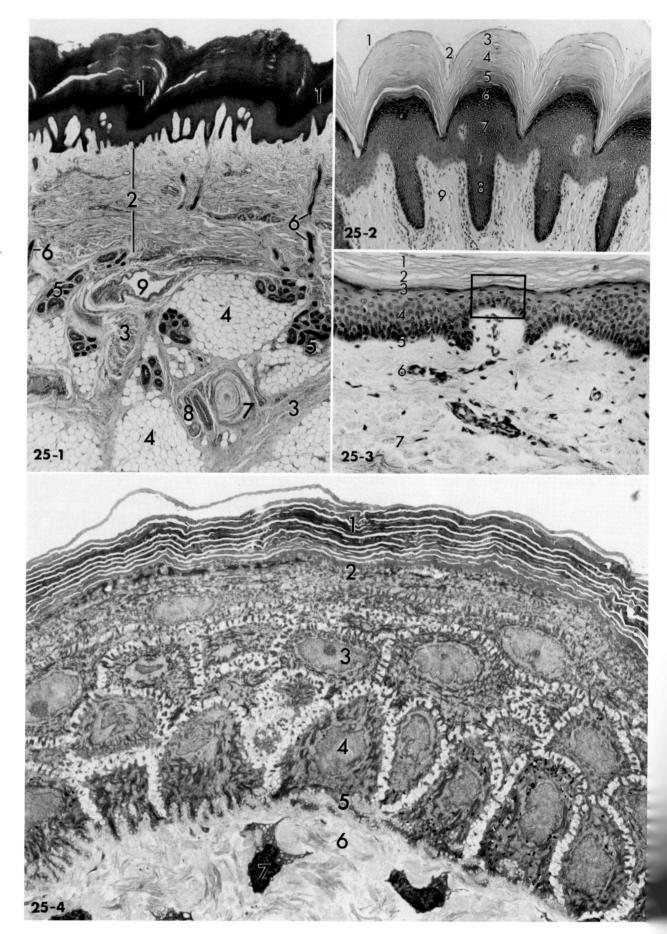

Fig. 25-1. Section through thick skin of palm of hand. Human. L.M. X 33. **1.** Epidermis with thick stratum corneum. **2.** Dermis.
3. Connective tissue septa of hypodermis.
4. Subcutaneous fat tissue. **5.** Sweat glands.
6. Ducts of sweat gland. **7.** Pacinian corpuscle.
8. Artery. **9.** Vein.

Fig. 25-2. Thick skin of palmar surface of finger. Monkey. L.M. X 85. **1.** Ridges. **2.** Grooves.
3. Stratum disjunctum. **4.** Stratum corneum.
5. Stratum lucidum. **6.** Stratum granulosum.
7. Stratum germinativum. **8.** Epidermal pegs and/or ridges. **9.** Dermal papillae.

Fig. 25-3. Thin skin of dorsal surface of hand. Human. L.M. X 210. **1.** Stratum disjunctum.
2. Stratum corneum. **3.** Thin stratum granulosum. **4.** Stratum germinativum.
5. Level of basal lamina. **6.** Papillary layer of dermis. **7.** Reticular layer of dermis.

Fig. 25-4. Epidermis. Enlargement of area similar to rectangle in Fig. 25-3. Axilla. Human. E.M. X 1900. **1.** Stratum corneum. Separation of layers accentuated by fixation and embedding procedures. **2.** Stratum granulosum (thin). **3.** Stratum spinosum.
4. Stratum basale. **5.** Level of basal lamina.
6. Collagenous fibrils of papillary layer.
7. Fibroblasts.

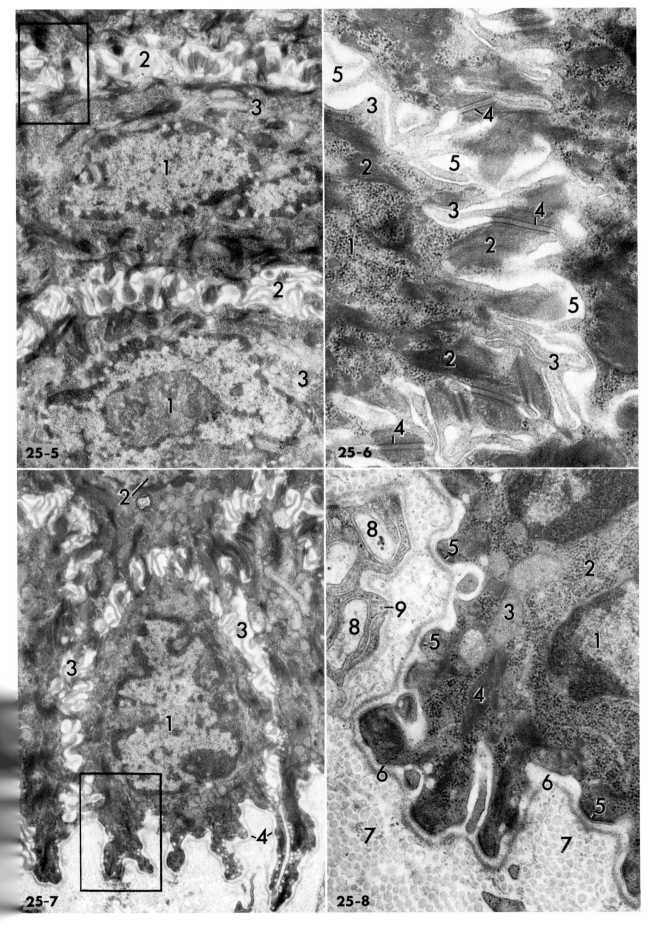

Fig. 25-5. Epidermis. Detail of stratum spinosum. Rat. E.M. X 9600. **1.** Nucleus. **2.** Intercellular space. **3.** Cytoplasm.

Fig. 25-6. Stratum spinosum of epidermis. Enlargement of area similar to rectangle in Fig. 25-5. Rat. E.M. X 30,000. **1.** Free ribosomes. **2.** Bundles of tonofilaments. **3.** Cytoplasmic processes. **4.** Desmosomes. **5.** Intercellular space.

Fig. 25-7. Epidermis. Detail of stratum basale. Rat. E.M. X 9000. **1.** Nucleus of basal cell. **2.** Nucleus of cell in stratum spinosum. **3.** Intercellular space. **4.** Basal lamina.

Fig. 25-8. Stratum basale of epidermis. Enlargement of area similar to rectangle in Fig. 25-7. Rat. E.M. X 29,000. **1.** Nucleus. **2.** Ribosomes. **3.** Mitochondria. **4.** Bundles of tonofilaments. **5.** Hemidesmosomes. **6.** Basal lamina. **7.** Collagenous fibrils in papillary layer of dermis. **8.** Nerve axons. **9.** Schwann cell cytoplasm.

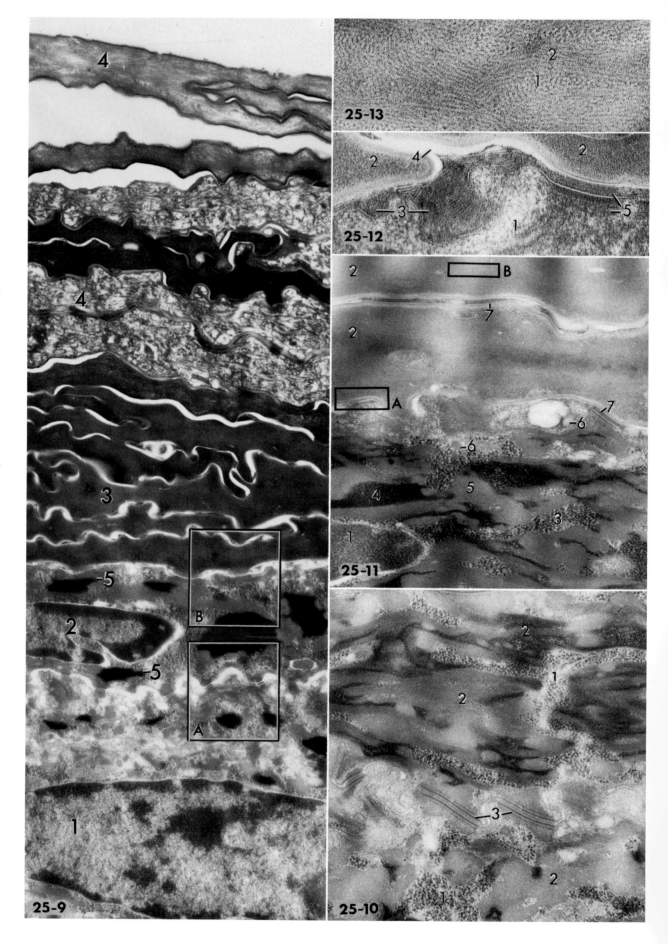

Fig. 25-9. Epidermis. Rat. E.M. X 12,000.
1. Nucleus of squamous cell in layer above stratum spinosum. **2.** Nucleus of cell in stratum granulosum. **3.** Stratum corneum. **4.** Stratum disjunctum. The cytoplasm of these cells is loosened up as part of a shedding process. **5.** Keratohyalin granules.

Fig. 25-10. Epidermis. Enlargement of area similar to square (A) in Fig. 25-9. Rat. E.M. X 31,000. **1.** Ribosomes. **2.** Masses of merging keratohyalin granules and tonofilaments. **3.** Desmosomes.

Fig. 25-11. Epidermis. Enlargement of area similar to square (B) in Fig. 25-9. Rat. E.M. X 32,000. **1.** Nucleus of cell in stratum granulosum. **2.** Squamous cells of stratum corneum. **3.** Ribosomes. **4.** Keratohyalin granules. **5.** Bundles of tonofilaments. **6.** Membrane-coating granules. **7.** Desmosomes.

Fig. 25-12. Epidermis. Enlargement of area similar to rectangle (A) in Fig. 25-11. Human. E.M. X 99,000. **1.** Cytoplasm of cell in stratum granulosum. **2.** Cells in stratum corneum. **3.** Multilamellar bodies (membrane-coating granules) at the moment of discharge. **4.** Intercellular space. **5.** Desmosomes.

Fig. 25-13. Epidermis. Stratum Corneum. Enlargement of area similar to rectangle (B) in Fig. 25-11. Rat. E.M. X 96,000. The fully keratinized cells of the epidermis are made up of bundles of densely packed keratin filaments. **1.** Cross-sectioned keratin filaments (80 Å). **2.** Longitudinally sectioned keratin filaments.

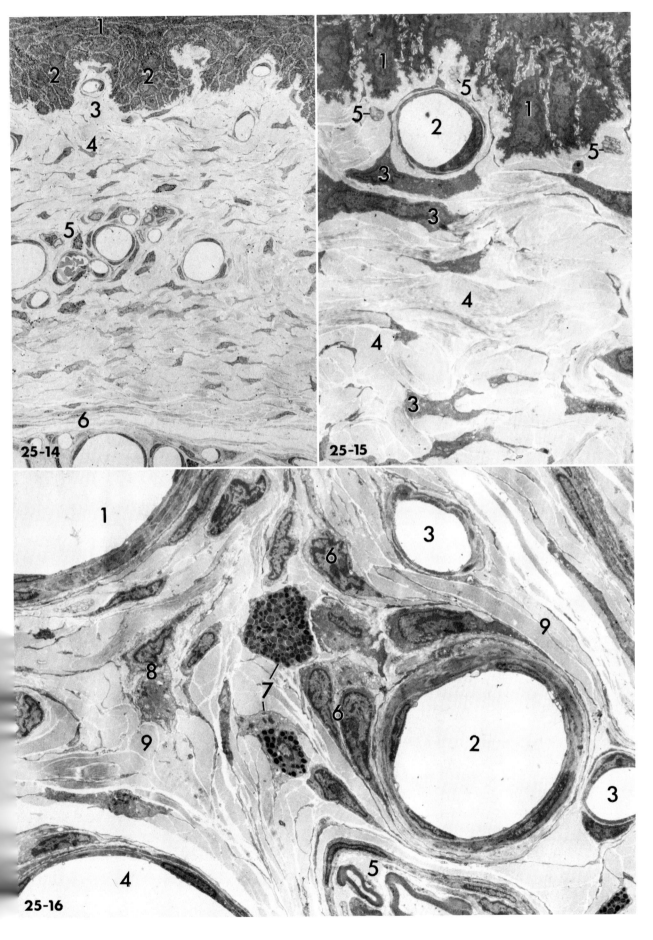

Fig. 25-14. Survey of dermis. Rat. E.M.X 590. **1.** Stratum germinativum of epidermis. **2.** Epidermal pegs. **3.** Dermal papillae. **4.** Papillary layer of dermis. **5.** Reticular layer of dermis with blood vessels and nerves. **6.** Hypodermis with blood vessels and nerves.

Fig. 25-15. Detail of papillary layer of dermis. Rat. E.M. X 1700. **1.** Stratum basale of epidermis. **2.** Capillary in dermal papilla (luminal diameter 11 μ). **3.** Fibroblasts. **4.** Bundles of collagenous fibrils. **5.** Non-myelinated nerves.

Fig. 25-16. Skin. Nerve-vascular bundle in the region between dermis and hypodermis. Rat. E.M. X 1900. **1.** Small artery. **2.** Arteriole, lumen 23 μ. **3.** Capillaries, lumen approx. 8 μ. **4.** Venule lumen 30 μ. **5.** Myelinated nerves. **6.** Fibroblasts. **7.** Mast cells. **8.** Macrophages. **9.** Bundles of collagenous fibrils.

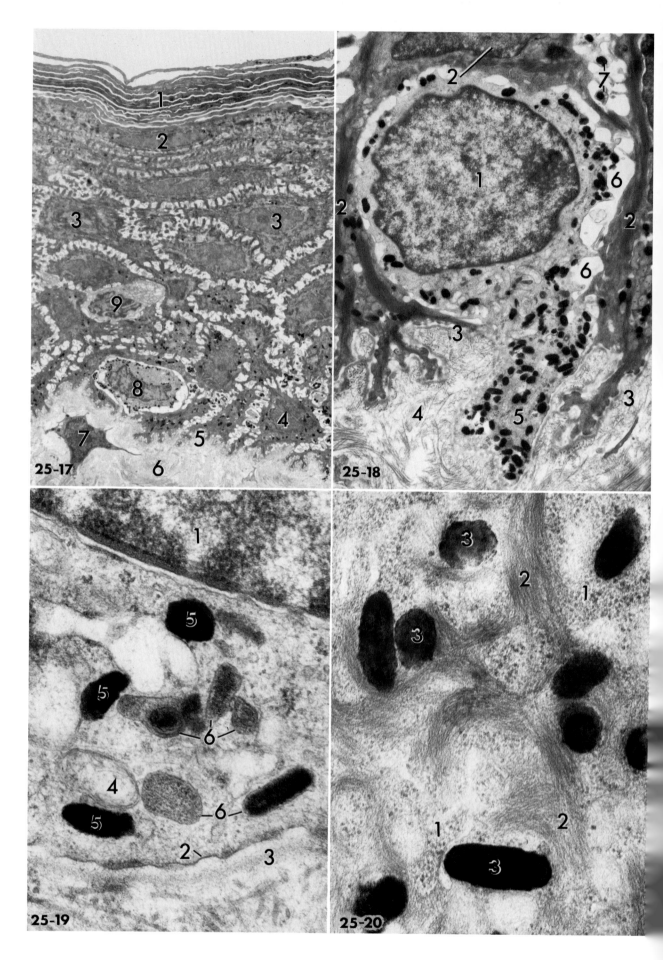

Fig. 25-17. Epidermis from axilla. Human. Negro. E.M. × 1800. **1.** Stratum corneum. **2.** Stratum granulosum. **3.** Stratum spinosum. **4.** Stratum basale. **5.** Basal lamina. **6.** Collagenous fibrils of papillary layer of dermis. **7.** Fibroblast. **8.** Melanocyte. **9.** Langerhans' cell (melanocyte without melanosomes.).

Fig. 25-18. Melanocyte. Epidermis. Human. Negro. E.M. × 10,000. **1.** Nucleus of melanocyte. **2.** Adjacent basal cells in the epidermis. **3.** Basal lamina. **4.** Collagenous fibrils. **5.** The "tail" of the melanocyte may indicate that the cell is in the process of moving from dermis to epidermis. **6.** Intercellular space. **7.** Narrow processes of melanocyte with melanosomes.

Fig. 25-19. Detail of melanocyte. Epidermis. Human. Negro. E.M. × 58,000. **1.** Nucleus of melanocyte. **2.** Cell membrane. **3.** Basal lamina of epidermis. **4.** Mitochondrion. **5.** Mature melanosomes. **6.** Pre-melanosomes in various stages of maturation. Each pre-melanosome is surrounded by a single trilaminar boundary membrane.

Fig. 25-20. Epidermis. Detail of basal cell. Human. Negro. E.M. × 60,000. **1.** Ribosomes. **2.** Bundles of tonofilaments. **3.** Mature melanosomes. Boundary membrane obscured by melanin pigmentation.

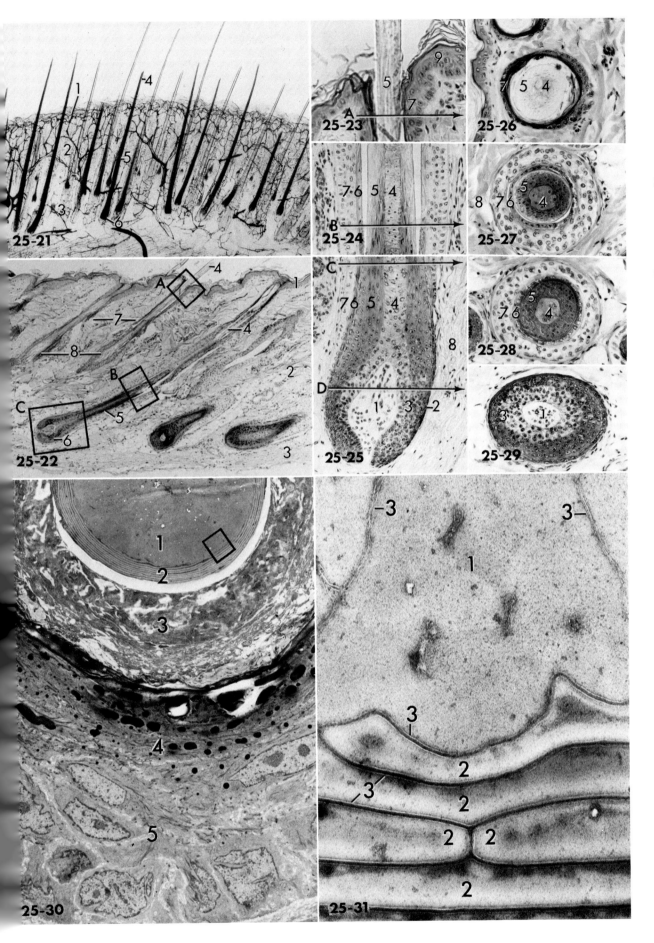

Fig. 25-21. Thick section of facial skin. Monkey. Preparation shows distribution of hairs and blood vessels. L.M. X 30.
1. Capillaries of papillary layer.
2. Subpapillary arterial plexus.
3. Cutaneous arterial plexus. 4. Hair shaft.
5. Hair follicle 6. Hair papilla.

Fig. 25-22. Thin section of skin. Scalp. Human. L.M. X 43. 1. Epidermis. 2. Dermis.
3. Hypodermis. 4. Hair shaft. 5. Hair follicle.
6. Hair papilla. 7. Resting hair follicles.
8. Club-hairs.

Figs. 25-23 to 25-25. Longitudinal sections of human hair: **Fig. 25-23** (L.M. X 200) corresponds to rectangle (A) in Fig. 25-22; **Fig. 25-24** (L.M. X 140) corresponds to rectangle (B); and **Fig. 25-25** (L.M. X 140) corresponds to rectangle (C). 1. Dermal papilla. 2. Hair papilla. 3. Hair matrix.
4. Hair medulla. 5. Hair cortex. 6. Inner root sheath. 7. Outer root sheath.
8. Connective tissue sheath. 9. Epidermis.

Fig. 25-26 to 25-29. Cross sections of human hair. L.M. X 145: **Fig. 25-26** corresponds to level A in Fig. 25-23; **Fig. 25-27** corresponds to level B in Fig. 25-24; **Fig. 25-28** corresponds to level C in Fig. 25-25; and **Fig. 25-29** corresponds to level D in Fig. 25-25. Legends to numerals 1–9 are identical to those in Fig. 25-25.

Fig. 25-30. Cross section of hair shaft at approximately the same level as Fig. 25-27. Vibrissa. Rat. E.M. X 1800. 1. Hair cortex.
2. Hair cuticle. 3. Remnants of keratinized inner root sheath. 4. Stratum granulosum of outer rooth sheath. 5. Stratum germinativum.

Fig. 25-31. Detail of cross-sectioned hair shaft. Enlargement of area similar to rectangle in Fig. 25-30. Vibrissa. Rat. E.M. X 39,000. 1. Cells of hair cortex fully keratinized (hard keratin). Individual keratin filaments are not resolved. 2. Cells of hair cuticle, fully keratinized. 3. Cell membranes with intercellular substance.

Fig. 25-32. Survey of hair root and papillae. Scalp. Human. L.M. X 320. **1.** Dermal papilla. **2.** Basal lamina. **3.** Hair matrix. **4.** Hair medulla. **5.** Hair cortex. **6.** Hair cuticles. **7.** Inner root sheath. **8.** Outer root sheath. **9.** Glassy membrane (basal lamina). **10.** Connective tissue sheath.

Fig. 25-33. Enlargement of area similar to rectangle in Fig. 25-32. Vibrissa. Rat. E.M. X 740. **1.** Dermal papilla. **2.** Basal lamina. **3.** Hair matrix. **4.** Hair cortex. **5.** Hair cuticle. **6.** Cuticle of inner root sheath. **7.** Huxley's layer. **8.** Henle's layer. **9.** Outer root sheath. **10.** Glassy membrane. **11.** Connective tissue sheath.

Fig. 25-34. Enlargement of area similar to rectangle in Fig. 25-33. Vibrissa. Rat. E.M. X 4500. **1.** Nuclei of cells forming the hair cuticle. **2.** Nuclei of cells forming cuticle of inner root sheath. **3.** Two layers of cells constitute Huxley's layer at this level. **4.** Trichohyalin granules. **5.** Cells of Henle's layer. **6.** Cells of outer root sheath. **7.** Basal lamina (glassy membrane).

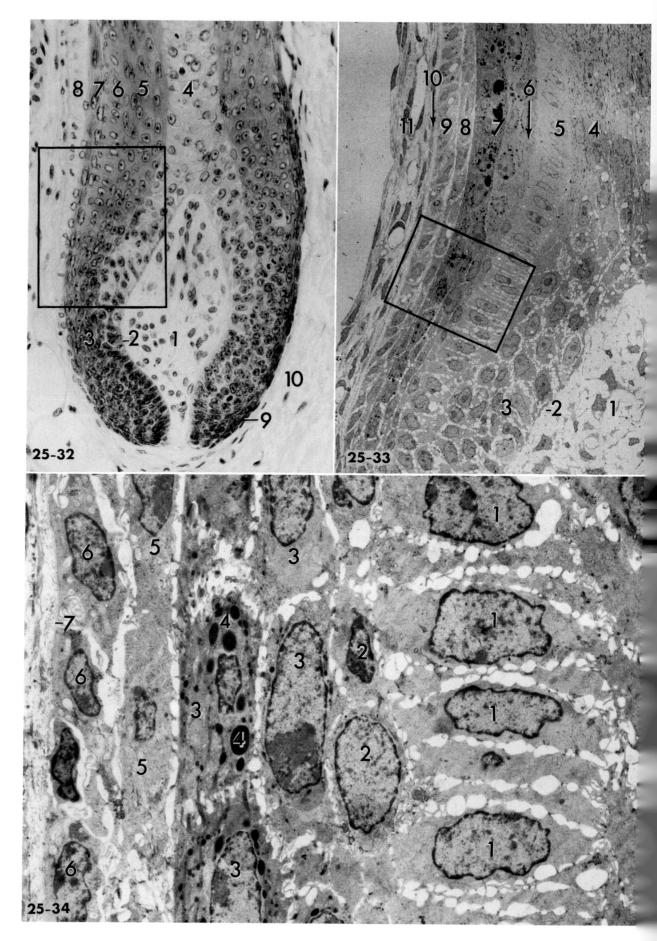

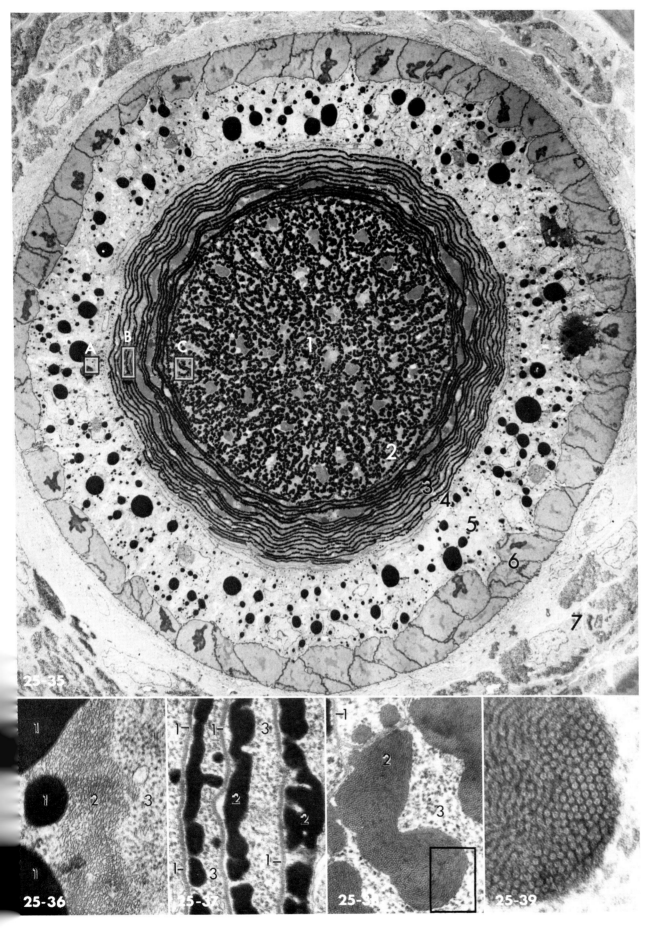

Fig. 25-35. Cross section of hair follicle at approximately the same level as Fig. 25-28. Vibrissa. Rat. E.M. X 1700. **1.** Center of hair. Medullary cells are not present in this particular hair. **2.** Hair cortex. Intensely black areas are cross-sectioned bundles of tonofibrils. Lighter areas are nuclei of hair cells. **3.** Layers of thin squamous hair cuticle cells. Dark lines represent beginning of keratinization. **4.** One thin layer of cells constitutes the cuticle of the inner root sheath. **5.** Huxley's layer is several cells deep. Abundant black trichohyalin granules indicate an approaching soft keratinization process. **6.** Cells of Henle's layer are keratinized at this level (soft keratin). Remnants of nuclei in some cells. **7.** Stratified epithelium of outer root sheath. Cells rich in particulate glycogen.

Fig. 25-36. Detail of cell in Huxley's layer. Enlargement of area similar to rectangle (A) in Fig. 25-35. Vibrissa. Rat. E.M. X 57,000. **1.** Trichohyalin granules. **2.** Cross-sectioned tonofilaments. **3.** Ribosomes.

Fig. 25-37. Detail of cells in hair cuticle. Enlargement of area similar to rectangle (B) in Fig. 25-35. Vibrissa. Rat. E.M. X 59,000. **1.** Cell borders. **2.** Amorphous keratin. **3.** Ribosomes.

Fig. 25-38. Detail of cell in hair cortex. Enlargement of area similar to rectangle (C) in Fig. 25-35. Vibrissa. Rat. E.M.X 59,000. **1.** Cell border. **2.** Cross-sectioned bundles of tonofibrils. **3.** Ribosomes.

Fig. 25-39. Detail of tonofibrillar bundle. Enlargement of area similar to rectangle in Fig. 25-38. Vibrissa. Rat. E.M. X 237,000. Each bundle of tonofibrils is composed of densely packed keratin filaments, referred to as α-filaments. Each filament is about 70 Å wide and has a lighter center with a dense filamentous subunit.

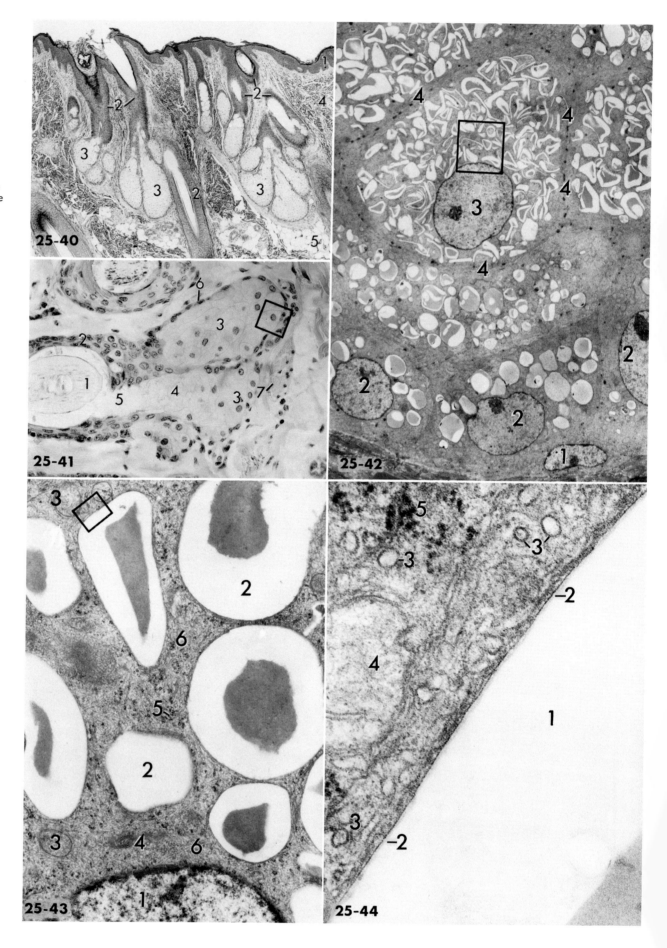

Fig. 25-40. Section of scalp. Human. L.M. X 31.
1. Epidermis. **2.** Hair follicles (hair shafts have fallen out during preparation). **3.** Sebaceous glands. **4.** Dermis. **5.** Subcutaneous fat.

Fig. 25-41. Section of scalp. Human. L.M. X 261. **1.** Hair shaft. (cross-sectioned). **2.** Outer root sheath. **3.** Alveoli of sebaceous glands. **4.** Sebum ready to be discharged. **5.** Duct of gland. **6.** Peripheral stem cells. **7.** Arrector pili muscle (cross-sectioned).

Fig. 25-42. Sebaceous gland. Enlargement of area similar to rectangle in Fig. 25-41. Monkey. E.M. X 1900. **1.** Nucleus of undifferentiated peripheral stem cell. **2.** Nuclei of cells with a limited number of droplets. **3.** Nucleus of a more central cell. Cytoplasm crowded with lipid droplets. **4.** Desmosomes along cell borders.

Fig. 25-43. Detail of secretory cell of sebaceous gland. Enlargement of area similar to rectangle in Fig. 25-42. Monkey. E.M. X 9300. **1.** Nucleus. **2.** Lipid droplets. Clear space and central dense mass indicate that some components have been removed in processing the tissue for microscopy. **3.** Mitochondria. **4.** Small Golgi zone. **5.** Free ribosomes. **6.** Cytoplasm filled with tubular profiles of the agranular endoplasmic reticulum.

Fig. 25-44. Enlargement of area similar to rectangle in Fig. 25-43. Monkey. E.M. X 92,000. **1.** Clear part of sebaceous droplet. **2.** Boundary membrane at interface of cytoplasm and sebaceous droplet. **3.** Cross-sectioned profiles of tubular agranular endoplasmic reticulum. **4.** Mitochondrion. **5.** Ribosomes.

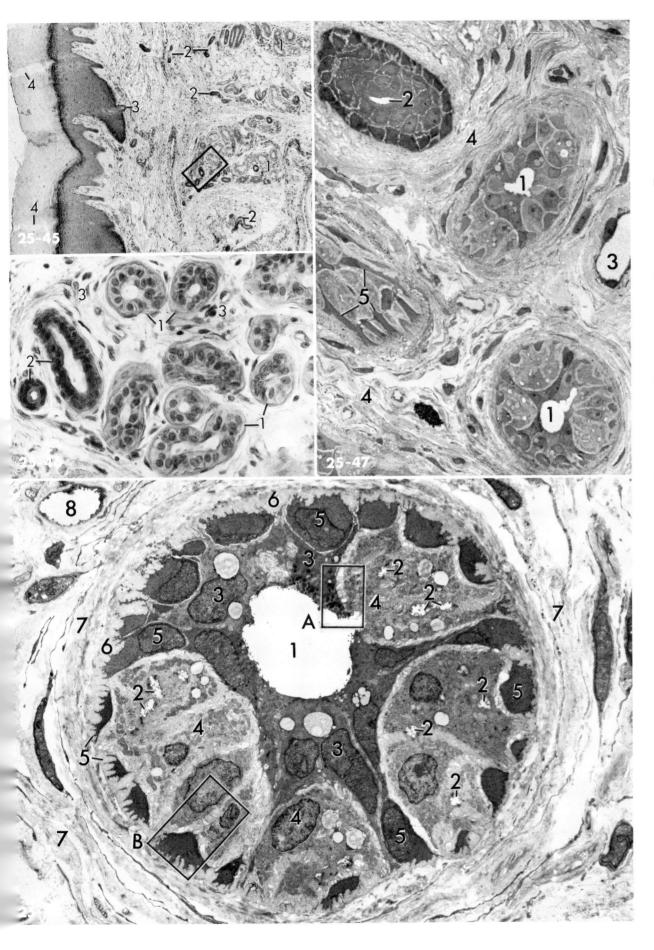

Fig. 25-45. Section through thick skin of palmar surface of finger. Monkey. L.M. X 55. **1.** Body of ordinary (eccrine) sweat gland in hypodermis. **2.** Excretory duct traversing dermis. **3.** Duct traversing stratum germinativum of epidermis. **4.** Ducts traversing stratum corneum.

Fig. 25-46. Ordinary (eccrine) sweat glands. Enlargement of area similar to rectangle in Fig. 25-45. Human. L.M. X 350. **1.** Sections of coiled body of ordinary sweat gland. **2.** Sections of excretory duct. The duct cells are smaller and stain more darkly than the cells of the gland itself. **3.** Connective tissue cells.

Fig. 25-47. Survey of ordinary (eccrine) sweat gland and excretory duct. Axilla. Human. E.M. X 600. **1.** Lumen of gland. **2.** Lumen of duct lined by a stratifed epithelium. **3.** Capillary. **4.** Connective tissue. **5.** Tangential section of gland in which the spread of the myoepithelial cells is clearly seen.

Fig. 25-48. Section of body of ordinary (eccrine) sweat gland. Axilla. Human. E.M. X 1700. **1.** Lumen. **2.** Intercellular canaliculi. **3.** Dark (mucoid) cells. **4.** Clear cells. **5.** Myoepithelial cells. **6.** Basal lamina (unusually thick). **7.** Connective tissue. **8.** Capillary.

Figs. 25-49 & 25-50. Ordinary (eccrine) sweat gland. Secretion granules of dark (mucoid) cells. Human. E.M. X 62,000. **1.** Secretion granules of some dark cells contain a highly electron-dense core and a loosely fitted boundary membrane. **2.** Other secretion granules are more electron-lucent with a tightly fitted boundary membrane. **3.** Ribosomes.

Fig. 25-51. Detail of ordinary (eccrine) sweat gland. Enlargement of area similar to rectangle (A) in Fig. 25-48. Human. E.M. X 9300. **1.** Lumen of sweat gland. **2.** Intercellular canaliculi. **3.** Dark (mucoid) cell with dense secretory granules. **4.** Light cells. **5.** Microvilli.

Fig. 25-52. Detail of ordinary (eccrine) sweat gland. Enlargement of area similar to rectangle (B) in Fig. 25-48. Human. E.M. X 9300. **1.** Nuclei of light cells. **2.** Intercellular space with numerous small cytoplasmic processes. **3.** Mitochondria. **4.** Myoepithelial cell (nucleus not in plane of section). **5.** Thick basal lamina.

Fig. 25-53. Cross section of excretory duct of sweat gland. Axilla. Human. E.M. X 1500. **1.** Lumen. **2.** Nuclei of cells in stratified epithelium. **3.** Intercellular space is wide in basal cell layer. **4.** Connective tissue.

Fig. 25-54. Apical part of cells in duct of sweat gland. Enlargement of area similar to rectangle in Fig. 25-53. Human. E.M. X 9300. **1.** Cytoplasm of cells bordering on duct lumen is filled with ribosomes, particulate glycogen, and scattered tonofilaments. **2.** Desmosomes hold cells together. **3.** This area has been referred to as "cuticle" in ordinary light microscopy.

Fig. 25-55. Enlargement of area similar to rectangle in Fig. 25-54. Human. E.M. X 62,000. **1.** The "cuticle" consists of numerous short and densely packed microvilli. **2.** Core of each villus contains microfilaments which descend into the apical cytoplasm. **3.** Small vacuole or vesicle.

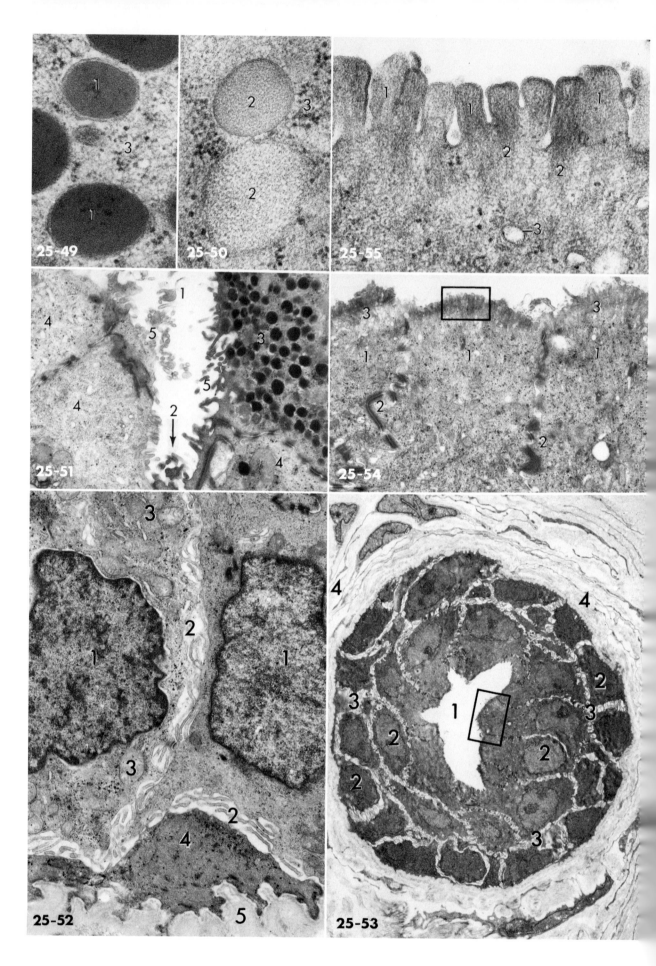

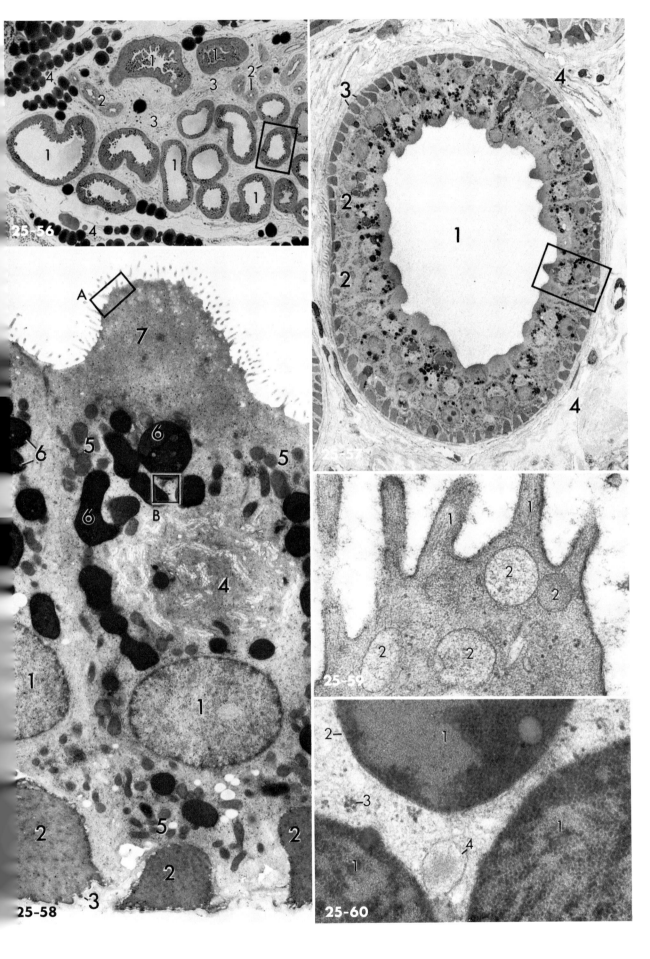

Fig. 25-56. Odoriferous (apocrine) sweat glands. Axilla. Human. L.M. X 57. **1.** Sections of coiled body of odoriferous sweat gland. **2.** Ordinary sweat glands. Cross-sectional diameter is far less than that of an odoriferous sweat gland. **3.** Connective tissue. **4.** Fat cells.

Fig. 25-57. Cross section of odoriferous (apocrine) sweat gland. Enlargement of area similar to rectangle in Fig. 25-56. Human. E.M. X 600. **1.** Lumen. **2.** Secretory, columnar cells. **3.** Myoepithelial cells. **4.** Connective tissue.

Fig. 25-58. Odoriferous (apocrine) sweat gland. Enlargement of area similar to rectangle in Fig. 25-57. Human. E.M. X 5600. **1.** Nuclei of epithelial cells. **2.** Myoepithelial cells. **3.** Thin basal lamina. **4.** Large Golgi zone. **5.** Mitochondria. **6.** Secondary lysosomes (or secretion granules). **7.** Apex of cell.

Fig. 25-59. Odoriferous sweat gland. Enlargement of area similar to rectangle (A) in Fig. 25-58. Human. E.M. X 60,000. **1.** Microvilli. **2.** Secretion droplets (granules).

Fig. 25-60. Odoriferous sweat gland. Enlargement of area similar to square (B) in Fig. 25-58. Human. E.M. X 60,000. **1.** Lysosomes (or secretion granules) with numerous small spheres or micelles inside. **2.** Boundary membrane. **3.** Ribosomes. **4.** Precursor of secretory granule (or primary lysosome).

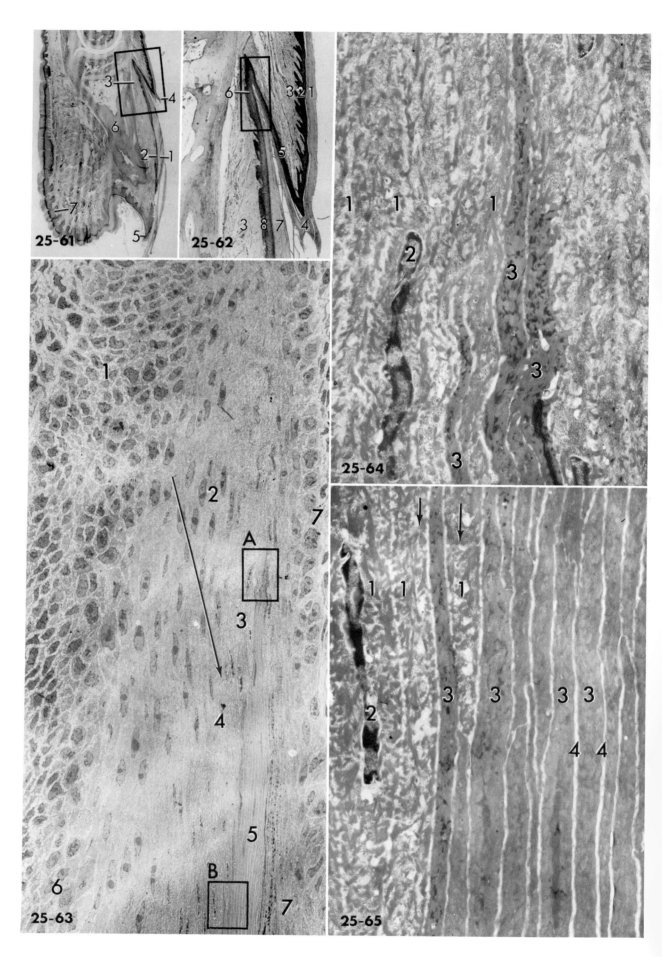

Fig. 25-61. Longitudinal section of finger tip. Monkey L.M. X 8. **1.** Nail plate. **2.** Nail bed. **3.** Nail root. **4.** Eponychium. **5.** Hyponychium. **6.** Bone of phalanx. **7.** Epidermis.

Fig. 25-62. Topography of proximal nail fold. Enlargement of rectangle in Fig. 25-61. Monkey. L.M. X 30. **1.** Stratum corneum of epidermis. **2.** Stratum germinativum of epidermis. **3.** Dermis. **4.** Eponychium. **5.** Epidermal nail fold. **6.** Nail matrix. **7.** Nail plate. **8.** Nail bed.

Fig. 25-63. Survey of claw matrix. Enlargement of area similar to rectangle in Fig. 25-62. Claw. Rat. E.M. X 630. **1.** Stem cells of nail (claw) matrix. Nuclei round. **2.** A continuous proliferation of stem cells make earlier generations of cells and their nuclei flatten out and move in the direction of the *arrow*. **3.** Cells become keratinized at this point. **4.** An increasing number of cells become keratinized and are added gradually to those previously keratinized. **5.** Beginning of nail (claw) plate. **6.** Cells of nail (claw) bed do not contribute to nail plate keratinization. **7.** Epidermal cells of nail (claw) fold give rise to eponychium (soft keratin).

Fig. 25-64. Enlargement of area similar to rectangle (A) in Fig. 25-63. Claw. Rat. E.M. X 5000. **1.** Cells with an increasingly large number of tonofibrils. **2.** Nucleus. **3.** Fully keratinized cells of claw (hard keratin).

Fig. 25-65. Enlargement of area similar to rectangle (B) in Fig. 25-63. Claw. Rat. E.M. X 5000. **1.** Squamous cells filled with tonofibrils just prior to becoming fully keratinized. **2.** Nucleus. **3.** Fully keratinized cells. **4.** Substance between cells remains unstained in this preparation.

References

Bell, M. A comparative study of sebaceous gland ultrastructure in subhuman primates. I. Anat. Rec. *166*: 213–224 (1970).

Bell, M. A comparative study of sebaceous gland ultrastructure in subhuman primates. III. Anat. Rec. *170*: 331–342 (1971).

Breathnach, A. S. The cell of Langerhans. Int. Rev. Cytol. *18*: 1–28 (1965).

Breathnach, A. S. An Atlas of the Ultrastructure of Human Skin. J. & A. Churchill, London, 1971.

Brody, I. An electron microscopic study of the fibrillar density in the normal human stratum corneum. J. Ultrastruct. Res. *30*: 209–217 (1970).

Brody, I. The ultrastructure of the tonofibrils in the keratinization process of normal human epidermis. J. Ultrastruct. Res. *4*: 264–297 (1960).

Brody, I. Variations in the differentiation of the fibrils in the normal human stratum corneum as revealed by electron microscopy. J. Ultrastruct. Res. *30*: 601–614 (1970).

Charles A. and Ingram, J. T. Electron microscope observations of the melanocytes of the human epidermis. J. Biophys. Biochem. Cytol. *6*: 41–44 (1959).

Chapman, R. E. and Gemmell, R. T. Stages in the formation and keratinization of the cortex of the wool fiber. J. Ultrastruct. Res. *36*: 342–354 (1971).

Ellis, R. A. Fine structure of the myoepithelium of the eccrine sweat glands of man. J. Cell Biol. *27*: 551–563 (1965).

Farbman, A. I. Plasma membrane changes during keratinization. Anat. Rec. *156*: 269–282 (1966).

Fukuyama, K., Wier, K. A. and Epstein, W. L. Dense homogeneous deposits of keratohyalin granules in newborn rat epidermis. J. Ultrastruct. Res. *38*: 16–26 (1972).

Hashimoto, K. Demonstration of the intercellular spaces of the human eccrine sweat gland by lanthanum. J. Ultrastruct. Res. *37*: 504–520 (1971).

Hashimoto, K. The ultrastructure of the skin of human embryos. VIII. Melanoblast and intrafollicular melanocyte. J. Anat. *108*: 99–108 (1971).

Hashimoto, K. Ultrastructure of the human toenail. J. Ultrastruct. Res. *36*: 391–410 (1971).

Hibbs, R. G. Electron microscopy of human axillary sebaceous glands. J. Investig. Derm. *38*: 329–336 (1962).

Jessen, H. Two types of keratohyalin granules. J. Ultrastruct. Res. *33*: 95–115 (1970).

Lavker, R. M. and Matoltsy, A. G. Formation of horny cells. The fate of organelles and differentiation products in ruminal epithelium. J. Cell Biol. *44*: 501–512 (1970).

Martinez, I. R. and Peters, A. Membrane-coating granules and membrane modifications in keratinizing epithelia. Am. J. Anat. *130*: 93–120 (1971).

Matoltsy, A. G. Membrane-coating granules of the epidermis. J. Ultrastruct. Res. *15*: 510–515 (1966).

Matoltsy, A. G. Keratinization of the avian epidermis. An ultrastructural study of the newborn chick skin. J. Ultrastruct. Res. *29*: 438–458 (1969).

Matoltsy, A. G. and Matoltsy, M. N. The chemical nature of keratohyalin granules of the epidermis. J. Cell Biol. *47*: 593–603 (1970).

Matoltsy, A. G. and Parakkal, P. F. Membrane-coating granules of keratinizing epithelia. J. Cell Biol. *24*: 297–307 (1965).

Matoltsy, A. G. and Parakkal, P. K. Keratinization. *In* Ultrastructure of Normal and Abnormal Skin. (Ed. A. Zelickson), pp. 76–104. Lea & Febiger, Philadelphia, 1967.

Menton, D. N. and Eisen, A. Z. Structure and organization of mammalian stratum corneum. J. Ultrastruct. Res. *35*: 247–264 (1971).

Millward, G. R. The substructure of α-keratin microfibrils. J. Ultrastruct. Res. *31*: 349–355 (1970).

Montagna, W. The Structure and Function of the Skin, 2nd ed. Academic Press, New York, 1962.

Munger, B. L. The cytology of apocrine sweat glands. 2. Human. Z. Zellforsch. *68*: 837–851 (1965).

Munger, B. L. and Brusilow, S. W. The histophysiology of rat plantar sweat glands. Anat Rec. *169*: 1–22 (1971).

Odland, G. F. A submicroscopic granular component in human epidermis. J. Invest. Derm. *34*: 11–15 (1960).

Odland, G. and Ross, R. Human wound repair. I. Epidermal regeneration. J. Cell Biol. *39*: 135–151 (1968).

Rawles, M. E. Origin of melanophores and their role in development of color pattern in vertebrates. Physiol. Rev. *28*: 383–408 (1948).

Rhodin, J. A. G. and Reith, E. J. Ultrastructure of keratin in oral mucosa, skin, esophagus, claw and hair. *In* Fundamentals of Keratinization, (Eds. E. O. Butcher and R. F. Sognaes), pp. 61–94. AAAS, Publication No. 70, Washington, D.C., 1962.

Robins, E. J. and Breathnach, A. S. Fine structure of the human foetal hair follicle at hair-peg stages of development. J. Anat. *104*: 553–569 (1969).

Robins, E. J. and Breathnach, A. S. Fine structure of bulbar end of human foetal hair follicle at stage of differentiation of inner root sheath. J. Anat. *107*: 131–146 (1970).

Roth, S. I. Hair and nail. *In* Ultrastructure of Normal and Abnormal Skin (Ed. A. Zelickson), pp. 105–131. Lea & Febiger, Philadelphia, 1967.

Roth, S. I. and Jones, W. A. The ultrastructure of epidermal maturation in the skin of the boa constrictor (Constrictor constrictor). J. Ultrastruct. Res. *32*: 69–93 (1970).

Snell, R. S. The fate of epidermal desmosomes in mammalian skin. Z. Zellforsch. *66*: 471–487 (1965).

Terzakis, J. A. The ultrastructure of monkey eccrine sweat glands. Z. Zellforsch. *64*: 493–509 (1964).

Ugel, A. R. Studies on isolated aggregating oligoribonucleoproteins of the epidermis with histochemical and morphological characteristics of keratohyalin. J. Cell Biol. *49*: 405–422 (1971).

Wier, K. A., Fukuyama, K. and Epstein, W. L. Nuclear changes during keratinization of normal human epidermis. J. Ultrastruct. Res. *37*: 138–145 (1971).

Wise, G. E. Origin of amphibian premelanosomes and their relation to microtubules. Anat. Rec. *165*: 185–196 (1969).

Zelickson, A. S. (Ed.). Ultrastructure of normal and abnormal skin. Lea & Febiger, Philadelphia, 1967.

26 Digestive system—mouth

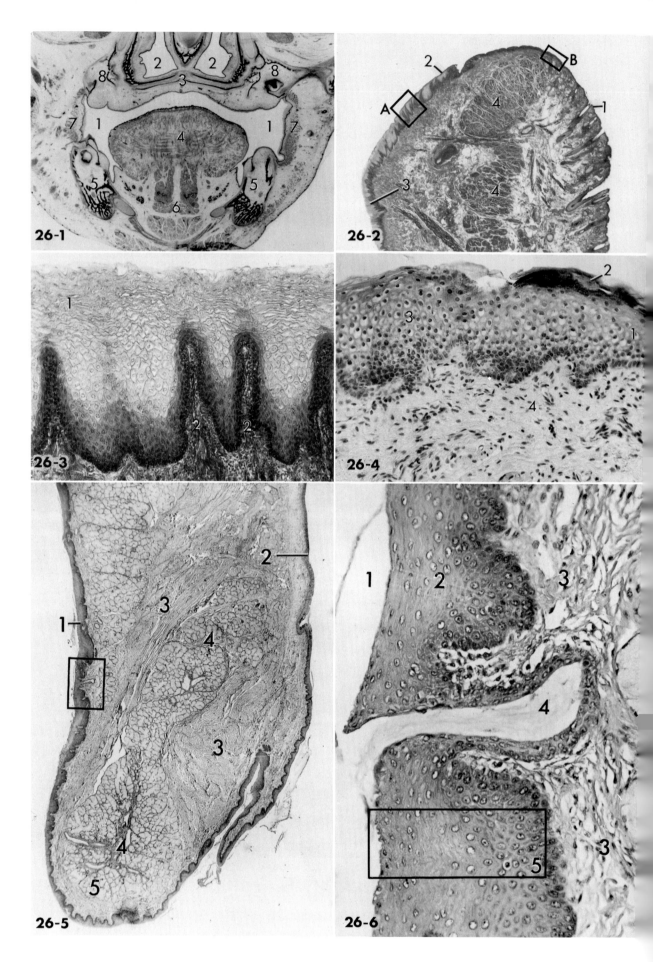

Fig. 26-1. Frontal section through oral cavity. Human fetus. L.M. × 6. **1.** Oral cavity. **2.** Nasal cavity. **3.** Palate. **4.** Tongue. **5.** Mandible. **6.** Floor of mouth with tongue muscles. **7.** Cheeks. **8.** Maxilla.

Fig. 26-2. Vertical section through lower lip. Human. L.M. × 5. **1.** Cutaneous area with hairs. **2.** Red border (vermilion). **3.** Oral surface. **4.** Orbicularis muscle.

Fig. 26-3. Enlargement of area similar to rectangle (A) in Fig. 26-2. Red border of lip. Human. L.M. × 110. **1.** Stratified squamous, non-keratinized epithelium. **2.** Deep connective tissue papillae.

Fig. 26-4. Enlargement of area similar to rectangle (B) in Fig. 26-2. Zone of transition between epidermis and red border. Lip. Human. L.M. × 190. **1.** Epidermis. **2.** Stratum corneum. **3.** Vermilion (red border) lacking stratum corneum. **4.** Connective tissue.

Fig. 26-5. Sagittal section through soft palate. Monkey. L.M. × 23. **1.** Oral surface. **2.** Nasal surface. **3.** Muscles. **4.** Salivary glands. **5.** Uvula.

Fig. 26-6. Enlargement of rectangle in Fig. 26-5. Oral epithelium of soft palate. Monkey. L.M. × 260. **1.** Oral cavity. **2.** Stratified squamous non-keratinized epithelium. **3.** Connective tissue. **4.** Excretory duct of salivary glands. **5.** Rectangle enlarged in Fig. 26-10.

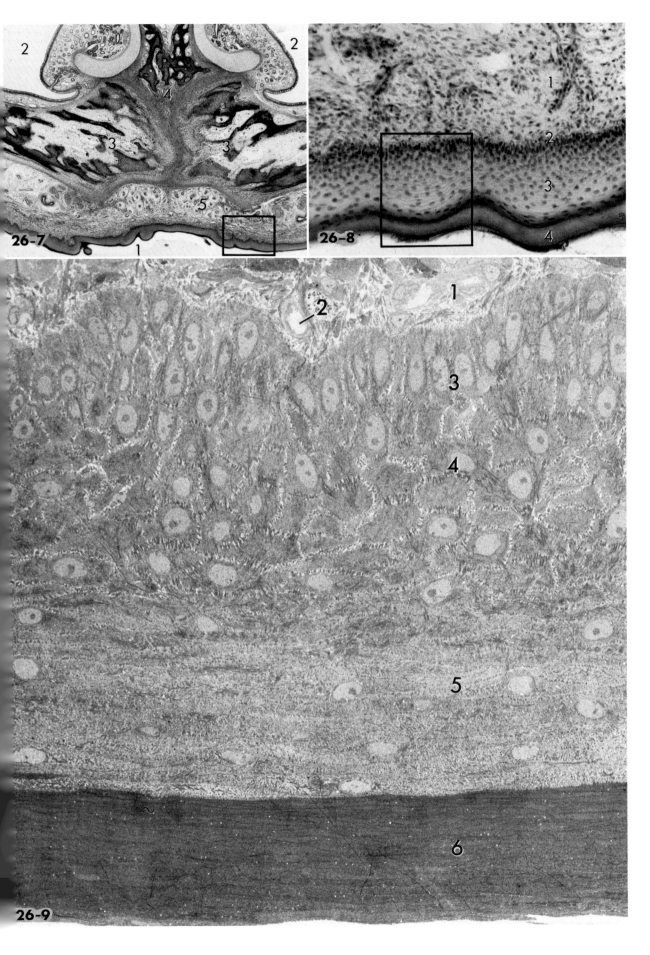

Fig. 26-7. Frontal section of hard palate. Kitten. L.M. X 23. **1.** Oral cavity. **2.** Nasal cavity. **3.** Lateral palatine processes (bone tissue). **4.** Nasal septum. **5.** Dense connective tissue and salivary glands.

Fig. 26-8. Enlargement of area similar to rectangle in Fig. 26-7. Hard palate. Kitten. L.M. X 200. **1.** Dense connective tissue. **2.** Level of basement membrane. **3.** Stratified squamous epithelium of hard palate. **4.** Stratum corneum.

Fig. 26-9. Enlargement of area similar to rectangle in Fig. 26-8. Stratified squamous keratinized epithelium. Hard palate. Cat. E.M. X 820. **1.** Subepithelial dense connective tissue. **2.** Capillary. **3.** Stratum basale. **4.** Stratum spinosum. **5.** This layer corresponds to stratum granulosum in the epidermis. However, keratohyalin granules are not present in this oral keratinized epithelium. **6.** Stratum corneum.

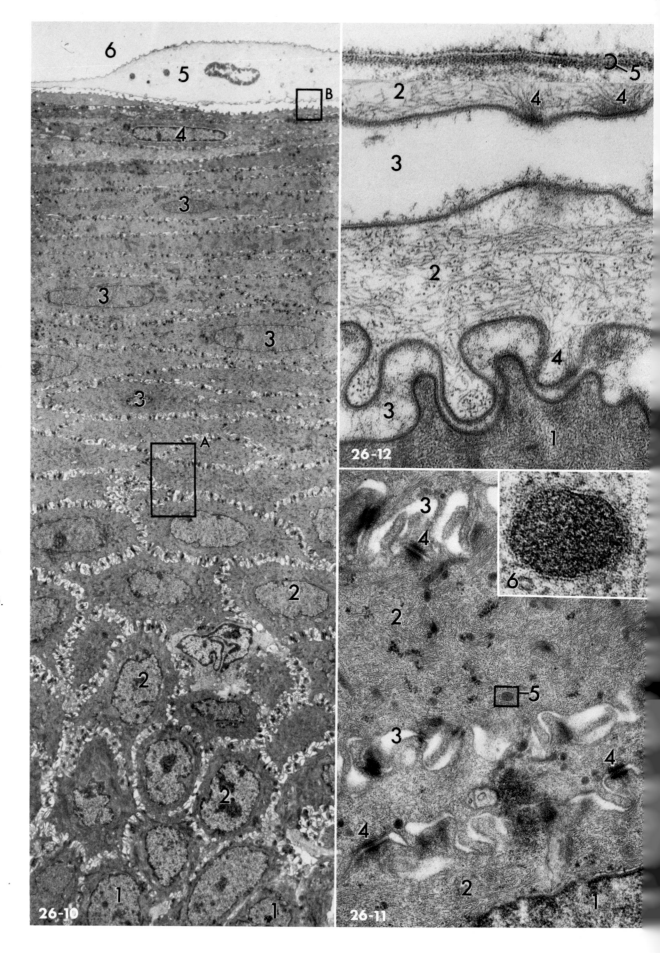

Fig. 26-10. Enlargement of area similar to rectangle (5) in Fig. 26-6. Stratified squamous non-keratinized epithelium. Soft palate. Cat. E.M. X 1800. **1.** Nuclei of basal cells. **2.** Nuclei of cells in stratum spinosum. **3.** Nuclei of cells becoming increasingly elongated as the cells move toward the epithelial surface. The elongated cells correspond to those forming the stratum granulosum in the epidermis. **4.** The more superficial cells become extremely long and flat. **5.** The most superficial cells tend to swell and lose their cytoplasmic density. **6.** Oral cavity.

Fig. 26-11. Enlargement of area similar to rectangle (A) in Fig. 26-10. Soft palate. Cat. E.M. X 31,000. **1.** Nucleus **2.** Cytoplasm with densely packed tonofilaments. **3.** Intercellular space. **4.** Desmosomes. **5.** Rectangle: membrane-coating granule. **6.** Inset: membrane-coating granule. Matrix finely granular. Boundary membrane 30 Å. X 186,000.

Fig. 26-12. Enlargement of area similar to rectangle (B) in Fig. 26-10. Soft palate. Cat. E.M. X 62,000. **1.** Part of cell with densely packed tonofilaments. **2.** Cells with loosely arranged tonofilaments. **3.** Intercellular space. **4.** Remnants of detached desmosomes. **5.** Inset: cell membrane of superficial cell. Of the two laminae forming the cell membrane, the innermost is greatly thickened. X 186,000.

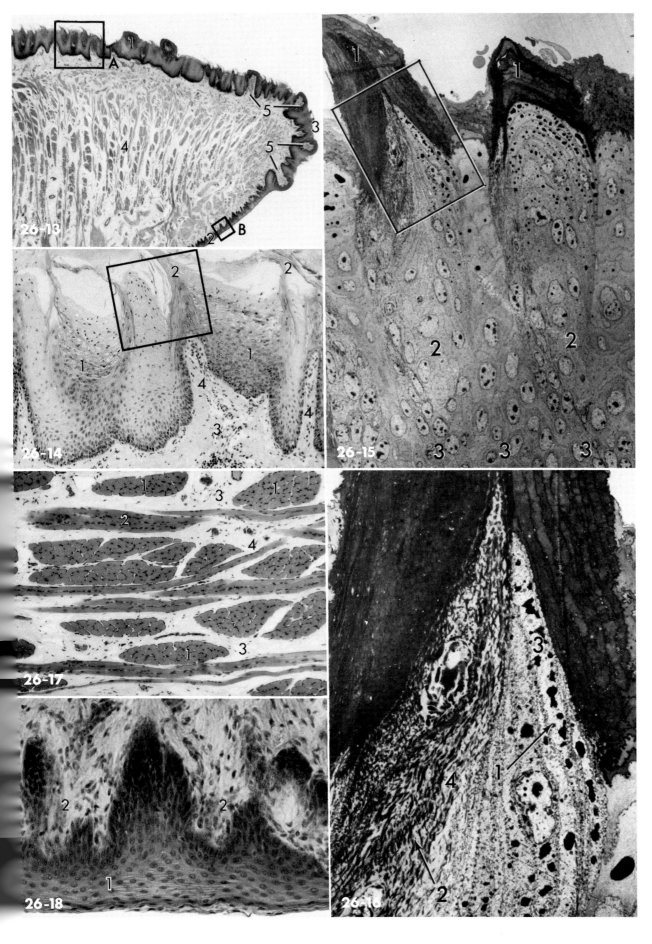

Fig. 26-13. Tongue. Cross section of lateral half. Monkey. L.M. X 13. **1.** Dorsal surface. **2.** Lower surface. **3.** Lateral edge. **4.** Intrinsic muscles. **5.** Fungiform papillae.

Fig. 26-14. Enlargement of area similar to rectangle (A) in Fig. 26-13. Monkey. L.M. X 89. **1.** Stratified squamous non-keratinized epithelium. **2.** Filiform papillae. **3.** Subepithelial connective tissue. **4.** Connective tissue papillae.

Fig. 26-15. Enlargement of area similar to rectangle in Fig. 26-14. Rat. E.M. X 620. **1.** Keratinized tips of filiform papillae. **2.** Cells of stratum intermedium. **3.** Basal cells.

Fig. 26-16. Enlargement of rectangle in Fig. 26-15. E.M. X 1900. **1.** Cells undergoing soft keratinization in the direction of the arrow. **2.** Cells undergoing hard keratinization in the direction of arrow. **3.** Keratohyalin granules. **4.** Bundles of tonofilaments.

Fig. 26-17. Bundles of intrinsic striated muscles of tongue. Monkey. L.M. X 100. **1.** Cross-sectioned bundles. **2.** Longitudinally sectioned bundles. **3.** Connective tissue core of tongue.

Fig. 26-18. Lower surface of tongue. Enlargement of area similar to rectangle (B) in Fig. 26-13. Monkey. L.M. X 430. **1.** Stratified squamous non-keratinized epithelium. **2.** Connective tissue papillae.

Fig. 26-19. Tongue. Dorsal surface. Monkey. L.M. × 43. **1.** Connective tissue core of fungiform papilla. **2.** Solitary taste bud. **3.** Filiform papillae. **4.** Partly keratinized surface epithelium.

Fig. 26-20. Tongue. Monkey. L.M. × 41. **1.** Connective tissue core of circumvallate papilla. **2.** Moat-like furrow. **3.** Numerous taste buds. **4.** Non-keratinized surface epithelium.

Fig. 26-21. Tongue. Monkey. L.M. × 41. **1.** Connective tissue core of foliate papillae. **2.** Clefts. **3.** Numerous taste buds. **4.** Non-keratinized surface epithelium. **5.** Lingual (mixed) salivary glands.

Fig. 26-22. Enlargement of area similar to rectangle in Fig. 26-21. Circumvallate papilla. Rat. E.M. × 660. **1.** Moat-like furrow. **2.** Taste buds. **3.** Superficial squamous cells of non-keratinized epithelium.

Fig. 26-23. Survey of a taste bud. Rat. E.M. × 2700. **1.** Furrow. **2.** Taste pore. **3.** Squamous surface epithelium. **4.** Nucleus of light cell. **5.** Nuclei of dark cells. **6.** Nuclei of basal (lateral) cells. **7.** Nucleus of tongue surface epithelial cell.

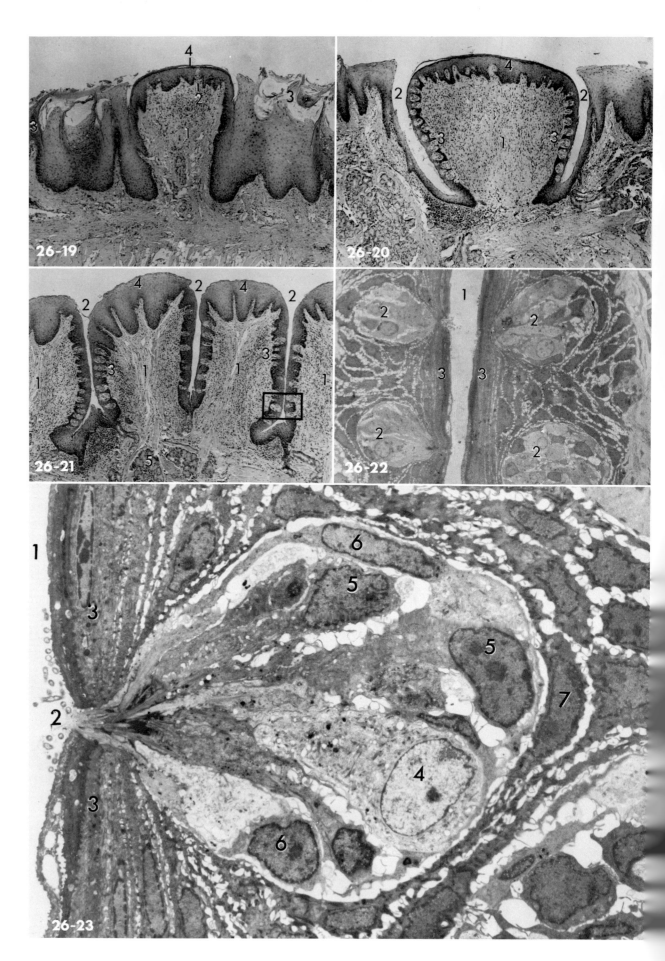

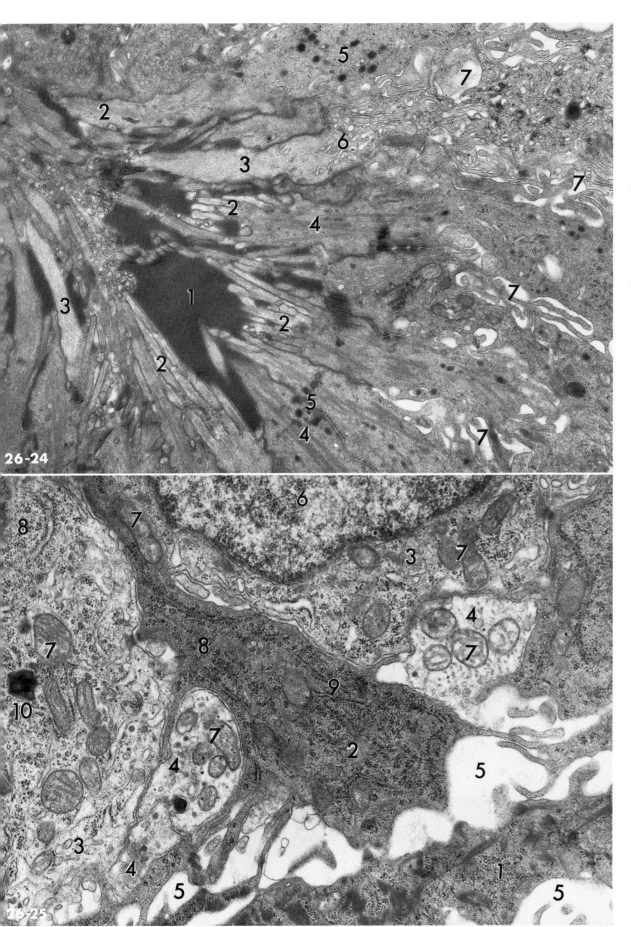

Fig. 26-24. Survey of structures forming the pit of a taste bud. Rat. E.M. X 31,000. **1.** Taste pit with darkly stained mucopolysaccharide substance. **2.** Villi of dark cells. **3.** Villi of light cells. **4.** Intracytoplasmic filaments. **5.** Secretory granules. **6.** Small vesicles. **7.** Intercellular space.

Fig. 26-25. Survey of the basal region of taste bud. Rat. E.M. X 43,000. **1.** Basal (lateral) cell. **2.** Dark cell. **3.** Light cells. **4.** Nerve endings. **5.** Intercellular space. **6.** Nucleus. **7.** Mitochondria. **8.** Ribosomes. **9.** Granular endoplasmic reticulum. **10** Lysosome.

References

ORAL MUCOSA

Farbman, A. I. Electron microscope study of a small cytoplasmic structure in rat oral epithelium. J. Cell Biol. *21*: 491–495 (1964).

Farbman, A. I. Morphological variability of keratohyalin. Anat. Rec. *154*: 275–286 (1966).

Farbman, A. I.: Plasma membrane changes during keratinization. Anat. Rec. *156*: 269–282 (1966).

Farbman, A. I. The dual pattern of keratinization in filiform papillae on rat tongue. J. Anat. *106*: 233–242 (1970).

Frithiof, L. Ultrastructural changes in the plasma membrane in human oral epithelium. J. Ultrastruct. Res. *32*: 1–17 (1970).

Hashimoto, K. Fine structure of horny cells of the vermilion border of the lip compared with skin. Arch. Oral Biol. *16*: 397–410 (1971).

Hashimoto, K., DiBella, R. J. and Shklar, G. Electron microscopic studies of the normal human buccal mucosa. J. Investig. Derm. *47*: 512–525 (1966).

Listgarten, M. A. The ultrastructure of human gingival epithelium. Am. J. Anat. *114*: 49–69 (1964).

Martinez, I. R., Jr. and Peters, A. Membrane-coating granules and membrane modifications in keratinizing epithelia. Am. J. Anat. *130*: 93–120 (1971).

Meyer, J. and Gerson, S. J. A comparison of human palatal and buccal mucosa. Periodontics *2*: 284–291 (1964).

Rhodin, J. A. G. and Reith, E. J. Ultrastructure of keratin in oral mucosa, skin, esophagus, claw and hair. *In* Fundamentals of Keratinization (Eds. E. O. Butcher and R. F. Sognaes), pp. 61–94. AAAS, Publication No. 70, Washington, D.C. 1962.

Scaletta, L. J. and MacCallum, D. K. A fine structural study of divalent cation-mediated epithelial union with connective tissue in human oral mucosa. Am. J. Anat. *133*: 431–454 (1972).

Silverman, S. Jr. Ultrastructure studies of oral mucosa. I. Comparison of normal and hyperkeratotic human buccal epithelium. J. Dent. Res. *46*: 1433–1443 (1967).

Silverman, S. Jr., Barbosa, J. and Kearns, G. Ultrastructural and histochemical localization of glycogen in human normal and hyperkeratotic oral epithelium. Arch. Oral Biol. *16*: 423–434 (1971).

Stern, I. B. Electron microscopic observations of oral epithelium. I. Basal cells and basement membrane. Periodontics *3*: 224–238 (1965).

Weinmann, J. P. The keratinization of the human oral mucosa. J. Dental Res. *19*: 57–71 (1940).

TASTE BUDS

Farbman, A. I. Fine structure of the taste bud. J. Ultrastruct. Res. *12*: 328–350 (1965).

Farbman, A. I. Fine structure of degenerating taste buds after denervation. J. Embryol. Exp. Morph. *22*: 55–68 (1969).

Fujimoto, S. and Murray, R. G. Fine structure of degeneration and regeneration in denervated rabbit vallate taste buds. Anat. Rec. *168*: 393–414 (1970).

Murray, R. G. and Murray, A. Fine structure of taste buds of rabbit foliate papillae. J. Ultrastruct. Res. *19*: 327–353 (1967).

Oakley, B. and Benjamin, R. M. Neural mechanisms of taste. Physiol. Rev. *46*: 173–211 (1966).

Scalzi, H. W. The cytoarchitecture of gustatory receptors from the rabbit foliate papillae. Z. Zellforsch. *80*: 413–435 (1967).

Uga, S. A study on the cytoarchitecture of taste buds of rat circumvallate papillae. Arch. Histol. Japan. *31*: 59–72 (1969).

27 Digestive system—salivary glands and teeth

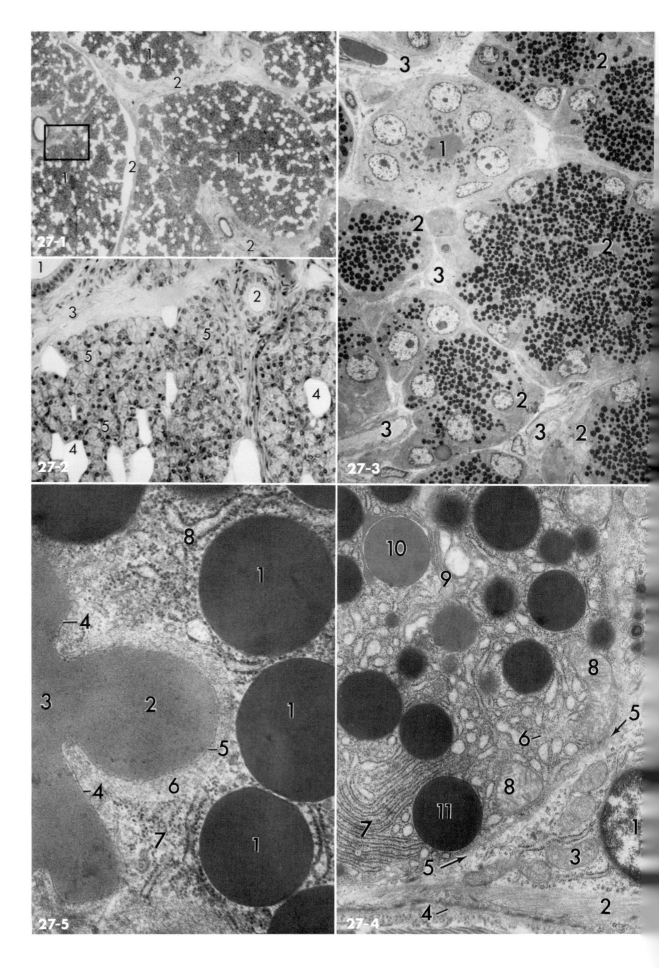

Fig. 27-1. Parotid (serous) gland. Human. L.M. X 28. **1.** Lobules with serous acini and fat cells (empty round spaces). **2.** Septa with ducts.

Fig. 27-2. Enlargement of rectangle in Fig. 27-1. Parotid. Human. L.M. X 200. **1.** Interlobular (excretory) duct. **2.** Intralobular (secretory) duct. **3.** Connective tissue septum. **4.** Fat cells. **5.** Serous acini.

Fig. 27-3. Survey of lingual (serous) gland. Rat. E.M. X 2500. **1.** Intralobular duct. **2.** Serous acini. **3.** Blood capillaries.

Fig. 27-4. Detail of serous acinus. Lingual gland. Rat. E.M. X 30,000. **1.** Nucleus of myoepithelial cell. **2.** Myofilaments. **3.** Mitochondria. **4.** Basal lamina. **5.** Cell borders. **6.** Ribosomes. **7.** Granular endoplasmic reticulum. **8.** Mitochondria. **9.** Golgi complex. **10.** Early secretory granule. **11.** Mature secretory granule.

Fig. 27-5. Detail of apical part of serous cell. Lingual salivary glands. Rat. E.M. X 61,000. **1.** Mature secretory granules approaching the apical cell surface. **2.** Secretory granule at the moment of discharge. **3.** Lumen of acinus with discharged content of secretory granules. **4.** Surface cell membrane. **5.** Boundary membrane of discharging secretory granule. **6.** Submembranous fine filaments. **7.** Ribosomes. **8.** Granular endoplasmic reticulum.

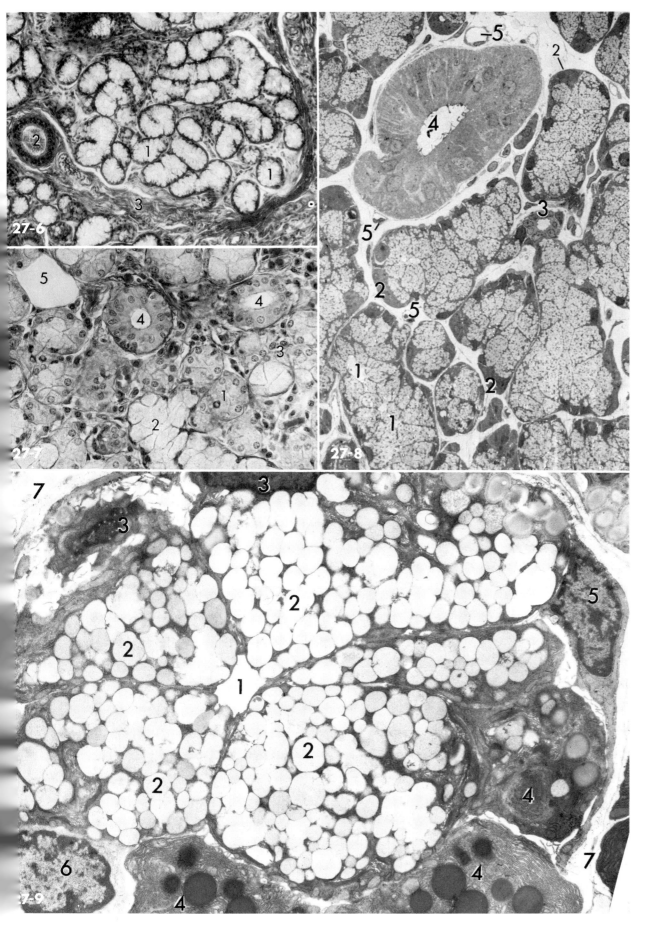

Fig. 27-6. Labial salivary (mucous) gland.
Human. L.M. X 110. **1.** Mucous acini.
2. Excretory duct. **3.** Connective tissue septum.

Fig. 27-7. Submandibular salivary (mixed)
gland. Human. L.M. X 333. **1.** Serous acinus.
2. Mucous acinus. **3.** Serous demilune.
4. Striated ducts. **5.** Fat cell.

Fig. 27-8. Sublingual salivary (mixed) gland.
Rat. E.M. X 580. **1.** Mucous acini. **2.** Serous
demilunes. **3.** Intercalated duct. **4.** Lumen of
striated ducts. **5.** Capillaries.

Fig. 27-9. Detail of a mixed acinus. Sublingual
salivary gland. Rat. E.M. X 4700. **1.** Lumen
of acinus. **2.** Mucous droplets. **3.** Nuclei of
mucous cells. **4.** Cells of serous demilunes with
secretory granules and granular endoplasmic
reticulum. **5.** Nucleus of myoepithelial cell.
6. Nucleus of small lymphocyte. **7.** Periacinar
connective tissue.

Fig. 27-10. Cross section of intercalated duct. Sublingual mixed salivary gland. Rat. E.M. X 4500. **1.** Lumen. **2.** Nuclei of lining cells; cytoplasm devoid of secretory granules. **3.** Myoepithelial cells.

Fig. 27-11. Cross section of striated duct. Sublingual mixed salivary gland. Rat. E.M. X 750. **1.** Lumen. **2.** Nuclei of lining cells. **3.** Blood capillaries.

Fig. 27-12. Detail of striated duct. Sublingual mixed salivary gland. Rat. E.M. X 4800. **1.** Lumen. **2.** Nucleus. **3.** Basal lamina. **4.** Mitochondria. **5.** Aggregation of particulate glycogen.

Fig. 27-13. Detail of transition between a striated duct and an excretory (interlobular) duct. Sublingual mixed salivary gland. Rat. E.M. X 4500. **1.** Lumen. **2.** Nuclei of columnar surface cells. **3.** Basal cell. **4.** Basal lamina. **5.** Interdigitations of surface cells and basal cells.

Fig. 27-14. Enlarged detail of area similar to rectangle (A) in Fig. 27-12. Rat. E.M. X 9300. **1.** Lumen of striated duct. **2.** Dense granules (whether secretory or absorptive is uncertain). **3.** Apical portion of duct cells. **4.** Microvilli.

Fig. 27-15. Enlarged detail of area similar to rectangle (B) in Fig. 27-12. Rat. E.M. X 39,000. **1.** Mitochondria. **2.** Narrow interdigitating cytoplasmic processes. **3.** Basal lamina. **4.** Connective tissue.

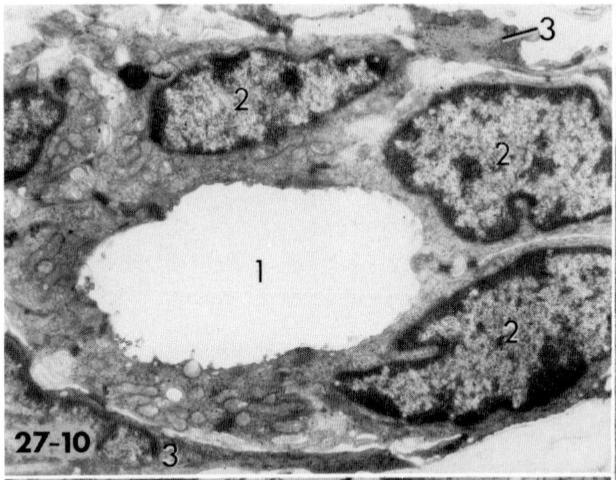

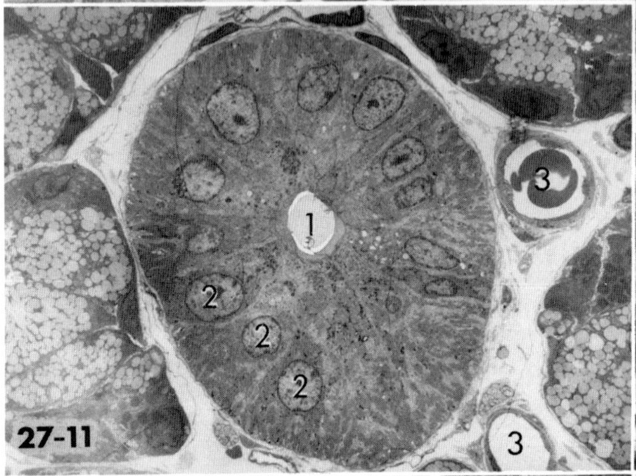

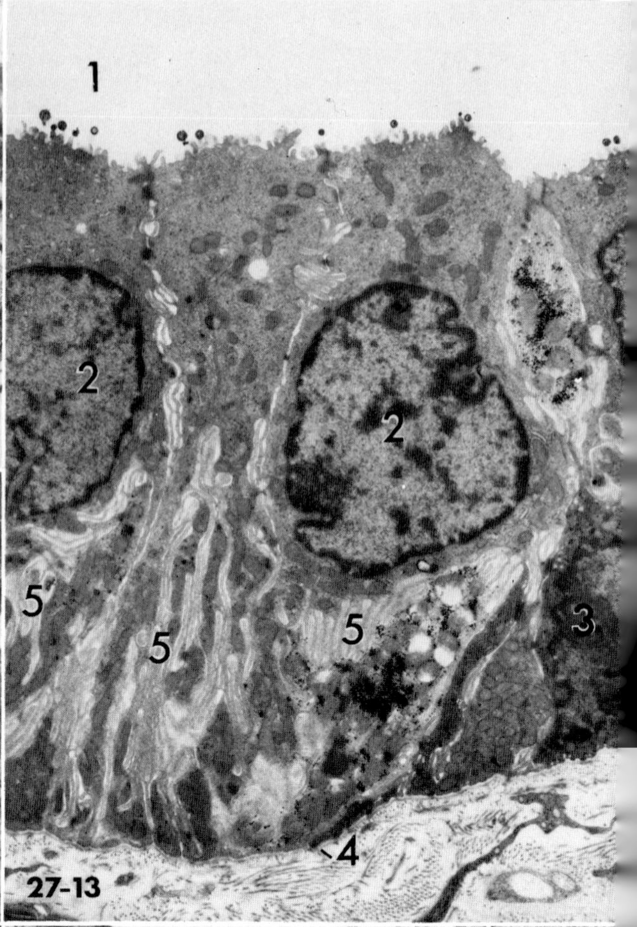

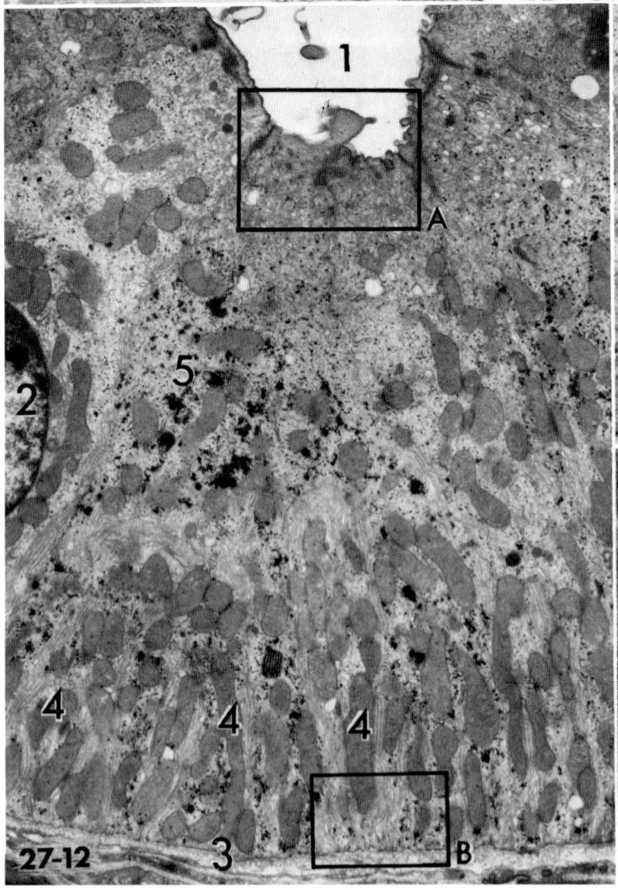

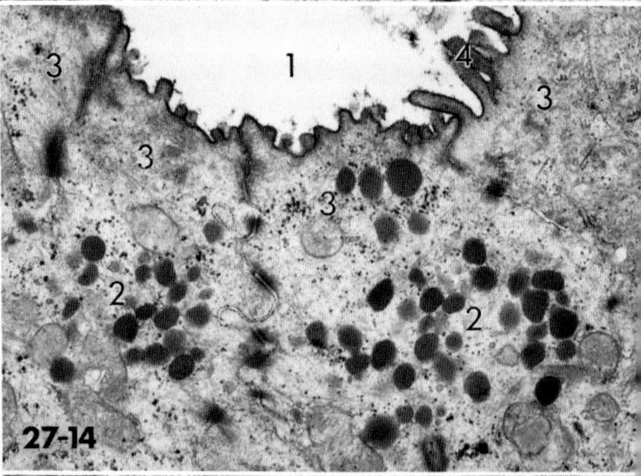

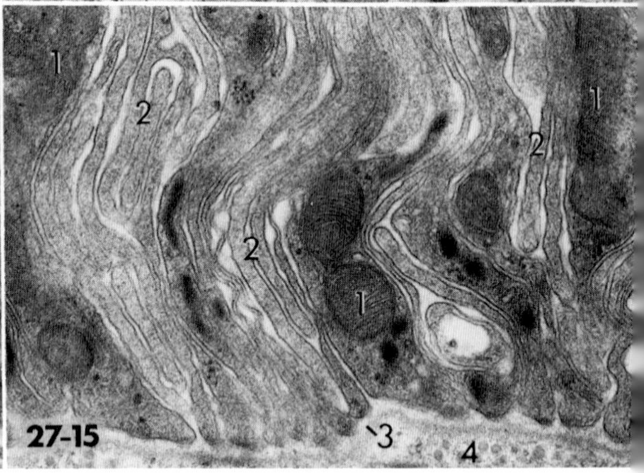

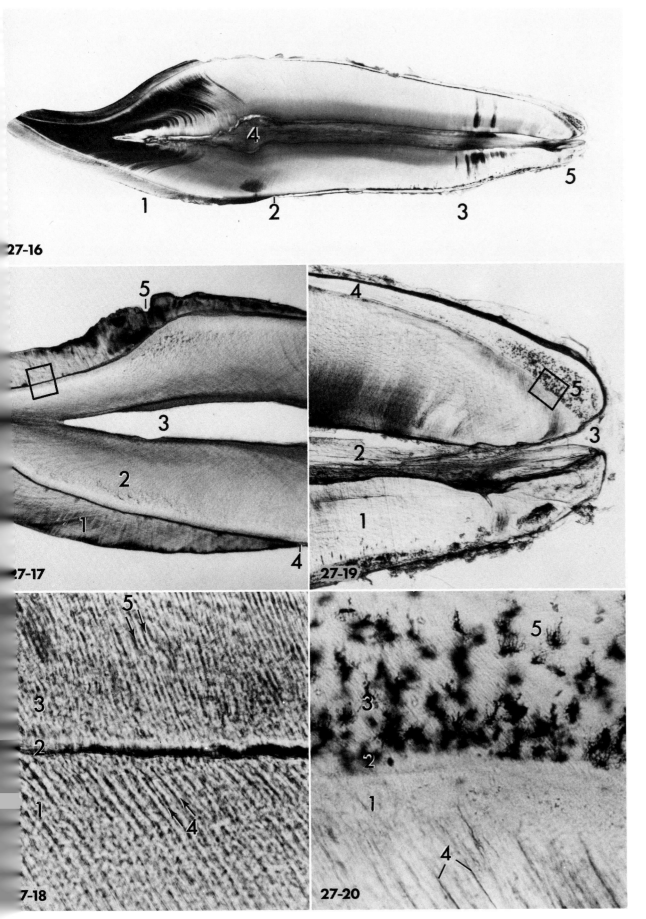

27-16

27-17

27-19

7-18

27-20

Fig. 27-16. Ground, longitudinal section of incisor. Human. L.M. X 6. **1.** Crown. **2.** Neck. **3.** Root. **4.** Pulp cavity. **5.** Apex of root. The lines and areas that appear black contain air-filled channels in this ground specimen.

Fig. 27-17. Detail of crown of incisor. Human. L.M. X 13. **1.** Enamel. **2.** Dentin. **3.** Pulp cavity. **4.** Neck. **5.** Erosion in enamel.

Fig. 27-18. Enlargement of area similar to rectangle in Fig. 27-17. Ground section. Human. L.M. X 300. **1.** Dentin. **2.** Dentino-enamel junction. **3.** Enamel. **4.** Dentinal tubules. **5.** Enamel prisms.

Fig. 27-19. Detail of root in Fig. 27-16. Human. L.M. X 23. **1.** Dentin. **2.** Radical pulp cavity. **3.** Apical foramen. **4.** Acellular cementum. **5.** Cellular cementum.

Fig. 27-20. Enlargement of rectangle in Fig. 27-19. L.M. X 220. **1.** Dentin. **2.** Dentino-enamel junction. **3.** Cementum. **4.** Dentinal tubules. **5.** Air-filled lacunae with canaliculi for cementocytes and their processes.

Fig. 27-21. Bicupsid in alveolar process. Decalcified. Monkey. L.M. X 35. **1.** Dissolved enamel. **2.** Dentin. **3.** Dental pulp. **4.** Bony socket. **5.** Bone marrow. **6.** Periodontal membrane.

Fig. 27-22. Detail of upper rectangle (A) in Fig. 27-21. Monkey. L.M. X 81. **1.** Dentin. **2.** Dissolved enamel. **3.** Epithelial attachment of gingiva. **4.** Free gingiva. **5.** Lamina propria. **6.** Oral cavity. **7.** Cementum.

Fig. 27-23. Enlargement of rectangle (B) in Fig. 27-21. L.M. X 420. **1.** Dental pulp. **2.** Blood vessels. **3.** Odontoblasts. **4.** Dentin. **5.** Odontoblastic processes in dentinal tubules.

Fig. 27-24. Detail of apex of root. Enlargement of area corresponding to rectangle (C) in Fig. 27-21. Monkey. L.M. X 72. **1.** Dentin. **2.** Cementum. **3.** Apical foramina. **4.** Periodontal membrane. **5.** Bony socket. **6.** Blood vessels.

Fig. 27-25. Detail of rectangle (D) in Fig. 27-21. L.M. X 260. **1.** Dentin. **2.** Acellular cementum. **3.** Principal collagenous fibers of periodontal membrane. **4.** Small blood vessel. **5.** Bone.

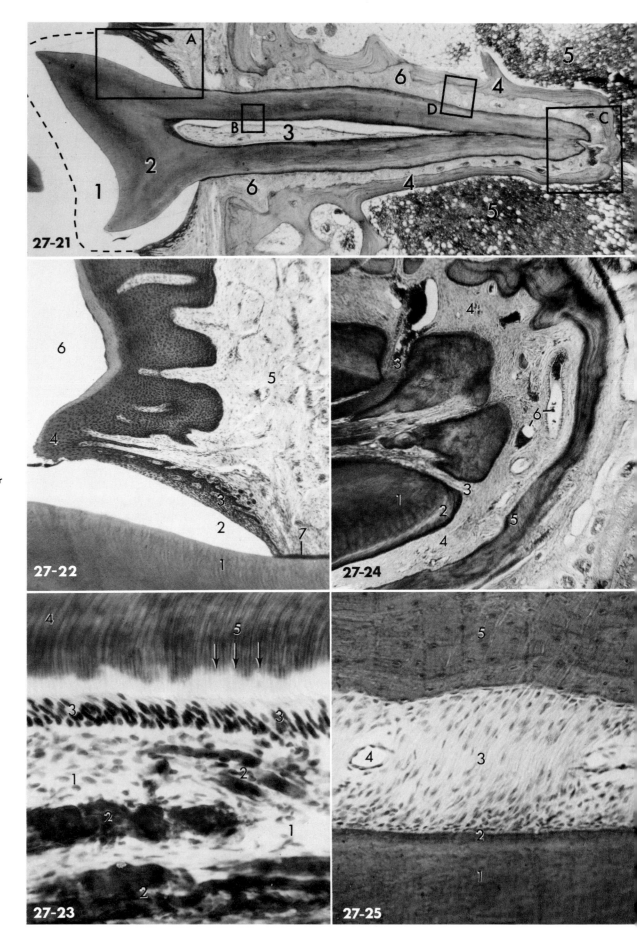

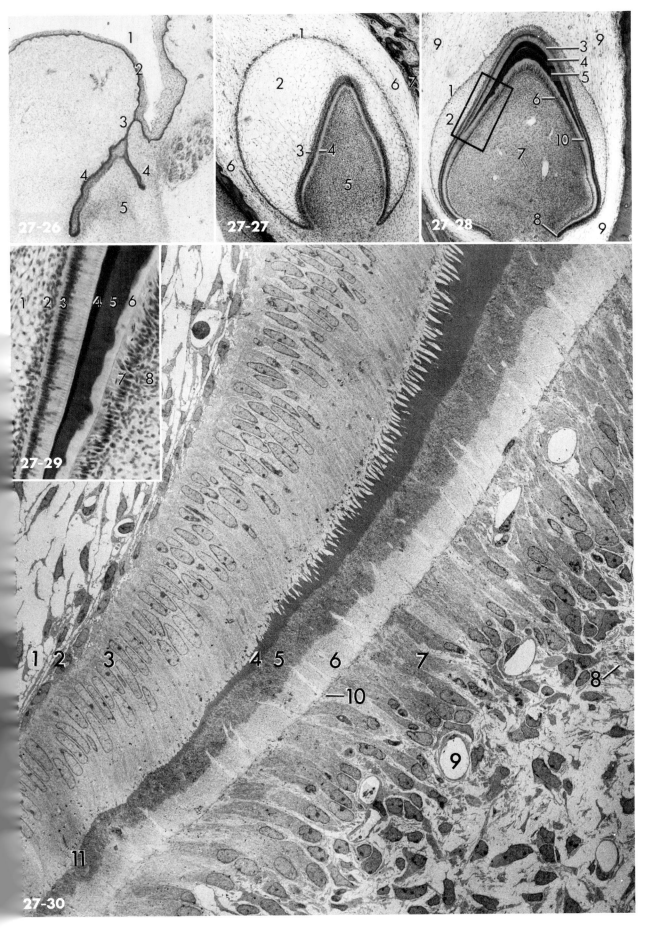

Fig. 27-26. Formation of enamel organ. Cap stage. Human embryo. L.M. X 40. **1.** Oral cavity. **2.** Oral epithelium. **3.** Dentinal lamina. **4.** Enamel organ in cap stage. **5.** Dental papilla.

Fig. 27-27. Formation of tooth germ. Bell stage of enamel organ. Kitten. L.M. X 40. **1.** Outer enamel epithelium. **2.** Stellate reticulum (enamel pulp). **3.** Inner enamel epithelium (ameloblasts). **4.** Odontoblasts. **5.** Dental papilla. **6.** Dental capsule (sac). **7.** Bony socket.

Fig. 27-28. Formation of tooth. Developing crown. Kitten. L.M. X 36. **1.** Outer enamel epithelium. **2.** Stellate reticulum. **3.** Ameloblasts. **4.** Enamel. **5.** Dentin. **6.** Odontoblasts. **7.** Dental papilla (future pulp). **8.** Epithelial root sheath (of Hertwig). **9.** Dental sac (capsule). **10.** Calcification front of dentin.

Fig. 27-29. Enlargement of rectangle in Fig. 27-28. L.M. X 180. Explanation, see Fig. 27-30.

Fig. 27-30. Area similar to Fig. 27-29. Rat molar. E.M. X 700. **1.** Stellate reticulum. **2.** Stratum intermedium. **3.** Ameloblasts. **4.** Enamel. **5.** Dentin. **6.** Predentin. **7.** Odontoblasts. **8.** Dental papilla with fibroblasts. **9.** Capillary. **10.** Attachment zone of odontoblasts. **11.** Calcification front of dentin.

Fig. 27-31. Detail of ameloblasts. Rat molar at the same stage of development as in Fig. 27-30. E.M.X 1800. **1.** Nuclei of ameloblasts. **2.** Distal ends of cells with granular endoplasmic reticulum. **3.** Ameloblastic processes. **4.** Enamel.

Fig. 27-32. Enlargement of an area similar to the rectangle in Fig. 27-31. Rat molar. E.M. X 28,000. **1.** Ameloblastic processes. **2.** Granular endoplasmic reticulum. **3.** Secretory granules. **4.** Discharging secretory granules. **5.** Extracellular space with pre-enamel matrix. **6.** Mineralized enamel prisms.

Fig. 27-33. Detail of odontoblasts from Fig. 27-30. Rat molar. E.M. X 1800. **1.** Nuclei of odontoblasts. **2.** Level of junctional complexes. **3.** Odontoblastic processes (wide part). **4.** Predentin. **5.** Odontoblastic processes (narrow part) in dentinal tubule. **6.** Dentin.

Fig. 27-34. Enlargement of an area similar to rectangle in Fig. 27-33. Rat molar. E.M. X 29,000. **1.** Odontoblastic processes (wide part). **2.** Coated vesicles. **3.** Collagenous fibrils in predentin. **4.** Odontoblastic processes (narrow part) in dentinal tubule. **5.** Mineralized dentin (decalcified specimen).

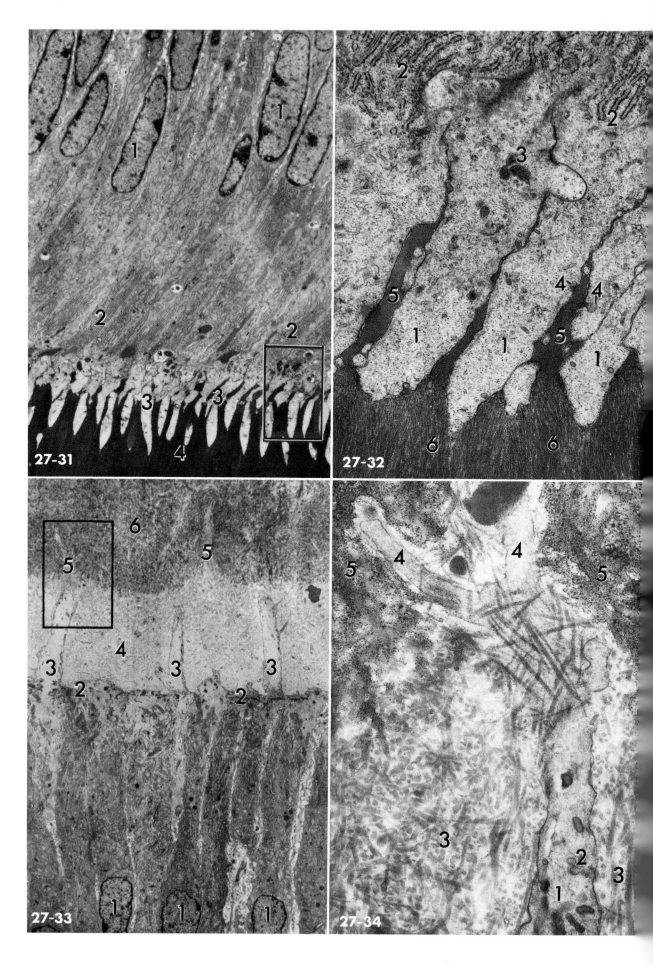

References

SALIVARY GLANDS

Amsterdam, A., Ohad, I. and Schramm, M. Dynamic changes in the ultrastructure of the acinar cells of the rat parotid gland during the secretory cycle. J. Cell Biol. *41*: 753–773 (1969).

Cowley, L. H. and Shackleford, J. M. An ultrastructural study of the submandibular glands of the squirrel monkey, Saimiri sciureus. J. Morph. *132*: 117–136 (1970).

Enomoto, S. and Scott, B. L. Intracellular distribution of mucosubstances in the major sublingual gland of the rat. Anat. Rec. *169*: 71–96 (1971).

Hand, A. R. The fine structure of von Ebner's gland of the rat. J. Cell Biol. *44*: 340–353 (1970).

Hand, A. R. Morphology and cytochemistry of the Golgi apparatus of rat salivary gland acinar cells. Am. J. Anat. *130*: 141–158 (1971).

Heap, P. F. and Bhoola, K. D. Ultrastructure of granules in the submaxillary gland of the guinea-pig. J. Anat. *107*: 115–130 (1970).

Hollmann, K. H. and Verley, J. M. La glande sous-maxillaire de la souris et du rat. Etude au microscope électronique Z. Zellforsch. *68*: 363–388 (1965).

Kagayama, M. The fine structure of the monkey sub-mandibular gland with a special reference to intra-acinar nerve endings. Am. J. Anat. *131*: 185–196 (1971).

Parks, H. F. Morphological study of the extrusion of secretory materials by the parotid glands of mouse and rat. J. Ultrastruct. Res. *6*: 449–465 (1962).

Rutberg, U. Ultrastructure and secretory mechanism of the parotid gland. Acta Odontol. Scand. *19*: Suppl. 30, 1–68 (1961).

Shackleford, J. M. and Wilborn, W. H. Ultrastructural aspects of calf submandibular glands. Am. J. Anat. *127*: 259–280 (1970).

Shackleford, J. M. and Wilborn, W. H. Ultrastructural aspects of cat submandibular glands. J. Morph. *131*: 253–276 (1970).

Tandler, B., Denning, C. R., Mandel, I. D. and Kutscher, A. H. Ultrastructure of human labial salivary glands. I. Acinar secretory cells. J. Morph. *127*: 382–408 (1969).

Tandler, B., Denning, C. R., Mandel, I. D. and Kutscher, A. H. Ultrastructure of human labial salivary glands. III. Myoepithelium and ducts. J. Morph. *130*: 227–246 (1970).

Yohro, T. Nerve terminals and cellular junctions in young and adult mouse submandibular glands. J. Anat. *108*: 409–417 (1971).

TEETH

Elwood, W. K. and Bernstein, M. H. The ultrastructure of the enamel organ related to enamel formation. Am. J. Anat. *122*: 73–94 (1968).

Garant, P. R., Szabo, G. and Nalbandian, J. The fine structure of the mouse odontoblast. Arch. Oral Biol. *13*: 857–876 (1968).

Harris, R. Fine structure of nerve endings in the human dental pulp. Arch. Oral Biol. *13*: 773–778 (1968).

Jande, S. S. and Bélanger, L. F. Fine structural study of rat molar cementum. Anat. Rec. *167*: 439–464 (1970).

Kallenbach, E. Cell architecture in the papillary layer of rat incisor enamel organ at the stage of enamel maturation. Anat. Rec. *157*: 683–698 (1967).

Kallenbach, E. Fine structure of rat incisor enamel organ during late pigmentation and regression stages. J. Ultrastruct. Res. *30*: 38–63 (1970).

Lester, K. S. The unusual nature of root formation in molar teeth of the laboratory rat. J. Ultrastruct. Res. *28*: 481–506 (1969).

Lester, K. S. The incorporation of epithelial cells by cementum. J. Ultrastruct. Res. *27*: 63–68 (1970).

Lester, K. S. On the nature of "fibrils" and tubules in developing enamel of the opossum, Didelphis marsupialis. J. Ultrastruct. Res. *30*: 64–77 (1970).

Levy, B. M. and Bernick, S. Studies on the biology of the periodontium of marmosets: II. Development and organization of the periodontal ligament of deciduous teeth in marmosets (Callithrix jacchus). J. Dental Res. *47*: 27–33 (1968).

Listgarten, M. A. Electron microscopic study of the gingivo-dental junction of man. Am. J. Anat. *119*: 147–178 (1966).

Matthiessen, M. E. and Bülow, F. A. von. The ultrastructure of human fetal odontoblasts. Z. Zellforsch. *105*: 569–578 (1970).

Moe, H. Morphological changes in the infranuclear portion of the enamel-producing cells during their life cycle. J. Anat. *108*: 43–62 (1971).

Reith, E. J. The ultrastructure of ameloblasts from the growing end of rat incisors. Arch. Oral Biol. *2*: 253–262 (1960).

Reith, E. J. The ultrastructure of ameloblasts during matrix formation and the maturation of enamel. J. Biophys. Biochem. Cytol. *9*: 825–840 (1961).

Reith, E. J. The early stage of amelogenesis as observed in molar teeth of young rats. J. Ultrastruct. Res. *17*: 503–526 (1967).

Reith, E. J. Collagen formation in developing molar teeth of rats. J. Ultrastruct. Res. *21*: 383–414 (1968).

Reith, E. J. The stages of amelogenesis as observed in molar teeth of young rats. J. Ultrastruct. Res. *30*: 111–151 (1970).

Reith, E. J. and Cotty, V. F. The absorptive activity of ameloblasts during the maturation of enamel. Anat. Rec. *157*: 577–588 (1967).

Stern, I. B. An electron microscopic study of the cementum, Sharpey's fibers and periodontal ligament in rat incisors. Am. J. Anat. *115*: 377–387 (1964).

Ten Cate, A. R., Melcher, A. H., Pudy, G. and Wagner, D. The non-fibrous nature of the von Korff fibres in developing dentine. A light and electron microscope study. Anat. Rec. *168*: 491–524 (1970).

Warshawsky, H. The fine structure of secretory ameloblasts in rat incisors. Anat. Rec. *161*: 211–230 (1968).

Warshawsky, H. A light and electron microscopic study of the nearly mature enamel of rat incisors. Anat. Rec. *169*: 559–584 (1971).

Watson, M. L. The extracellular nature of enamel in the rat. J. Biophys. Biochem. Cytol. *7*: 489–492 (1960).

Weinstock, A. and Leblond, C. P. Elaboration of the matrix glycoprotein of enamel by the secretory ameloblasts of the rat incisor as revealed by radio-autography after galactose-^{3}H injection. J. Cell Biol. *51*: 26–51 (1971).

28 Digestive system—esophagus and stomach

Fig. 28-1. Cross section of mid-portion of esophagus. Cat. L.M. X 15. **1.** Lumen with heavily folded mucous membrane. **2.** Lamina mucosae. **3.** Stratified squamous epithelium. **4.** Lamina propria. **5.** Muscularis mucosae. **6.** Submucosa. **7.** Muscularis externa: inner circular layer. **8.** Muscularis externa: outer longitudinal layer. **9.** Adventitia.

Fig. 28-2. Esophageal mucous membrane. Enlargement of area similar to rectangle (A) in Fig. 28-1. Cat. L.M. X 200. **1.** Lumen. **2.** Stratified squamous non-keratinized epithelium. **3.** Lamina propria. **4.** Connective tissue papillae.

Fig. 28-3. Esophageal musculature: lamina muscularis externa. Enlargement of area similar to rectangle (B) in Fig. 28-1. Middle third of esophagus. Cat. L.M. X 820. **1.** Nuclei of smooth muscle cells. Cell borders are not seen. **2.** Striated skeletal muscle cell. **3.** Connective tissue.

Fig. 28-4. Stratified squamous non-keratinized epithelium. Enlargement of area similar to rectangle in Fig. 28-2. Esophagus. Cat. E.M. X 1700. **1.** Basal cell nucleus. **2.** Spinous cell nucleus. **3.** Nucleus of cell which has started to become squamous. **4.** Nuclei of squamous cells. **5.** Superficial squamous cells in the process of being sloughed. **6.** Bacteria on the epithelial surface. **7.** Lumen of esophagus.

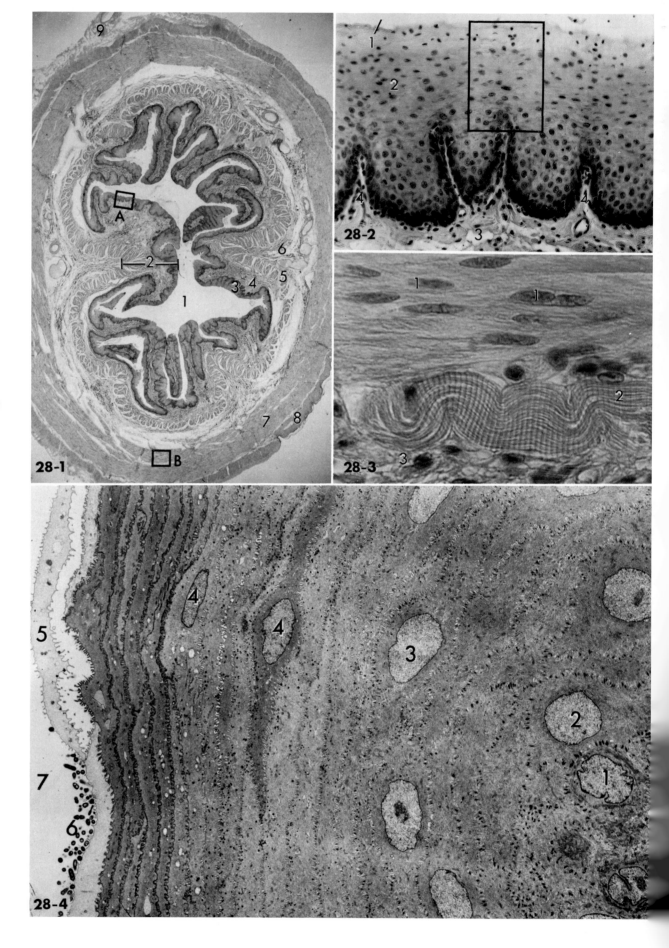

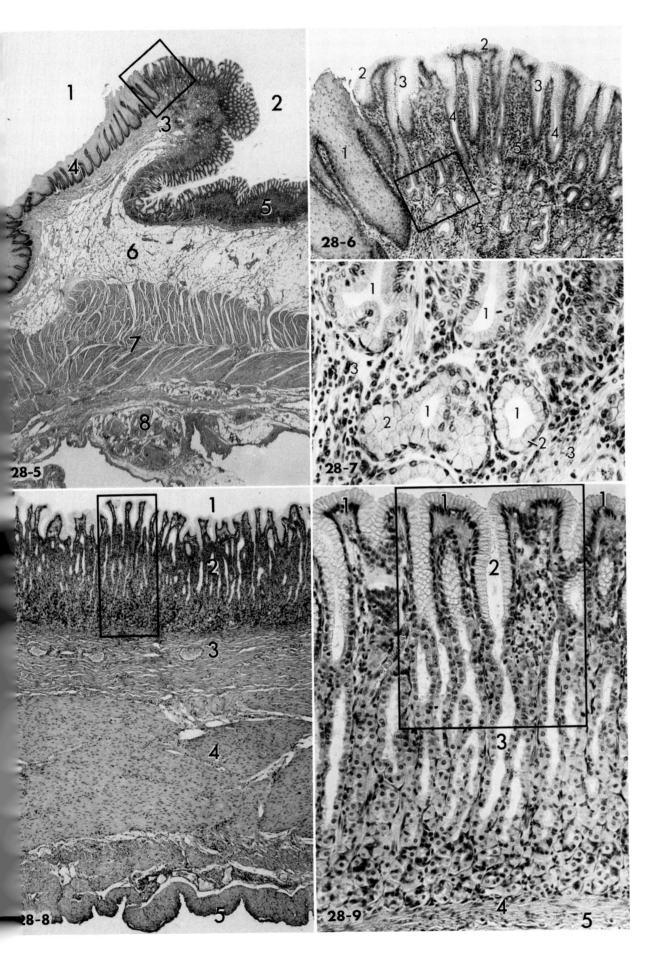

Fig. 28-5. Longitudinal section of cardia. Monkey. Esophagogastric junction. L.M. X 15. **1.** Lumen of esophagus. **2.** Lumen of stomach. **3.** Mucosal flap (fold). **4.** Esophageal epithelium. **5.** Cardiac mucosa. **6.** Submucosa. **7.** Lamina muscularis externa. **8.** Adventitia.

Fig. 28-6. Enlargement of rectangle in Fig. 28-5. L.M. X 74. **1.** Stratified squamous epithelium of esophagus. **2.** Simple columnar surface epithelium of cardia. **3.** Cardiac pits. **4.** Cardiac glands. **5.** Lamina propria.

Fig. 28-7. Enlargement of rectangle in Fig. 28-6. L.M. X 300. **1.** Lumina of cardiac mucous glands. **2.** Mucous cells with flattened nuclei at the base of the cells. **3.** Lamina propria.

Fig. 28-8. Section of entire wall of stomach (body). Monkey. L.M. X 48. **1.** Lumen of stomach. **2.** Lamina mucosae. **3.** Submucosa. **4.** Lamina muscularis externa. **5.** Serosa.

Fig. 28-9. Enlargement of rectangle in Fig. 28-8. L.M. X 210. **1.** Surface epithelium. **2.** Gastric pit. **3.** Gastric gland proper. **4.** Muscularis mucosae. **5.** Submucosa.

309

Fig. 28-10. Gastric mucosa (body of stomach). Enlargement of rectangle in Fig. 28-9. Monkey. L.M. × 363. **1.** Lumen of stomach. **2.** Gastric pit. **3.** Lumina of gastric glands. **4.** Neck of glands. **5.** Surface mucous epithelium. **6.** Lamina propria. **7.** Mucous neck cells.

Fig. 28-11. Enlargement of area similar to rectangle in Fig. 28-10. Body of stomach. Cat. E.M. × 610. **1.** Lumen. **2.** Entrances to gastric pits. **3.** Simple columnar mucous epithelium. **4.** Lamina propria. **5.** Level of basal lamina. **6.** Capillary. **7.** Smooth muscle cells. **8.** Epithelial cells of pits sectioned tangentially.

Fig. 28-12. Surface mucous cell. Enlargement of area similar to rectangle in Fig. 28-11. Stomach. Cat. E.M. × 8900. **1.** Lumen. **2.** Nucleus. **3.** Intercellular space. **4.** Accumulation of highly electron-dense mucous droplets. **5.** Junctional complexes.

Fig. 28-13. Surface of mucous cell. Enlargement of area similar to rectangle in Fig. 28-12. Stomach. Cat. E.M. × 92,000. **1.** Glycocalyx. **2.** Trilaminar cell membrane. **3.** Ground substance of the cytoplasm. **4.** Mucous droplets with dense matrix. **5.** Trilaminar boundary membrane.

Fig. 28-14. Mucous neck cell. Gastric gland proper. E.M. × 92,000. **1.** Mucoid droplets with light matrix. **2.** Trilaminar boundary membrane. **3.** Small vacuoles, probably precursors of mucoid droplets.

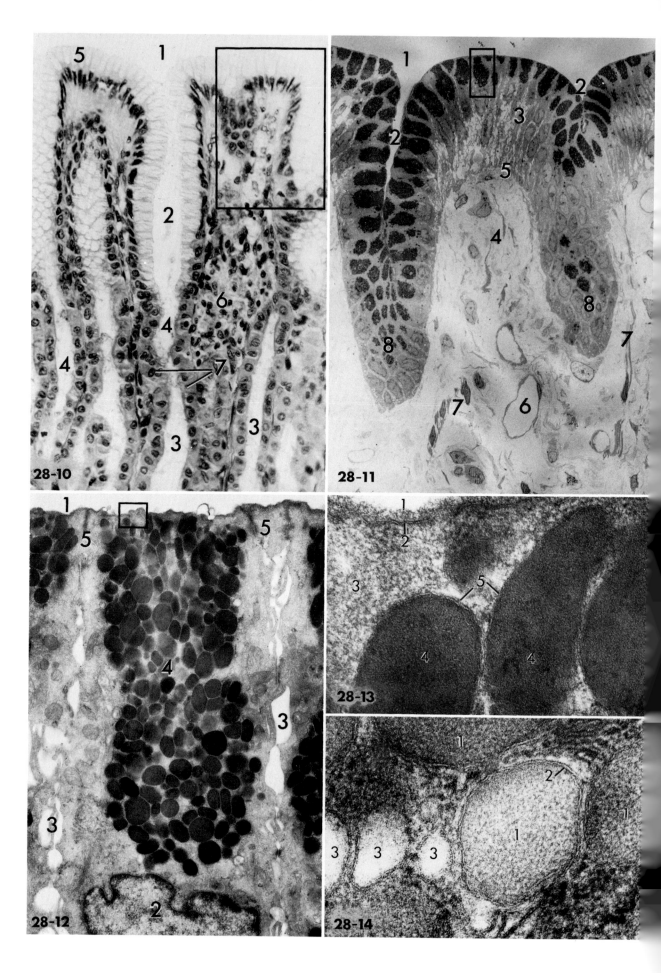

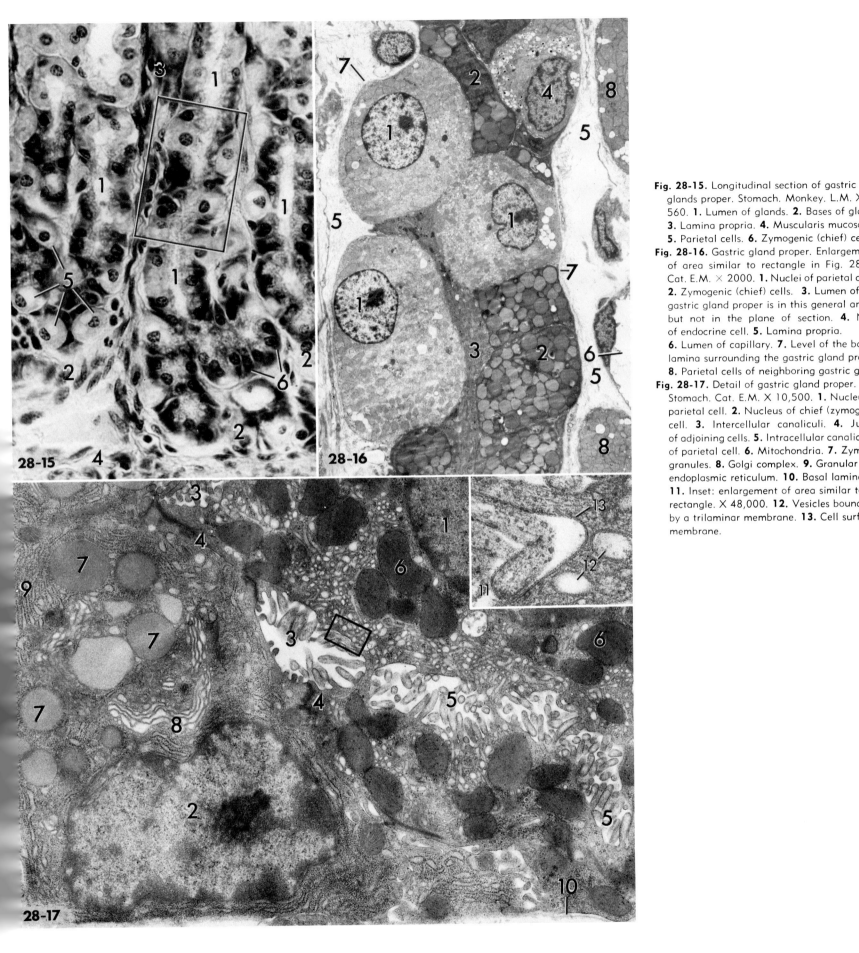

Fig. 28-15. Longitudinal section of gastric glands proper. Stomach. Monkey. L.M. X 560. **1.** Lumen of glands. **2.** Bases of glands. **3.** Lamina propria. **4.** Muscularis mucosae. **5.** Parietal cells. **6.** Zymogenic (chief) cells.

Fig. 28-16. Gastric gland proper. Enlargement of area similar to rectangle in Fig. 28-15. Cat. E.M. X 2000. **1.** Nuclei of parietal cells. **2.** Zymogenic (chief) cells. **3.** Lumen of gastric gland proper is in this general area, but not in the plane of section. **4.** Nucleus of endocrine cell. **5.** Lamina propria. **6.** Lumen of capillary. **7.** Level of the basal lamina surrounding the gastric gland proper. **8.** Parietal cells of neighboring gastric gland.

Fig. 28-17. Detail of gastric gland proper. Stomach. Cat. E.M. X 10,500. **1.** Nucleus of parietal cell. **2.** Nucleus of chief (zymogenic) cell. **3.** Intercellular canaliculi. **4.** Junctions of adjoining cells. **5.** Intracellular canaliculi of parietal cell. **6.** Mitochondria. **7.** Zymogen granules. **8.** Golgi complex. **9.** Granular endoplasmic reticulum. **10.** Basal lamina. **11.** Inset: enlargement of area similar to rectangle. X 48,000. **12.** Vesicles bounded by a trilaminar membrane. **13.** Cell surface membrane.

Fig. 28-18. Section of pyloric mucosa. Stomach. Monkey. L.M. X 127. **1.** Lumen of pyloric channel. **2.** Lumina of pyloric glands. **3.** Lamina propria. **4.** Muscularis mucosae.

Fig. 28-19. Enlargement of area similar to rectangle in Fig. 28-18. Stomach. Cat. E.M. X 580. **1.** Lumen of cross-sectioned pyloric gland. **2.** Lumen of arteriole. **3.** Lamina propria. **4.** Muscularis mucosae. **5.** Capillary.

Fig. 28-20. Cross-sectioned pyloric gland. Stomach. Cat. E.M. X 1800. **1.** Lumen of pyloric gland. **2.** Nuclei of mucous cells. **3.** Nuclei of endocrine cells. The upper endocrine cell borders on the lumen of the gland. **4.** Lamina propria.

Fig. 28-21. Detail of pyloric gland. Stomach. Cat. E.M. X 9200. **1.** Nucleus of mucous cell. **2.** Nucleus of endocrine (argyrophil) cell, probably Type V, synthesizing gastrin or histamine. **3.** Lumen of pyloric gland. **4.** Microvilli. **5.** Basal lamina. **6.** Mitochondria. **7.** Secretory granules. **8.** Mucous droplets. **9.** Golgi zone. **10.** Lipid droplets. **11.** Lysosomes.

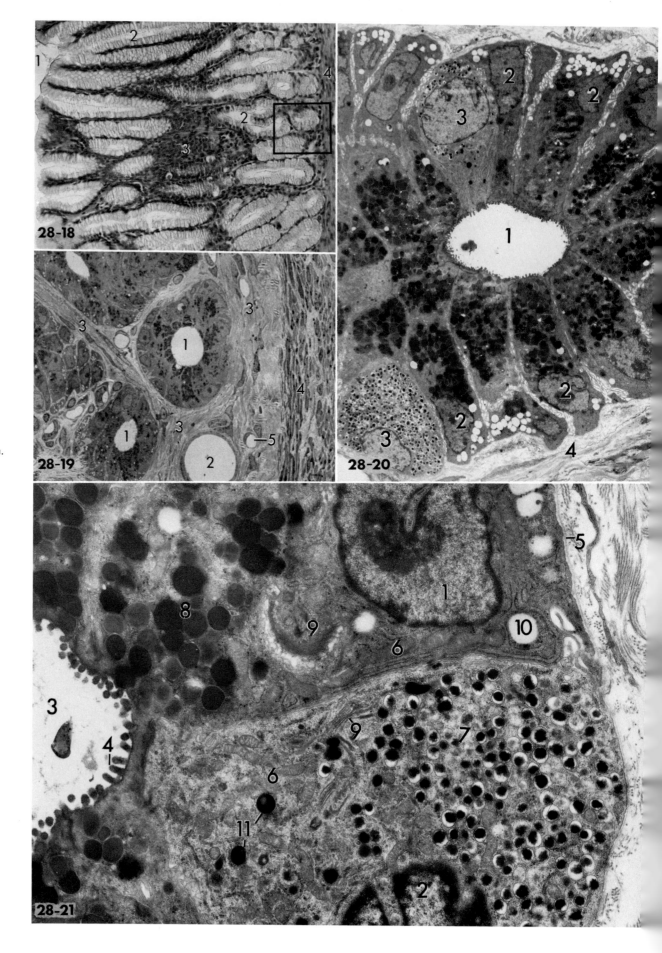

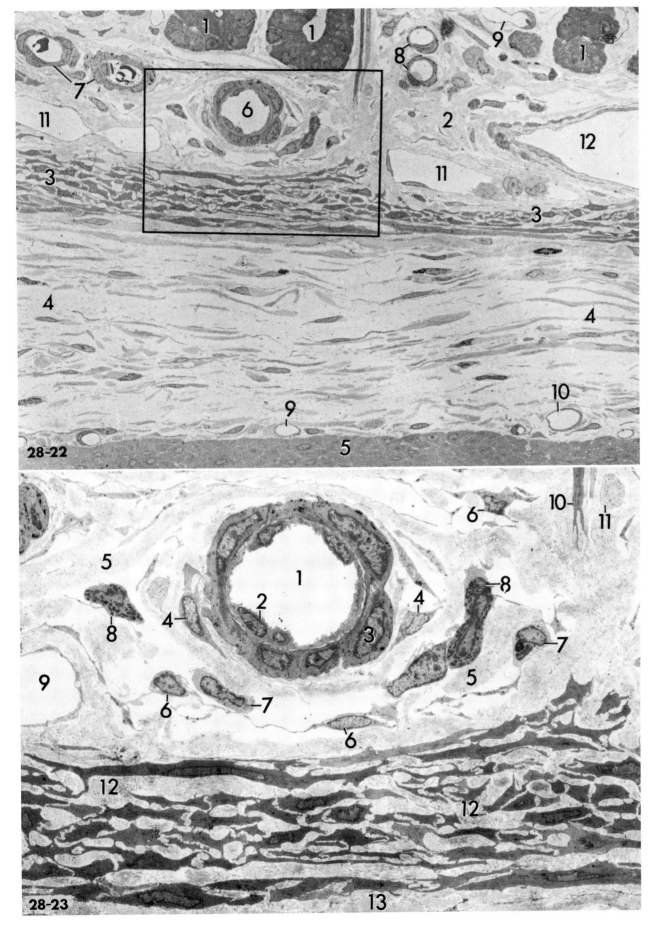

Fig. 28-22. Survey of the middle layers of the wall of the stomach. Cat. E.M. X 680. **1.** Bases of gastric glands proper. **2.** Lamina propria. **3.** Lamina muscularis mucosae. **4.** Submucosa. **5.** Part of lamina muscularis externa. **6.** Arteriole. **7.** Terminal arterioles. **8.** Precapillary sphincters. **9.** Blood capillaries. **10.** Postcapillary venule. **11.** Lymphatic capillary. **12.** Lymphatic vessel.

Fig. 28-23. Topography of lamina muscularis mucosae. Enlargement of rectangle in Fig. 28-22. Stomach. Cat. E.M. X 1600. **1.** Lumen of slightly constricted arteriole; luminal diameter 18 μ. **2.** Endothelial nucleus. **3.** Nucleus of vascular smooth muscle cells. **4.** Nucleus of adventitial fibroblasts. **5.** Bundles of fine collagenous fibrils of lamina propria. **6.** Fibroblasts. **7.** Macrophages. **8.** Eosinophil leukocytes. **9.** Lumen of lymphatic capillary. **10.** Part of smooth muscle cells ascending the lamina propria. **11.** Cross-sectioned non-myelinated nerve. **12.** Lamina muscularis mucosae is composed of a loose skein of delicate smooth muscle cells. The muscle cells contact each other via thin cytoplasmic processes. There is a large amount of collagenous fibrils between the smooth muscle cells of the muscularis mucosae. **13.** Connective tissue of the submucosa.

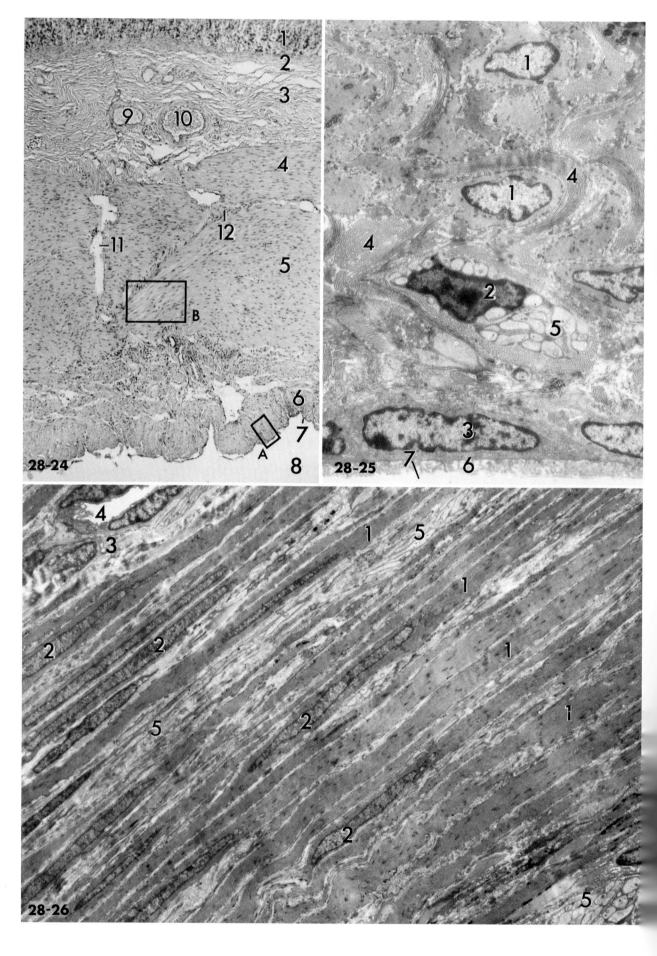

Fig. 28-24. Survey of outer part of wall of stomach. Monkey. L.M. X 60. **1.** Bases of gastric glands proper. **2.** Muscularis mucosae. **3.** Submucosa. **4.** Muscularis externa: inner oblique layer. **5.** Muscularis externa: middle circular layer. **6.** Muscularis externa: outer longitudinal layer. **7.** Visceral peritoneum. **8.** Peritoneal cavity. **9.** Small vein. **10.** Small artery. **11.** Venule. **12.** Thin connective tissue septum.

Fig. 28-25. Enlargement of area similar to rectangle (A) in Fig. 28-24. Stomach. Cat. E.M. X 4700. **1.** Nuclei of smooth muscle cells in outer longitudinal layer of muscularis externa. **2.** Nucleus of Schwann cell. **3.** Nucleus of mesothelial cell. **4.** Bundles of densely packed collagenous fibrils. **5.** Non-myelinated nerves. **6.** Microvilli. **7.** Peritoneal cavity.

Fig. 28-26. Enlargement of area similar to rectangle (B) in Fig. 28-24. Stomach. Cat. E.M. X 1900. **1.** Densely packed smooth muscle cells in middle circular layer of muscularis externa. **2.** Nuclei of smooth muscle cells. **3.** Connective tissue septa. **4.** Lumen of venule. **5.** Non-myelinated nerve fibers.

References

ESOPHAGUS

Goetsch, E. The structure of the mammalian esophagus. Am. J. Anat. *10*: 1–40 (1910).

Johns, B. A. E. Developmental changes in the oesophageal epithelium in man. J. Anat. *86*: 431–442 (1952).

Mottet, N. K. Mucin biosynthesis by chick and human oesophagus during ontogenic metaplasia. J. Anat. *107*: 49–66 (1970).

Parakkal, P. F. An electron microscopic study of esophageal epithelium in the newborn and adult mouse. Am. J. Anat. *121*: 175–196 (1967).

Rhodin, J. A. G. and Reith, E. J. Ultrastructure of keratin in oral mucosa, skin, esophagus, claw and hair. *In*: Fundamentals of Keratinization (Eds. E. O. Butcher and R. F. Sognaes), pp. 61–94. AAAS, Publication No. 70, Washington, D.C., 1962.

STOMACH

Corpron, R. E. The ultrastructure of the gastric mucosa in normal and hypophysectomized rats. Am. J. Anat. *118*: 53–90 (1966).

Forssmann, W. G. and Orci, L. Ultrastructure and secretory cycle of the gastrin-producing cell. Z. Zellforsch. *101*: 419–432 (1969).

Forssmann, W. G., Orci, L., Pictet, R., Renold, A. E. and Rouiller, C. The endocrine cells in the epithelium of the gastrointestinal mucosa of the rat. An electron microscope study. J. Cell Biol. *40*: 692–715 (1969).

Hammond, J. B. and LaDeur, L. Fibrovesicular cells in the fundic glands of the canine stomach: evidence for a new cell type. Anat. Rec. *161*: 393–412 (1968).

Hayward, A. F. The ultrastructure of developing gastric parietal cells in the foetal rabbit. J. Anat. *101*: 69–81 (1967).

Hayward, A. F. The fine structure of gastric epithelial cells in the suckling rabbit with particular reference to the parietal cell. Z. Zellforsch. *78*: 474–483 (1967).

Helander, H. F. Ultrastructure of fundus glands of the mouse gastric mucosa. J. Ultrastruct. Res. *4*: 1–123 Suppl. (1962).

Helander, H. F. Ultrastructure of gastric fundus glands of refed mice. J. Ultrastruct. Res. *10*: 160–175 (1964).

Helander, H. F. Ultrastructure and function of gastric mucoid and zymogen cells in the rat during development. Gastroenterology *56*: 53–70 (1969).

Ito, S. Anatomic structure of the gastric mucosa. *In*: Handbook of Physiology, Alimentary Canal, Secretion (Eds. C. F. Code and W. Heidel). American Physiol. Soc., Washington, D.C. Sect. 6, *2*: 705–741 (1967).

Ito, S. and Winchester, R. J. The fine structure of the gastric mucosa in the bat. J. Cell Biol. *16*: 541–577 (1963).

Jacobson, E. D. The circulation of the stomach. Progress in Gastroenterology *48*: 85–109 (1965).

Johnson, F. R. and McMinn, R. M. H. Microscopic structure of pyloric epithelium of the cat. J. Anat. *107*: 67–86 (1970).

Lillibridge, C. B. The fine structure of normal human gastric mucosa. Gastroenterology *47*: 269–290 (1964).

Pfeiffer, C. J. Surface topology of the stomach in man and the laboratory ferret. J. Ultrastruct. Res. *33*: 252–262 (1970).

Rohrer, G. V., Scott, J. R., Joel, W. and Wolf, S. The fine structure of human gastric parietal cells. Am. J. Dig. Dis. *10*: 13–21 (1965).

Rubin, W. Enzyme cytochemistry of gastric parietal cells at a fine structure level. Cytochemical separation of the endoplasmic reticulum from the "tubulovesicles." J. Cell Biol. *42*: 332–338 (1969).

Rubin, W. Endocrine cells in the normal human stomach. A fine structural study. Gastroenterology *62*: 784–800 (1972).

Rubin, W., Ross, L. L., Sleisenger, M. H. and Jeffries, G. H. The normal human gastric epithelia. A fine structural study. Lab. Investig. *19*: 598–626 (1968).

Sedar, A. W. The fine structure of the oxyntic cell in relation to the functional activity of the stomach. Ann. N.Y. Acad. Sci. *99*: 9–29 (1962).

Sedar, A. W. Stomach and intestinal mucosa. *In*: Electron Microscopic Anatomy (Ed. S. M. Kurtz), pp. 123–148. Academic Press, New York, 1964.

Sedar, A. W. Fine structure of the stimulated oxyntic cell. Fed. Proc. *24*: 1360–1367 (1965).

Sedar, A. W. Electron microscopic demonstration of polysaccharides associated with acid-secreting cells of the stomach after "inert dehydration." J. Ultrastruct. Res. *28*: 112–124 (1969).

Sedar, A. W. and Friedman, M. H. F. Correlation of the fine structure of the gastric parietal cell (dog) with functional activity of the stomach. J. Biophys. Biochem. Cytol. *11*: 349–363 (1961).

29 Digestive system—intestines

Fig. 29-1. Duodenum. Cross section. Cat. L.M.
X 8. 1. Lumen. 2. Mucosa. 3. Brunner's
glands in submucosa. 4. Muscularis externa
(exceptionally thick in cat). 5. Plica circularis,
obliquely cut. 6. Villi intestinales. 7. Pancreas.
8. Pancreatic duct.

Fig. 29-2. Ileum. Cross section. Monkey. L.M.
X 16. 1. Lumen. 2. Mucosa. 3. Submucosa.
4. Muscularis externa. 5. Plicae circulares.
6. Villi intestinales. 7. Aggregated nodules
(Peyer's patch).

Fig. 29-3. Jejunum. Longitudinal section.
Human. L.M. X 18. 1. Lumen. 2. Villi
intestinales. 3. Submucosa. 4. Muscularis
externa (inner circular layer). 5. Muscularis
externa (outer longitudinal layer). 6. Primary
plicae circulares. 7. Secondary fold. 8. Tertiary
fold.

Fig. 29-4. Jejunum. Cross section. Kitten. L.M.
X 81. 1. Lumen. 2. Intestinal villus.
3. Intestinal glands. 4. Lamina propria.
5. Muscularis mucosae. 6. Submucosa.
7. Muscularis externa.

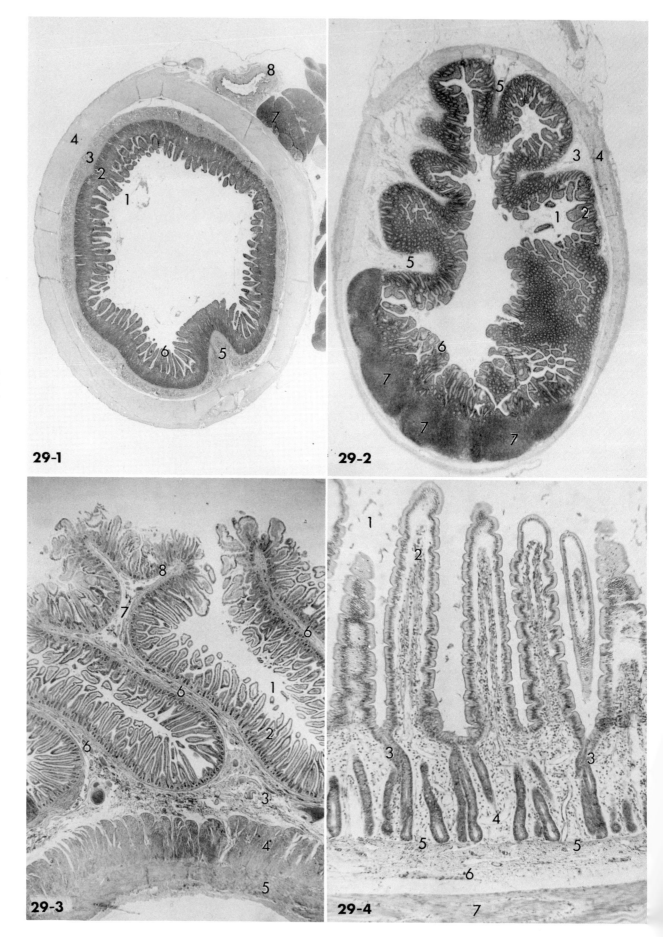

29-1

29-2

29-3

29-4

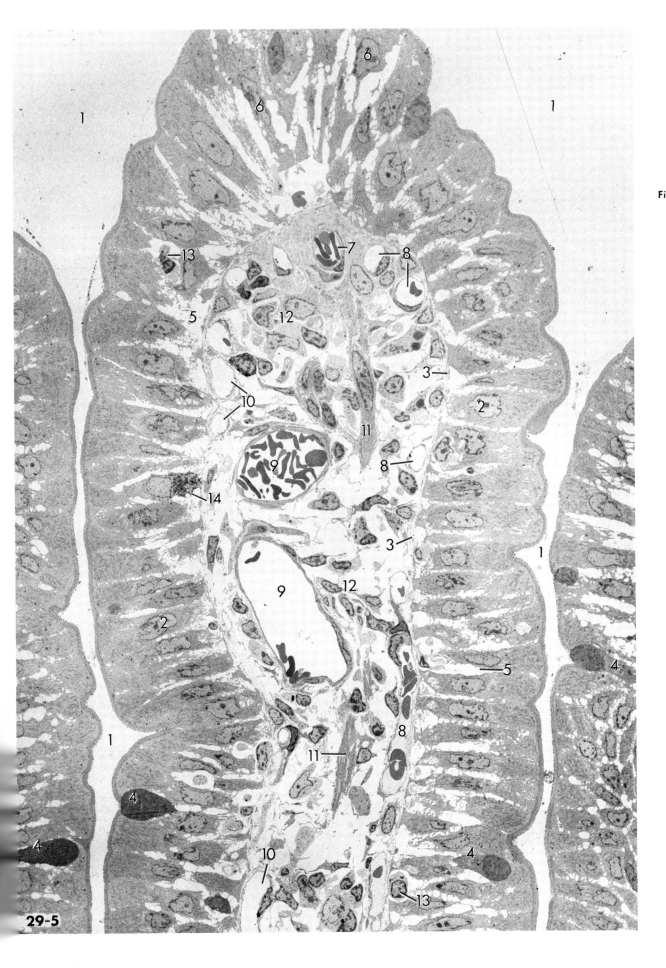

Fig. 29-5. Intestinal villus from duodenum. Tip region. Longitudinal section through the middle of the core. Rat. E.M. X 860. **1.** Intestinal lumen. **2.** Nuclei of absorptive cells in the surface epithelium. **3.** Basal lamina. **4.** Mucous (goblet) cells. **5.** Intercellular space. **6.** Nuclei of absorptive cells, apparently being shed into the intestinal lumen. **7.** Cross section of ateriole. **8.** Blood capillaries. **9.** Postcapillary venules. **10.** Lymphatic capillary (lacteal). **11.** Smooth muscle cells. **12.** The core of the villus (lamina propria) is made up of loose connective tissue with a multitude of assorted cell elements. **13.** Lymphocytes en route through the surface epithelium. **14.** Endocrine cell (argyrophil cell).

29-5

Fig. 29-6. Surface epithelium of intestinal villus. Duodenum. Rat. E.M. X 1830. **1.** Intestinal lumen. **2.** Nuclei of absorptive cells. **3.** Basal part of mucous cell. **4.** Lymphocytes. **5.** Microvilli. **6.** Mitochondria. **7.** Intercellular space. **8.** Blood capillaries in lamina propria. **9.** Lymphatic capillary. **10.** Many cells in the connective tissue cannot be identified at this magnification.

Fig. 29-7. Enlargement of area similar to rectangle in Fig. 29-6. Duodenum. Rat. E.M. X 6000. **1.** Lumen. **2.** Microvilli. **3.** Rootlets in terminal web. **4.** Mitochondria. **5.** Granular endoplasmic reticulum. **6.** Lateral cell borders. **7.** Secondary lysosome.

Fig. 29.8. Detail of basal part of surface epithelium. Duodenum. Rat. E.M. X 4900. **1.** Base of absorptive cell with mitochondria. **2.** Intercellular space. **3.** Lymphocyte. **4.** Basal lamina. **5.** Thin collagenous fibrils. **6.** Blood capillary. **7.** Part of macrophage.

Fig. 29-9. Longitudinally sectioned microvilli of absorptive cells in duodenal intestinal villus. Rat. E.M. X 52,000. **1.** Lumen. **2.** Filaments in core of microvillus. **3.** Rootlets. **4.** Pits.

Fig. 29-10. Cross section of microvilli at level (A) in Fig. 29-9. Rat. X 86,000. **1.** Filaments in core of microvillus. **2.** Surface coat (glycocalyx). **3.** Trilaminar cell membrane.

Fig. 29-11. Cross section of rootlets at level (B) in Fig. 29-9. Rat. X 70,000. **1.** Rootlets. **2.** Pits. **3.** Coated vesicle.

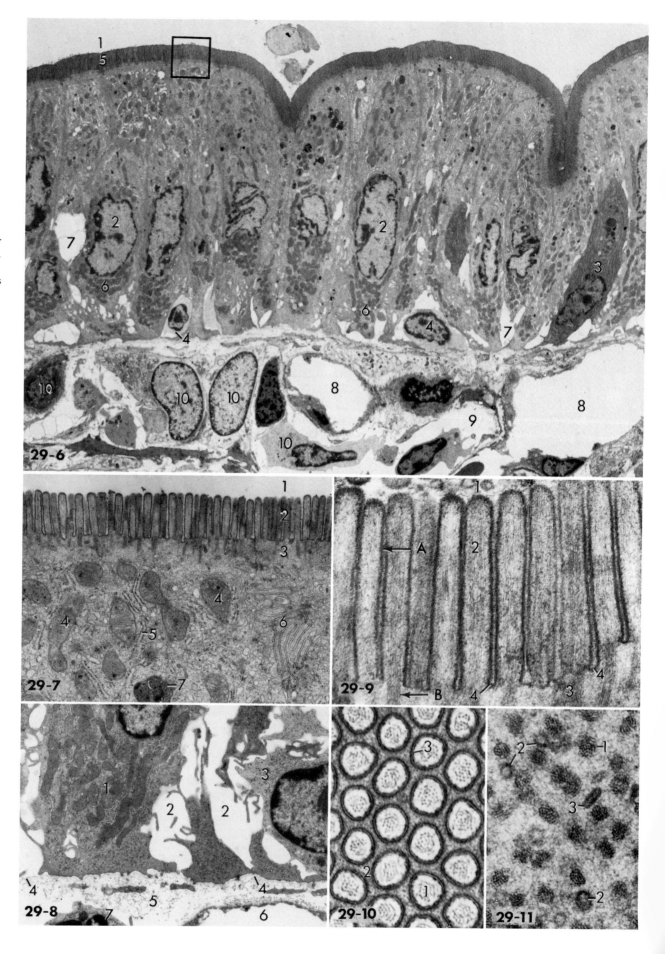

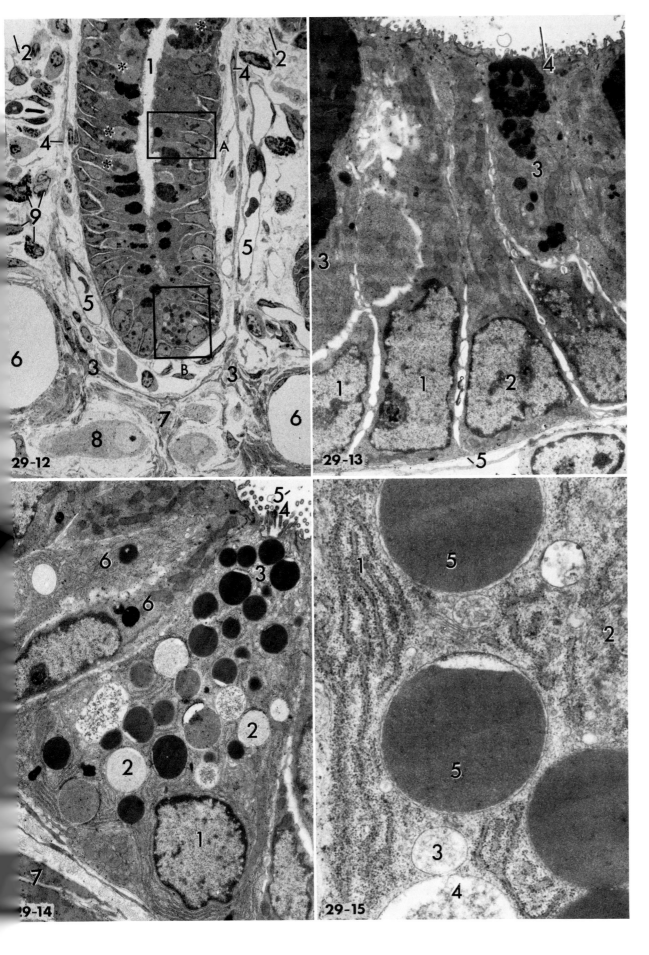

Fig. 29-12. Survey of the deep part of the intestinal wall. Jejunum. Rat. E.M. X 580. **1.** Lumen of intestinal gland. **2.** Lamina propria. **3.** Muscularis mucosae. **4.** Ascending smooth muscle cells. **5.** Blood capillaries. **6.** Lymph vessels. **7.** Submucosa. **8.** Ganglion cell (plexus of Meissner). **9.** Connective tissue cells. **10.** *Asterisks:* mitoses among undifferentiated cells in glandular epithelium.

Fig. 29-13. Enlargement of area similar to rectangle (A) in Fig. 29-12. Rat. X 4800. **1.** Nuclei of undifferentiated cells. **2.** Nucleus of apparent absorptive cell. **3.** Mucous cells. **4.** Lumen. **5.** Basal lamina.

Fig. 29-14. Enlargement of area similar to rectangle (B) in Fig. 29-12. Rat. E.M. X 4800. **1.** Nucleus of Paneth cell. **2.** Presecretory granules. **3.** Mature secretory granules. **4.** Microvilli. **5.** Lumen. **6.** Paneth precursor cells. **7.** Smooth muscle cells of muscularis mucosae.

Fig. 29-15. Detail of Paneth cell. Jejunum. Rat. X 26,000. **1.** Granular endoplasmic reticulum. **2.** Vesicular (small) Golgi complex. **3.** Vacuole. **4.** Presecretory granule. **5.** Maturing secretory granules with distinct boundary membrane and dense core.

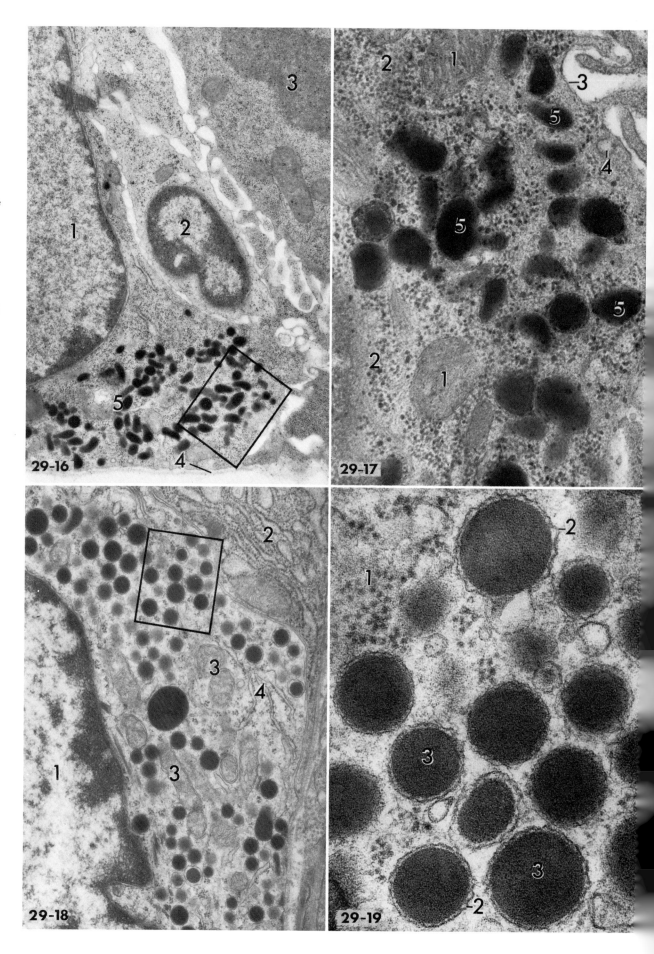

Fig. 29-16. Detail of intestinal crypt. Jejunum. Rat. E.M. X 17,000. **1.** Nucleus of endocrine cell (type I). **2.** Nucleus of undifferentiated cell. **3.** Undifferentiated cell in mitosis. **4.** Basal lamina. **5.** Secretory granules.

Fig. 29-17. Enlargement of area similar to rectangle in Fig. 29-16. Endocrine cell (type I). Jejunum. Rat. E.M. X 48,000. **1.** Mitochondria. **2.** Ribosomes. **3.** Cell membrane. **4.** Pinocytotic invagination. **5.** Oval and irregularly shaped secretory granules with tightly fitted boundary membrane and highly electron-dense core. Based on the appearance of the secretory granules, this cell is referred to as type I, and it is suggested that the secretory granules contain serotonin (5-hydroxytryptamine) or its precursor.

Fig. 29-18. Detail of gastric gland proper. Stomach. Rat. E.M. X 18,000. **1.** Nucleus of endocrine cell (type IV). **2.** Cytoplasm of neighboring chief cell. **3.** Mitochondria. **4.** Granular endoplasmic reticulum.

Fig. 29-19. Enlargement of area similar to rectangle in Fig. 29-18. Endocrine cell (type IV). Stomach. Rat. E.M. X 93,000. **1.** Ribosomes. **2.** Granule boundary membrane. **3.** Core of spherical secretory granule. Based on the appearance of the secretory granules, this cell is referred to as type IV, and it is suggested that the secretory granules contain noradrenaline or its precursor.

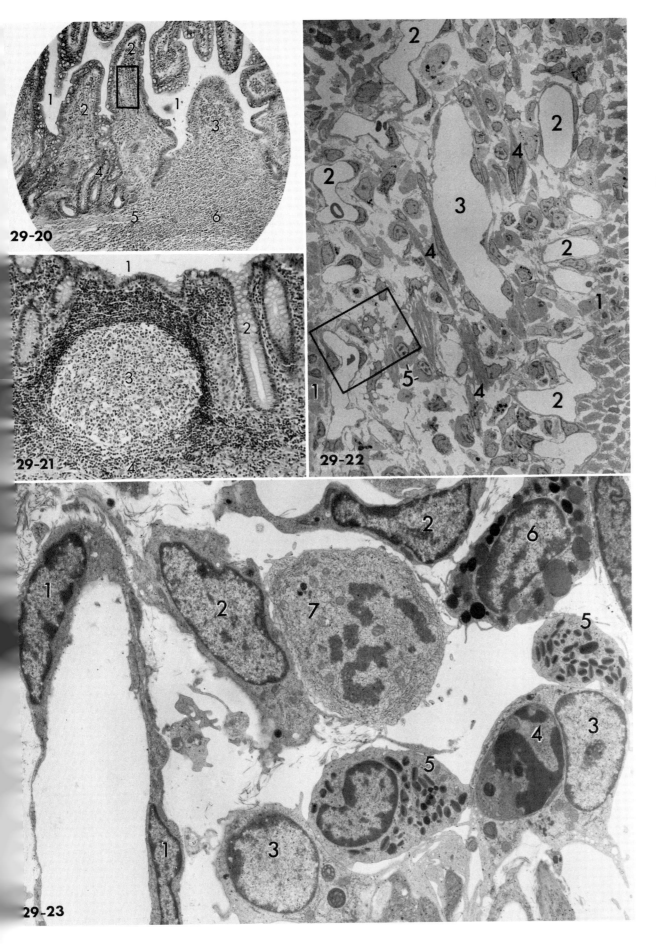

Fig. 29-20. Diffuse lymphocyte aggregation. Jejunum. Cat. L.M. × 60. **1.** Intestinal lumen. **2.** Intestinal villi with normal amount of scattered lymphocytes in the lamina propria. **3.** Villus with diffuse lymphocyte aggregation. **4.** Intestinal glands. **5.** Muscularis mucosae. **6.** Lymphocyte aggregation obliterating intestinal glands and muscularis mucosae.

Fig. 29-21. Solitary lymphatic nodule. Appendix. Human. L.M. × 120. **1.** Lumen. **2.** Intestinal gland. **3.** Germinal center. **4.** Muscularis mucosae is obliterated.

Fig. 29-22. Survey of longitudinal section of intestinal villus. Area similar to rectangle in Fig. 29-20. Jejunum. Rat. E.M. × 640. This demonstrates the general architecture of loose connective tissue in the intestinal lamina propria. Identification of specific cell types is difficult at this magnification but is greatly aided by the use of a hand lens. **1.** Surface epithelium. **2.** Loops of blood capillaries. **3.** Central lacteal. **4.** Smooth muscle cells. **5.** Plasma cells.

Fig. 29-23. Enlargement of area similar to rectangle in Fig. 29-22. Core of intestinal villus. Jejunum. Rat. E.M. × 4700. **1.** Nuclei of capillary endothelial cells. **2.** Nuclei of fibroblasts. **3.** Nuclei of macrophages. **4.** Phagocytosed lymphocyte. **5.** Eosinophil leukocytes. **6.** Mast cell nucleus. **7.** Dividing lymphocyte.

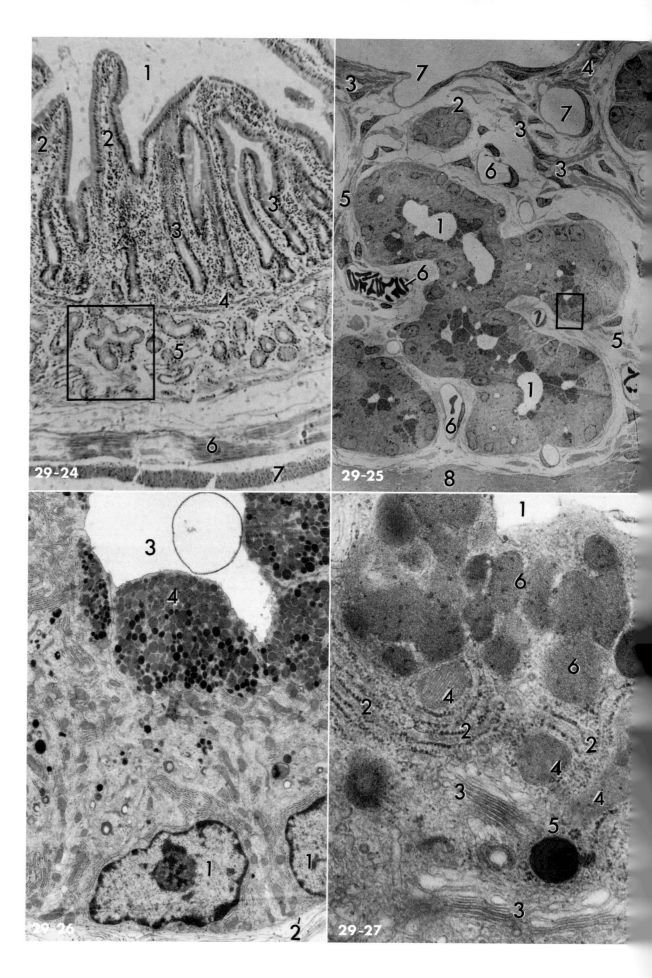

Fig. 29-24. Duodenum. Cross section. Monkey. L.M. × 94. **1.** Intestinal lumen. **2.** Intestinal villi. **3.** Intestinal glands. **4.** Muscularis mucosae. **5.** Submucosa with duodenal (Brunner's) glands. **6.** Muscularis externa (inner circular layer). **7.** Muscularis externa (outer longitudinal layer).

Fig. 29-25. Enlargement of area similar to rectangle in Fig. 29-24. Duodenum. Rat. E.M. × 600. **1.** Lumen of duodenal (Brunner's) gland. **2.** Cross-sectioned excretory duct of Brunner's gland. **3.** Thin strands of muscularis mucosae. **4.** Lamina propria. **5.** Connective tissue of submucosa. **6.** Blood capillaries. **7.** Lymphatic capillaries. **8.** Muscularis externa.

Fig. 29-26. Enlargement of area similar to rectangle in Fig. 29-25. Duodenum. Rat. E.M. × 5000. **1.** Nuclei of secretory cells of Brunner's gland. **2.** Basal lamina. **3.** Lumen of gland. **4.** Apical accumulation of secretory droplets.

Fig. 29-27. Enlargement of secretory cells of Brunner's gland. Duodenum. Rat. E.M. × 40,000. **1.** Lumen of gland. **2.** Granular endoplasmic reticulum and free ribosomes. **3.** Golgi complexes. **4.** Mitochondria. **5.** Lysosome. **6.** Secretory droplets (their boundary membrane is poorly defined).

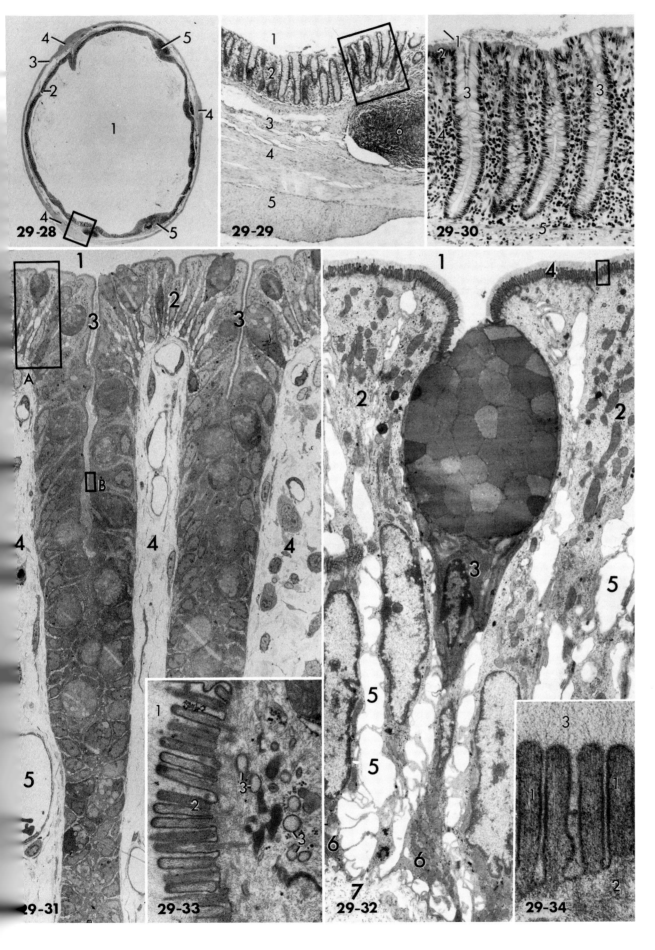

Fig. 29-28. Cross section of colon. Cat. L.M. X 3. **1.** Lumen. **2.** Mucous membrane. **3.** Muscularis externa. **4.** Teniae coli. **5.** Solitary lymphatic nodules.

Fig. 29-29. Enlargement of area similar to rectangle in Fig. 29-28. Colon. Cat. L.M. X 36. **1.** Lumen. **2.** Mucous membrane. **3.** Submucosa. **4.** Muscularis externa, circular layer. **5.** Muscularis externa: one band (tenia coli) of longitudinal fibers. **6.** Solitary lymphatic nodule.

Fig. 29-30. Enlargement of area similar to rectangle in Fig. 29-29. Colon. Monkey. L.M. X 148. **1.** Lumen. **2.** Surface epithelium. **3.** Intestinal glands (crypts of Lieberkühn). **4.** Lamina propria. **5.** Muscularis mucosae.

Fig. 29-31. Survey of two intestinal glands. Colon. Rat. E.M. X 660. **1.** Lumen. **2.** Surface epithelium. **3.** Entrance to lumen of intestinal gland. **4.** Lamina propria. **5.** Venule.

Fig. 29-32. Enlargement of area similar to rectangle (A) in Fig. 29-31. Colon. Rat. E.M. X 4900. **1.** Lumen. **2.** Columnar absorptive cells. **3.** Mucous (goblet) cell. **4.** Microvilli. **5.** Intercellular space. **6.** Base of absorptive cells. **7.** Basal lamina.

Fig. 29-33. Enlargement of area similar to rectangle (B) in Fig. 29-31. Apical part of columnar cell in intestinal gland. Colon. Rat. E.M. X 28,000. **1.** Lumen. **2.** Microvilli. **3.** Secretory granules.

Fig. 29-34. Enlargement of rectangle in Fig. 29-32. Colon. Rat. E.M. X 74,000. **1.** Microvilli with central core of filaments. **2.** Rootlets. **3.** Surface coat (glycocalyx).

Fig. 29-35. Cross section of appendix. Human. L.M. X 9. **1.** Lumen. **2.** Lamina mucosae. **3.** Submucosa. **4.** Muscularis externa. **5.** Serosa. **6.** Mesoappendix.

Fig. 29-36. Cross section of appendix. Human. L.M. X 35. **1.** Lumen. **2.** Intestinal glands. **3.** Lymphatic nodule. **4.** Submucosa.

Fig. 29-37. Longitudinal section of rectum and anal canal. Monkey. L.M. X 7. **1.** Lumen of rectum proper. **2.** Anal canal. **3.** Anus (cutaneous zone of anal canal). **4.** Plicae transversales. **5.** Lymphatic nodules in submucosa. **6.** Muscularis externa. **7.** Inner anal sphincter (smooth muscle). **8.** Outer anal sphincter (striated muscle).

Fig. 29-38. Enlargement of part of Fig. 29-37. Monkey. L.M. × 23. **1.** Mucosa. **2.** Lymphatic follicles. **3.** These folds correspond to the anal valves in human. **4.** Intermediate zone of anal canal. **5.** Cutaneous zone of anal canal. **6.** Inner sphincter muscle. **7.** Outer sphincter muscle.

Fig. 29-39. Rectal lamina mucosae. Enlargement of area similar to rectangle. (A) in Fig. 29-38. Monkey. L.M. X 148. **1.** Lumen. **2.** Columnar surface epithelium. **3.** Intestinal gland. **4.** Lamina propria. **5.** Muscularis mucosae.

Fig. 29-40. Enlargement of rectangle (B) in Fig. 29-38. L.M. × 40. **1.** Lumen. **2.** Columnar surface epithelium. **3.** Stratified cuboidal epithelium. **4.** Subepithelial connective tissue.

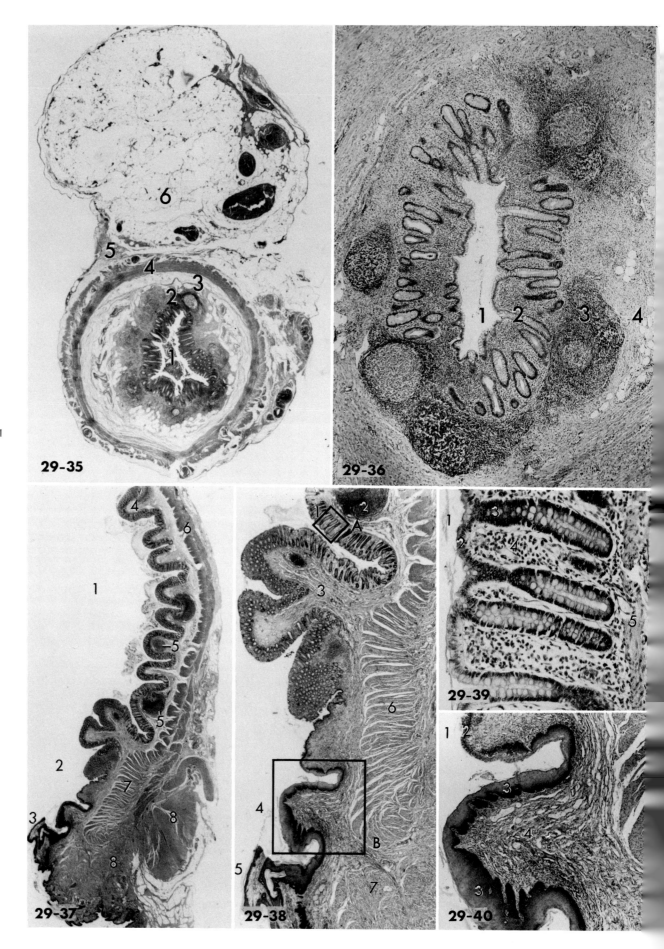

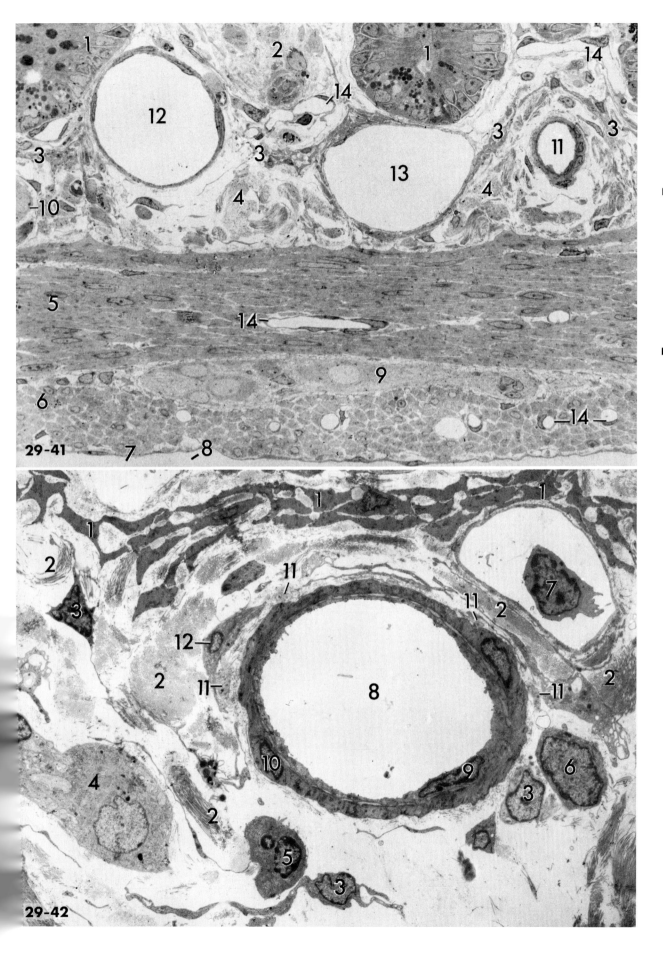

Fig. 29-41. Survey of peripheral segment of intestinal wall. Cross section. Jejunum. Rat. E.M. X 600. **1.** Base of intestinal glands. **2.** Lamina propria. **3.** Muscularis mucosae. **4.** Submucosa. **5.** Muscularis externa: inner circular layer. **6.** Muscularis externa: outer longitudinal layer. **7.** Serosa with mesothelium. **8.** Peritoneal cavity. **9.** Ganglion cells of myenteric (Auerbach's) nerve plexus. **10.** Ganglion cell of submucous (Meissner's) nerve plexus. **11.** Arteriole. **12.** Venule. **13.** Lymphatic vessel. **14.** Blood capillaries.

Fig. 29-42. Detail of submucosa. Jejunum. Rat. E.M. X 1800. **1.** Chain of cross-sectioned smooth muscle cells in the muscularis mucosae. **2.** Collagenous bundles in the submucosa. **3.** Fibroblasts. **4.** Ganglion nerve cell in Meissner's plexus. **5.** Plasma cell. **6.** Macrophage. **7.** Lymphocyte in lymphatic capillary (lacteal). **8.** Lumen of arteriole; diameter 30 μ. **9.** Nucleus of endothelial cell. **10.** Nucleus of smooth muscle cells. **11.** Non-myelinated, sympathetic and parasympathetic, nerve fibers. **12.** Schwann cell nucleus.

Fig. 29-43. Mesentery of the large intestine. Rat. L.M. X 64. **1.** Intestinal mucosa. **2.** Muscularis externa. **3.** Core of mesentery. **4.** Peritoneal cavity. **5.** Artery. **6.** Vein. **7.** Adipose tissue. **8.** Small vein.

Fig. 29-44. Enlargement of area similar to rectangle (A) in Fig. 29-43. Large intestine. Rat. E.M. X 4600. **1.** Peritoneal cavity. **2.** Visceral peritoneum. **3.** Muscularis externa. **4.** Nucleus of mesothelial cell. **5.** Bundles of collagenous fibrils in connective tissue part of serosa. **6.** Nucleus of smooth muscle cell. **7.** Microvilli.

Fig. 29-45. Enlargement of rectangle (B) in Fig. 29-43. Mesentery of the large intestine. Rat. E.M. X 610. **1.** Lumen of artery. **2.** Muscular media of artery. **3.** Loose connective tissue core of mesentery. **4.** Sheet of serous membrane. **5.** Peritoneal cavity. **6.** Cross-sectioned non-myelinated nerve bundles. **7.** Blood capillaries. **8.** Lymph capillary.

Fig. 29-46. Enlargement of area similar to rectangle in Fig. 29-45. Mesentery of large intestine. Rat. E.M. X 1800. **1.** Mesothelium. **2.** Elastic membrane. **3.** Bundles of collagenous fibrils. **4.** Cytoplasmic strands of fibroblast. **5.** Lymphocyte.

Fig. 29-47. Enlargement similar to rectangle in Fig. 29-46. Detail of mesenterial surface. Large intestine. Rat. E.M. X 61,000. **1.** Peritoneal cavity. **2.** Mesothelial cell cytoplasm. **3.** Basal lamina. **4.** Collagenous fibrils in submesothelial connective tissue. **5.** Microvilli. **6.** Junctional complex. **7.** Mitochondrion. **8.** Granular endoplasmic reticulum. **9.** Ribosomes. **10.** Micropinocytotic vesicles.

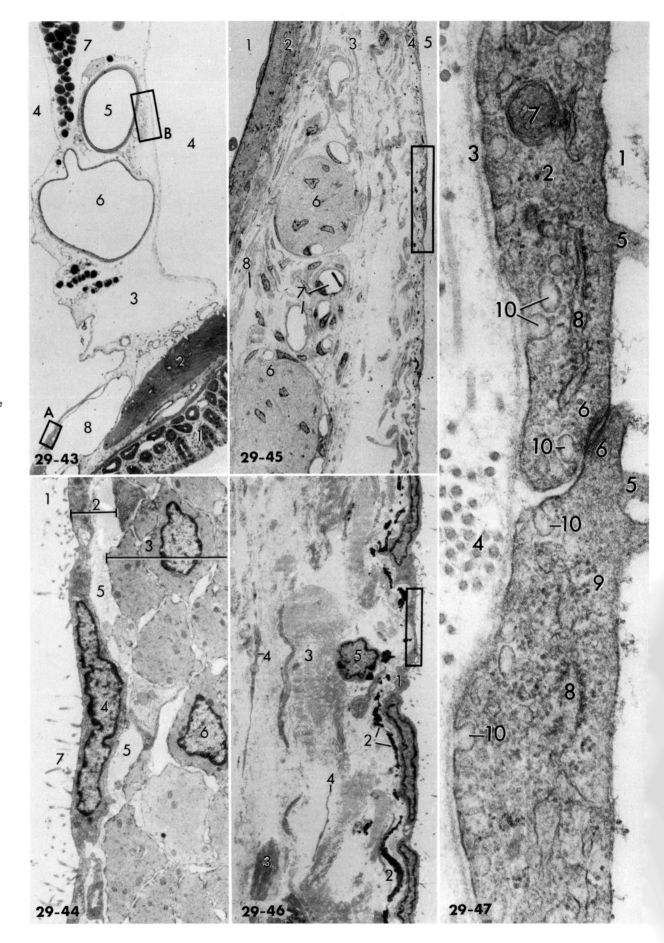

References

Atkins, A. M., Schofield, G. C., and Reeders, T. Studies on the structure and distribution of immunoglobulin A-containing cells in the gut of the pig. J. Anat. *109*: 385–395 (1971).

Baradi, A. F. and Hope, J. Observations on ultrastructure of rabbit mesothelium. Exp. Cell Res. *34*: 33–44 (1964).

Behnke, O. and Moe, H. An electron microscope study of mature and differentiating Paneth cells in the rat, especially of their endoplasmic reticulum and lysosomes. J. Cell Biol. *22*: 633–652 (1964).

Bennett, G. Migration of glycoprotein from Golgi apparatus to cell coat in the columnar cells of the duodenum epithelium. J. Cell Biol. *45*: 668–673 (1970).

Bonneville, M. A. and Weinstock, M. Brush border development in the intestinal absorptive cells of Xenopus during metamorphosis. J. Cell Biol. *44*: 151–171 (1970).

Brunser, O. and Luft, J. H. Fine structure of the apex of absorptive cells from rat small intestine. J. Ultrastruct. Res. *31*: 291–311 (1970).

Cardell, R. R., Jr., Badenhausen, S. and Porter, K. R. Intestinal triglyceride absorption in the rat. An electron microscopic study. J. Cell Biol. *34*: 123–155 (1967).

Cheng, H., Merzel, J. and Leblond, C. P. Renewal of Paneth cells in the small intestine of the mouse. Am. J. Anat. *126*: 507–526 (1969).

Cornell, R. and Padykula, H. A. A cytological study of intestinal absorption in the suckling rat. Am. J. Anat. *125*: 291–316 (1969).

Cotran, R. S. and Karnovsky, M. J. Ultrastructural studies on the permeability of the mesothelium to horseradish peroxidase. J. Cell Biol. *37*: 123–137 (1968).

Dawson, I. The endocrine cells of the gastrointestinal tract. Histochemical J. *2*: 527–549 (1970).

Deschner, E. E. Observations on the Paneth cell in human ileum. Exp. Cell Res. *47*: 624–628 (1967).

Dobbins, W. O., III and Rollins, E. L. Intestinal mucosal lymphatic permeability: an electron microscopic study of endothelial vesicles and cell junctions. J. Ultrastruct. Res. *33*: 29–59 (1970).

Forsmann, W. G., Orci, L., Pictet, R., Renold, A. E. and Rouiller, C. The endocrine cells in the epithelium of the gastrointestinal mucosa of the rat. J. Cell Biol. *40*: 692–715 (1969).

Freeman, J. A. Goblet cell fine structure. Anat. Rec. *154*: 121–148 (1966).

Freeman, J. A. and Geer, J. C. Intestinal fat and iron transport, goblet cell mucus secretion, and cellular changes in protein deficiency observed with the electron microscope. Am. J. Digest. Dis. *10*: 1004–1023 (1965).

Friend, D. The fine structure of Brunner's glands in the mouse. J. Cell Biol. *25*: 563–576 (1965).

Hertzog, A. J. The Paneth cell. Am. J. Path. *13*: 351–360 (1937).

Hollmann, K. H. Über den Feinbau des Rectumepithels. Z. Zellforsch. *68*: 502–542 (1965).

Ingelfinger, F. J. Gastrointestinal absorption. Nutrition Today *2*: 2–10 (1967).

Ingelfinger, F. J. For want of an enzyme. Nutrition Today *3*: 2–10 (1968).

Ito, S. The enteric surface coat on cat intestinal microvilli. J. Cell Biol. *27*: 475–491 (1965).

Jersild, R. A., Jr. A time sequence study of fat absorption in the rat jejunum. Am. J. Anat. *118*: 135–162 (1966).

Johnson, F. R. and Young, B. A. Undifferentiated cells in gastric mucosa. J. Anat. *102*: 541–551 (1968).

Krause, W. J. and Leeson, C. R. Studies of Brunner's glands in opossum. I. Adult morphology. Am. J. Anat. *126*: 255–274 (1969).

Lacy, D. and Taylor, A. B. Fat absorption by epithelial cells of the small intestine of the rat. Am. J. Anat. *110*: 155–186 (1962).

Ladman, A. J., Padykula, H. A. and Strauss, E. W. A morphological study of fat transport in the normal human jejunum. Am. J. Anat. *112*: 387–394 (1963).

Laguens, R. and Briones, M. Fine structure of the microvillus of columnar epithelial cells of human intestine. Lab. Investig. *14*: 1616–1623 (1965).

Leeson, T. S. and Leeson, C. R. The fine structure of Brunner's glands in man. J. Anat. *103*: 263–276 (1968).

Meader, R. and Landers, D. Electron and light microscopic observations on relationships between lymphocytes and intestinal epithelium. Am. J. Anat. *121*: 763–774 (1967).

Merzel, J. and Leblond, C. P. Origin and renewal of goblet cells in the epithelium of the mouse small intestine. Am. J. Anat. *124*: 281–306 (1969).

Moe, H. The ultrastructure of Brunner's glands of the cat. J. Ultrastruct. Res. *4*: 58–72 (1960).

Moe, H. The goblet cells, Paneth cells, and basal granular cells of the epithelium of the intestine. Int. Rev. Gen. Exp. Zool. *3*: 241–287 (1968).

Mukherjee, T. M. and Staehelin, L. A. The fine-structural organization of the brush border of intestinal epithelial cells. J. Cell Sci. *8*: 573–599 (1971).

Palay, S. L. and Karlin, L. J. An electron microscopic study of the intestinal villus. II. The pathway of fat absorption. J. Biophys. Biochem. Cytol. *5*: 373–384 (1959).

Palay, S. L. and Revel, J. P. The morphology of fat absorption. *In* Proceedings of an International Symposium on Lipid Transport (Ed. H. C. Meng). Charles C. Thomas, Springfield, pp. 33–43 (1964).

Pratt, S. A. and Napolitano, L. Osmium binding to the surface coat of intestinal microvilli in the cat under various conditions. Anat. Rec. *165*: 197–210 (1969).

Reynolds, D. S., Brim, J. and Sheehy, T. W. The vascular architecture of the small intestinal mucosa of the monkey (Macaca mulatta). Anat. Rec. *159*: 211–218 (1967).

Schofield, G. C. Columnar cells with secretory granules in the large intestine of the macaque (Cynamolgus iris). J. Anat. *106*: 1–14 (1970).

Schofield, G. C. and Atkins, A. Secretory immunoglobulin in columnar epithelial cells of the large intestine. J. Anat. *107*: 491–504 (1970).

Schofield, G. C. and Silva, D. The fine structure of enterochromaffin cells in the mouse colon. J. Anat. *103*: 1–13 (1968).

Singh, I. On argyrophile and argentaffin reactions in individual granules of enterochromaffin cells of the human gastro-intestinal tract. J. Anat. *98*: 497–500 (1964).

Staley, T. E., Jones, E. W. and Marshall, A. E. The jejunal absorptive cell of the newborn pig: an electron microscopic study. Anat. Rec. *161*: 497–516 (1968).

Strauss, E. W. Electron microscopic study of intestinal fat absorption in vitro from mixed micelles containing linolenic acid, monoolein, and bile salt. J. Lipid Res. *7*: 307–323 (1966).

Thrasher, J. D. and Greulich, R. C. The duodenal progenital population. III. The progenitor cell cycle of principal, goblet and Paneth cells. J. Exp. Zool. *161*: 9–19 (1966).

Toner, P. G. Cytology of intestinal epithelial cells. Int. Rev. Cytol. *24*: 233–243 (1968).

Toner, P. G. and Ferguson, A. Intraepithelial cells in the human intestinal mucosa. J. Ultrastruct. Res. *34*: 329–344 (1971).

Trier, J. S. Studies on small intestinal crypt epithelium. I. The fine structure of the crypt epithelium of the proximal small intestine of fasting humans. J. Cell Biol. *18*: 599–620 (1963).

Trier, J. S. Morphology of the epithelium of the small intestine. *In* Handbook of Pyhsiology: Sect. 6. Alimentary Canal, Vol. 32 (Ed. C. F. Code), American Physiological Society, Washington, D.C. pp. 1125–1175 (1968).

Trier, J. S., Lorenzsonn, V. and Groehler, K. Pattern of secretion of Paneth cells of the small intestine of mice. Gastroenterology *53*: 240–249 (1967).

Troughton, W. D., and Trier, J. S. Paneth and goblet cell renewal in mouse duodenal crypts. J. Cell Biol. *41*: 251–268 (1969).

Vassallo, G., Solcia, E. and Capella, C. Light and electron microscopic identification of several types of endocrine cells in the gastrointestinal mucosa of the cat. Z. Zellforsch. *98*: 333–356 (1969).

Wissig, S. L. and Graney, D. O. Membrane modifications in the apical endocytic complex of ileal epithelial cells. J. Cell Biol. *39*: 564–579 (1968).

30 Liver and pancreas

Fig. 30-1. Liver. Human. L.M. X 10. **1.** Capsule.
2. Rectangle: hepatic lobule. **3.** Portal areas.
4. Central venules. **5.** Sublobular hepatic vein.

Fig. 30-2. Hepatic lobule. Cross section.
Enlargement of area similar to rectangle in
Fig. 30-1. Liver. Human. L.M. X 130.
1. Portal areas. **2.** Hepatic sinusoids. **3.** Plates
of hepatic cells. **4.** Central venule.
5. Sublobular vein.

Fig. 30-3. Hepatic lobule. Longitudinal section.
Liver. Rat. L.M. X 253. **1.** Plates of hepatic
cells. Nuclei of hepatic cells stained black.
2. Hepatic sinusoids. **3.** Central venule.
Arrows indicate direction of blood flow.

Fig. 30-4. Diagram of cross-sectioned hepatic
lobules. **1.** Portal areas. **2.** Central venules.
3. Hexagonal, classical **hepatic lobule.** Lines
depict plates of hepatic cells and sinusoids
converging on the central venule.
4. Triangular **portal lobule. 5.** Diamond-shaped
liver acinus.

Fig. 30-5. Three-dimensional diagram of the
classical hepatic lobule. (Redrawn and
modified from L. C. Junqueira & J. Carneiro,
Histologia Basica, 2nd Ed., Guanabara
Koogan, S.A., Rio de Janeiro, 1971).
1. Interlobular portal veins. **2.** Interlobular
hepatic arteries. **3.** Hepatic sinusoids. **4.** Plates
of hepatic cells. **5.** Central venule.
6. Sublobular hepatic vein. *Arrows* indicate
direction of blood flow. **7.** Bile canaliculi.
8. Bile ductules. **9.** Bile ducts. *Arrows*
indicate direction of bile flow. **10.** Perilobular
surfaces of adjoining hepatic lobules.

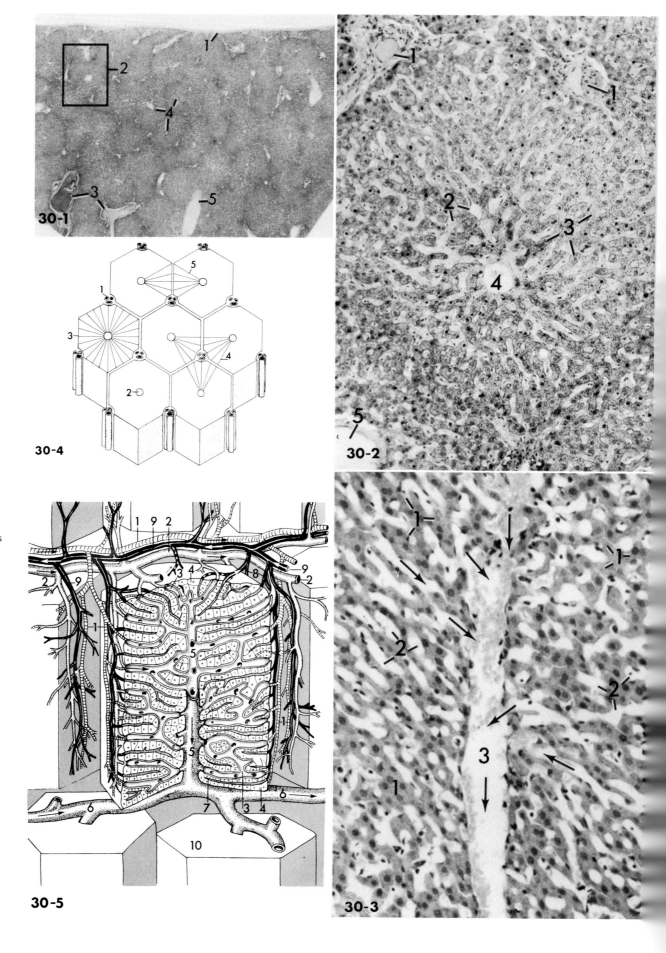

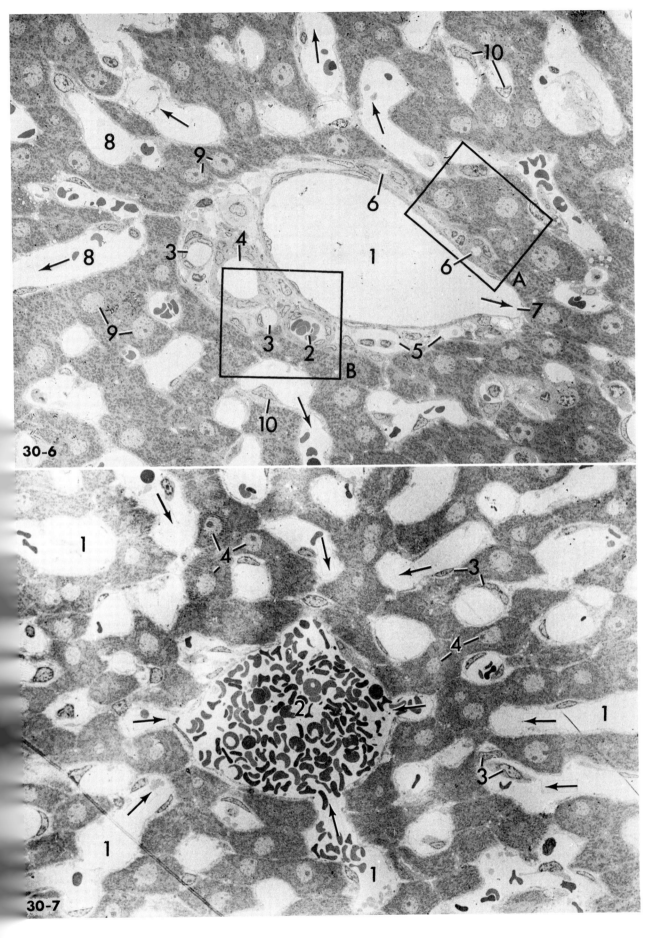

Fig. 30-6. Portal area. Liver. Rat. E.M. X 640.
1. Portal vein. **2.** Small hepatic artery.
3. Peribiliary blood capillaries. **4.** Bile duct.
5. Lymphatic capillaries. **6.** Bile ductules.
7. Inlet venule. *Arrows* indicate direction of
blood flow. **8.** Hepatic sinusoids, some with
erythrocytes. **9.** Nuclei of hepatic cells.
10. Nuclei of sinusoidal endothelial cells.
Rectangle (A) is enlarged in Fig. 30-8 and
rectangle (B) is enlarged in Fig. 30-16.

Fig. 30-7. Central part of hepatic lobule. Liver.
Rat. E.M. X 640. **1.** Hepatic sinusoids.
Arrows indicate direction of blood flow.
2. Central venule with numerous erythrocytes
and connecting hepatic sinusoids. **3.** Nuclei of
sinusoidal endothelial cells. **4.** Nuclei of
hepatic cells.

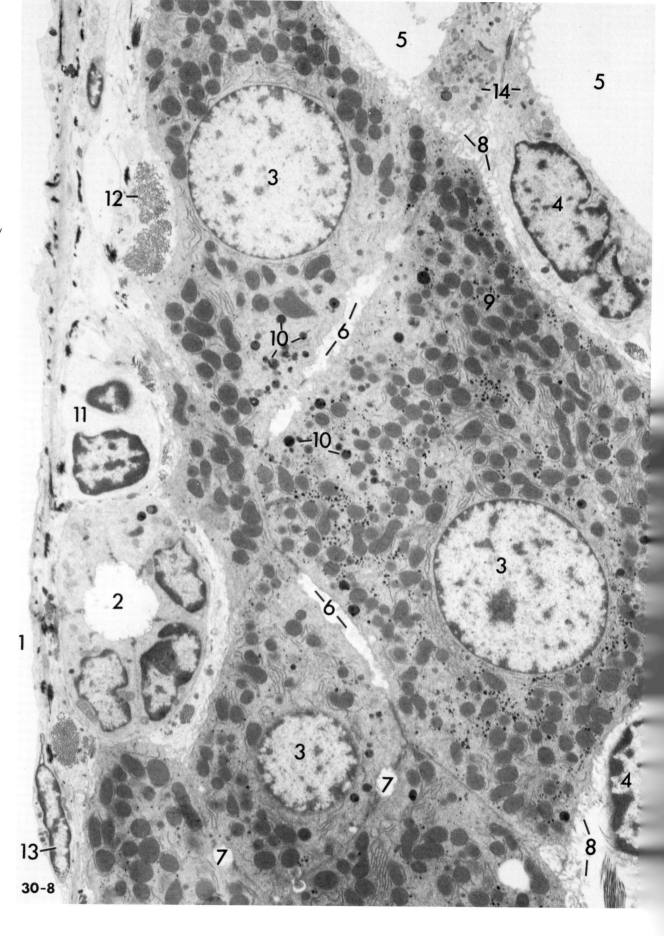

Fig. 30-8. Survey of part of perilobular area and peripheral portion of hepatic lobule. Enlargement of rectangle (A) in Fig. 30-6. Liver. Rat. E.M. X 1900. 1. Lumen of portal vein lined by a squamous endothelium. 2. Lumen of bile ductule, lined by low cuboidal epithelial cells. 3. Nuclei of hepatic cells. 4. Nucleus of sinusoidal endothelial (Kupffer) cell. 5. Lumen of hepatic sinusoids. 6. Longitudinally sectioned bile canaliculi. 7. Cross-sectioned bile canaliculi. 8. Perisinusoidal space of Disse. 9. Mitochondria. 10. Lysosomes (peribiliary dense bodies). 11. Lymphocyte. 12. Bundle of collagenous fibrils. 13. Nucleus of endothelial cell lining the inlet venule. 14. Numerous lysosomes in endothelial and Kupffer cells.

30-8

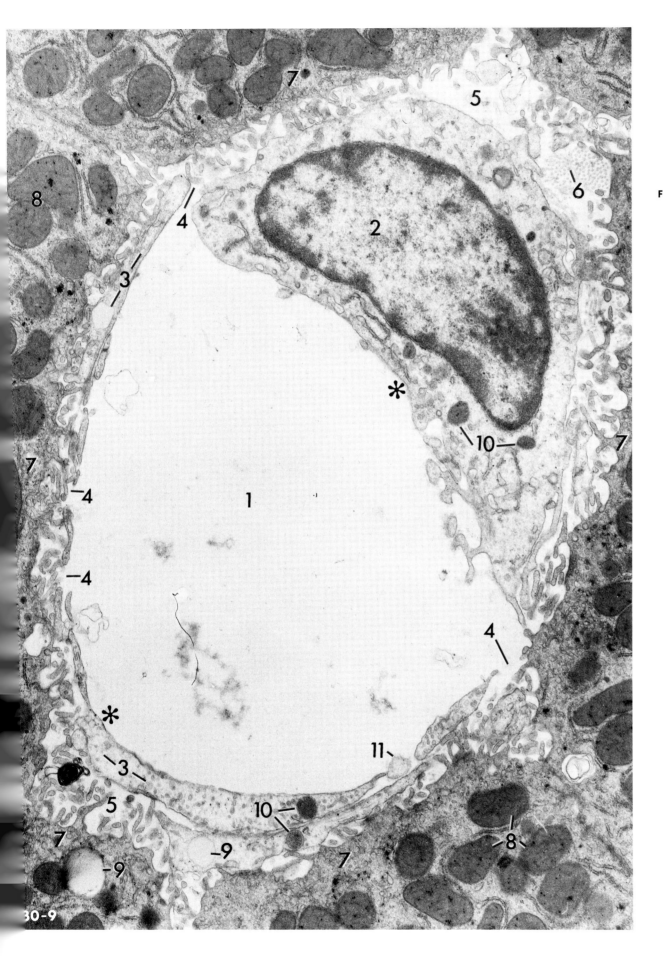

Fig. 30-9. Cross section of hepatic sinusoid. Liver. Rat. E.M. × 12,000. **1.** Lumen of sinusoid. Distance between *asterisks* is 10 μ. **2.** Nucleus of sinusoidal endothelial cell. **3.** Squamous endothelium. **4.** Endothelial gaps. **5.** Perisinusoidal space of Disse. **6.** Bundles of collagenous fibrils. **7.** Bases of hepatic cells with microvilli projecting into the space of Disse. **8.** Mitochondria. **9.** Lipid droplets. **10.** Lysosomes. **11.** Chylomicron. Lipids, absorbed by the intestinal mucosa, are passed on to intestinal lacteals and capillary network of the core of the intestinal villus. The lipids, referred to as chylomicra, reach the liver via the portal vein.

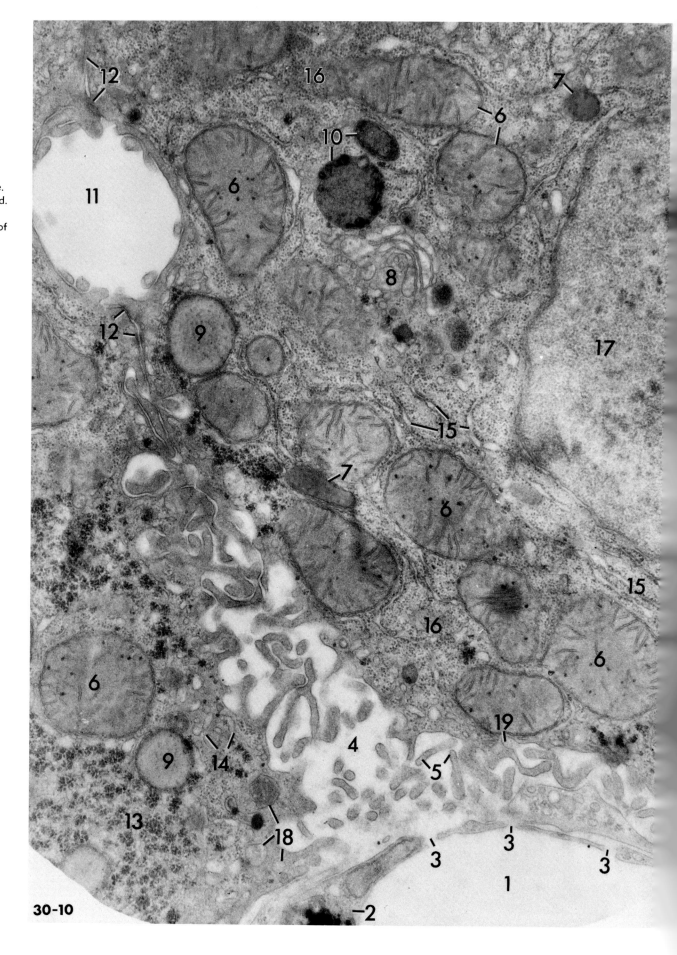

Fig. 30-10. Detail of hepatic cell. Liver. Mouse. E.M. X 26,000. **1.** Lumen of hepatic sinusoid. **2.** Cytoplasm of endothelial (Kupffer) cell. **3.** Endothelial gaps. **4.** Perisinusoidal space of Disse. **5.** Microvilli. **6.** Mitochondria. **7.** Microbodies (peroxisomes). **8.** Golgi zone. **9.** Lipid droplets. **10.** Lysosomes (peribiliary dense bodies). **11.** Bile canaliculus (bile capillary). **12.** Junctional complexes. **13.** Glycogen particles. **14.** Agranular endoplasmic reticulum. **15.** Granular endoplasmic reticulum. **16.** Free monoribosomes and polysomes. **17.** Nucleus. **18.** Vacuoles with amorphous granules of "very low density lipoproteins." **19.** Micropinocytotic invagination.

30-10

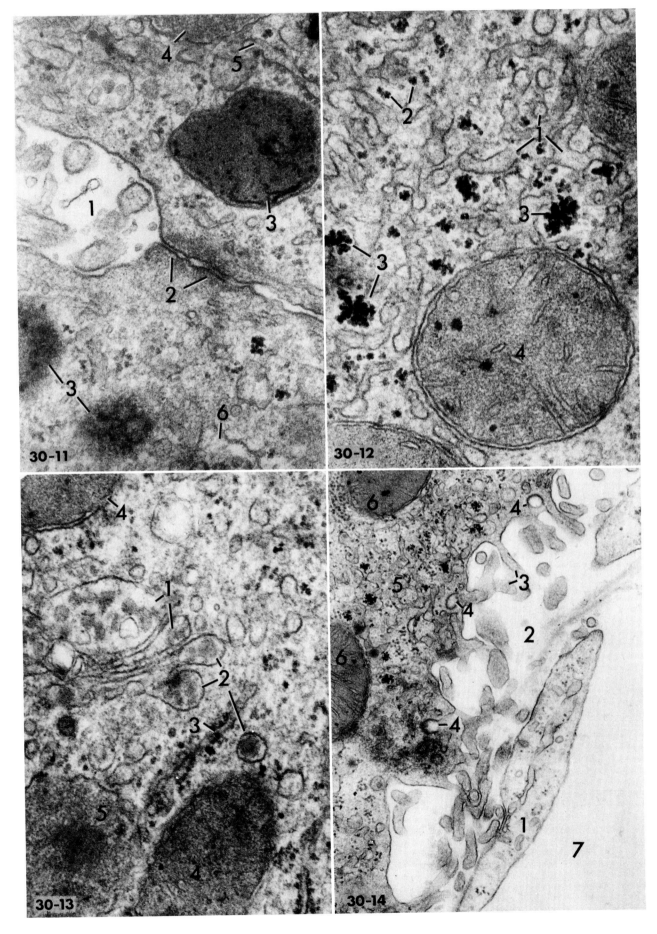

Fig. 30-11. Peribiliary region. Hepatic cell. Liver. Rat. E.M. X 70,000. **1.** Bile canaliculus with microvilli projecting into it. **2.** Junctional complex. **3.** Lysosomes (peribiliary dense bodies). **4.** Part of microbody (peroxisome). **5.** Cisterna of granular endoplasmic reticulum. **6.** Part of multivesicular body.

Fig. 30-12. Central region. Hepatic cell. Liver. Rat. E.M. X 83,000. **1.** Tubules of agranular endoplasmic reticulum. **2.** Glycogen particles (beta particles). **3.** Glycogen particles (alpha particles). **4.** Mitochondrion.

Fig. 30-13. Golgi region. Hepatic cell. Liver. Rat. E.M. X 75,000. **1.** Saccules of Golgi zones. **2.** Dilated, bulbous ends of Golgi saccules, containing very low density lipoprotein granules. **3.** Cisterna of granular endoplasmic reticulum. **4.** Mitochondria. **5.** Microbody (peroxisome).

Fig. 30-14. Perisinusoidal region. Hepatic cell. Liver. Rat. E.M. X 83,000. **1.** Part of sinusoidal endothelial cell. **2.** Perisinusoidal space of Disse. **3.** Microvilli. **4.** Coated micropinocytotic invaginations. **5.** Tubules of agranular endoplasmic reticulum among ribosomes and glycogen particles. **6.** Mitochondria. **7.** Lumen of sinusoid.

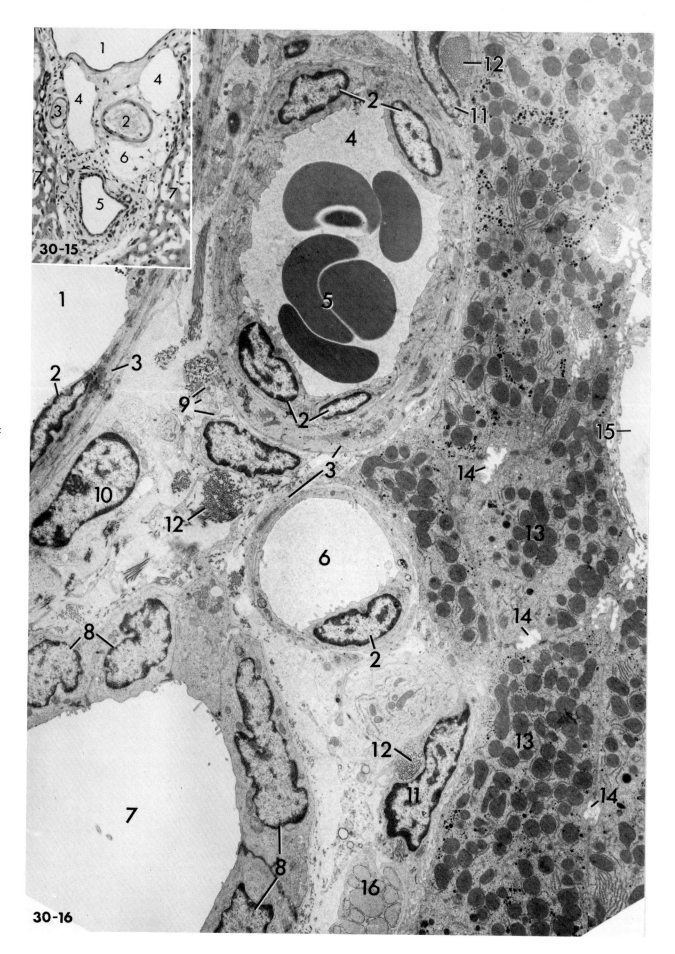

Fig. 30-15. Large portal area. Liver. Rat. L.M. X 160. **1.** Portal vein. **2.** Hepatic artery. **3.** Hepatic arteriole. **4.** Lymphatics. **5.** Biliary duct. **6.** Portal area connective tissue. **7.** Hepatic sinusoids and plates of hepatic cells.

Fig. 30-16. Small portal area. Enlargement of rectangle (B) in Fig. 30-6. Liver. Rat. E.M. X 4700. **1.** Lumen of portal vein. **2.** Nuclei of endothelial cells. **3.** Vascular smooth muscle cells. **4.** Lumen of small hepatic artery. **5.** Erythrocytes. **6.** Lumen of precapillary arteriole. **7.** Lumen of interlobular biliary duct. **8.** Nuclei of epithelial duct cells. **9.** Non-myelinated nerve fibers (require higher magnification for positive identification). **10.** Nucleus of lymphocyte. **11.** Nucleus of fibroblast. **12.** Bundles of collagenous fibrils. **13.** Mitochondria in hepatic cells. **14.** Cross-sectioned bile canaliculi. **15.** Lumen of hepatic sinusoid. **16.** Part of plasma cell with dilated cisternae of the granular endoplasmic reticulum.

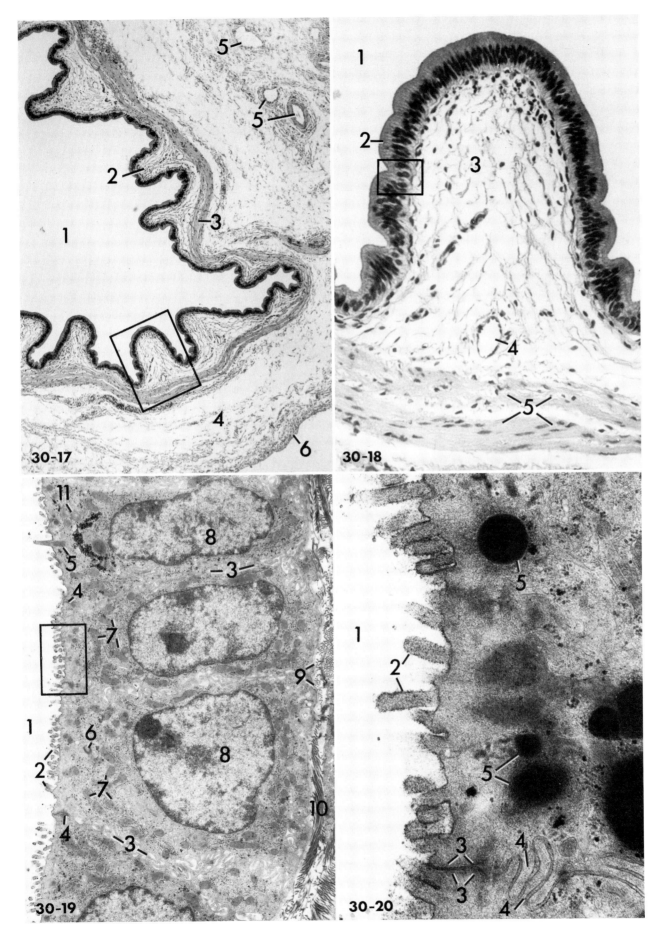

Fig. 30-17. Gallbladder. Monkey. L.M. X 56.
1. Lumen. **2.** Mucous membrane. **3.** Lamina muscularis. **4.** Adventitia. **5.** Blood vessels. **6.** Serosa.

Fig. 30-18. Gallbladder. Enlargement of rectangle in Fig. 30-17. L.M. X 315.
1. Lumen. **2.** Simple columnar epithelium. **3.** Stroma of connective tissue ("lamina propria"). **4.** Venule. **5.** Smooth muscle cells of lamina muscularis.

Fig. 30-19. Gallbladder epithelium. Enlargement of area similar to rectangle in Fig. 30-18. Rat. E.M. X 7,000. **1.** Lumen of gallbladder. **2.** Microvilli. **3.** Cell borders. **4.** Junctional complexes. **5.** Basal body of cilium. **6.** Centriole. **7.** Mitochondria. **8.** Nuclei. **9.** Basal lamina. **10.** Collagenous fibrils of stroma. **11.** Accumulation of glycogen particles.

Fig. 30-20. Surface of epithelial cells. Gallbladder. Enlargement of area similar to rectangle in Fig. 30-19. Rat. E.M. X 34,000. **1.** Lumen of gallbladder. **2.** Microvilli. **3.** Junctional complex. **4.** Cell to cell interdigitations. **5.** Mucoid granules.

Fig. 30-21. Pancreas. Human. L.M. X 12.
  1. Thin capsule. **2.** Septa. **3.** Lobes. **4.** Lobules.
  5. Islets of Langerhans.
Fig. 30-22. Pancreas. Enlargement of area
  similar to rectangle in Fig. 30-21. Monkey.
  L.M. X 305. **1.** Arterioles. **2.** Acini (alveoli).
  3. Interlobular duct. **4.** Intralobular duct.
Fig. 30-23. Two acini and interlobular connective
  tissue septum. Enlargement of area similar to
  rectangle in Fig. 30-22. Pancreas. Rat. E.M.
  X 1800. **1.** Nuclei of acinar epithelial cells.
  2. Lumen (secretory capillary) of acinus,
  surrounded by intracellular zymogen
  (secretory) granules. **3.** Centroacinar cells.
  4. Lumen of intralobular (intercalated) duct,
  lined by low cuboidal duct cells. *Arrow*
  indicates position of duct cells which connect
  centroacinar cells with intercalated
  (intralobular) duct. **5.** Lumina of blood
  capillaries. **6.** Nucleus of Schwann cell with
  associated non-myelinated nerve fibers.
  7. Nuclei of lymphocytes. **8.** Connective
  tissue fibrils and fibroblasts of interlobular
  septum. **9.** Delicate interacinar connective
  tissue septum. **10.** Lumen of arteriole.
  11. Lumen of interlobular duct. **12.** Epithelial
  duct cells. Area corresponding to rectangle
  is enlarged in Fig. 30-24.

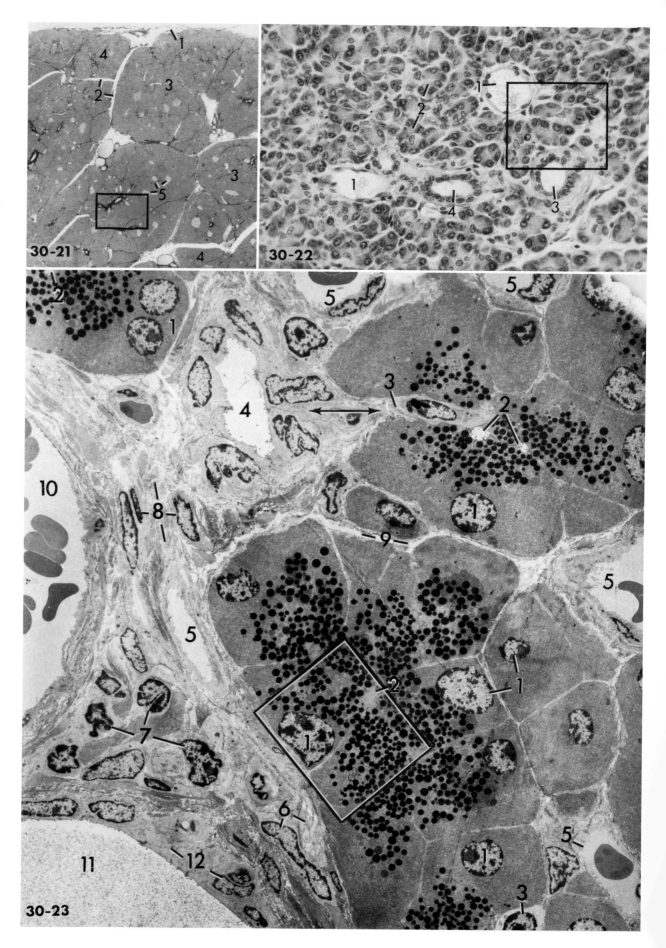

340

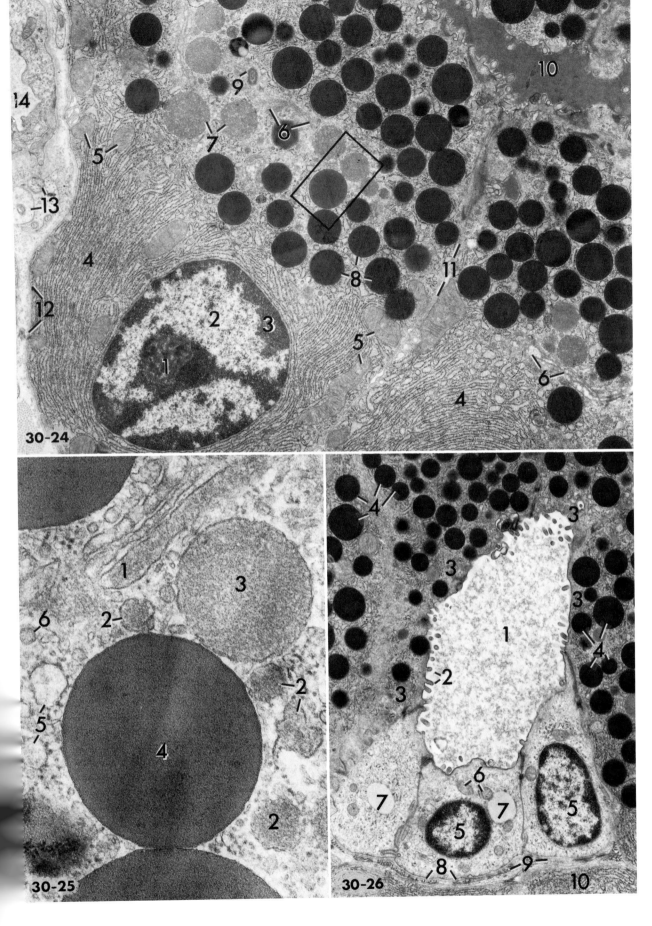

Fig. 30-24. Acinar epithelial cells. Enlargement of area corresponding to rectangle in Fig. 30-23. Pancreas. Rat. E.M. X 9000.
1. Nucleolus. **2.** Euchromatin.
3. Heterochromatin. **4.** Granular endoplasmic reticulum. **5.** Mitochondria. **6.** Golgi zones.
7. Prezymogen granules. **8.** Zymogen granules.
9. Centriole. **10.** Acinar lumen filled with dense secretory material. **11.** Cell border.
12. Basal lamina. **13.** Non-myelinated nerve fibers. **14.** Lumen of blood capillary.

Fig. 30-25. Secretory granules. Acinar cell. Enlargement of area similar to rectangle in Fig. 30-24. Pancreas. Rat. E.M. X 62,000. **1.** Saccule of Golgi zone containing medium electron-dense amorphous material.
2. Condensing Golgi vacuoles. **3.** Prezymogen granule. **4.** Zymogen granule. **5.** Vacuolar profile of granular endoplasmic reticulum.
6. Transfer vesicle.

Fig. 30-26. Center of acinus. Pancreas. Rat. E.M. X 8000. **1.** Lumen of acinus with flocculent secretory material. **2.** Microvilli.
3. Apices of acinar cells. **4.** Zymogen granules.
5. Nuclei of centroacinar cells.
6. Mitochondria. **7.** Lipid droplets in cytoplasm of centroacinar cells. **8.** Basal lamina. **9.** Interacinar connective tissue fibrils. **10.** Basal cytoplasm of acinar cells in adjacent acinus.

Fig. 30-27. Islet of Langerhans. Pancreas. Human. L.M. X 190. **1.** Cords of cells in islet. **2.** Collapsed blood capillaries. **3.** Acini of exocrine portion of pancreas. **4.** Plane of section to obtain Fig. 30-28.

Fig. 30-28. Edge of islet of Langerhans. Plane of section indicated by 4—4 in Fig. 30-27. Pancreas. Rat. E.M. X 4500. **1.** Lumina of blood capillaries. **2.** Nuclei of endothelial cells. **3.** Nucleus of pericyte. **4.** Nuclei of fibroblasts. **5.** Bundles of collagenous fibrils. **6.** Nuclei of alpha (glucagon) cells. **7.** Nuclei of beta (insulin) cells. **8.** Nucleus of delta cell. **9.** Nuclei of C-cells. Identification of cell types is based on analysis of this field at higher magnifications.

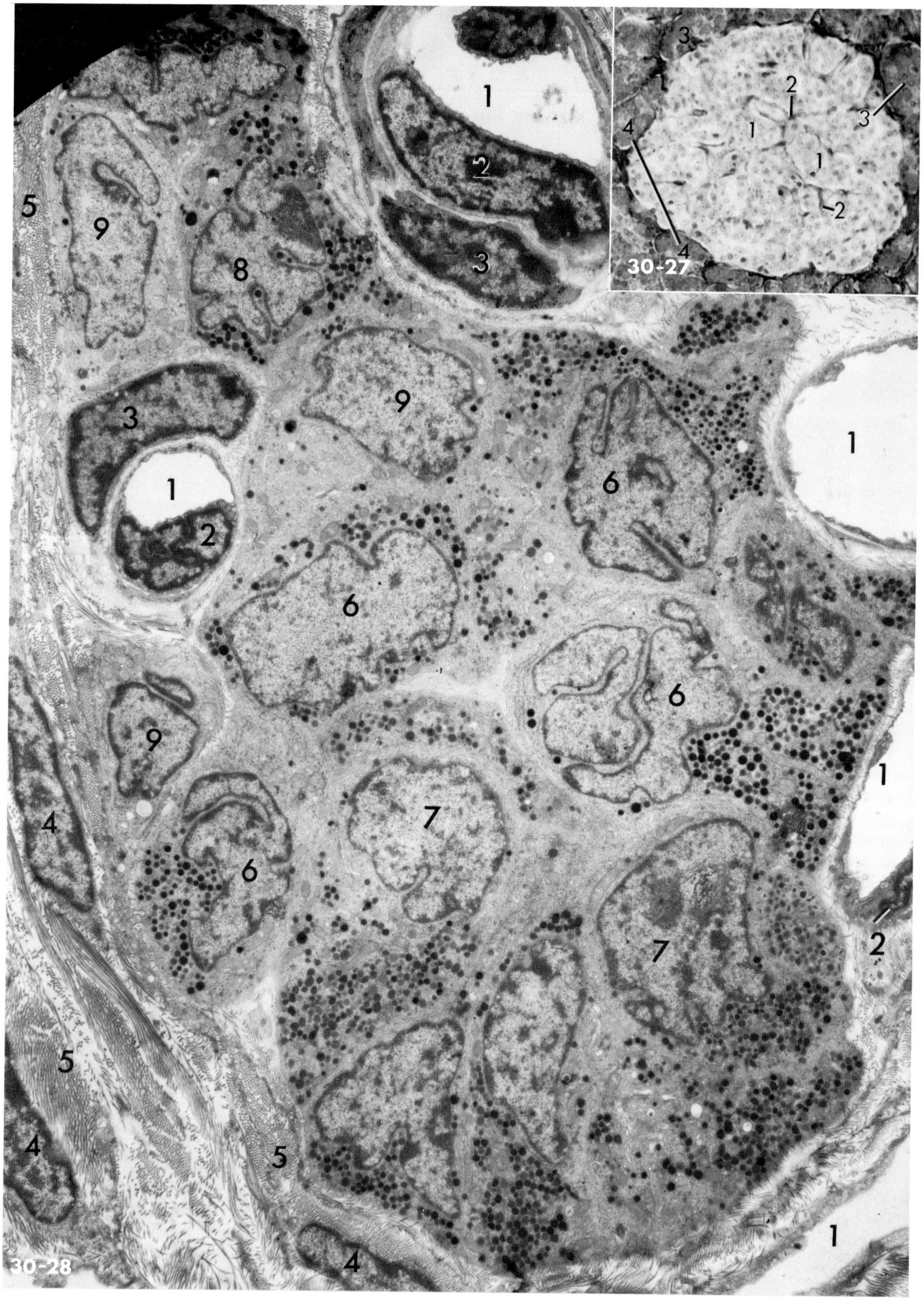

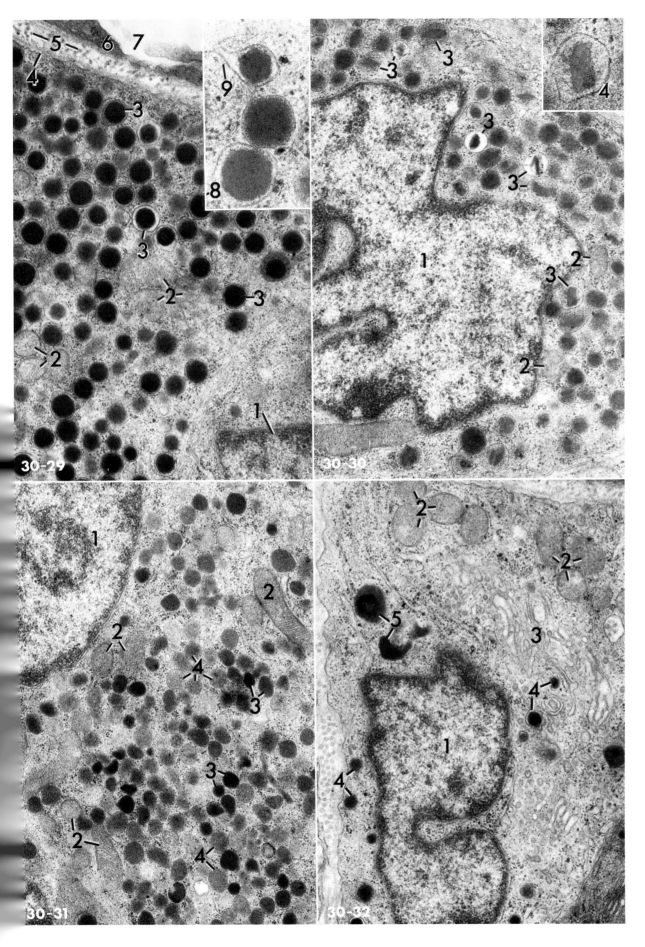

Fig. 30-29. Detail of alpha (glucagon) cell. Islet of Langerhans. Pancreas. Rat. E.M. X 17,000. **1.** Nucleus. **2.** Mitochondria. **3.** Secretory granules with loosely fitting boundary membrane. **4.** Cell membrane. **5.** Collagenous fibrils. **6.** Capillary endothelium. **7.** Capillary lumen. **8.** Inset: secretory granules; X 60,000. **9.** Discharging secretory granule, boundary membrane fused with surface membrane.

Fig. 30-30. Detail of beta (insulin) cell. Islet of Langerhans. Pancreas. Rat. E.M. X 17,000. **1.** Nucleus. **2.** Mitochondria. **3.** Secretory granules with angular core. **4.** Inset: secretory granule with rectangular crystalline core; X 60,000.

Fig. 30-31. Detail of delta cell. Islet of Langerhans. Pancreas. Rat. E.M. X 17,000. **1.** Nucleus. **2.** Mitochondria. **3.** Dense secretory granule. **4.** Electron-lucent secretory granules.

Fig. 30-32. Detail of C-cell. Islet of Langerhans. Pancreas. Rat. E.M. X 17,000. **1.** Nucleus. **2.** Mitochondria. **3.** Golgi zone. **4.** Limited number of small secretory granules. **5.** Lysosome.

343

References

LIVER

Amakawa, T. Electron microscopic studies on lysosomes in human hepatic parenchymal cells. J. Electron Micr. *16*: 154–168 (1967).

Bassi, M., Cajone, F. and Bernelli-Zazzera, A. Agranular endoplasmic reticulum in liver cells during glycogen loss and glycogen accumulation. J. Submicr. Cytol. *1*: 143–158 (1969).

Biempica, L. Human hepatic microbodies with crystalloid cores. J. Cell Biol. *29*: 383–386 (1966).

Boler, R. K. Fine structure of canine Kupffer cells and their microtubule-containing cytosomes. Anat. Rec. *163*: 483–496 (1969).

Brown, W. R., Grodsky, G. M. and Carbone, J. V. Intracellular distribution of tritiated bilirubin during hepatic uptake and excretion. Am. J. Physiol. *207*: 1237–1244 (1965).

Bruni, C. and Porter, K. R. The fine structure of the parenchymal cell of the normal rat liver. Am. J. Path. *46*: 691–755 (1965).

Burkel, W. E. The fine structure of the terminal branches of the hepatic arterial system of the rat. Anat. Rec. *167*: 329–350 (1970).

Burkel, W. E. and Low, F. N. The fine structure of rat liver sinusoids, space of Disse and associated tissue space. Am. J. Anat. *118*: 769–784 (1966).

Cardell, R. R., Jr. Action of metabolic hormones on the fine structure of rat liver cells. I. Effects of fasting on the ultrastructure of hepatocytes. Am. J. Anat. *131*: 21–54 (1971).

Chapman, G. B., Chiarodo, A. J., Coffey, R. J. and Wieneke, K. The fine structure of mucosal epithelial cells of a pathological human gallbladder. Anat. Rec. *154*: 579–616 (1966).

Cossel, L. Die menschliche Leber im Elektronenmikroskop. Gustav Fischer, Jena, 1964.

DeMann, J. C. H. and Blok, A. P. R. Relationship between glycogen and agranular endoplasmic reticulum in rat hepatic cells. J. Histochem. Cytochem. *14*: 135–146 (1966).

Elias, H. Liver morphology. Biological Reviews *30*: 263–310 (1955).

Elias, H. and Sherrick, J. C. Morphology of the Liver. Academic Press, New York, 1969.

Essner, E. Endoplasmic reticulum and the origin of microbodies in fetal mouse liver. Lab. Investig. *17*: 71–87 (1967).

Fawcett, D. W. Observations on the cytology and electron microscopy of hepatic cells. J. Nat. Cancer Inst. *15*: Supp. 1475–1503 (1955).

Flaks, B. Observations on the fine structure of the normal porcine liver. J. Anat. *108*: 563–577 (1971).

Fox, H. Ultrastructure of the human gallbladder epithelium in cholelithiasis and chronic cholecystitis. J. Path. *108*: 157–164 (1972).

Goldfischer, S., Novikoff, A. B., Albala, A. and Biempica, L. Hemoglobin uptake by rat hepatocytes and its breakdown within lysosomes. J. Cell Biol. *44*: 513–529 (1970).

Grubb, D. J. and Jones, A. L. Ultrastructure of hepatic sinusoids in sheep. Anat. Rec. *170*: 75–80 (1971).

Hamilton, R. L., Regen, D. M., Gray, M. E. and LeQuire, V. S. Lipid transport in liver. I. Electron microscopic identification of very low density lipoproteins in perfused rat liver. Lab. Investig. *16*: 305–319 (1967).

Hampton, J. C. Liver. *In* Electron Microscopic Anatomy. (Ed. S. M. Kurtz), Chapter 2, pp. 41–58, Academic Press, New York, 1964.

Hayward, A. F. The fine structure of the gallbladder epithelium of the sheep. Z. Zellforsch. *65*: 331–339 (1965).

Hayward, A. F. The structure of gallbladder epithelium. Int. Rev. Gen. Exp. Zool. *3*: 205–239 (1968).

Ito, T. and Nemoto, M. Über die kupfferschen Sternzellen und die "Fettspeicherungszellen" in der Blutkapillarwand der menschlichen Leber. Okajimas Folia Anat. Japan. *24*: 243–258 (1952).

Ito, T. and Nemoto, M. Über die kupfferschen Sternthe hepatic sinusoidal wall and the fat-storing cells in the normal human liver. Arch. Histol. Japon. *29*: 137–192 (1968).

Kaye, G. I., Wheeler, H. O., Whitlock, R. T. and Lane, N. Fluid transport in rabbit gallbladder. J. Cell Biol. *30*: 237–268 (1966).

Kugler, J. H. Correlation of the glycogen concentration in rat liver and the appearance of glycogen and agranular endoplasmic reticulum. J. Roy. Microsc. Soc. *86*: 285–296 (1966).

Laschi, R. and Casanova, S. Fenestrae closed by a diaphragm in the endothelium of liver sinusoids. J. Microscopie *8*: 1037–1040 (1969).

Leeson, T. S. and Melax, H. Fine structure of the common bile duct in adult rats. Can. J. Zool. *47*: 33–35 (1969).

Loud, A. V. A quantitative stereological description of the ultrastructure of normal rat liver parenchymal cells. J. Cell Biol. *37*: 27–46 (1968).

Luciano, L. Die Feinstruktur der Gallenblase und der Gallengänge. I. Das Epithel der Gallenblase der Maus. Z. Zellforsch. *135*: 87–102 (1972).

Luciano, L. Die Feinstruktur der Gallenblase und der Gallengänge. II. Das Epithel der extrahepatischen Gallengänge der Maus und der Ratte. Z. Zellforsch. *135*: 103–114 (1972).

McCuskey, R. S. A dynamic and static study of hepatic arterioles and hepatic sphincters. Am. J. Anat. *119*: 455–477 (1966).

McCuskey, R. S. Dynamic microscopic anatomy of the fetal liver. I. Microcirculation. Angiology *18*: 648–653 (1967).

Ma, M. H. and Biempica, L. The normal human liver cell. Am. J. Path. *62*: 353–376 (1971).

Nicolescu, P. and Rouiller, C. Beziehungen zwischen den Endothelzellen der Lebersinusoide und den von Kupfferschen Sternzellen. Z. Zellforsch. *76*: 313–338 (1967).

Novikoff, A. B. and Essner, E. The liver cell; some new approaches to its study. Am. J. Med. *29*: 102–131 (1960).

Novikoff, A. B. and Shin, W. Y. The endoplasmic reticulum in the Golgi zone and its relations to microbodies, Golgi apparatus and autophagic vacuoles in rat liver cells. J. Microscopie *3*: 187–206 (1964).

Oudea, P. and Domart-Oudea, M.-C. L'ultrastructure hépatique. I. Le foie normal. Rev. fr. Étud. Clin. biol. *12*: 527–543 (1967).

Parks, H. F. On the uptake of chylomicrons by hepatic cells of mice. Anat. Rec. *142*: 320 (1962).

Parks, H. F. An experimental study of microscopic and submicroscopic lipid inclusions in hepatic cells of the mouse. Am. J. Anat. *120*: 253–280 (1967).

Parks, H. F. Notes on membrane-enclosed lipid spherules in hepatic cells of the mouse. Anat. Rec. *151*: 397 (1965).

Rappaport, A. M. Acinar units and the pathophysiology of the liver. *In* The Liver, Morphology, Biochemistry, Physiology (Ed. C. Rouiller). Vol. 1, pp. 265–328. Academic Press, New York, 1965.

Rhodin, J. A. G. Ultrastructure and function of liver sinusoids. Proc. IV. Intern. Symp. of R. E. S. Kyoto, Japan, pp. 108 –124. 1964.

Riches, D. J. and Palfrey, A. J. The ultrastructure of the bile duct epithelium of the rat. J. Anat. *100*: 429–430 (1966).

Rouiller, C. and Jezequel, A. M. Electron microscopy of the liver. *In* The Liver, Morphology, Biochemistry, Physiology (Ed. C. Rouiller), Vol. I, pp. 195–264. Academic Press, New York, 1965.

Steiner, J. W. and Carruthers, J. S. Studies on the fine structure of the terminal branches of the biliary tree. I. The morphology of normal bile canaliculi, bile pre-ductules (ducts of Hering) and bile ductules. Am. J. Path. *38*: 639–661 (1961).

Sternlieb, I. Electron microscopic study of intrahepatic biliary ductules. J. Microscopie *4*: 71–80 (1965).

Sternlieb, I. Mitochondrion desmosome complexes in human hepatocytes. Z. Zellforsch. *93*: 249–253 (1969).

Svoboda, D., Grady, H. and Azarnoff, D. Microbodies in experimentally altered cells. J. Cell Biol. *35*: 127–152 (1967).

Trotter, N. L. A fine structure study of lipid in mouse liver regeneration after partial hepatectomy. J. Cell Biol. *25*: 233–244 (1964).

Vrensen, G. F. J. M. and Kuyper, Ch. M. A. Involvement of rough endoplasmic reticulum and ribosomes in early stages of glycogen repletion in rat liver. J. Microscopie *8*: 599–614 (1969).

Weibel, E. D., Stäubli, W., Gnägi, H. R. and Hess, F. A. Correlated morphometric and biochemical studies on the liver cell. I. Morphometric model, stereologic methods, and normal morphometric data for rat liver. J. Cell Biol. *42*: 68–91 (1969).

Widman, J.-J., Cotran, R. S. and Fahimi, H. D. Mononuclear phagocytes (Kupffer cells) and endothelial cells. Identification of two functional cell types in rat liver sinusoids by endogenous peroxidase activity. J. Cell Biol. *52*: 159–170 (1971).

Willis, E. J. Crystalline structures in the mitochondria of normal human liver parenchymal cells. J. Cell Biol. *24*: 511–514 (1965).

Wisse, E. An electron microscopic study of the fenestrated endothelial lining of rat liver sinusoids. J. Ultrastruct. Res. *31*: 125–150 (1970).

Wisse, E. An ultrastructural characterization of the endothelial cell in the rat liver sinusoid under normal and various experimental conditions, as a contribution to the distinction between endothelial and Kupffer cells. J. Ultrastruct. Res. *38*: 528–562 (1972).

Wisse, E. and Daems, T. Fine structural study on the sinusoidal lining cells of rat liver. *In* Mononuclear Phagocytes (Ed. R. van Furth), pp. 200–210. Blackwell Scientific Publications, Oxford, 1970.

Wood, R. L. Evidence of species differences in the ultrastructure of the hepatic sinusoid. Z. Zellforsch. *58*: 679–692 (1963).

Wood, R. L. Development of peribiliary dense bodies in embryonic rat. Anat. Rec. *166*: 635–658 (1970).

Yamada, E. The fine structure of the gallbladder epithelium of the mouse. J. Biophys. Biochem. Cytol. *1*: 445–458 (1955).

Yamada, K. Aspects of the fine structure of the intrahepatic bile duct epithelium in normal and cholecystectomized mice. J. Morph. *124*: 1–22 (1968).

Yamada, K. Fine structure of rodent common bile duct epithelium. J. Anat. *105*: 511–523 (1969).

PANCREAS

Caramia, F., Munger, B. L. and Lacy, P. E. The ultrastructural basis for the identification of cell types in the pancreatic islets. I. Guinea pig. Z. Zellforsch. *67*: 533–546 (1965).

Caro, L. G. and Palade, G. E. Protein synthesis, storage, and discharge in the pancreatic exocrine cell. J. Cell Biol. *20*: 473–495 (1964).

Ekholm, R. and Edlund, Y. Ultrastructure of the human endocrine pancreas. J. Ultrastruct. Res. *2*: 453–481 (1959).

Ekholm, R., Zelander, T. and Edlund, Y. The ultrastructural organization of the rat exocrine pancreas. 1. Acinar cells. J. Ultrastruct. Res. *7*: 61–72 (1962).

Ekholm, R., Zelander, T. and Edlund, Y. The ultrastructural organization of the rat exocrine pancreas. 2. Centroacinar cells. Intercalary and intralobular ducts. J. Ultrastruct. Res. *7*: 73–83 (1962).

Greider, M. H., Bencosme, S. A. and Lechago, J. The human pancreatic islet cells and their tumors. I. The normal pancreatic islets. Lab. Investig. *22*: 344–354 (1970).

Ichikawa, A. Fine structural changes in response to hormonal stimulation of the perfused canine pancreas. J. Cell Biol. *24*: 369–385 (1965).

Jamieson, J. D. and Palade, G. E. Condensing vacuole conversion and zymogen granule discharge in pancreatic exocrine cells: metabolic studies. J. Cell Biol. *48*: 503–522 (1971).

Jamieson, J. D. and Palade, G. E. Intracellular transport of secretory proteins in the pancreatic exocrine cell. I. Role of the peripheral elements of the Golgi complex. J. Cell Biol. *34*: 577–596 (1967).

Jamieson, J. D. and Palade, G. E. Intracellular transport of secretory proteins in the pancreatic exocrine cell. II. Transport to condensing vacuoles and zymogen granules. J. Cell Biol. *34*: 597–615 (1967).

Jamieson, J. D. and Palade, G. E. Intracellular transport of secretory proteins in the pancreatic exocrine cell. III. Dissociation of intracellular transport from protein synthesis. J. Cell Biol. *39*: 580–588 (1968).

Jamieson, J. D. and Palade, G. E. Intracellular transport of secretory proteins in the pancreatic exocrine cell.

IV. Metabolic requirements. J. Cell Biol. *39*: 589–603 (1968).

Kern, H. F. and Ferner, H. Die Feinstruktur des exokrinen Pankreasgewebes vom Menschen. Z. Zellforsch. *113*: 322–343 (1971).

Lacy, P. E. Electron microscopy of the islets of Langerhans. Diabetes *11*: 509–513 (1962).

Lacy, P. E. The pancreatic beta cell. Structure and function. New Eng. J. Med. *276*: 187–195 (1967).

Lacy, P. E. and Greider, M. H. Ultrastructural organization of mammalian pancreatic islets. *In* Handbook of Physiology, Section 7, Vol. I, Digestion, 1970, pp. 77–000.

Like, A. A. The ultrastructure of the secretory cells of the islets of Langerhans in man. Lab. Investig. *16*: 937–951 (1967).

Merlini, D. and Caramia, F. G. Electron microscopic study of the cells of the human pancreatic islets. Rev. Int. Hepat. *16*: 687–694 (1966).

Munger, B. L., Caramia, F. and Lacy, P. E. The ultrastructural basis for the identification of cell types in the pancreatic islets. II. Rabbit, dog and opossum. Z. Zellforsch. *67*: 776–798 (1965).

Palade, G. E., Siekevitz, P. and Caro, L. G. Structure, chemistry and function of the pancreatic exocrine cell. Ciba Foundation Symp. Exocrine Pancreas, pp. 23–55 (1963).

Sjöstrand, F. S. and Hanzon, V. Membrane structures of cytoplasm and mitochondria in exocrine cells of mouse pancreas as revealed by high resolution electron microscopy. Exp. Cell Res. *7*: 393–414 (1954).

Sjöstrand, F. S. and Hanzon, V. Ultrastructure of Golgi apparatus of exocrine cells of mouse pancreas. Exp. Cell Res. *7*: 415–429 (1954).

31 Respiratory system

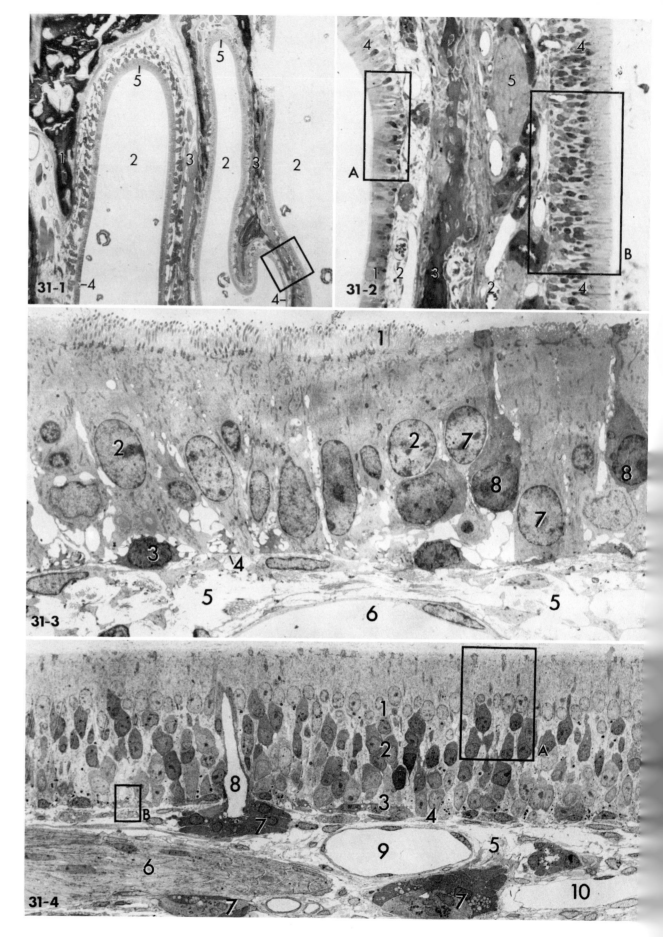

Fig. 31-1. Frontal section of olfactory region of the nasal cavity. Cat. L.M. X 25. **1.** Nasal septum. **2.** Nasal cavities. **3.** Nasal conchae (cat has several more than man). **4.** Respiratory epithelium. **5.** Olfactory epithelium.

Fig. 31-2. Section of nasal concha. Enlargement of rectangle in Fig. 31-1. Cat. L.M. X 235. **1.** Respiratory epithelium. **2.** Lamina propria. **3.** Bone. **4.** Olfactory epithelium. **5.** Olfactory nerve bundle.

Fig. 31-3. Transition between respiratory and olfactory epithelia. Enlargement of area similar to rectangle (A) in Fig. 31-2. Cat. E.M. X 1600. **1.** Cilia. **2.** Nuclei of ciliated cells in respiratory epithelium. **3.** Basal cell. **4.** Basal lamina. **5.** Lamina propria. **6.** Sinusoidal capillary. **7.** Nuclei of sustentacular cell in olfactory epithelium. **8.** Nuclei of olfactory bipolar nerve cells.

Fig. 31-4. Olfactory epithelium. Enlargement of area similar to rectangle (B) in Fig. 31-2. Cat. E.M. X 580. **1.** Level of nuclei of sustentacular cells. **2.** Nuclei of olfactory bipolar nerve cells. **3.** Basal cells. **4.** Level of basal lamina. **5.** Lamina propria. **6.** Olfactory nerve bundle. **7.** Bowman's glands. **8.** Lumen of excretory duct of Bowman's gland. **9.** Postcapillary venule. **10.** Lymphatic capillary.

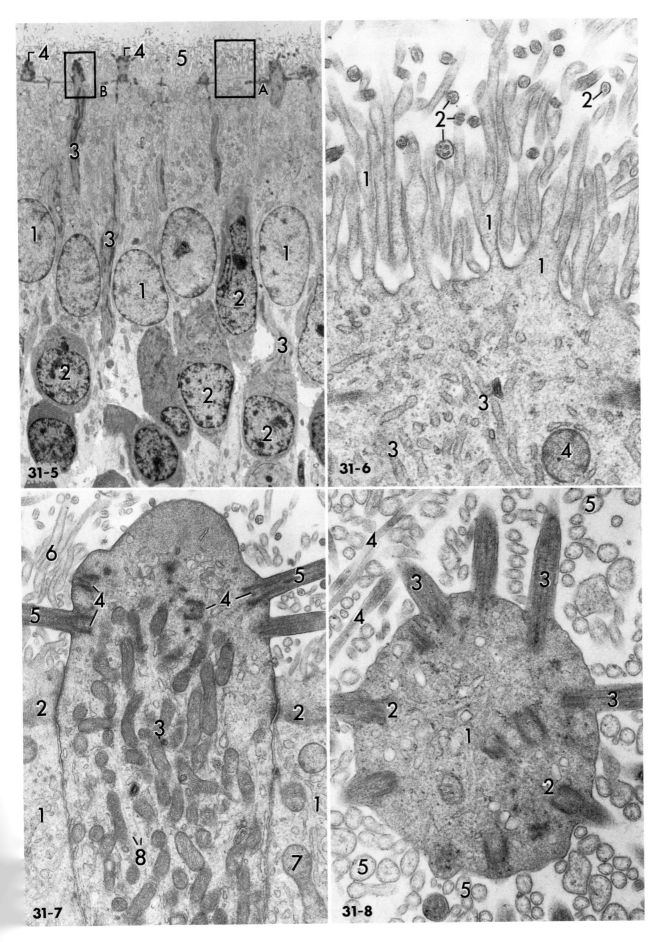

Fig. 31-5. Olfactory epithelium. Enlargement of area similar to rectangle (A) in Fig. 31-4. Cat. E.M. × 1900. **1.** Nuclei of sustentacular cells. **2.** Nuclei of olfactory bipolar nerve cells. **3.** Peripheral dendritic processes of olfactory bipolar nerve cells. **4.** Olfactory vesicle. **5.** Microvilli of sustentacular cells.

Fig. 31-6. Detail of free surface of sustentacular cell of olfactory epithelium. Enlargement of area similar to rectangle (A) in Fig. 31-5. Cat. E.M. × 80,000. **1.** Thin, branching microvilli. **2.** Cross-sectioned peripheral parts of cilia from adjacent olfactory bipolar nerve cells containing two or three microtubules. **3.** Profiles of agranular endoplasmic reticulum. **4.** Mitochondrion.

Fig. 31-7. Detail of olfactory vesicle. Enlargement of area similar to rectangle (B) in Fig. 31-5. Cat. E.M. × 48,000. **1.** Parts of sustentacular cells. **2.** Junctional complexes. **3.** Mitochondria in olfactory vesicle. **4.** Basal bodies. **5.** Olfactory cilia. **6.** Microvilli. **7.** Mitochondria in sustentacular cell. **8.** Microtubules.

Fig. 31-8. Cross section of olfactory vesicle (sectioned parallel to the epithelial surface). Rat. E.M. × 87,000. **1.** Center of olfactory vesicle. **2.** Basal bodies. **3.** Olfactory cilia **4.** Longitudinally sectioned peripheral parts of olfactory cilia from adjacent olfactory vesicles. **5.** Cross-sectioned microvilli ascending from sustentacular cells.

Fig. 31-9. Detail of basal part of olfactory epithelium. Enlargement of area similar to rectangle (B) in Fig. 31-4. Cat. E.M. X 39,000. **1.** Nucleus of olfactory bipolar nerve cell. **2.** Basal part of sustentacular cells. **3.** Tonofibrils. **4.** Central processes (axons) of bipolar nerve cells. **5.** Basal lamina. **6.** Bundle of olfactory nerves in lamina propria. **7.** Collagenous fibrils. **8.** Lipofuscin granules.

Fig. 31-10. Detail of basal part of olfactory epithelium. Enlargement of area similar to rectangle in Fig. 31-9. Cat. E.M. X 128,000. **1.** Cytoplasm of sustentacular cell. **2.** Cytoplasmic processes of basal cells. **3.** Cross-sectioned central processes (axons) of olfactory bipolar nerve cells. **4.** Microtubules. **5.** Mitochondria. **6.** Desmosomes. **7.** Basal lamina. **8.** Collagenous fibrils in lamina propria.

Fig. 31-11. Olfactory epithelium. Enlargement of duct of Bowman's gland seen in Fig. 31-4. Cat. E.M. X 1200. **1.** Lumen of duct. **2.** Nuclei of secretory cells of Bowman's gland. **3.** Nucleus of secretory duct cell. **4.** Nucleus of squamous duct cell. **5.** Nuclei of basal cells. **6.** Nuclei of olfactory bipolar nerve cells.

Fig. 31-12. Olfactory epithelium. Detail of Bowman's gland in lamina propria. Cat. E.M. X 25,000. **1.** Nuclei of serous cells. **2.** Nucleus of mucous cell. **3.** Mucous droplets. **4.** Discharging mucous droplets containing a dense granular substance. **5.** Lumen of gland. **6.** Golgi zone. **7.** Serous secretory granules. **8.** Granular endoplasmic reticulum. **9.** Agranular endoplasmic reticulum.

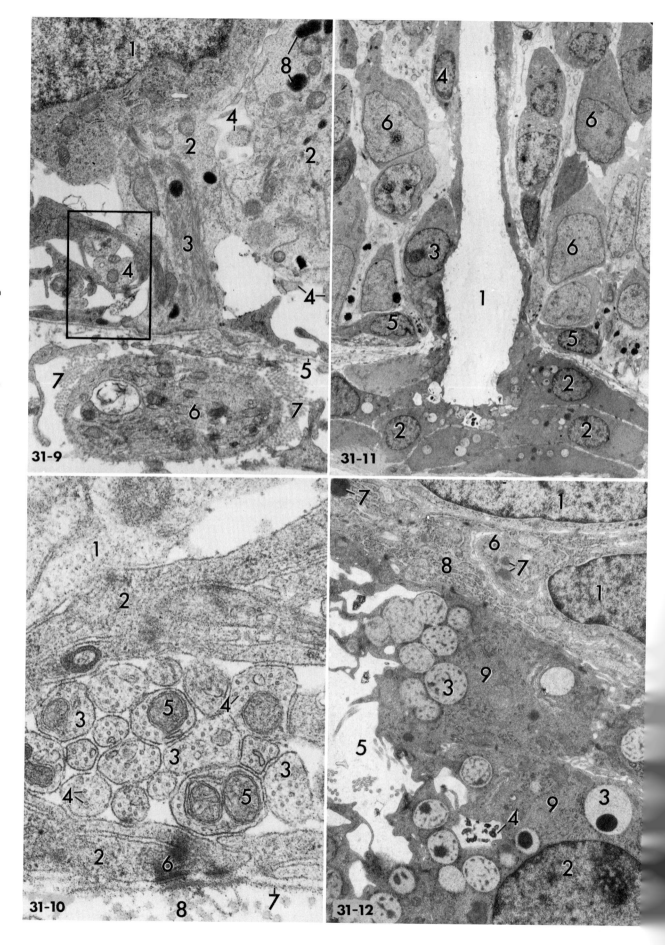

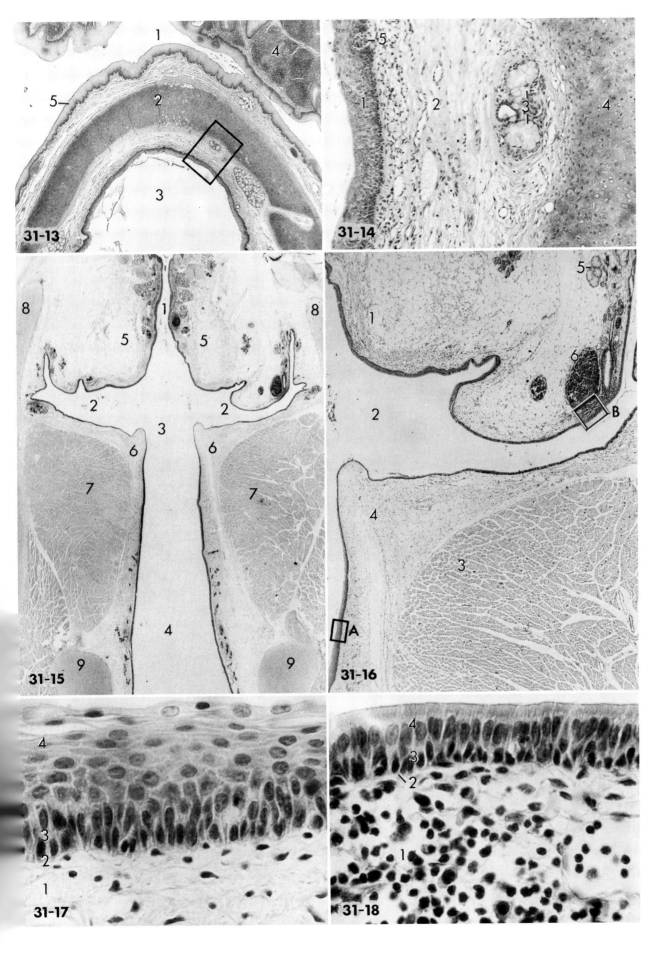

Fig. 31-13. Frontal section of epiglottis. Monkey. L.M. X 15. **1.** Hypopharynx. **2.** Cartilage of epiglottis. **3.** Vestibule of laryngeal cavity. **4.** Pharyngeal tonsils. **5.** Stratified squamous non-keratinized epithelium.

Fig. 31-14. Epiglottis. Enlargement of rectangle in Fig. 31-13. Monkey. L.M. X 105. **1.** Stratified squamous non-keratinized epithelium. **2.** Lamina propria with elastic fibers. **3.** Mucous glands. **4.** Elastic cartilage of epiglottis. **5.** Single taste bud.

Fig. 31-15. Frontal section of larynx. Monkey. L.M. X 10. **1.** Vestibule. **2.** Ventricles. **3.** Rima glottidis. **4.** Infraglottic cavity. **5.** Ventricular folds (false vocal cords). **6.** Vocal folds (true vocal cords). **7.** Vocal (thyroarytenoid) muscle. **8.** Thyroid cartilage. **9.** Cricoid cartilage.

Fig. 31-16. Enlargement of larynx in Fig. 31-15. Monkey. L.M. X 31. **1.** False cords. **2.** Laryngeal ventricle. **3.** Vocal muscle. **4.** Vocal ligament. **5.** Mucous glands. **6.** Lymph nodule.

Fig. 31-17. Stratified squamous non-keratinized epithelium. Vocal folds. Larynx. Enlargement of rectangle (A) in Fig. 31-16. Monkey. L.M. X 600. **1.** Lamina propria. **2.** Basal lamina. **3.** Stratum germinativum. **4.** Nuclei are retained in squamous superficial layers.

Fig. 31-18. Stratified or pseudostratified columnar epithelium. Ventricle of larynx. Enlargement of rectangle (B) in Fig. 31-16. Monkey. L.M. X 600. **1.** Diffuse lymphoid infiltration in lamina propria. **2.** Basal lamina. **3.** Basal cells. **4.** Columnar non-ciliated cells.

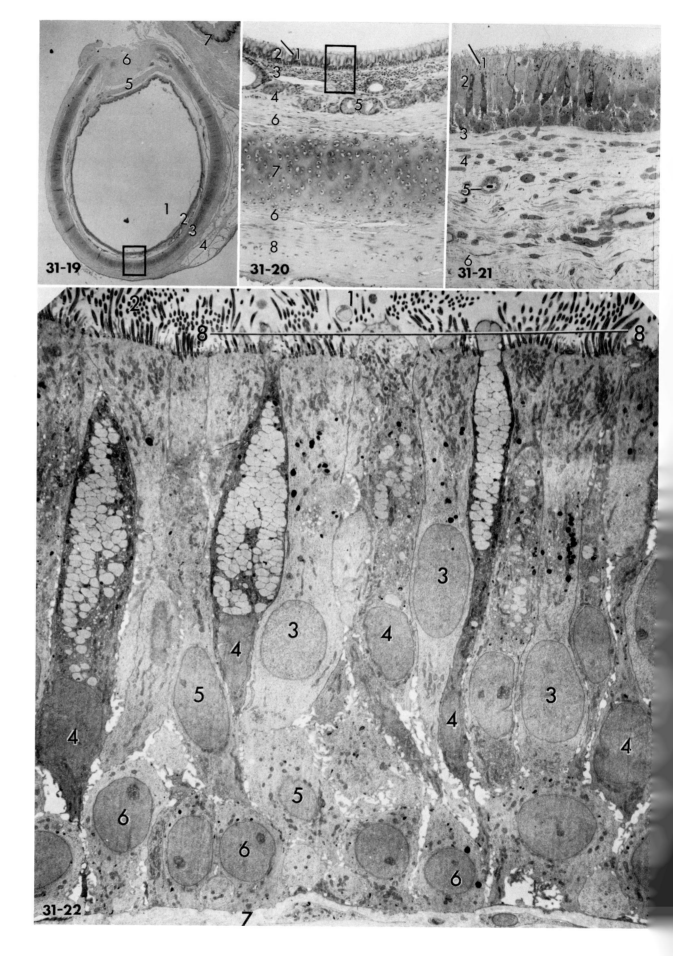

Fig. 31-19. Cross section of trachea. Monkey. L.M. X 10. **1.** Lumen. **2.** Mucous membrane. **3.** C-shaped cartilage. **4.** Adventitia. **5.** Trachealis muscle. **6.** Fibroelastic membrane. This part of the trachea faces posteriorly. **7.** Part of adjacent esophagus.

Fig. 31-20. Wall of trachea. Enlargement of area similar to rectangle in Fig. 31-19. Monkey. L.M. X 80. **1.** Lumen. **2.** Epithelium. **3.** Lamina propria. **4.** Submucosa. **5.** Mucous glands. **6.** Fibrous perichondrium. **7.** Hyaline tracheal cartilage. **8.** Outer fibroelastic membrane.

Fig. 31-21. Wall of trachea. Enlargement of area similar to rectangle in Fig. 31-20. Human. E.M. X 320. **1.** Lumen of trachea. **2.** Pseudostratified, columnar ciliated (respiratory) epithelium. **3.** Level of basement membrane. **4.** Lamina propria. **5.** Blood vessel. **6.** Submucosa.

Fig. 31-22. Pseudostratified, columnar ciliated (respiratory) epithelium. Trachea. Human. E.M. X 1800. **1.** Lumen of trachea. **2.** Cilia. **3.** Nuclei of ciliated cells. **4.** Nuclei of goblet (mucous) cells. **5.** Nuclei of intermediate cells. **6.** Nuclei of basal cells. **7.** Basement membrane. **8.** See Fig. 31-25.

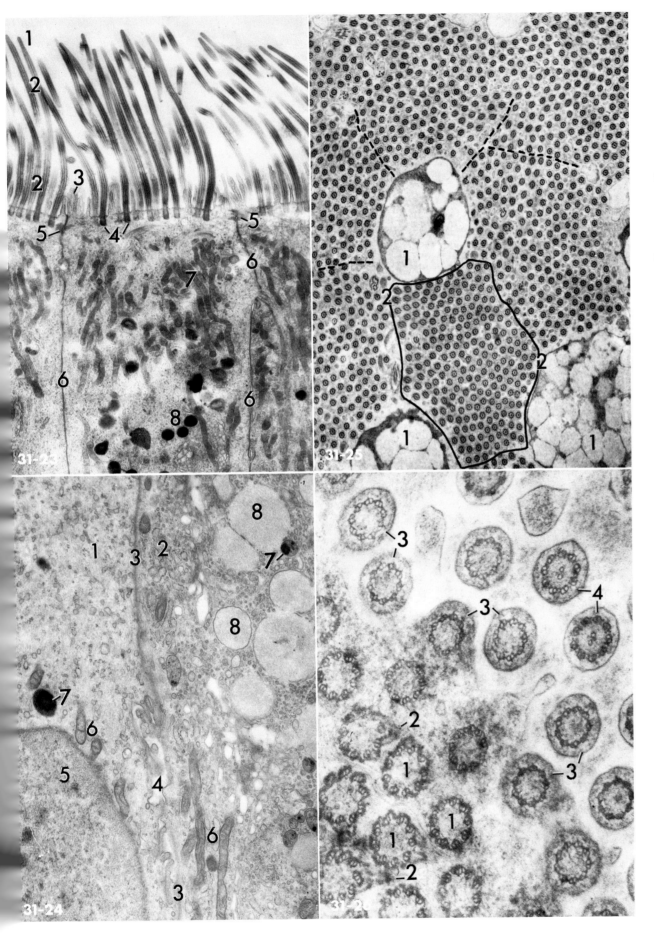

Fig. 31-23. Detail of free surface of ciliated cells. Respiratory epithelium. Trachea. Human. E.M. X 7000. **1.** Lumen. **2.** Cilia. **3.** Short microvilli. **4.** Basal bodies. **5.** Junctional complexes. **6.** Cell borders. **7.** Mitochondria. **8.** Lysosomes.

Fig. 31-24. Detail of respiratory epithelium Trachea. Human. E.M. X 15,000. **1.** Cytoplasm of ciliated cell. **2.** Cytoplasm of mucous (goblet) cell. **3.** Cell borders. **4.** Intercellular space. **5.** Nucleus. **6.** Mitochondria. **7.** Lysosomes.

Fig. 31-25. Cross section of cilia and mucous cells at the level indicated by line 8–8 in Fig. 31-22. Trachea. Human. E.M. X 15,000. **1.** Domes of mucous cells with secretory droplets, protruding above surface level of adjacent ciliated cells. **2.** The line indicates the group of cilia (about 250) that belongs to one ciliated cell. The demarcation lines of groups of cilia indicating other cells are more difficult to see. They are indicated by incompletely drawn dotted lines.

Fig. 31-26. Cross section of cilia and basal bodies. Respiratory epithelium. Trachea. Human. E.M. X 60,000. **1.** Basal bodies with 9 triplets of microtubules. **2.** Lateral spurs. **3.** At a level above the basal bodies, the 9 triplets become 9 doublets of microtubules. **4.** At a slightly higher level, a central pair of microtubules takes its origin and runs the entire length of the cilium.

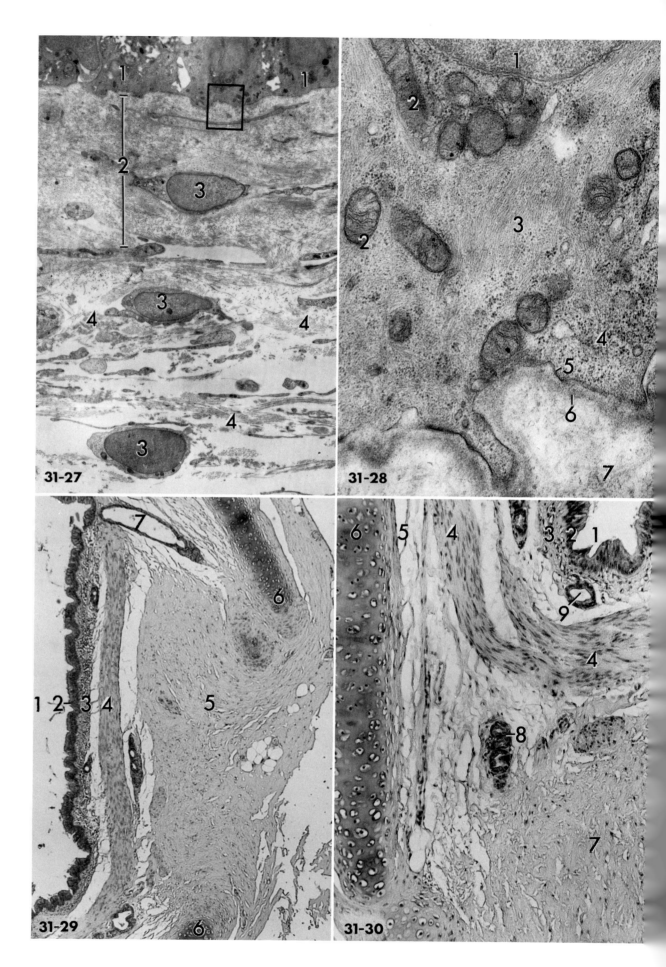

Fig. 31-27. Survey of basement membrane. Respiratory epithelium. Trachea. Human. E.M. X 3000. **1.** Basal cells of pseudostratified columnar ciliated (respiratory) epithelium. **2.** Basement membrane is made up of densely packed fine collagenous fibrils. **3.** Nuclei of fibroblasts. **4.** Loose connective tissue of lamina propria.

Fig. 31-28. Detail of basal cell. Respiratory epithelium. Trachea. Enlargement of area similar to rectangle in Fig. 31-27. Human. E.M. X 30,000. **1.** Nucleus of basal cell. **2.** Mitochondria. **3.** Tonofilaments. **4.** Ribosomes. **5.** Basal cell membrane. **6.** Basal lamina forms a thin part of the basement membrane of the respiratory epithelium. **7.** Delicate collagenous fibrils of basement membrane.

Fig. 31-29. Posterior wall of trachea. Cross section. Monkey. L.M. X 56. **1.** Lumen of trachea. **2.** Respiratory epithelium. **3.** Lamina propria. **4.** Trachealis muscle. **5.** Fibroelastic membrane. **6.** Free ends of C-shaped tracheal cartilage. **7.** Excretory duct of tracheal glands.

Fig. 31-30. Detail of posterior wall of trachea. Monkey. L.M. X 120. **1.** Lumen of trachea. **2.** Respiratory epithelium. **3.** Lamina propria. **4.** Trachealis muscle. **5.** Perichondrium. **6.** Tracheal cartilage (hyaline). **7.** Fibroelastic membrane. **8.** Serous glands. **9.** Excretory duct.

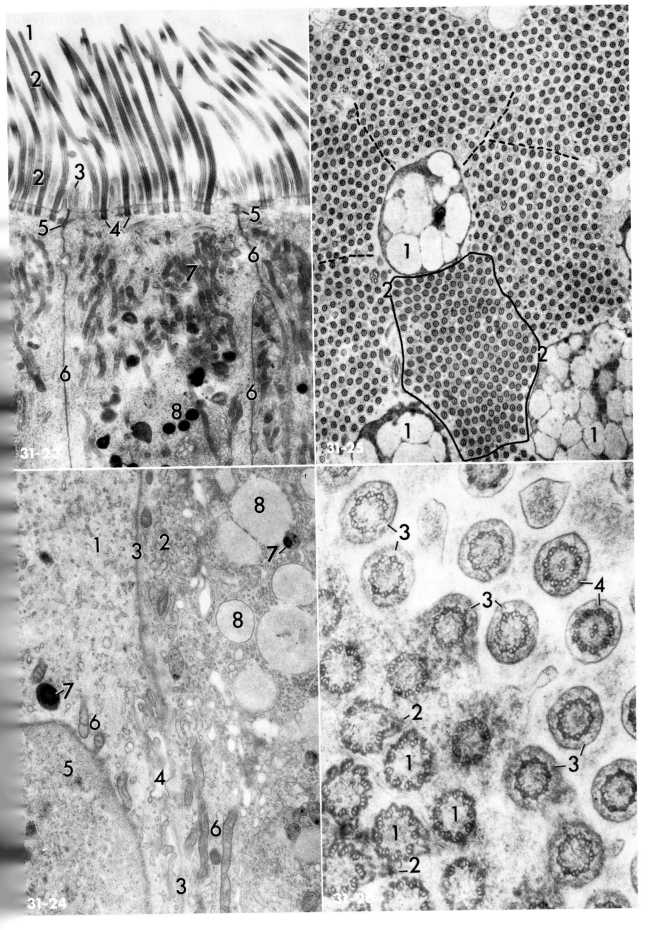

Fig. 31-23. Detail of free surface of ciliated cells. Respiratory epithelium. Trachea. Human. E.M. X 7000. **1.** Lumen. **2.** Cilia. **3.** Short microvilli. **4.** Basal bodies. **5.** Junctional complexes. **6.** Cell borders. **7.** Mitochondria. **8.** Lysosomes.

Fig. 31-24. Detail of respiratory epithelium Trachea. Human. E.M. X 15,000. **1.** Cytoplasm of ciliated cell. **2.** Cytoplasm of mucous (goblet) cell. **3.** Cell borders. **4.** Intercellular space. **5.** Nucleus. **6.** Mitochondria. **7.** Lysosomes.

Fig. 31-25. Cross section of cilia and mucous cells at the level indicated by line 8—8 in Fig. 31-22. Trachea. Human. E.M. X 15,000. **1.** Domes of mucous cells with secretory droplets, protruding above surface level of adjacent ciliated cells. **2.** The line indicates the group of cilia (about 250) that belongs to one ciliated cell. The demarcation lines of groups of cilia indicating other cells are more difficult to see. They are indicated by incompletely drawn dotted lines.

Fig. 31-26. Cross section of cilia and basal bodies. Respiratory epithelium. Trachea. Human. E.M. X 60,000. **1.** Basal bodies with 9 triplets of microtubules. **2.** Lateral spurs. **3.** At a level above the basal bodies, the 9 triplets become 9 doublets of microtubules. **4.** At a slightly higher level, a central pair of microtubules takes its origin and runs the entire length of the cilium.

Fig. 31-27. Survey of basement membrane. Respiratory epithelium. Trachea. Human. E.M. X 3000. **1.** Basal cells of pseudostratified columnar ciliated (respiratory) epithelium. **2.** Basement membrane is made up of densely packed fine collagenous fibrils. **3.** Nuclei of fibroblasts. **4.** Loose connective tissue of lamina propria.

Fig. 31-28. Detail of basal cell. Respiratory epithelium. Trachea. Enlargement of area similar to rectangle in Fig. 31-27. Human. E.M. X 30,000. **1.** Nucleus of basal cell. **2.** Mitochondria. **3.** Tonofilaments. **4.** Ribosomes. **5.** Basal cell membrane. **6.** Basal lamina forms a thin part of the basement membrane of the respiratory epithelium. **7.** Delicate collagenous fibrils of basement membrane.

Fig. 31-29. Posterior wall of trachea. Cross section. Monkey. L.M. X 56. **1.** Lumen of trachea. **2.** Respiratory epithelium. **3.** Lamina propria. **4.** Trachealis muscle. **5.** Fibroelastic membrane. **6.** Free ends of C-shaped tracheal cartilage. **7.** Excretory duct of tracheal glands.

Fig. 31-30. Detail of posterior wall of trachea. Monkey. L.M. X 120. **1.** Lumen of trachea. **2.** Respiratory epithelium. **3.** Lamina propria. **4.** Trachealis muscle. **5.** Perichondrium. **6.** Tracheal cartilage (hyaline). **7.** Fibroelastic membrane. **8.** Serous glands. **9.** Excretory duct.

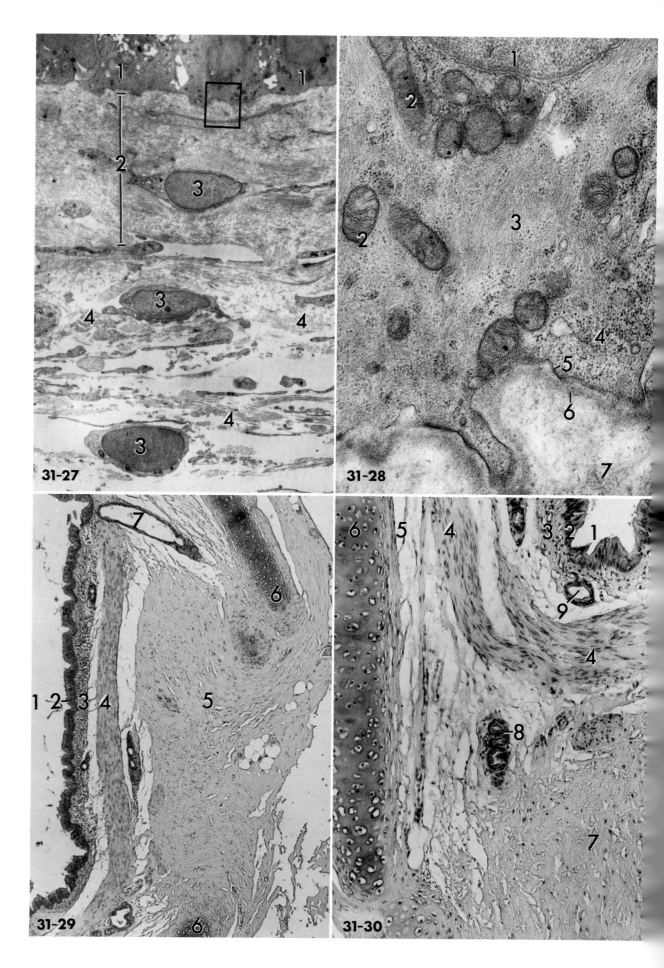

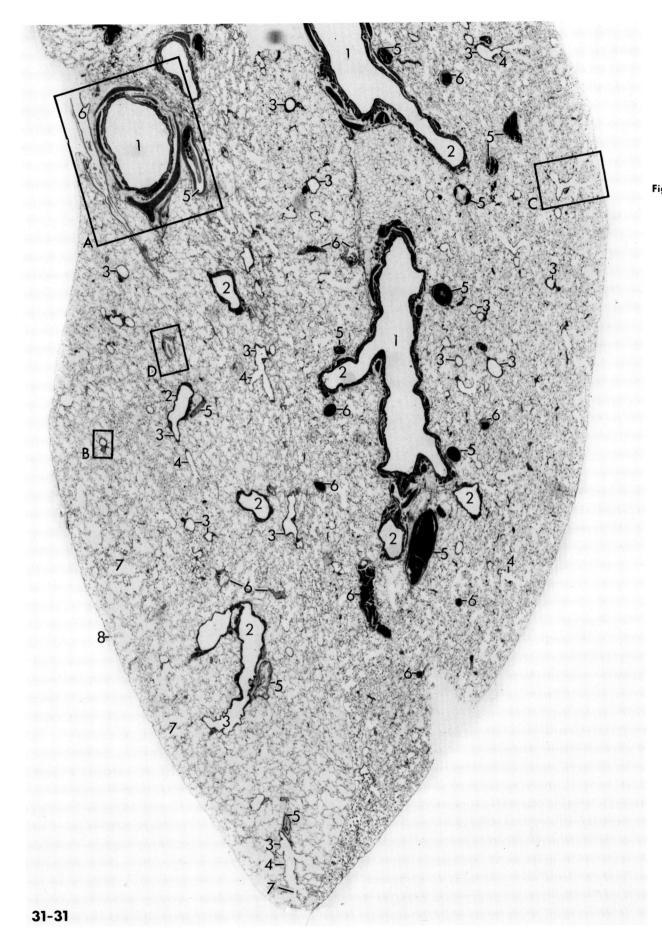

Fig. 31-31. Survey of lung. Monkey. L.M. X 7.
1. Secondary bronchi. **2.** Tertiary bronchi and their subdivisions. **3.** Bronchioles.
4. Respiratory bronchioles. **5.** Branches of pulmonary artery. **6.** Branches of pulmonary vein. **7.** Alveolar ducts and alveoli.
8. Pleura visceralis. *Rectangles:* **A** is enlarged in Fig. 31-32. **B** is enlarged in Fig. 31-38; it contains a bronchiole and a branch of the pulmonary artery. **C** is enlarged in Fig. 31-41; it contains bronchioles, respiratory bronchioles, alveolar ducts, and alveoli. **D** is enlarged in Fig. 31-62; it contains a branch of the pulmonary vein.

31-31

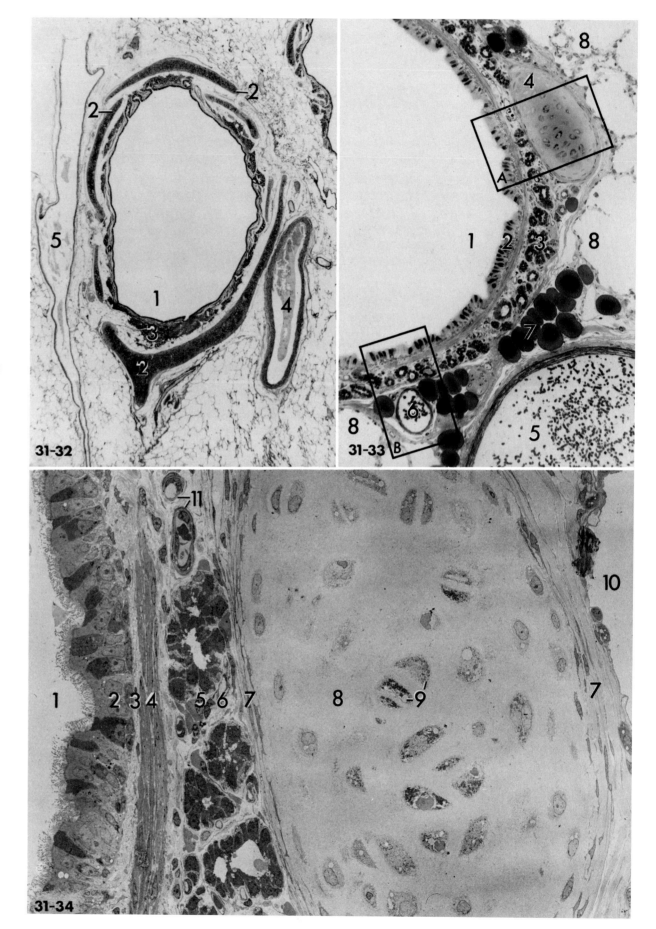

Fig. 31-32. Cross section of secondary bronchus. Enlargement of rectangle (A) in Fig. 31-31. Monkey. L.M. X 16. **1.** Lumen of bronchus, 4 mm wide. **2.** Cartilage. **3.** Bronchial glands. **4.** Pulmonary artery. **5.** Pulmonary vein.

Fig. 31-33. Cross section of tertiary bronchus (or ramification thereof). Cat. L.M. X 120. **1.** Lumen of bronchus, 0.9 mm wide. **2.** Mucous membrane. **3.** Bronchial glands. **4.** Bronchial cartilage. **5.** Branch of pulmonary artery. **6.** Bronchial artery. **7.** Fat cells. **8.** Alveoli.

Fig. 31-34. Detail of wall of tertiary bronchus. Enlargement of rectangle (A) in Fig. 31-33. Cat. E.M. X 590. **1.** Lumen. **2.** Pseudostratified columnar ciliated (respiratory) epithelium. **3.** Narrow lamina propria. **4.** Bronchial muscle. **5.** Glands. **6.** Submucosa. **7.** Perichondrium. **8.** Matrix of hyaline cartilage. **9.** Chondrocytes. **10.** Pulmonary alveoli. **11.** Arterioles in submucosa.

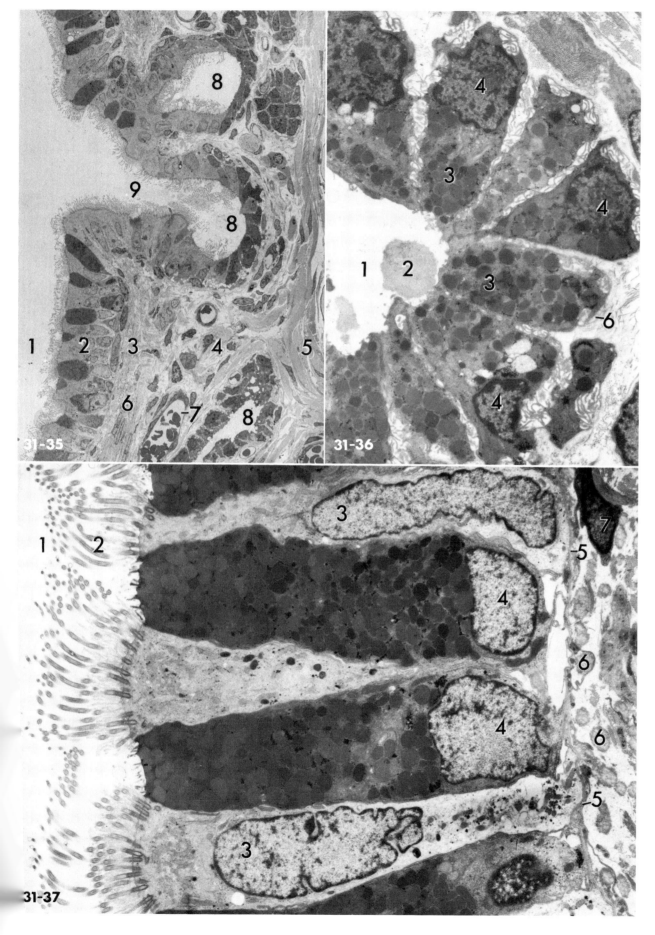

Fig. 31-35. Wall of tertiary bronchus. Lung. Cat. E.M. X 590. **1.** Lumen of bronchus. **2.** Pseudostratified columnar ciliated epithelium. **3.** Lamina propria. **4.** Submucosa. **5.** Adventitia with dense connective tissue. **6.** Edge of bronchial smooth muscle, interrupted by excretory ducts. **7.** Venule. **8.** Acini of mixed glands. **9.** Excretory ducts of serous and mucous bronchial glands.

Fig. 31-36. Detail of bronchial gland. Tertiary bronchus. Cat. E.M. × 4400. **1.** Lumen of gland. **2.** Discharged mucus. **3.** Intracellular mucous droplets. **4.** Nuclei of mucous cells. **5.** Intercellular space with narrow lateral cell processes. **6.** Thin basal lamina.

Fig. 31-37. Detail of simple columnar ciliated epithelium of small bronchus. Cat. E.M. X 4800. **1.** Lumen. **2.** Cilia. **3.** Nuclei of ciliated cells. **4.** Nuclei of mucous cells. **5.** Basal lamina. **6.** Cross-sectioned elastic fibers of lamina propria. **7.** Nucleus of fibroblast.

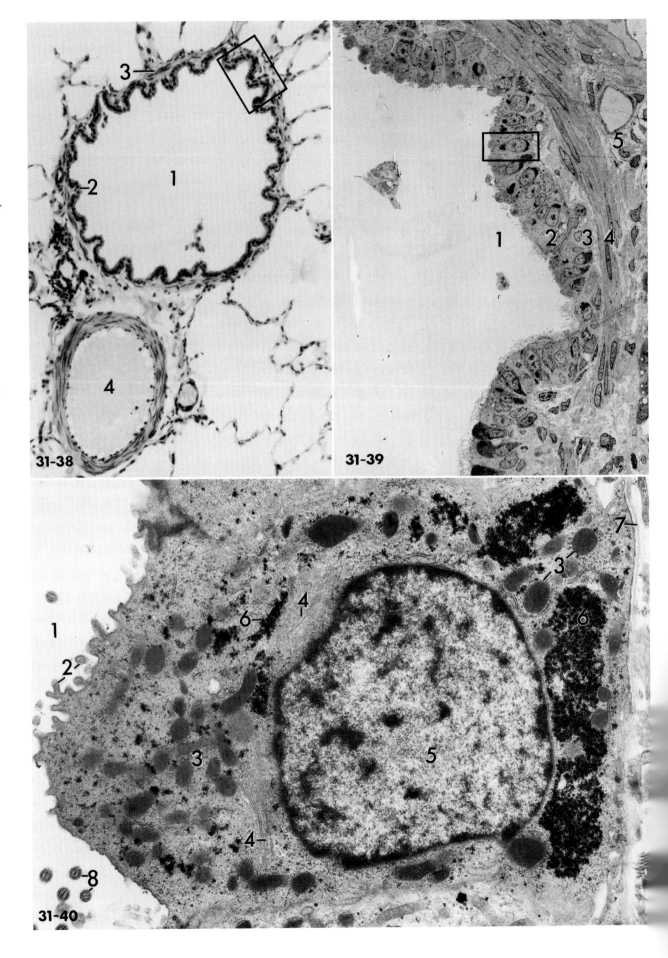

Fig. 31-38. Bronchiole and pulmonary artery. Enlargement of rectangle (B) in Fig. 31-31. Monkey. L.M. X 185. **1.** Bronchiole, lumen 300 μ (0.3 mm) wide. **2.** Epithelium, its scalloped appearance caused by slightly contracted bronchial muscle. Note the absence of cartilage in the bronchiolar wall. **3.** Bronchiolar smooth muscle. **4.** Branch of pulmonary artery, lumen 120 μ wide.

Fig. 31-39. Part of bronchiole. Enlargement of area similar to rectangle in Fig. 31-38. Cat. E.M. X 600. **1.** Lumen 200 μ wide. **2.** Simple low columnar respiratory epithelium with several ciliated cells, many Clara cells, and occasional mucous cells. **3.** Lamina propria. **4.** Bronchiolar smooth muscle. **5.** Submucosa.

Fig. 31-40. Clara cell. Respiratory epithelium. Bronchiole. Enlargement of area similar to rectangle in Fig. 31-39. Cat. E.M. X 10,000. **1.** Lumen. **2.** Microvilli. **3.** Mitochondria. **4.** Small Golgi areas. **5.** Nucleus. **6.** Accumulations of particulate glycogen. **7.** Basal lamina. **8.** Cilia of adjacent ciliated cell.

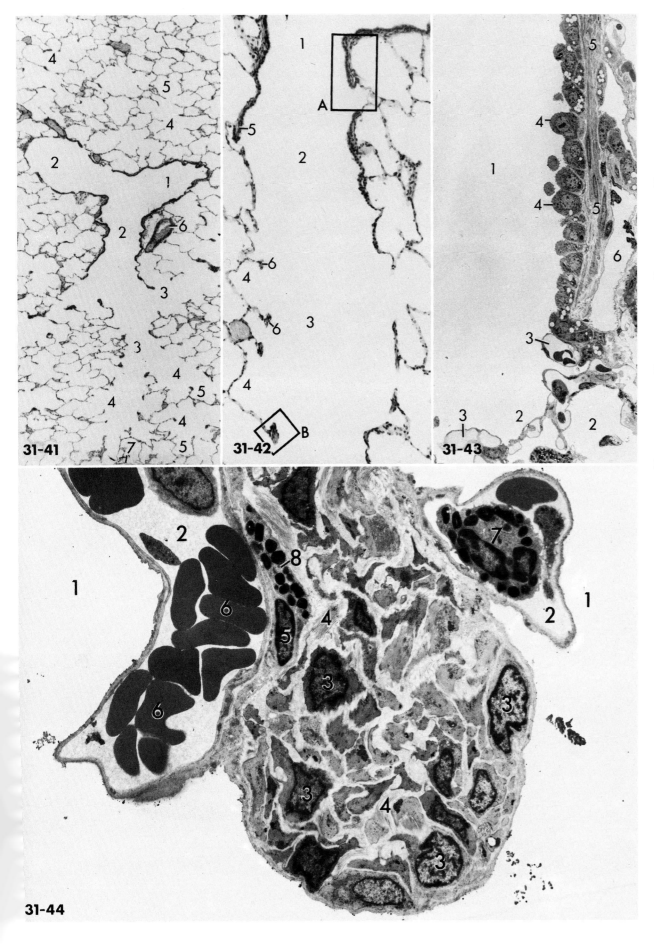

Fig. 31-41. Terminal ramification of air passages. Lung. Enlargement of rectangle (C) in Fig. 31-31. Monkey. L.M. X 40. **1.** Terminal bronchiole. **2.** Respiratory bronchioles. **3.** Alveolar ducts. **4.** Alveolar sacs. **5.** Alveoli. **6.** Branch of pulmonary artery. **7.** Visceral pleura.

Fig. 31-42. Detail of terminal air passages. Lung. Monkey. L.M. X 110. **1.** Terminal bronchiole. **2.** Respiratory bronchiole. **3.** Alveolar duct. **4.** Alveoli. **5.** Wall of respiratory bronchiole. **6.** Knob-like swelling at the entrance to alveolus of an alveolar duct.

Fig. 31-43. Wall of respiratory bronchiole. Lung. Enlargement of area similar to rectangle (A) in Fig. 31-42. Cat. E.M. X 600. **1.** Lumen of respiratory bronchiole. **2.** Alveoli. **3.** Alveolar capillaries. **4.** Clara cells make up the simple cuboidal epithelium. **5.** Bronchiolar smooth muscle cells. **6.** Lymphatic capillary.

Fig. 31-44. Knob-like swelling at the entrance to alveolus of an alveolar duct. Enlargement of area similar to rectangle (B) in Fig. 31-42. Cat. E.M. X 3000. **1.** Alveoli. **2.** Pulmonary capillaries. **3.** The knob-like swelling contains smooth muscle cells. **4.** Bundles of collagen. **5.** Occasional fibroblasts. **6.** Erythrocytes. **7.** Leukocyte in capillary. **8.** Leukocyte in connective tissue.

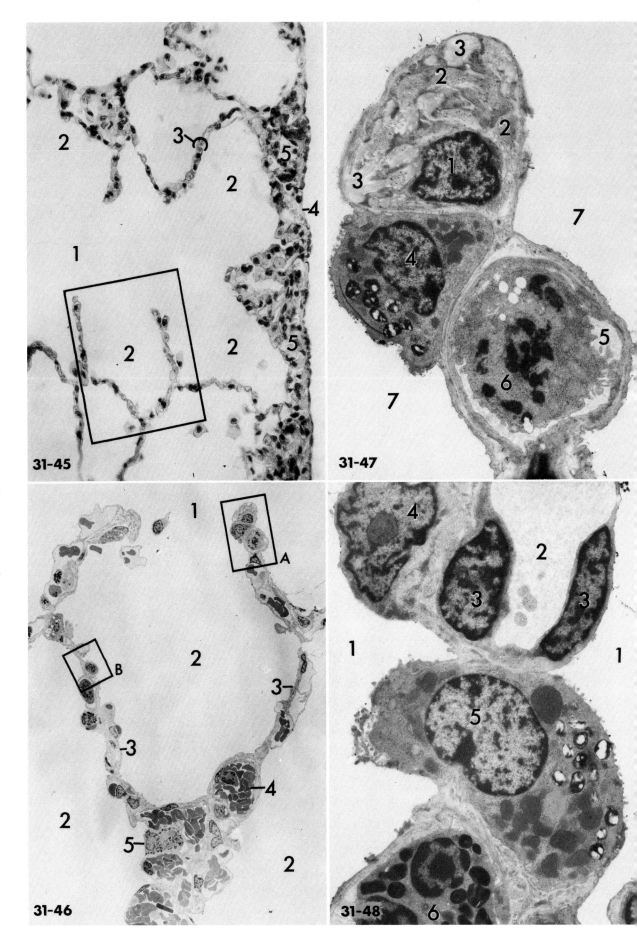

Fig. 31-45. Pulmonary alveoli. Lung. Monkey. L.M. X 290. **1.** Alveolar sac. **2.** Alveoli. **3.** Alveolar septum (wall). **4.** Visceral pleura. **5.** Subpleural connective tissue.

Fig. 31-46. Survey of pulmonary alveolus. Lung. Enlargement of area similar to rectangle in Fig. 31-45. Cat. E.M. X 440. **1.** Entrance to pulmonary alveolus (atrium). **2.** Center of pulmonary alveoli. **3.** Alveolar septa with pulmonary capillaries. **4.** Pulmonary venule. **5.** Alveolar phagocyte in a niche of alveolar septum.

Fig. 31-47. Edge of entrance to pulmonary alveolus. Lung. Enlargement of rectangle (A) in Fig. 31-46. Cat. E.M. X 4000. **1.** Nucleus of fibroblast in core of alveolar edge. **2.** Bundles of collagenous fibrils. **3.** Elastic fibers. **4.** Nucleus of great alveolar cell (type II cell). **5.** Lumen of pulmonary capillary. **6.** Lymphocyte in mitosis. **7.** Pulmonary alveoli.

Fig. 31-48. Detail of alveolar septum. Lung. Enlargement of area similar to rectangle (B) in Fig. 31-46. Cat. E.M. X 5400. **1.** Pulmonary alveoli. **2.** Lumen of pulmonary capillary. **3.** Nuclei of capillary endothelial cells. **4.** Nucleus of squamous alveolar cell (type I cell). **5.** Nucleus of great alveolar cell. This particular cell borders on both pulmonary alveoli. **6.** Leukocyte in lumen of pulmonary capillary.

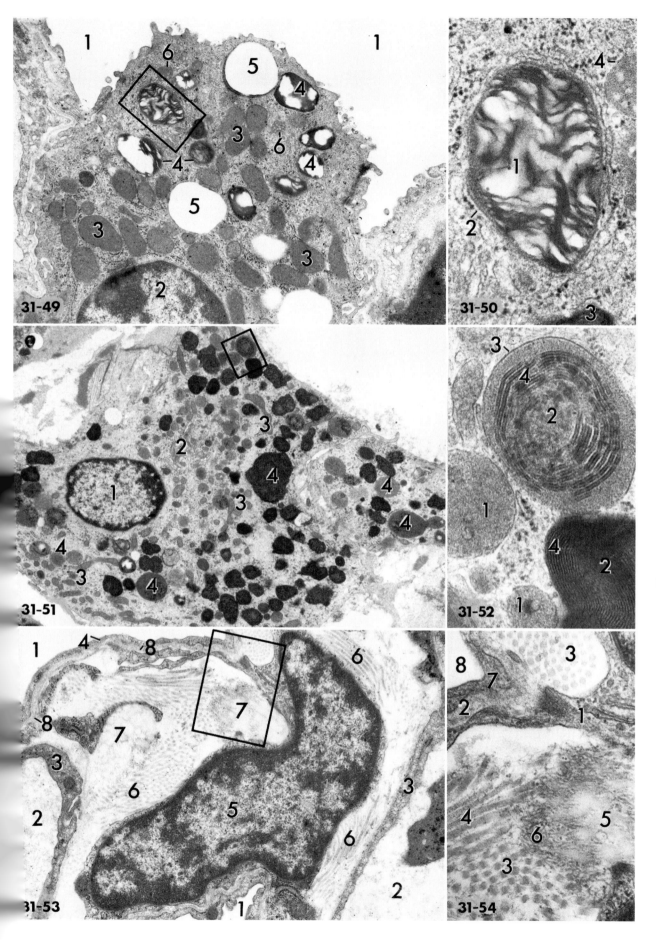

Fig. 31-49. Detail of great alveolar cell. Lung. Cat. E.M. X 25,000. **1.** Pulmonary alveolus. **2.** Nucleus of great alveolar cell. **3.** Mitochondria. **4.** Lamellar bodies. **5.** Lipid droplets. **6.** Multivesicular bodies.

Fig. 31-50. Lamellar body. Enlargement of rectangle in Fig. 31-49. Cat. E.M. X 85,000. **1.** Typical appearance of lamellar body in the great alveolar cell of the pulmonary alveoli. The electron-lucent areas have probably been dissolved during preparation. **2.** 40 Å-thick trilaminar boundary membrane. **3.** Part of early lamellar body. **4.** Part of multivesicular body.

Fig. 31-51. Alveolar phagocyte in pulmonary alveolus. Cat. E.M. × 4400. **1.** Nucleus **2.** Golgi region. **3.** Mitochondria. **4.** Numerous primary and secondary lysosomes.

Fig. 31-52. Lysosomes. Enlargement of rectangle in Fig. 31-51. Cat. E.M. X 58,000. **1.** Primary lysosomes. **2.** Secondary lysosomes. **3.** Trilaminar boundary membrane. **4.** Lipoprotein layering.

Fig. 31-53. Detail of connective tissue core of the alveolar septum. Lung. Cat. E.M. X 20,000. **1.** Alveolar lumen. **2.** Capillary lumen. **3.** Capillary endothelium. **4.** Alveolar epithelium. **5.** Nucleus of fibroblast (septal cell). **6.** Collagenous fibrils. **7.** Elastic fibers. **8.** Basal lamina.

Fig. 31-54. Enlargement of rectangle in Fig. 31-53. E.M. X 53,000. **1.** Cytoplasmic strand of fibroblast. **2.** Basal lamina. **3.** Cross-sectioned collagenous fibrils. **4.** Longitudinal section of collagenous fibrils. **5.** Amorphous part of elastic fiber. **6.** Filamentous part of elastic fiber. **7.** Alveolar epithelium. **8.** Alveolar lumen.

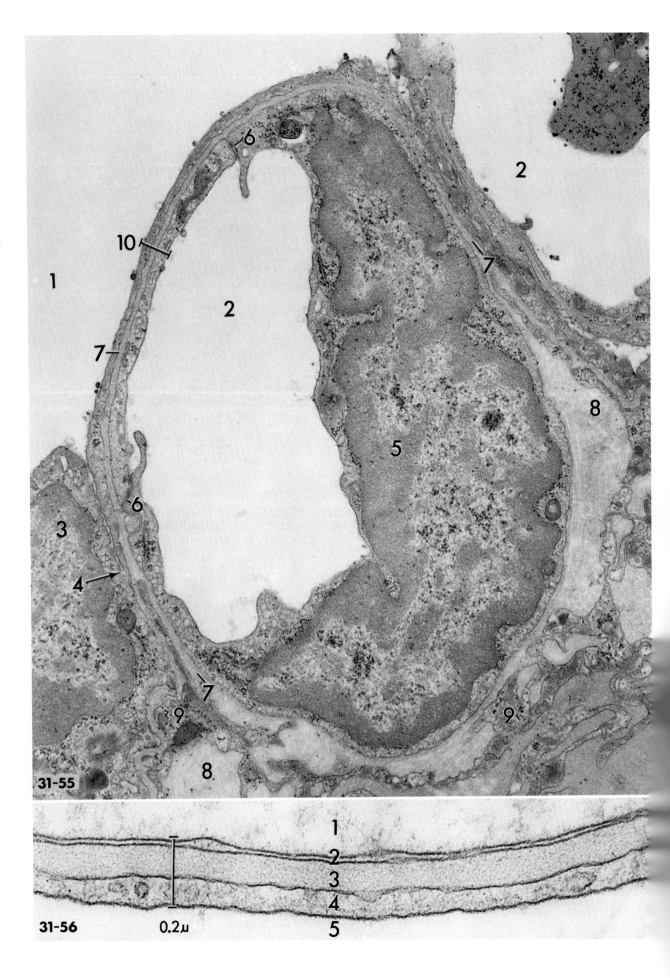

Fig. 31-55. Pulmonary capillary. Rat. E.M. X 23,000. **1.** Pulmonary alveolus. **2.** Lumina of capillaries. **3.** Nucleus of squamous alveolar cell (type I cell). **4.** Arrow marks point where the squamous cytoplasm of type I cell begins its stretch around the pulmonary capillary. **5.** Nucleus of capillary endothelial cell. **6.** Junctions of strands of endothelial cytoplasm. **7.** Basal lamina. **8.** Collagenous fibrils in connective tissue core of alveolar septum. **9.** Thin cytoplasmic strands of fibroblasts. **10.** Blood-air barrier (0.2–0.3 μ).

Fig. 31-56. Detail of blood-air barrier (0.2 μ). Lung. Mouse. E.M. X 84,000. **1.** Lumen of pulmonary capillary. **2.** Thin sheet of endothelial cytoplasm (200 Å). **3.** Basal lamina (900 Å). **4.** Thin sheet of squamous alveolar epithelial cell (900 Å). **5.** Pulmonary alveolus.

31-55

31-56   0.2μ

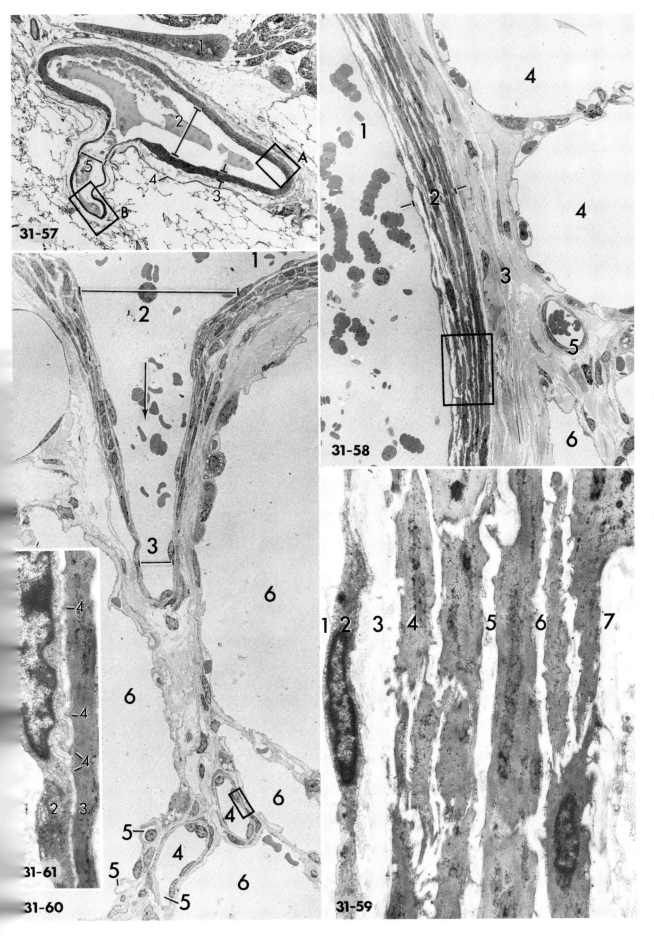

Fig. 31-57. Pulmonary artery. Same artery as that in Fig. 31-32, several sections deeper. Lung. Monkey. L.M. X 25. **1.** Cartilage of nearby bronchus. **2.** Lumen of artery, 565 μ wide at site indicated. **3.** Thickness of arterial wall (intima and media) is 70 μ. **4.** Adventitia. **5.** Branch of pulmonary artery, 265 μ wide at site indicated.

Fig. 31-58. Branch of pulmonary artery, mostly muscular type. Enlargement of area similar to rectangle (A) in Fig. 31-57. Cat. E.M. X 620. **1.** Lumen of artery, 640 μ wide. **2.** Thickness of arterial wall (intima and media) is 20 μ. **3.** Dense connective tissue adventitia. **4.** Pulmonary alveoli. **5.** Venule. **6.** Lymphatic vessel.

Fig. 31-59. Wall of pulmonary artery. Enlargement of area similar to rectangle in Fig. 31-58. Cat. E.M. X 8300. **1.** Lumen of artery, 640 μ wide. **2.** Nucleus of endothelial cell. **3.** Internal elastic membrane. **4.** Smooth muscle cells. **5.** Central elastic membrane. **6.** Mostly collagenous fibrils in the narrow intermuscular spaces. **7.** External elastic membrane.

Fig. 31-60. Terminal ramifications of pulmonary artery. Enlargement of area similar to rectangle (B) in Fig. 31-57. Cat. E.M. X 670. **1.** Lumen of pulmonary artery, 360 μ wide. **2.** Branch of pulmonary artery, entrance of which is 68 μ wide at site indicated by bar. **3.** The branch rapidly decreases in size and the lumen of the pulmonary arteriole is 13 μ at site indicated by bar. Observe the gradual reduction in number of smooth muscle layers with decreasing luminal diameter. Arrow indicates direction of blood flow. **4.** Terminal arterioles, luminal diameter averaging 10 μ. **5.** Pulmonary capillaries. **6.** Alveoli.

Fig. 31-61. Enlargement of area similar to rectangle in Fig. 31-60. Cat. E.M. X 13,000. **1.** Lumen. **2.** Endothelium. **3.** Smooth muscle cell. **4.** Myoendothelial junctions.

Fig. 31-62. Branch of pulmonary vein. Enlargement of rectangle (D) in Fig. 31-31. Monkey. L.M. X 30. **1.** Branch of pulmonary vein. These vessels always occur singly in the pulmonary tissue. **2.** Alveolar ducts. **3.** Alveolar sacs.

Fig. 31-63. Enlargement of pulmonary vein in Fig. 31-61. Monkey. L.M. X 89. **1.** Lumen, 500 μ wide at site indicated. **2.** Thickness of venous wall (intima and media) is 12 μ. **3.** Adventitia and perivascular loose connective tissue. **4.** Pulmonary alveoli.

Fig. 31-64. Detail of branch of pulmonary vein. Enlargement of area similar to rectangle in Fig. 31-63. Cat. E.M. X 600. **1.** Lumen, 400 μ wide. **2.** Endothelial cells. **3.** Media consists of scattered smooth muscle cells. **4.** Adventitia with dense connective tissue. **5.** Lymphoid infiltration in perivascular loose connective tissue. **6.** Pulmonary alveoli.

Fig. 31-65. Wall of pulmonary vein. Enlargement of area similar to rectangle in Fig. 31-64. Cat. E.M. X 12,000. **1.** Lumen, 400 μ wide. **2.** Nucleus of endothelial cell. **3.** Fine collagenous and reticular fibrils. Note the absence of basal lamina and internal elastic membrane. **4.** Nucleus of smooth muscle cell. **5.** Bundles of medium-size collagenous fibrils. **6.** Elastic fibers form an incomplete outer elastic membrane. **7.** Myoendothelial junction.

Fig. 31-66. Wall of pulmonary vein. Enlargement of area similar to rectangle in Fig. 31-65. Rat. E.M. X 47,000. **1.** Smooth muscle cell with myofilaments sectioned longitudinally. **2.** Endothelial cell. **3.** Myoendothelial junction. In rat pulmonary veins these junctions continue for up to 20 μ or more without an interposed basal lamina. **4.** Specific endothelial granules. **5.** Mitochondrion. **6.** Granular endoplasmic reticulum. **7.** Pinocytotic vesicles. **8.** Lumen of pulmonary vein.

Fig. 31-67. Specific endothelial granules. Pulmonary vein. Rat. E.M. X 120,000. **1.** Core of granule, finely stippled. In some species, this core may contain microtubules. See Fig. 2-57 (p. 35). **2.** Single boundary membrane.

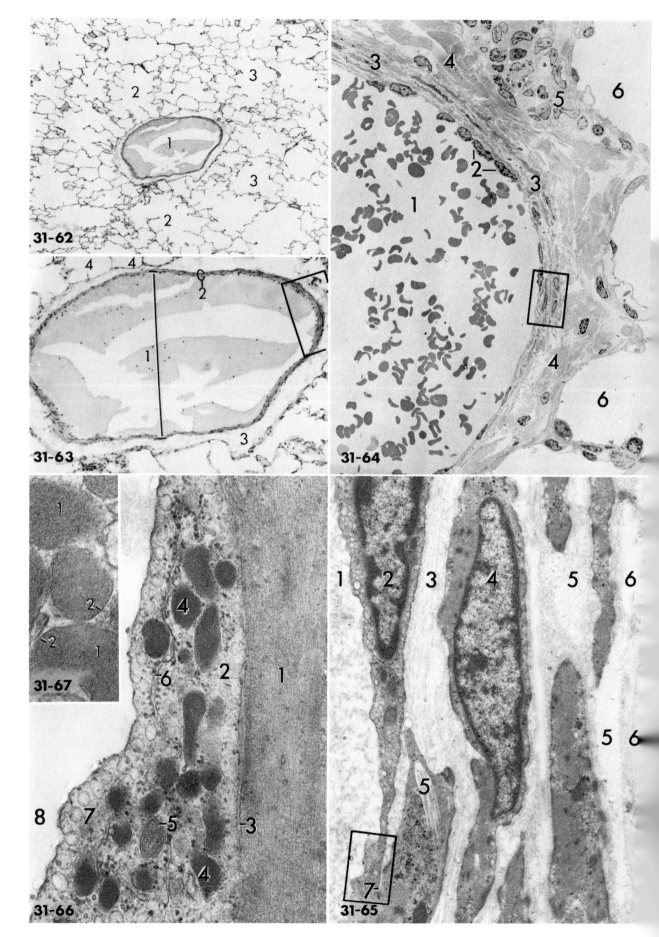

364

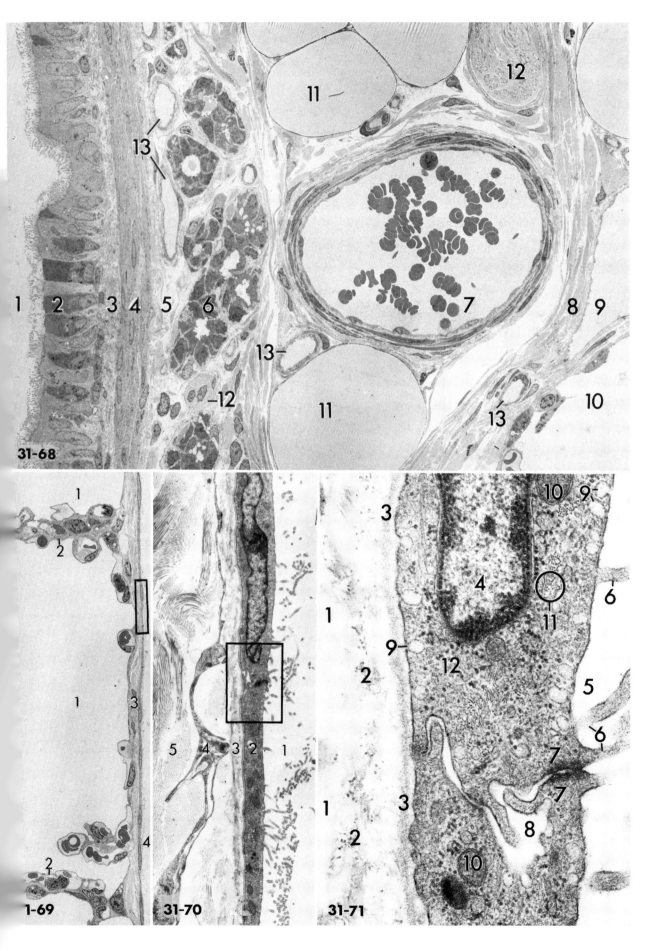

Fig. 31-68. Survey of peribronchial space. Tertiary bronchus. Enlargement of rectangle (B) in Fig. 31-33. Cat. E.M. X 700. **1.** Lumen of bronchus. **2.** Pseudostratified columnar ciliated (respiratory) epithelium. **3.** Lamina propria. **4.** Bronchial smooth muscle. **5.** Submucosa. **6.** Mixed (seromucous) bronchial glands. **7.** Lumen of bronchial arteriole, 70 μ wide. **8.** Peribronchial dense connective tissue. **9.** Lymphatic vessel. **10.** Pulmonary alveolus. **11.** Fat cells. **12.** Non-myelinated nerve bundle. **13.** Blood capillaries.

Fig. 31-69. Periphery of lung. Cat. E.M. X 580. **1.** Pulmonary alveoli. **2.** Alveolar septa. **3.** Visceral pleura. **4.** Pleural cavity.

Fig. 31-70. Visceral pleura. Enlargement of area similar to rectangle in Fig. 31-69. Cat. E.M. X 4500. **1.** Pleural cavity. **2.** Mesothelial cell with numerous microvilli. **3.** Elastic membrane. **4.** Cytoplasmic strands of fibroblasts. **5.** Bundles of collagenous fibrils.

Fig. 31-71. Pleural mesothelium. Enlargement of area similar to rectangle in Fig. 31-70. Cat. E.M. X 60,000. **1.** Amorphous part of elastic membrane. **2.** Filamentous part of elastic membrane. **3.** Basal lamina. **4.** Nucleus of mesothelial cell. **5.** Pleural cavity. **6.** Microvilli. **7.** Junctional complex. **8.** Intercellular space. **9.** Micropinocytotic vesicles. **10.** Mitochondria. **11.** Tonofilaments. **12.** Ribosomes.

References

NASAL CAVITY

Adams, D. R. Olfactory and non-olfactory epithelia in the nasal cavity of the mouse. Am. J. Anat. *133*: 37–50 (1972).

Andres, K. H. Der Feinbau der Regio olfactoria von Makrosmatikern. Z. Zellforsch. *69*: 140–154 (1966).

Andres, K. H. Der olfaktorische Saum der Katze Z. Zellforsch. *96*: 250–275 (1969).

Breipohl, W. Licht- und elektronenmikroskopische Befunde zur Struktur de Bowmanschen Drüsen im Riechepithel der weissen Maus. Z. Zellforsch. *131*: 329–346 (1972)..

Cauna, N., Hinderer, K. H. and Wentges, R. T. Sensory receptor organs of the human nasal respiratory mucosa. Am. J. Anat. *124*: 187–210 (1969).

Frisch, D. Ultrastructure of mouse olfactory mucosa. Am. J. Anat. *121*: 87–120 (1967).

Gemne, G. and Doving, K. B. Ultrastructural properties of primary olfactory neurones in fish (Lota lota L.). Am. J. Anat. *126*: 457–476 (1969).

Matulionis, D. H. and Parks, H. F. Ultrastructural morphology of the normal nasal respiratory epithelium in the mouse. Anat. Rec. *176*: 65–83 (1973).

Mozell, M. M. The spatiotemporal analysis of odorants at the level of the olfactory receptor sheet. J. Gen. Physiol. *50*: 25–41 (1969).

Mulvaney, B. D. Chemography of lysosome-like structures in olfactory epithelium. J. Cell Biol. *51*: 568–574 (1971).

Okano, M., Weber, A. F. and Frommes, S. P. Electron microscopic studies of the distal border of the canine olfactory epithelium. J. Ultrastruct. Res. *17*: 487–502 (1967).

Pinching, A. J. and Powell, T. P. S. The neuropil of the periglomerular region of the olfactory bulb. J. Cell Sci. *9*: 379–409 (1971).

Price, J. L. and Powell, T. P. S. The morphology of the granule cells of the olfactory bulb. J. Cell Sci. *7*: 91–123 (1970).

Thornhill, R. A. The ultrastructure of the olfactory epithelium of the lamprey Lampreta fluviatilis. J. Cell Sci. *2*: 591–602 (1967).

Zotterman, Y. (Ed.). Olfaction and Taste. Pergamon, Oxford, 1963.

TRACHEA AND BRONCHI

Baskerville, A. Ultrastructure of the bronchial epithelium of the pig. Souder. Zentra. Veter. *17*: 796–802 (1970).

Bensch, K. G., Gordon, C. B. and Miller, L. R. Studies on the bronchial counterpart of the Kultschitzky (argentaffin) cell and innervation of bronchial glands. J. Ultrastruct. Res. *12*: 668–686 (1965).

Clara, M. Histologie des Bronchialepithels. Z. mikr.-anat. Forsch. *41*: 321–347 (1937).

Cutz, E. and Conen, P. E. Ultrastructure and cytochemistry of Clara cells. Am. J. Path. *62*: 127–134 (1971).

Frasca, J. M., Auerbach, O., Parks, V. R. and Jamieson, J. D. Electron microscopic observations of the bronchial epithelium of dogs. Exp. Molec. Path. *9*: 363–379 (1968).

Hansell, M. M. and Moretti, R. L. Ultrastructure of the mouse tracheal epithelium. J. Morphol. *128*: 159–170 (1969).

Luciano, L., Reale, E. and Ruska, H. Über eine "chemorezeptive" Sinneszelle in der Trachea der Ratte. Z. Zellforsch. *85*: 350–375 (1968).

Meyrick, B. and Reid, L. Ultrastructure of cells in the human bronchial submucosal glands. J. Anat *107*: 281–299 (1970).

Miani, A., Pizzini, G. and DeGasperis, C. "Special type cells" in human tracheal epithelium. J. Submicroscop. Cytol. *3*: 81–84 (1971).

Rhodin, J. A. G. Ultrastructure and function of the human tracheal mucosa. Am. Rev. Resp. Dis. *93*: 1–15 (1966).

Rhodin, J. A. G. and Dalhamn, T. Electron microscopy of the tracheal ciliated mucosa in rat. Z. Zellforsch. *44*: 345–412 (1956).

Watson, J. H. L. and Brinkman, G. L. Electron microscopy of the epithelial cells of normal and bronchitic human bronchus. Am. Rev. Resp. Dis. *90*: 851–866 (1964).

LUNG

Askin, F. B. and Kuhn, C. The cellular origin of pulmonary surfactant. Lab. Investig. *25*: 260–268 (1971).

Basset, F., Poirier, J., Le Crom, M. and Turiaf, J. Étude ultrastructurale de l'épithélium bronchiolaire humain. Z. Zellforsch. *116*: 425–442 (1971).

Blümcke, S., Kessler, W. D., Niedorf, H. R., Becker, N. H. and Veith, F. J. Ultrastructure of lamellar bodies of type II pneumocytes after osmium-zinc impregnation. J. Ultrastruct. Res. *42*: 417–433 (1973).

Boyden, E. A. Segmental Anatomy of the Lungs. A study of the patterns of the segmental bronchi and related pulmonary vessels. The Blakiston Div. McGraw-Hill, New York, 1955.

Brooks, R. E. Ultrastructural evidence for a non-cellular lining layer of lung alveoli: a critical review. Arch. Intern. Med. *127*: 426–428 (1971).

Collet, A. J. Fine structure of the alveolar macrophage of the cat and modifications of its cytoplasmic components during phagocytosis. Anat. Rec. *167*: 277–290 (1970).

Curry, R. H., Simon, G. T. and Ritchie, A. C. An electron microscopic study of normal mouse lung and the early diffuse changes following uracil mustard administration. J. Ultrastruct. Res. *28*: 335–352 (1969).

Clements, J. A. Pulmonary surfactant. Am. Rev. Resp. Dis. *101*: 984–990 (1970).

Dermer, G. B. The fixation of pulmonary surfactant for electron microscopy. I. The alveolar surface lining layer. J. Ultrastruct. Res. *27*: 88–104 (1969).

Dermer, G. G. The fixation of pulmonary surfactant for electron microscopy. II. Transport of surfactant through the air-blood barrier. J. Ultrastruct. Res. *31*: 229–246 (1970).

Dermer, G. B. The pulmonary surfactant content of the inclusion bodies found within type II alveolar cell. J. Ultrastruct. Res. *33*: 306–317 (1970).

Divertie, M. B. and Brown, A. L. The fine structure of the normal human alveolocapillary membrane. J. A. M.A. *187*:938–41 (1964).

Gil, J. and Weibel, E. R. Extracellular lining of bronchioles after perfusion-fixation of rat lungs for electron microscopy. Anat Rec. *169*: 185–200 (1971).

Heinemann, H. O. and Fishman, A. P. Nonrespiratory functions of mammalian lung. Physiol. Rev. *49*: 1–47 (1969).

Kalifat, S. R., Dupuy-Coin, A. M. and Delarue, J. Démonstration ultrastructurale des polysaccharides dont certains acides dans le film de surface de l'alvéole pulmonaire. J. Ultrastruct. Res. *32*: 572–589 (1970).

Karrer, H. E. Electron microscopic study of bronchiolar epithelium of normal mouse lung. Exp. Cell Res. *10*: 237–241 (1956).

Kikkawa, Y. Morphology of alveolar lining layer. Anat. Rec. *167*: 389–400 (1970).

Kikkawa, Y. and Spitzer, R. Inclusion bodies of type II alveolar cells: species differences and morphogenesis. Anat. Rec. *163*: 525–542 (1969).

Krasno, J. R., Kneslon, J. H. and Dalldorf, F. G. Changes in the alveolar lining with onset of breathing. Am. J. Path. *66*: 471–476 (1972).

Lambson, R. O. and Cohn, J. E. Ultrastructure of the lung of the goose and its lining of surface material. Am. J. Anat. *122*: 631–650 (1968).

Lauweryns, J. M. and Boussauw, L. The ultrastructure of pulmonary lymphatic capillaries of newborn rabbits and of human infants. Lymphology *2*: 108–129 (1969).

Liebow, A. A. and Smith, D. E. (Eds.). The Lung. Int. Acad. Path. Monograph, Williams & Wilkins, Baltimore, 1968.

Ludatscher, R. M. Fine structure of the muscular wall of rat pulmonary veins. J. Anat. *103*: 345–357 (1968).

Mann, P. E. G., Cohen, A. B., Finley, T. N. and Ladman, A. J. Alveolar macrophages. Structural and functional differences between nonsmokers and smokers of marijuana and tobacco. Lab. Investig. *25*: 111–120 (1971).

Meyrick, B. and Reid, L. The alveolar brush-cell in rat lung—a third pneumocyte. J. Ultrastruct. Res. *23*: 71–80 (1968).

Miller, W. S. The Lung. Charles C. Thomas, Springfield, Ill., 1947.

O'Hare, K. H. and Sheridan, M. N. Electron microscopic observations on the morphogenesis of the albino rat lung with special reference to pulmonary epithelial cells. Am. J. Anat. *127*: 181–206 (1970).

Petrik, P. Fine structural identification of peroxisomes in mouse and rat bronchiolar and alveolar epithelium. J. Histochem. Cytochem. *19*: 339–348 (1971).

Petrik, P. and Collet, A. J. Infrastructure descellules bronchiolaires non ciliées chez la souris. Rev. Canad. Biol. *29*: 141–152 (1970).

Policard, A., Collet, A. and Giltaire-Ralyte, L. Observations micro-électronique sur l'infrastructure des cellules bronchiolaires. Bronches *5*: 187–196 (1955).

Pratt, S. A., Finley, T. N., Smith, M. H. and Ladman, A. J. A comparison of alveolar macrophages and pulmonary surfactant (?) obtained from the lungs of human smokers and nonsmokers by endobronchial lavage. Anat. Rec. *163*: 497–508 (1969).

Pump, K. K. Morphology of the acinus of the human lung. Dis. Chest *56*: 126–134 (1969).

Ryan, S. F. The structure of the interalveolar septum of the mammalian lung. Anat. Rec. *165*: 467–484 (1965).

Ryan, S. F., Ciannella, A. and Dumais, C. The structure of the interalveolar septum of the mammalian lung. Anat. Rec. *165*: 467–484 (1969).

Schneeberger-Keeley, E. E. and Karnovsky, M. J. The ultrastructural basis of alveolar-capillary membrane permeability to peroxidase used as a tracer. J. Cell Biol. *37*: 781–793 (1968).

Schultz, von H. The Submicroscopic Anatomy and Pathology of the Lung. Springer-Verlag, Berlin, 1959.

Smith, U., Smith, D. S. and Ryan, J. W. Tubular myelin assembly in type II alveolar cells: freeze-fracture studies. Anat. Rec. *176*: 125–128 (1973).

Sobin, S. S., Intaglietta, M., Frasher, W. G. and Tremer, H. M. The geometry of the pulmonary microcirculation. Angiology *17*: 24–30 (1966).

Sorokin, S. P. A morphologic and cytochemical study on the great alveolar cell. J. Histochem. Cytochem. *14*: 884–897 (1967).

Verity, M. A. and Bevan, J. A. Fine structural study of the terminal effector plexus, neuromuscular and intermuscular relationships in the pulmonary artery. J. Anat. *103*: 49–63 (1968).

Wang, N. S., Huang, S. N., Sheldon, H. and Thurlbeck, W. M. Ultrastructural changes of Clara and type II alveolar cells in adrenalin-induced pulmonary edema in mice. Am. J. Pathol. *62*: 237–252 (1971).

Weibel, E. R. The ultrastructure of the alveolar-capillary membrane or barrier. *In* The Pulmonary Circulation and Interstitial Space (Eds. A. P. Fishman and H. H. Hecht), pp. 9–27. University of Chicago Press, Chicago, 1969.

Weibel, E. R. The mystery of "non-nucleated plates" in the alveolar epithelium of the lung explained. Acta Anat. *78*: 425–443 (1971).

Weibel, E. R. and Knight, B. W. A morphometric study on the thickness of the pulmonary air-blood barrier. J. Cell Biol. *21*: 367–384 (1964).

32 Urinary system

Fig. 32-1. Section of unilobar kidney. Rabbit. L.M. X 14. **1.** Capsule. **2.** Cortex. **3.** Medulla. **4.** Pyramid. **5.** Papilla. **6.** Renal pelvis. **7.** Adipose tissue. **8.** Surface epithelium of ureter. See also Fig. 1-1, p. 4.

Fig. 32-2. Enlargement of rectangle in Fig. 32-1. Kidney. Rabbit. L.M. X 40. **1.** Capsule. **2.** Cortex. **3.** Cortical labyrinth. **4.** Medullary rays. **5.** Outer zone of medulla. **6.** Inner zone of medulla. Dotted lines indicate approximate levels of zonal borders.

Fig. 32-3. Enlargement of area similar to rectangle in Fig. 32-2. Kidney. Rat. E.M. X 620. **1.** Renal corpuscle. **2.** Proximal convoluted segment. **3.** Distal convoluted segment. **4.** Cortical collecting tubule. **5.** Afferent arteriole. **6.** Peritubular capillaries.

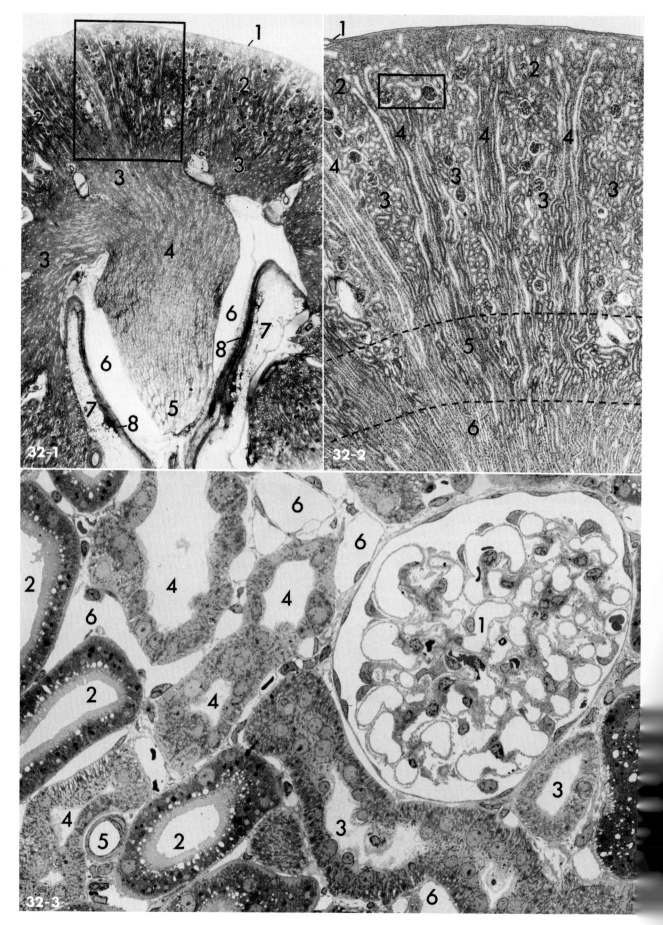

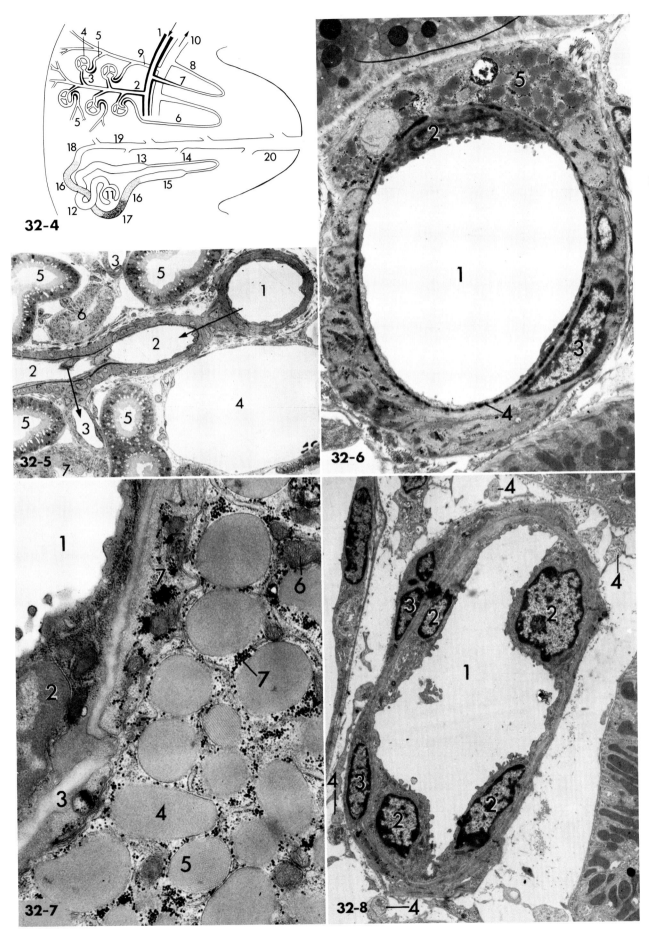

Fig. 32-4. Diagram of vasculature and nephron in a unilobular kidney. **1.** Arcuate artery. **2.** Interlobular artery. **3.** Afferent arteriole. **4.** Glomerulus. **5.** Efferent arteriole. **6.** Arterial vasa recta (spuria). **7.** Arterial vasa recta (vera). **8.** Venous vasa recta. **9.** Cortical vein. **10.** Arcuate vein. **11.** Bowman's capsule (of the renal corpuscle). **12.** Proximal convoluted segment. **13.** Straight descending limb of Henle's loop. **14.** Thin segment of Henle's loop. **15.** Thick ascending limb of Henle's loop. **16.** Distal convoluted segment. **17.** Macula densa of distal convoluted segment. **18.** Cortical collecting tubule. **19.** Straight collecting tubule. **20.** Collecting duct.

Fig. 32-5. Survey of kidney cortex. Rat. E.M. X 380. **1.** Arcuate artery (cross-sectioned). **2.** Interlobular artery. **3.** Afferent (glomerular) arteriole. Arrows indicate direction of blood flow. **4.** Arcuate vein (thin-walled in rat). **5.** Proximal convoluted segment. **6.** Distal convoluted segment. **7.** Cortical collecting tubule.

Fig. 32-6. Cross section of afferent arteriole. Kidney. Rat. E.M. X 4000. **1.** Lumen, 16 μ wide. **2.** Nucleus of endothelial cell. **3.** Nucleus of smooth muscle cell. **4.** Remnants of elastic membrane. **5.** Juxtaglomerular cell.

Fig. 32-7. Detail of efferent arteriole. Kidney. Rat. E.M. X 27,000. **1.** Lumen. **2.** Nucleus of endothelial cell. **3.** Basal lamina. **4.** Secretory granules of JG-cell. **5.** Secretory granule with crystalline core. **6.** Mitochondrion. **7.** Particulate glycogen.

Fig. 32-8. Cross section of efferent arteriole. Kidney. Rat. E.M. X 4000. **1.** Lumen. **2.** Nuclei of endothelial cells. **3.** Nuclei of smooth muscle cells. **4.** Non-myelinated nerves.

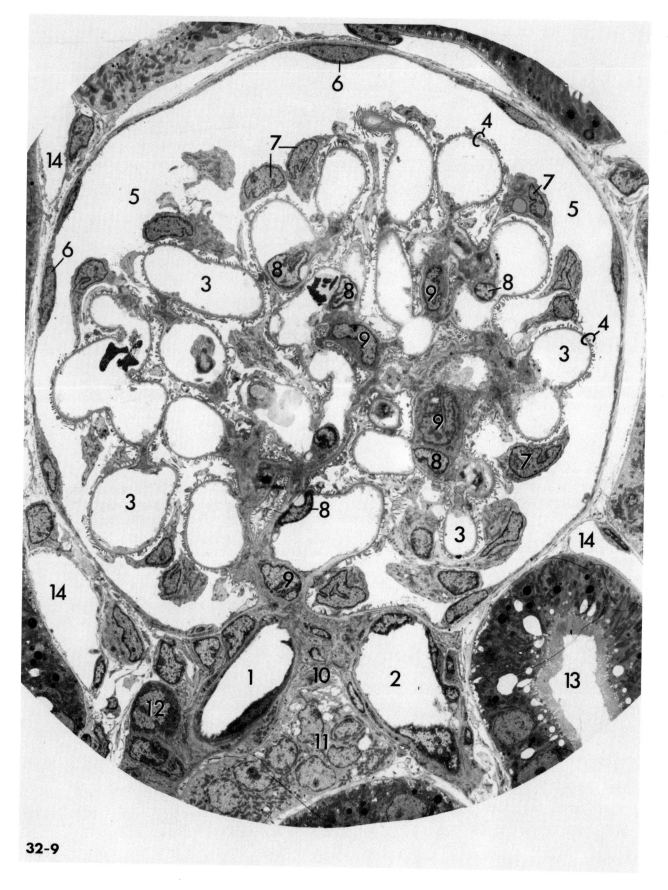

Fig. 32-9. Renal corpuscle. Kidney. Fixed by vascular perfusion. Rat. E.M. X 1200.
1. Afferent arteriole. **2.** Efferent arteriole.
3. Lumina of glomerular capillaries.
4. Glomerular filtration membrane. **5.** Urinary space of Bowman's capsule. **6.** Nuclei of cells of parietal layer of Bowman's capsule.
7. Nuclei of cells of visceral layer of Bowman's capsule; glomerular epithelial cells; podocytes. **8.** Nuclei of endothelial cells.
9. Nuclei of mesangial cells. **10.** Vascular pole of renal corpuscle. Urinary pole is not in plane of section. **11.** Cells of macula densa.
12. Nucleus of JG-cell. **13.** Proximal convoluted segment of the nephron.
14. Peritubular capillaries.

32-9

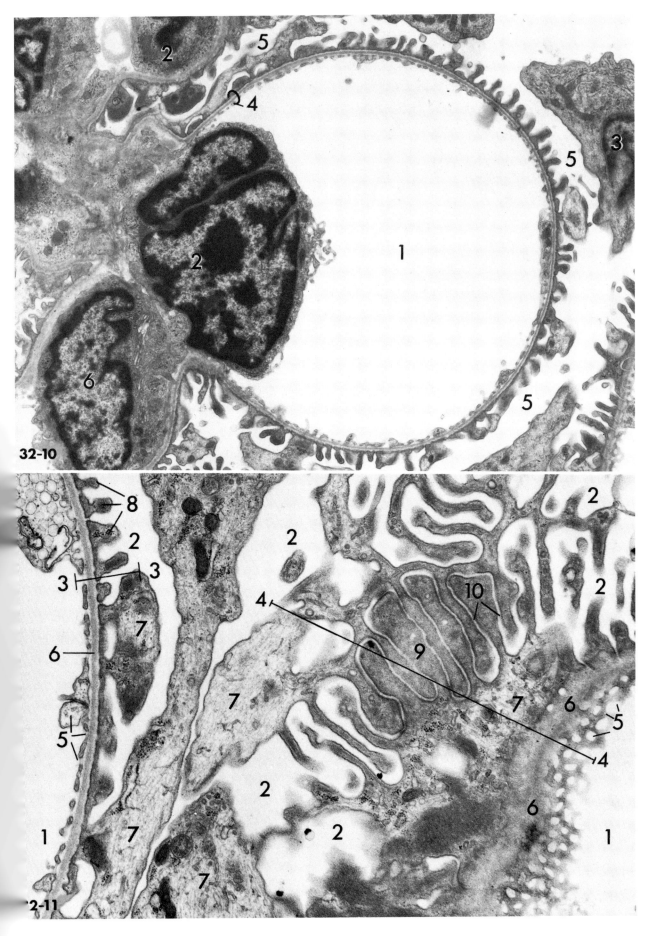

Fig. 32-10. Glomerular capillary. Kidney. Rat. E.M X 10,000. **1.** Lumen, 10 μ wide. **2.** Nuclei of endothelial cells. **3.** Nucleus of epithelial cell (podocyte). **4.** Glomerular filtration membrane. **5.** Urinary space. **6.** Nucleus of mesangial cell.

Fig. 32-11. Detail of architecture of glomerular filtration membrane. Kidney. Rat. E.M. X 20,500. **1.** Lumina of glomerular capillaries. **2.** Urinary space. **3.** Cross section of filtration membrane. **4.** Oblique to tangential section of filtration membrane. **5.** Endothelium with fenestrae. **6.** Basal lamina. **7.** Large cytoplasmic processes of podocytes. **8.** Small cytoplasmic foot processes (pedicles) of podocytes. **9.** Interlocking of pedicles. **10.** Slit-pore.

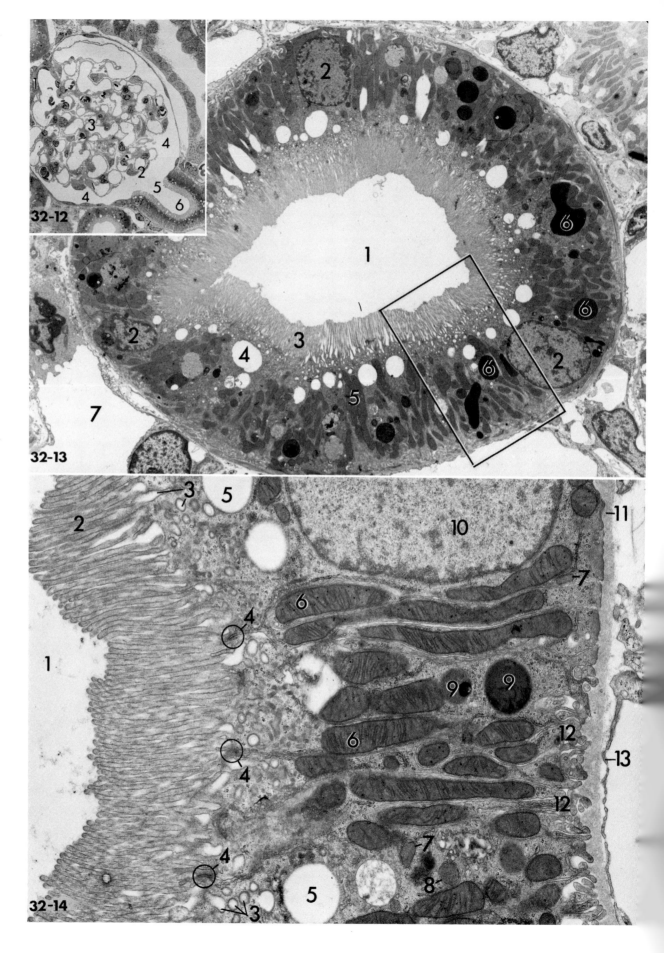

Fig. 32-12. Renal corpuscle. Kidney. Rat. E.M. X 300. **1.** Vascular pole. **2.** Urinary pole. **3.** Glomerular capillaries. **4.** Urinary space. **5.** Entrance to proximal convoluted segment. **6.** Lumen of proximal tubule.

Fig. 32-13. Cross section of proximal convoluted segment. Kidney. Rat. E.M. X 2500. **1.** Lumen of tubule. **2.** Nuclei of epithelial cells. **3.** Microvilli (brush border). **4.** Apical vacuole (phagosome). **5.** Mitochondria. **6.** Dense granules (secondary lysosomes). **7.** Peritubular capillaries.

Fig. 32-14. Enlargement of area similar to rectangle in Fig. 32-13. Kidney. Rat. E.M. X 12,000. **1.** Lumen of tubule. **2.** Microvilli. **3.** Tubular invaginations. **4.** Circles: junctional complexes. **5.** Apical vacuoles (phagosomes). **6.** Mitochondria. **7.** Microbodies. **8.** Primary lysosomes. **9.** Secondary lysosomes (dense granules). **10.** Nucleus. **11.** Basal lamina. **12.** Basal infoldings of cell membrane. **13.** Fenestrated endothelium of peritubular capillary.

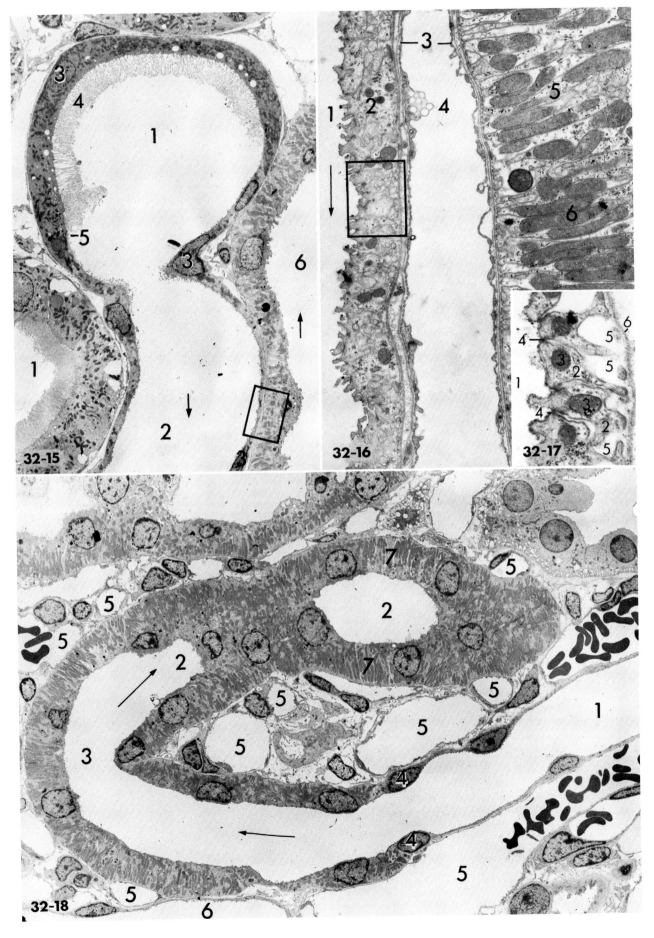

Fig. 32-15. Part of descending limb of Henle's loop. Kidney. Rat. E.M. X 1650. **1.** Lumen of straight descending limb. **2.** Lumen of thin segment of Henle's loop. **3.** Nuclei of epithelial cells. **4.** Microvilli. **5.** Termination of long microvilli, marking point of transition between thick descending and thin segments. **6.** Lumen of thick ascending limb. Arrows indicate direction of urine flow.

Fig. 32-16. Detail of area similar to rectangle in Fig. 32-15. Kidney. Rat. E.M. X 9000. **1.** Lumen of thin descending limb. Arrow indicates direction of urine flow. **2.** Epithelium of thin descending limb. **3.** Endothelium of peritubular capillary. **4.** Lumen of capillary. **5.** Epithelium of thick ascending limb. **6.** Mitochondria.

Fig. 32-17. Enlargement of area similar to rectangle in Fig. 32-16. Kidney. Rat. E.M. X 28,000. **1.** Lumen of thin segment. **2.** Interdigitating processes of epithelial cytoplasm. **3.** Mitochondria. **4.** Junctional complexes. **5.** Intercellular space. **6.** Basal lamina.

Fig. 32-18. Hairpin turn of Henle's loop. Kidney. Rat. E.M. X 1100. **1.** Lumen of thin segment. **2.** Lumen of thick ascending limb. **3.** Hairpin turn. Arrows indicate direction of urine flow. **4.** Nuclei of cells at point of transition between thin descending and thick ascending segments of Henle's loop. **5.** Peritubular capillaries of differing diameters. **6.** Adjoining thin segment. **7.** Cells of thick ascending limb are provided with numerous mitochondria.

Fig. 32-19. Cross section of distal convoluted segment. Kidney. Rat. E.M. X 4500. **1.** Lumen of tubule. **2.** Nuclei of epithelial cells. **3.** Short microvilli. **4.** Vacuoles. **5.** Mitochondria. **6.** Peritubular blood capillaries.

Fig. 32-20. Enlargement of area similar to rectangle in Fig. 32-19. Kidney. Rat. E.M. X 19,000. **1.** Lumen of tubule. **2.** Very short microvilli. **3.** Junctional complexes. **4.** Mitochondria. **5.** Nucleus. **6.** Basal infoldings of cell membrane. **7.** Basal lamina. **8.** Fenestrated endothelium of peritubular capillary.

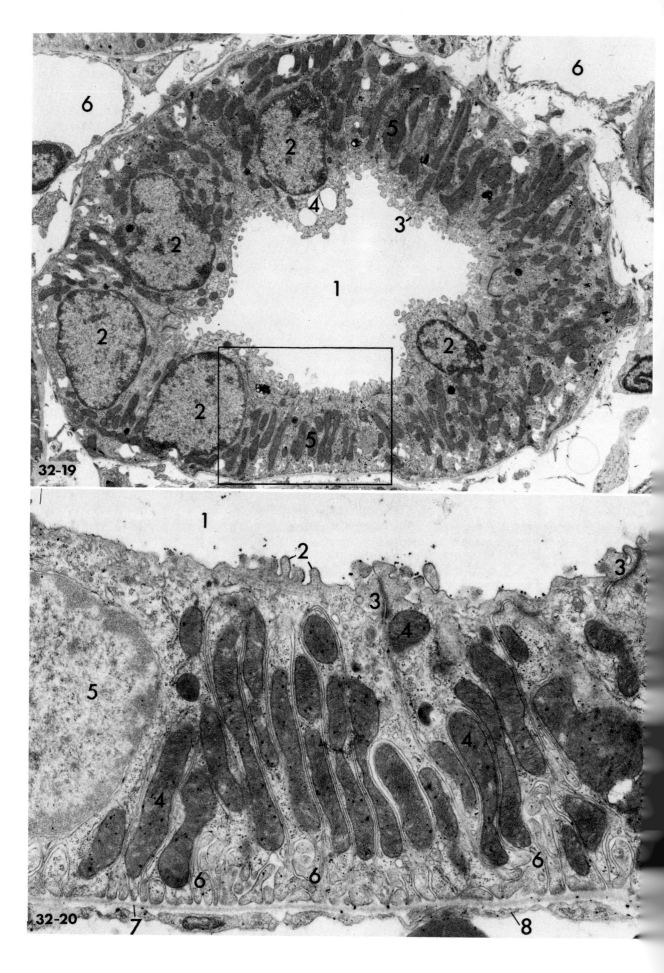

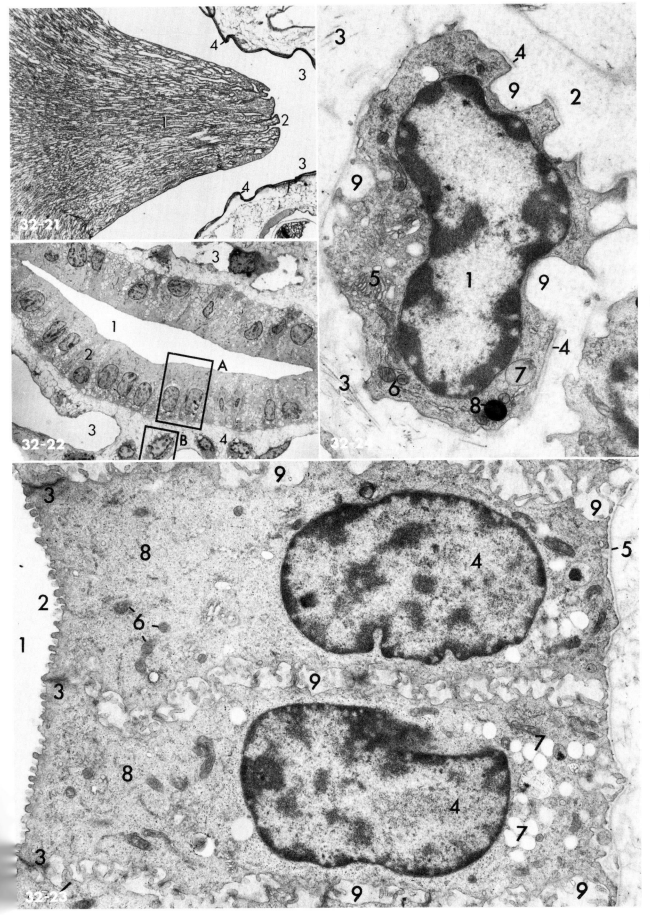

Fig. 32-21. Longitudinal section of renal papilla. Kidney. Rat. L.M. X 30. **1.** Papilla. **2.** Tip of papilla with openings of papillary ducts. **3.** Renal pelvis. **4.** Transitional epithelium of renal pelvis.

Fig. 32-22. Survey of collecting duct. Longitudinal section. Kidney. Rat. E.M. X 720. **1.** Lumen of duct. **2.** Columnar epithelial cells. **3.** Peritubular capillaries. **4.** Connective tissue cells.

Fig. 32-23. Enlargement of area similar to rectangle (A) in Fig. 32-22. Kidney. Rat. E.M. X 9300. **1.** Lumen of duct. **2.** Short microvilli. **3.** Junctional complexes. **4.** Nuclei. **5.** Basal lamina. **6.** Mitochondria. **7.** Lipid droplets. **8.** Ribosomes form the finely stippled background. **9.** Intercellular space.

Fig. 32-24. Enlargement of area similar to rectangle (B) in Fig. 32-22. Kidney. Rat. E.M. X 9300. **1.** Nucleus of fibroblast-like cell. **2.** Matrix of connective tissue. **3.** Collagenous fibrils. **4.** External lamina. **5.** Golgi complex. **6.** Mitochondria. **7.** Lysosome. **8.** Lipid droplet. **9.** Pit-like depressions of unknown nature.

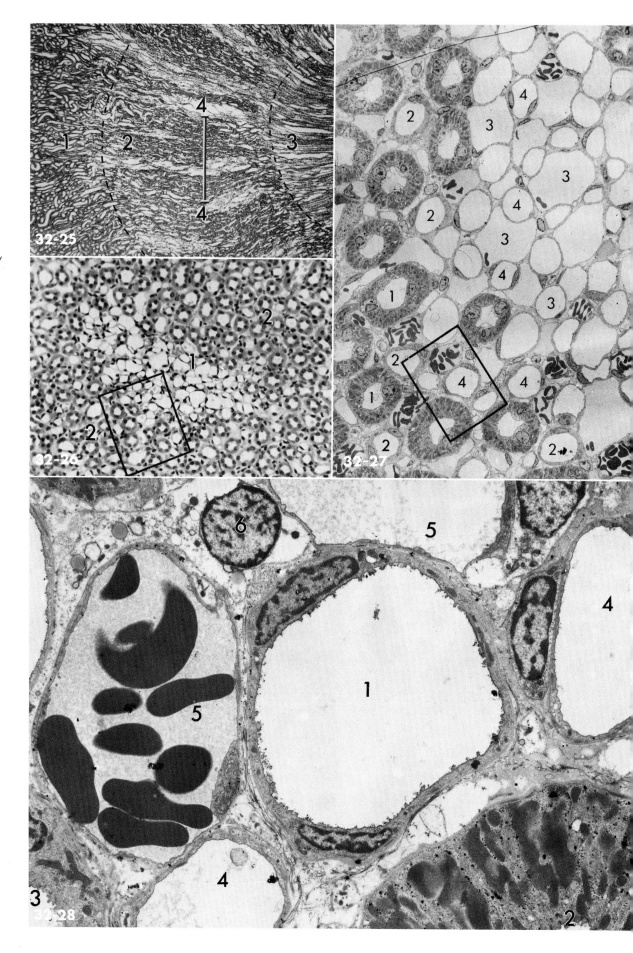

Fig. 32-25. Longitudinal section of the renal medulla. Kidney. Rat. L.M. X 27. **1.** Cortex. **2.** Outer zone of medulla. **3.** Inner zone of medulla. **4.** Plane of section to produce Fig. 32-26.

Fig. 32-26. Cross section of the outer medullary zone in the plane indicated by 4—4 in Fig. 32-15. Kidney. Rat. L.M. X 175. **1.** Rete or bundle of vasa recta and some thin segments of Henle's loop. **2.** Mostly collecting tubules and thick ascending loops of Henle.

Fig. 32-27. Enlargement of area similar to rectangle in Fig. 32-26. Kidney. Rat. E.M. X 580. **1.** Thick ascending limbs. **2.** Straight collecting tubules. **3.** Vasa recta. **4.** Thin segments.

Fig. 32-28. Enlargement of rectangle in Fig. 32-27. Kidney. Rat. E.M. X 17,500. **1.** Thin segment. **2.** Thick ascending limb. **3.** Collecting tubule. **4.** Arterial vasa recta. **5.** Venous vasa recta. **6.** Nucleus of connective tissue cell

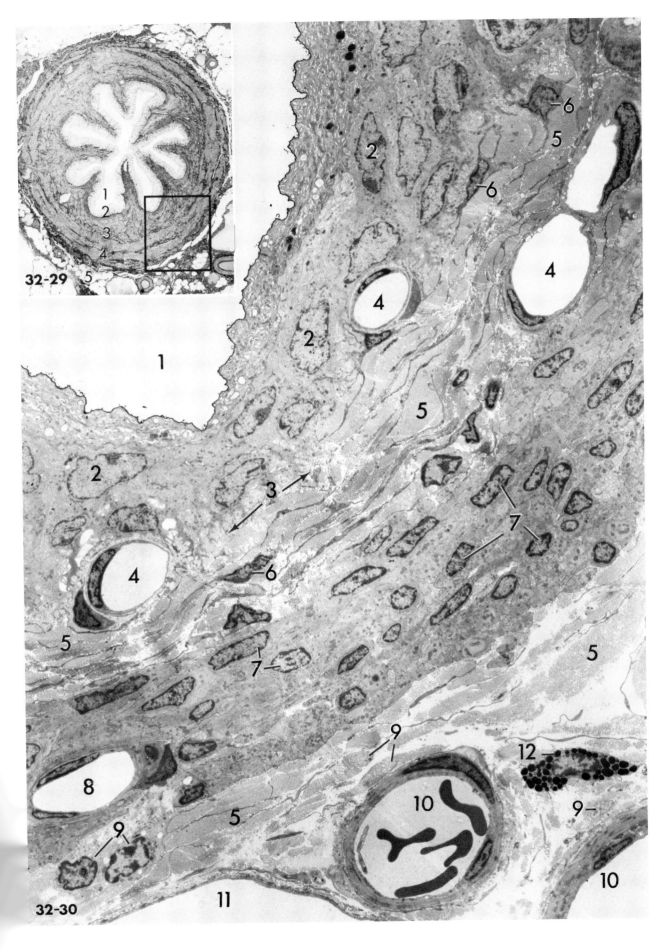

Fig. 32-29. Ureter. Cross section. Human. L.M. X 26. **1.** Lumen. **2.** Transitional epithelium. **3.** Connective tissue. **4.** Smooth muscle. **5.** Loose connective tissue with adipose tissue and blood vessels.

Fig. 32-30. Enlargement of area similar to rectangle in Fig. 32-29. Ureter. Cross section. Rat. E.M. X 1860. **1.** Lumen. **2.** Nuclei of cells of transitional epithelium. **3.** Level of basal lamina. **4.** Lumina of subepithelial blood capillaries. **5.** Bundles of collagenous fibrils. **6.** Fibroblasts. **7.** Nuclei of smooth muscle cells. **8.** Lumen of capillary in smooth muscle layer. **9.** Non-myelinated nerves. **10.** Arterioles. **11.** Venule. **12.** Mast cell.

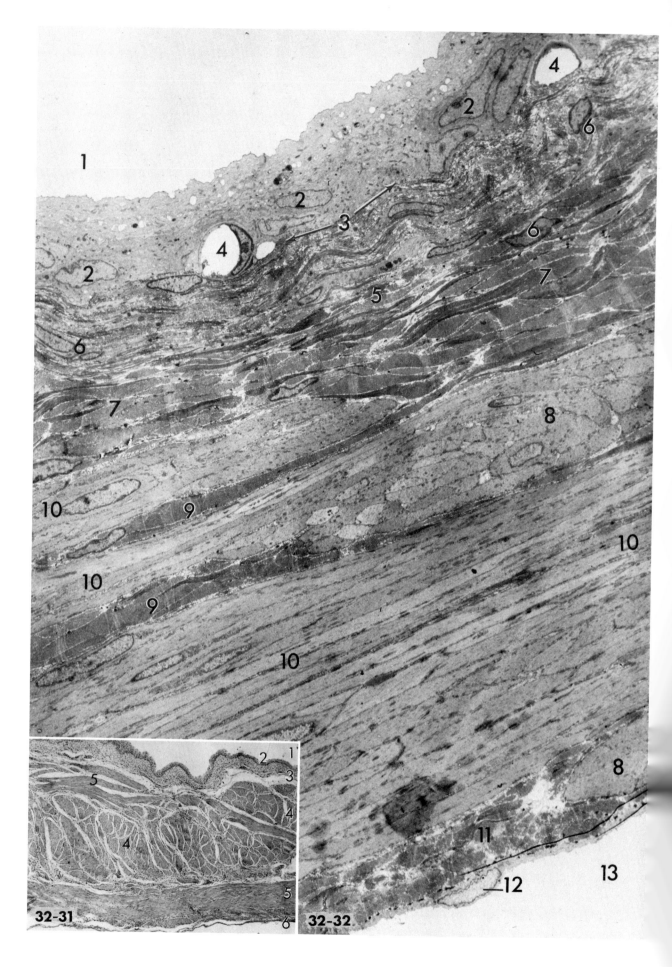

Fig. 32-31. Wall of partly collapsed urinary bladder. Human. L.M. X 24. **1.** Lumen. **2.** Transitional surface epithelium. **3.** Submucosa. **4.** Cross-sectioned bundles of smooth muscle cells. **5.** Longitudinally sectioned bundles of smooth muscle cells. **6.** Serosa.

Fig. 32-32. Wall of distended urinary bladder. Rat. E.M. X 1900. **1.** Lumen. **2.** Nuclei of cells in transitional epithelium. **3.** Plane of basal lamina. **4.** Subepithelial capillaries indenting the base of the epithelium. **5.** Submucosa. **6.** Nuclei of fibroblasts. **7.** Bundles of collagen. **8.** Cross-sectioned smooth muscle cells. **9.** Bundles of collagen between layers of smooth muscle cells. **10.** Longitudinally sectioned smooth muscle cells. **11.** Submesothelial connective tissue of the serosa. **12.** Mesothelial cell nucleus. **13.** Peritoneal cavity.

380

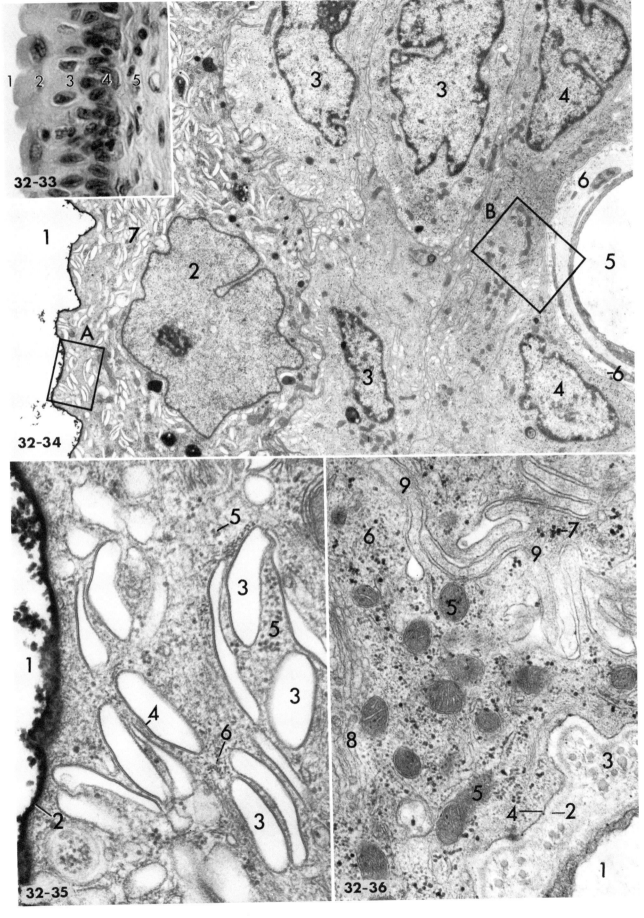

Fig. 32-33. Transverse section of transitional epithelium. Urinary bladder. Monkey. L.M. X 550. **1.** Lumen. **2.** Superficial cells. **3.** Intermediate cells. **4.** Basal cells. **5.** Submucosa.

Fig. 32-34. Transverse section of transitional epithelium. Ureter. Rat. E.M. X 5300. **1.** Lumen. **2.** Nucleus of superficial cell. **3.** Nuclei of intermediate cells. **4.** Nuclei of basal cells. **5.** Lumen of subepithelial capillary. **6.** Collagen of submucosa. **7.** Discoid vesicles. **8.** Lysosomes.

Fig. 32-35. Enlargement of rectangle (A) in Fig. 32-34. Transitional epithelium. Ureter. Rat. E.M. X 60,000. **1.** Lumen. **2.** Surface cell membrane. Dense material attached to luminal aspect is of unknown nature. **3.** Flat discoid vesicles. **4.** Trilaminar membrane. **5.** Particulate glycogen. **6.** Ribosomes.

Fig. 32-36. Enlargement of area similar to rectangle (B) in Fig. 32-34. Detail of basal region of transitional epithelium. Ureter. Rat. E.M. X 44,000. **1.** Lumen of capillary. **2.** Basal lamina. **3.** Collagenous fibrils. **4.** Basal cell membrane. **5.** Mitochondria. **6.** Ribosomes. **7.** Particulate glycogen. **8.** Golgi complex.

Fig. 32-37. Cross section of male urethra (pars cavernosa). Child. L.M. X 40. **1.** Lumen of urethra. **2.** Subepithelial connective tissue. **3.** Trabeculae. **4.** Lacunae. **5.** Small arteries.

Fig. 32-38. Cross section of female urethra. Human. L.M. X 27. **1.** Lumen, lined by stratified squamous epithelium. **2.** Subepithelial connective tissue. **3.** Thin-walled veins. **4.** Arteries. **5.** Smooth muscle cells. **6.** Striated muscle fibers of urethral sphincter.

Fig. 32-39. Enlargement of area similar to rectangle in Fig. 32-37. Detail of male urethra and corpus cavernosum (spongiosum). Rat. E.M. X 1800. **1.** Lumen of urethra. **2.** Stratified epithelium. **3.** Subepithelial connective tissue with some capillaries. **4.** Narrow trabeculae of corpus spongiosum. **5.** Lacunae. **6.** Wide trabeculae.

Fig. 32-40. Enlargement of area similar to rectangle (A) in Fig. 32-39. Detail of a wide trabeculum of corpus spongiosum. Rat. E.M. X 1800. **1.** Lumen of lacuna. **2.** Endothelium. **3.** Fibroblasts. **4.** Smooth muscle cells. **5.** Bundles of collagen. **6.** Schwann cell nucleus.

Fig. 32-41. Enargement of area similar to rectangle (B) in Fig. 32-39. Detail of stratified epithelium. Male urethra. Pars cavernosa. Rat. E.M. X 4700. **1.** Lumen of urethra. **2.** Nuclei of cuboidal, basal cells. **3.** Nuclei of cuboidal cells in the middle of the epithelium. **4.** Squamous and/or cuboidal surface cells. **5.** Basal lamina. **6.** Particulate glycogen. **7.** Microvilli.

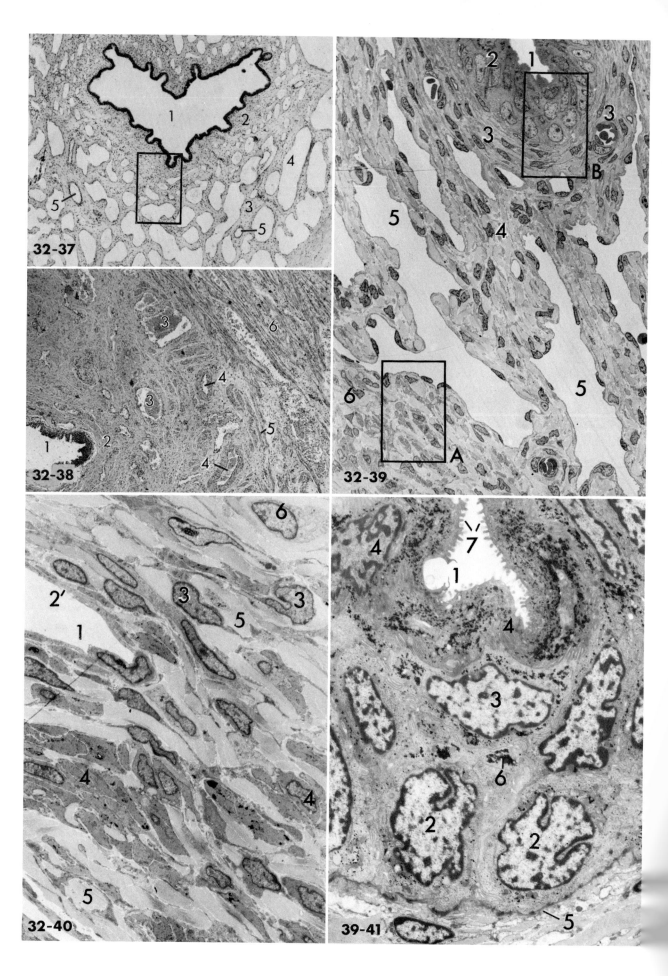

382

References

KIDNEY

Bulger, R. E. The shape of rat kidney tubular cells. Am. J. Anat. *116*: 237–255 (1965).

Bulger, R. E. and Trump, B. F. Fine structure of the rat renal papilla. Am. J. Anat. *118*: 685–721 (1966).

Bulger, R. E., Tisher, C. C., Myers, C. H. and Trump, B. F. Human renal ultrastructure. II. The thin limb of Henle's loop and the interstitium in healthy individuals. Lab. Investig. *16*: 124–141 (1967).

Dieterich, H. J. Die Ultrastruktur des Gefässbündel im Mark der Rattenniere. Z. Zellforsch. *84*: 350–371 (1968).

Ericsson, J. L. E. Transport and digestion of hemoglobin in the proximal tubule. II. Electron microscopy. Lab. Investig. *14*: 16–39 (1965).

Ericsson, J. L. E. and Trump, B. F. Electron microscopic studies of the epithelium of the proximal tubule of the rat kidney. Lab. Investig. *11*: 1427–1456 (1964).

Farquhar, M. G. and Palade, G. E. Functional evidence for the existence of a third cell type in the renal glomerulus. J. Cell Biol. *13*: 55–87 (1962).

Forster, R. P. Kidney cells. *In* The Cell, Vol. 5 (Eds. J. Brachet and A. E. Mirsky), pp. 89–161. Academic Press, New York, 1961.

Gottschalk, C. W. and Mylle, M. Micropuncture study of the mammalian urinary concentrating mechanism: evidence for the countercurrent hypothesis. Am. J. Physiol. *196*: 927–936 (1959).

Griffith, L. D., Bulger, R. E. and Trump, B. F. Fine structure and staining of mucosubstances on "intercalated cells" from the rat distal convoluted tubule and collecting duct. Anat. Rec. *160*: 643–662 (1968).

Johnson, F. R. and Darnton, S. J. Ultrastructural observations on the renal papilla of the rabbit. Z. Zellforsch. *81*: 390–406 (1967).

Jorgensen, F. The Ultrastructure of the Normal Human Glomerulus. Munksgaard, Copenhagen, 1966.

Jorgensen, F. Electron microscopic studies of normal visceral epithelial cells (human glomerulus). Lab. Investig. *17*: 225–242 (1967).

Latta, H., Maunsbach, A. B. and Madden, S. C. The centrolobular region of the renal glomerulus studied by electron microscopy. J. Ultrastruct. Res. *4*: 455–472 (1960).

Miller, F. Hemoglobin absorption by the cells of the proximal convoluted tubule in mouse kidney. J. Biophys. Biochem. Cytol. *8*: 689–718 (1960).

Moffat, D. B. and Fourman, J. The vascular pattern of the rat kidney. J. Anat. *97*: 543–553 (1963).

Mueller, C. B. The structure of the renal glomerulus. Am. Heart J. *55*: 304–322 (1958).

Myers, C. H., Bulger, R. E., Tisher, C. C. and Trump, B. F. Human renal ultrastructure. IV. Collecting ducts of healthy individuals. Lab. Investig. *15*: 1921–1950 (1966).

Nissen, H. M. On lipid droplets in renal interstitial cells. IV. Isolation and identification. Z. Zellforsch. *97*: 274–284 (1969).

Oliver, J. New directions in renal morphology. Harvey Lectures Series *40*: 102–155 (1944–45).

Osvaldo, L. and Latta, H. Interstitial cells of the renal medulla. J. Ultrastruct. Res. *15*: 589–613 (1966).

Rhodin, J. Correlation of ultrastructural organization and function in normal and experimentally changed proximal convoluted tubule cells of the mouse kidney. Thesis. Karolinska Institutet, Stockholm. pp. 1–76, 1954.

Rhodin, J. Anatomy of kidney tubules. Int. Rev. Cytol. *7*: 485–534 (1958).

Rhodin, J. Electron microscopy of the kidney. Am. J. Med. *24*: 661–675 (1958).

Rhodin, J. A. G. Electron microscopy of the kidney. *In* Renal Disease (Ed. D. A. K. Black), pp. 117–156. Blackwell, Oxford, 1962.

Rhodin, J. A. G. The structure of the kidney. *In* Diseases of the Kidney (Eds. M. B. Strauss and L. G. Welt), pp. 10–55. Little, Brown, Boston, 1963.

Ross, M. H. and Reith, E. J. Myoid elements in the mammalian nephron and their relationship to other specializations in the basal part of the kidney tubule cells. Am. J. Anat. *129*: 399–416 (1970).

Tisher, C. C., Bulger, R. E. and Valtin, H. Morphology of renal medulla in water diuresis and vasopressin-induced antidiuresis. Am. J. Physiol. *220*: 87–94 (1971).

Tisher, C. C., Bulger, R. E. and Trump, B. F. Human renal ultrastructure. I. Proximal tubule of healthy individuals. Lab. Investig. *15*: 1357–1394 (1966).

Waugh, D., Prentice, R. S. A. and Yadav, D. The structure of the proximal tubule: a morphological study of basement membrane cristae and their relationships in the renal tubule of the rat. Am. J. Anat. *121*: 775–786 (1967).

URETER AND URINARY BLADDER

Dixon, J. S. and Gosling, J. A. Electron microscopic observations of the renal caliceal wall in the rat. Z. Zellforsch. *103*: 328–340 (1970).

Dixon, J. S. and Gosling, J. A. Histochemical and electron microscopical observations on the innervation of the upper segment of the mammalian ureter. J. Anat. *110*: 57–66 (1971).

Hicks, R. M. The fine structure of the transitional epithelium of rat ureter. J. Cell Biol. *26*: 25–48 (1965).

Hicks, R. M. The function of the Golgi complex in transitional epithelium. Synthesis of the thick cell membrane. J. Cell Biol. *30*: 623–643 (1966).

Monis, B. and Zambrano, D. Transitional epithelium of urinary tract in normal and dehydrated rats. Z. Zellforsch. *85*: 165–182 (1968).

Porter, K. R., Kenyon, K. and Badenhausen, S. Specializations of the unit membrane. Protoplasma *63*: 262–274 (1967).

Richter, W. R. and Moize, S. M. Electron microscopic observations on the collapsed and distended mammalian urinary bladder. J. Ultrastruct. Res. *9*: 1–9 (1963).

33 Male reproductive system

Fig. 33-1. Section of testis. Rabbit. L.M. X 5.
1. Testis. **2.** Efferent ductules. **3.** Head of epididymis. **4.** Tunica albuginea.

Fig. 33-2. Enlargement of area similar to rectangle in Fig. 33-1. Section of four segments of seminiferous tubules. Testis. Human. L.M. X 168. **1.** Lumen of seminiferous tubule. **2.** Stratified epithelium of spermatogenic cells. **3.** Interstitial tissue. **4.** Cells of Leydig.

Fig. 33-3. Enlargement of area similar to rectangle in Fig. 33-2. Cross section of seminiferous tubule. Testis. Rat. E.M. X 580. **1.** Lumen of seminiferous tubule. **2.** Sertoli cells. **3.** Spermatogonia type B or very early primary spermatocytes. **4.** Primary spermatocytes in the pachytene stage of chromosomal rearrangement (late prophase of meiotic division). **5.** Early spermatids. **6.** Interstitial cells of Leydig. **7.** Peritubular capillaries and venules. **8.** Arteriole. **9.** Peritubular lymphatic space.

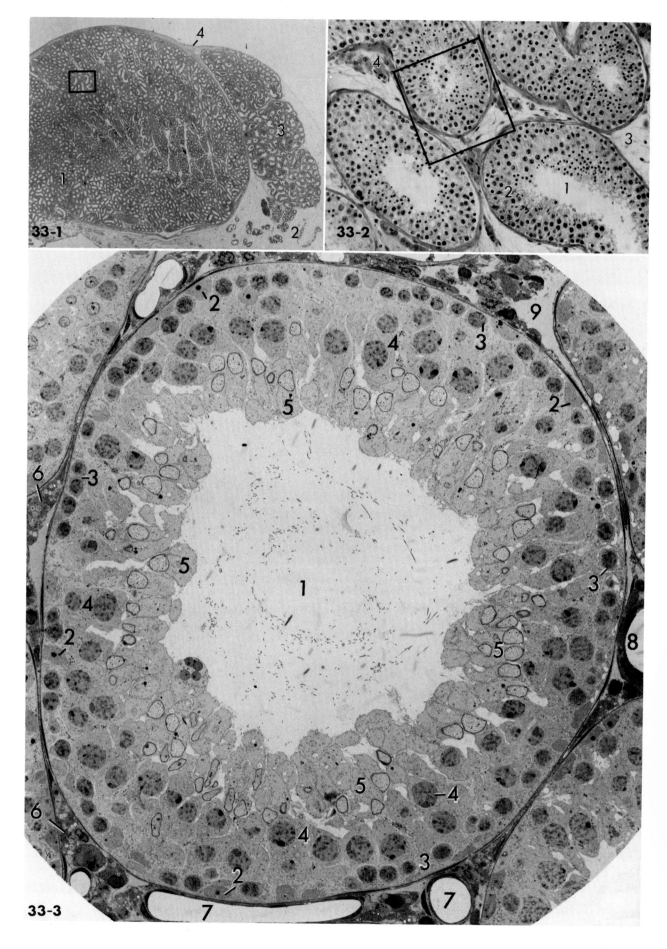

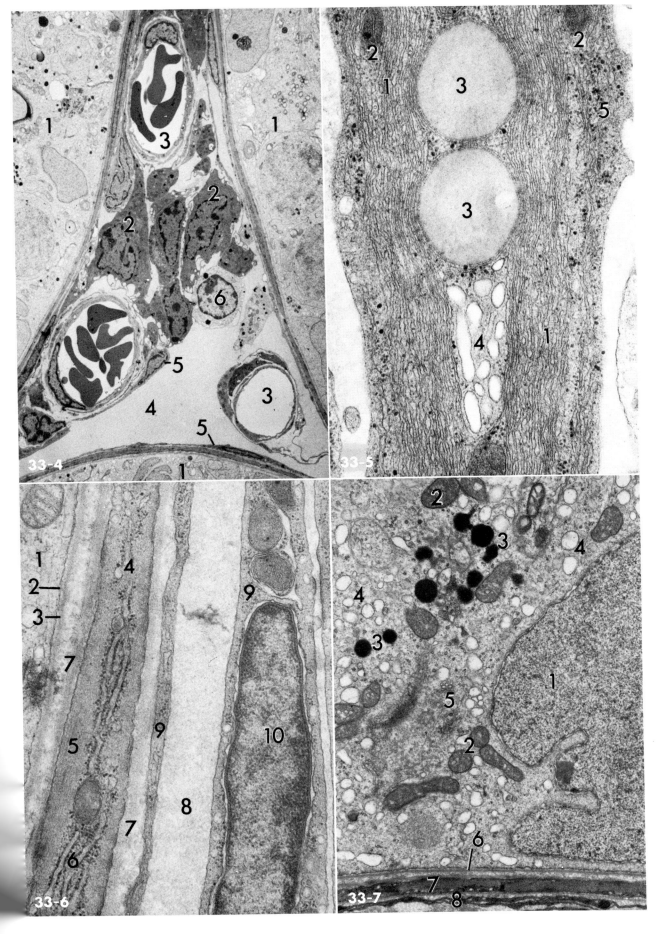

Fig. 33-4. Survey of the interstitial space of the testis. Rat. E.M. X 1800. **1.** Base of spermatogenic epithelium. **2.** Interstitial cells of Leydig. **3.** Capillaries and venules. **4.** Lymphatic space. **5.** Lymphatic endothelium. **6.** Lymphocyte.

Fig. 33-5. Detail of Leydig cell. Testis. Rat. E.M. X 37,000. **1.** Agranular endoplasmic reticulum. **2.** Small mitochondria. **3.** Lipid droplets. **4.** Golgi vacuoles. **5.** Ribosomes.

Fig. 33-6. Detail of the base of the seminiferous tubule and adjacent structures. Testis. Rat. E.M. X 27,000. **1.** Part of Sertoli cell. **2.** Cell membrane. **3.** Basal lamina. **4.** Part of squamous smooth muscle cell. **5.** Myofilaments. **6.** Granular endoplasmic reticulum. **7.** Basal (external) lamina surrounding smooth muscle cell. **8.** Lumen of lymphatic space. **9.** Endothelial cytoplasm. **10.** Endothelial nucleus.

Fig. 33-7. Part of Sertoli cell. Seminiferous tubule. Testis. Rat. E.M. X 15,000. **1.** Nucleus. **2.** Mitochondria. **3.** Lipid droplets. **4.** Agranular endoplasmic reticulum. **5.** Golgi zone. **6.** Basal lamina. **7.** Smooth muscle cell. **8.** Lymphatic endothelium.

Fig. 33-8. Cross section of seminiferous tubule. Testis. Rat. E.M. X 600. **1.** Lumen of tubule with tails of late spermatids. **2.** Sertoli cells. **3.** Primary spermatocytes (leptotene stage of prophase). **4.** Early spermatids. **5.** Middle piece of late spermatids.

Fig. 33-9. Cross section of seminiferous tubule. Testis. Rat. E.M. X 600. **1.** Lumen of tubule. **2.** Sertoli cells. **3.** Spermatogonia type B. **4.** Dividing primary spermatocytes (meiotic division). **5.** Secondary spermatocytes. **6.** Spermatids in midstage of their development.

Fig. 33-10. Survey of the stratified spermatogenic epithelium. Testis. Rat. E.M. X 1800. **1.** Smooth muscle sheath surrounding the seminiferous tubule. **2.** Sertoli cell nucleus. **3.** Type A spermatogonia with oval nuclei and a broad cytoplasmic base resting on the basal lamina. **4.** Nuclei of primary spermatocytes (leptotene stage of prophase of meiotic division). **5.** Nuclei of early spermatids with rows of marginated small mitochondria. **6.** Vesiculated vertical cytoplasm of Sertoli cell with heads of late spermatids. **7.** Vesiculated horizontal stretch of Sertoli cell cytoplasm.

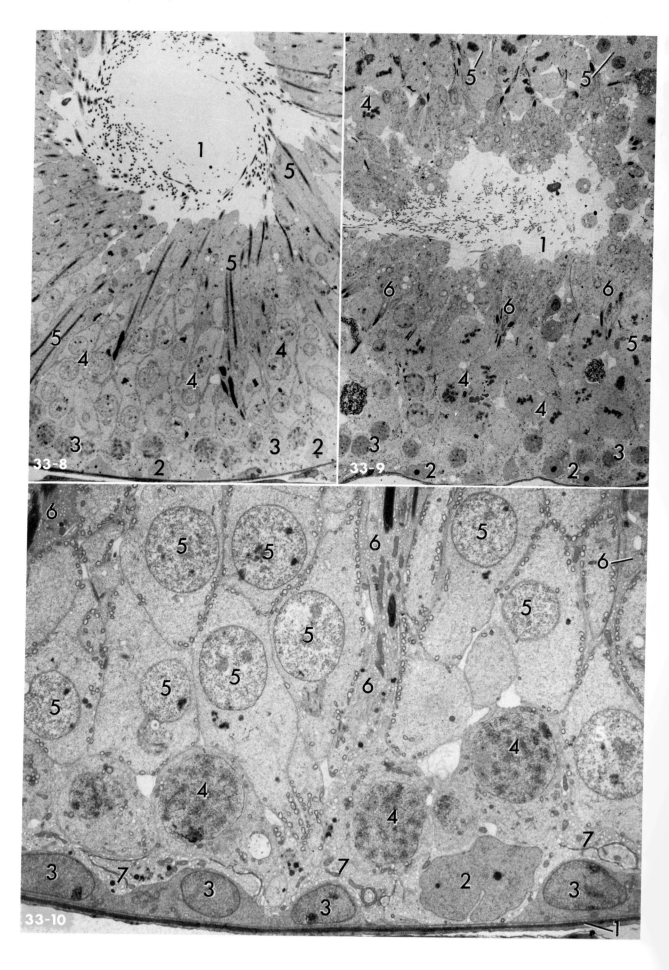

388

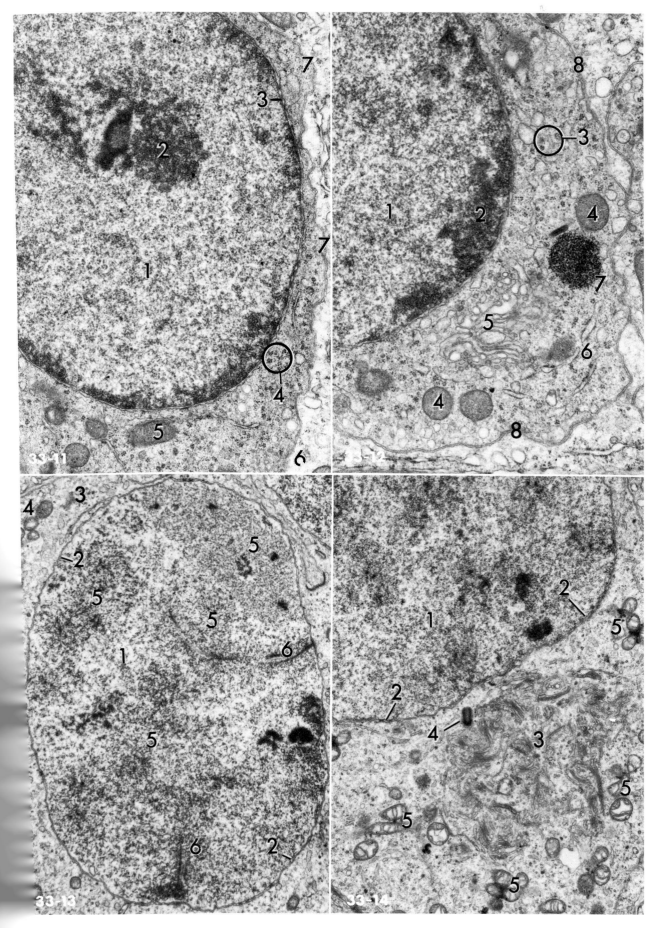

Fig. 33-11. Spermatogonium type A. Seminiferous tubule. Testis. Rat. E.M. X 15,000. **1.** Oval nucleus. **2.** Nucleolus. **3.** Nuclear envelope. **4.** Circle: polysomes in dense cytoplasm. **5.** Mitochondrion. **6.** Light cytoplasm of Sertoli cell. **7.** Cell borders.

Fig. 33-12. Spermatogonium type B. Seminiferous tubule. Testis. Rat. E.M. X 18,000. **1.** Round nucleus. **2.** Chromatin masses. **3.** Circle: polysomes. **4.** Mitochondrion. **5.** Golgi zone. **6.** Granular endoplasmic reticulum. **7.** Chromatoid body. **8.** Cell borders.

Fig. 33-13. Primary spermatocyte. Seminiferous tubule. Testis. Rat. E.M. X 10,000. **1.** Nucleus in late pachytene stage of chromosomal rearrangement during prophase of first meiotic division. **2.** Nuclear envelope. **3.** Narrow rim of cytoplasm. **4.** Mitochondria. **5.** Masses of delicate granules represent chromosomes, sectioned at varied angles. **6.** Fibrillar core in chromosomes (transient structure).

Fig. 33-14. Early spermatid. Seminiferous tubule. Testis. Rat. E.M. X 10,000. **1.** Nucleus. **2.** Nuclear envelope. **3.** Large Golgi zone. **4.** Centriole. **5.** Aggregations of mitochondria.

389

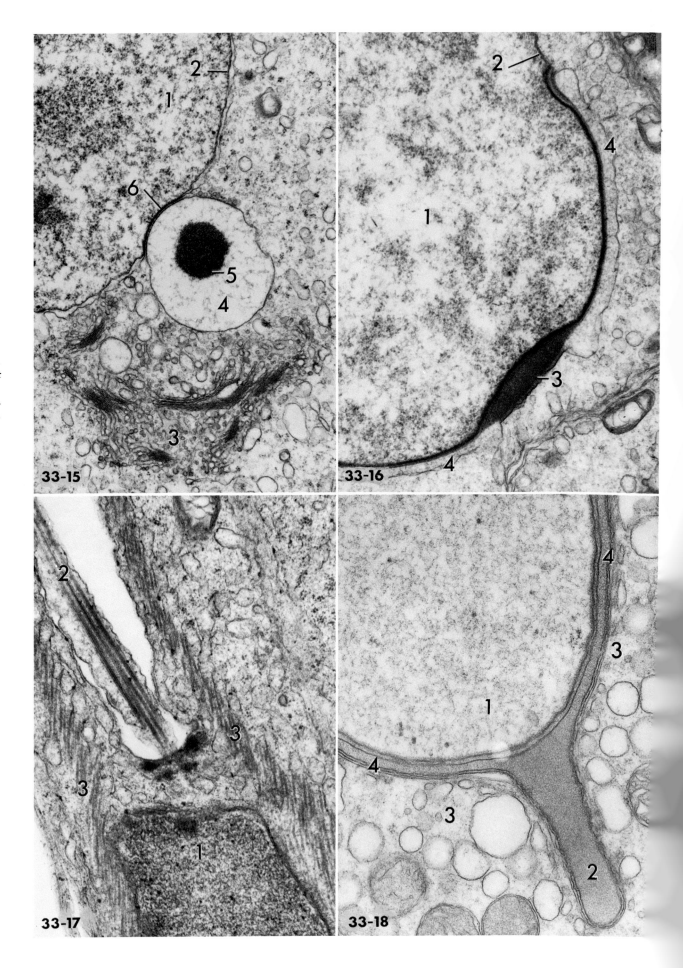

Fig. 33-15. Early spermatid. Seminiferous tubule. Testis. Rat. E.M. X 17,000. **1.** Nucleus. **2.** Nuclear envelope. **3.** Golgi zone. **4.** Acrosomal vesicle. **5.** Acrosomal granule. **6.** Point of adherence between acrosomal vesicle and nuclear envelope, marking future tip of the sperm nucleus.

Fig. 33-16. Spermatid in a developmental stage subsequent to that seen in Fig. 33-15. Seminiferous tubule. Testis. Rat. E.M. X 17,000. **1.** Nucleus. **2.** Nuclear envelope. **3.** Acrosome. **4.** Acrosomal head cap.

Fig. 33-17. Late spermatid. Seminiferous tubule. Testis. Mouse. E.M. X 16,000. **1.** Caudal, flat end of nucleus. **2.** Axoneme. **3.** Manchette: transient structure, composed of microtubules.

Fig. 33-18. Late spermatid. Seminiferous tubule. Testis. Mouse. E.M. X 30,000. **1.** Frontal end of nucleus. **2.** Acrosome. **3.** Cytoplasm of Sertoli cell. **4.** Head cap.

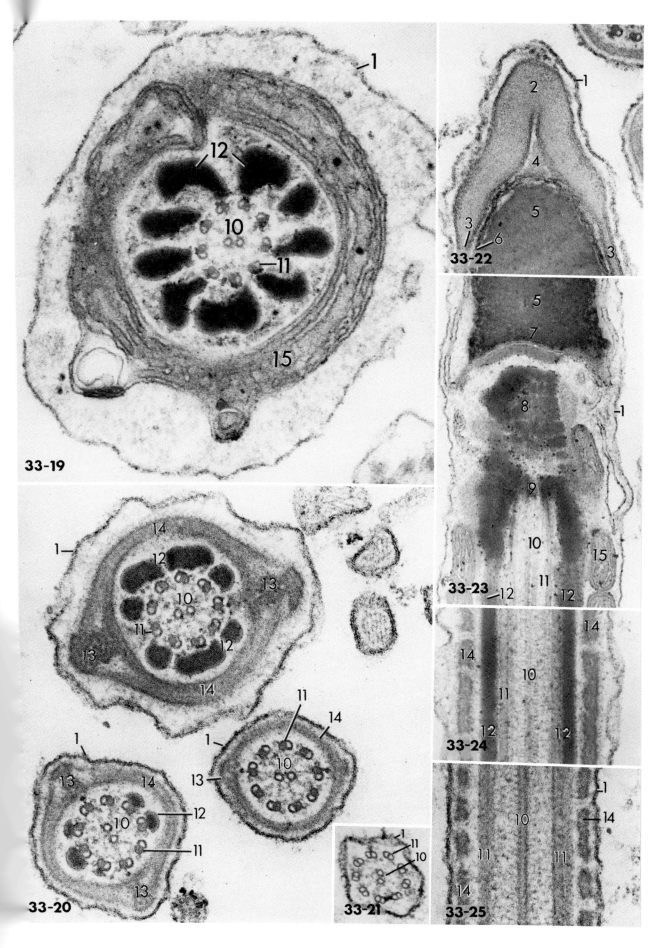

Cross and longitudinal sections of rat spermatozoon.

Fig. 33-19. Cross section of **middle piece.** E.M. × 108,000.

Fig. 33-20. Cross sections at varied levels of **principal piece.** E.M. × 80,000.

Fig. 33-21. Cross section of **end piece.** E.M. × 72,000.

Fig. 33-22. Longitudinal section of frontal end of **head.** E.M. × 70,000.

Fig. 33-23. Longitudinal section of **head, neck** and beginning of **middle piece.** E.M. × 51,000.

Fig. 33-24. Longitudinal section of **principal piece.** E.M. × 64,000.

Fig. 33-25. Longitudinal section of **principal piece,** near its end. E.M. × 96,000.

1. Cell membrane. **2.** Acrosome. **3.** Acrosomal cap. **4.** Subacrosomal space. **5.** Nucleus. **6.** Nuclear membrane. **7.** Caudal end of nucleus. **8.** Modified proximal centriole. **9.** Distal centriole. **10.** Central microtubules. **11.** Peripheral microtubules. **12.** Outer dense fibrils. **13.** Longitudinal column. **14.** Rib of fibrous sheath. **15.** Mitochondrial sheath.

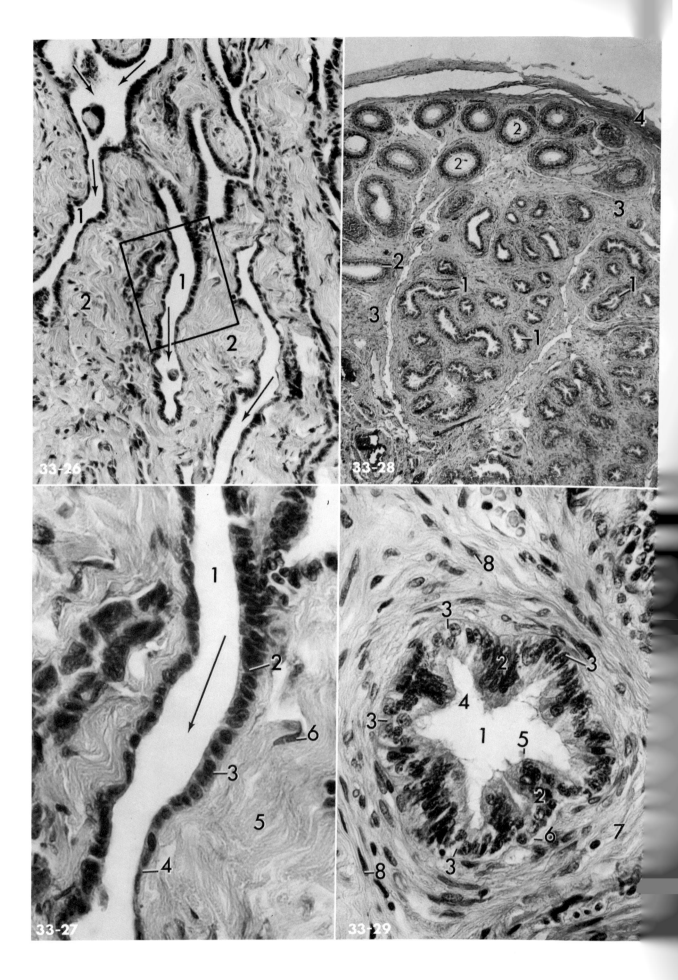

Fig. 33-26. General architecture of rete testis. Human. L.M. X 300. **1.** Interconnected tubules; arrows indicate direction in which sperm moves from testis to epididymis. **2.** Irregular dense connective tissue of the mediastinum testis.

Fig. 33-27. Enlargement of rectangle in Fig. 33-26. Testis. Human. L.M. X 630. **1.** Tubular lumen. **2.** Columnar epithelial cells. **3.** Cuboidal cells. **4.** Squamous cells. **5.** Dense bundles of collagenous fibrils. **6.** Nucleus of fibroblast.

Fig. 33-28. Section through head of epididymis. Human. L.M. X 42. **1.** Efferent ductules. **2.** Sections of the convoluted duct of epididymis. **3.** Loose connective tissue. **4.** Capsule of caput epididymidis.

Fig. 33-29. Enlargement of a cross-sectioned efferent ductule. Human. L.M. X 510. **1.** Lumen. **2.** Pseudostratified columnar epithelium. **3.** Area with simple cuboidal epithelium. **4.** Cilia. **5.** Secretory cell with coarse cytoplasmic processes extending into the lumen. **6.** Basal lamina. **7.** Collagenous bundles. **8.** Nuclei of fibroblasts.

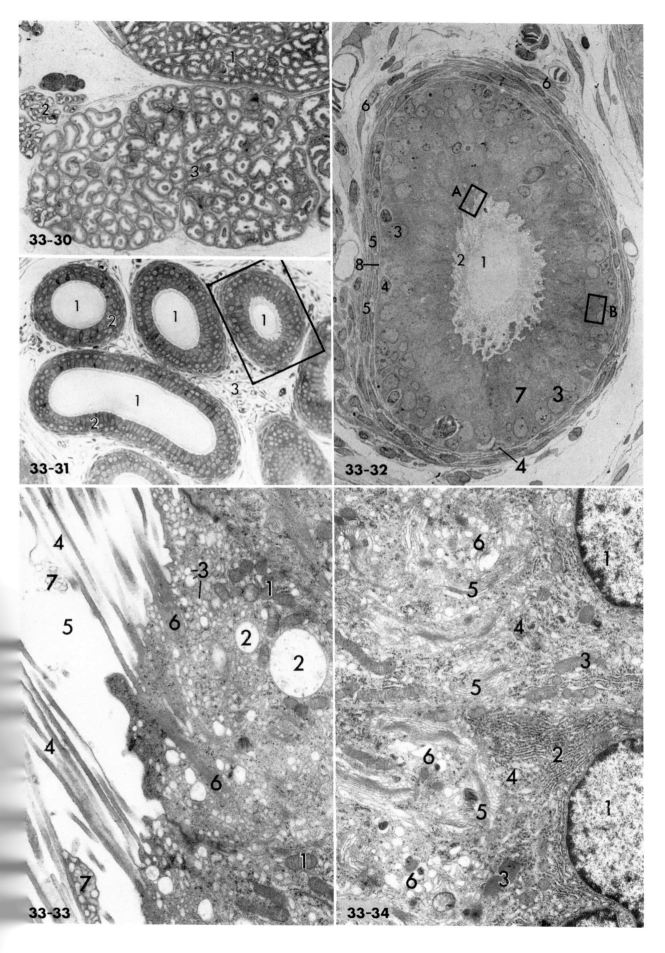

Fig. 33-30. Section of epididymis. Rabbit. L.M. X 14. **1.** Part of testis. **2.** Efferent ductules. **3.** Convoluted ductus epididymidis.

Fig. 33-31. Ductus epididymidis. Rat. L.M. X 170. **1.** Lumen of the duct. **2.** Pseudostratified columnar epithelium. **3.** Loose connective tissue.

Fig. 33-32. Enlargement of an area similar to rectangle in Fig. 33-31. Epididymis. Rat. E.M. X 600. **1.** Lumen of the duct. **2.** Stereocilia. **3.** Nuclei of columnar cells. **4.** Nuclei of basal cells. **5.** Nuclei of smooth muscle cells. **6.** Fibroblasts of loose connective tissue. **7.** Prominent Golgi complexes in columnar cells. **8.** Basal lamina.

Fig. 33-33. Enlargement of rectangle (A) in Fig. 33-32. Epididymis. Rat. E.M. X 8400. **1.** Mitochondria. **2.** Large and medium size secretory droplets. **3.** Vesicles. **4.** Stereocilia. **5.** Lumen. **6.** Filaments of stereocilia continue down into the cell. **7.** Vesicular cytoplasm along stereocilia.

Fig. 33-34. Enlargement of rectangle (B) in Fig. 33-32. Epididymis. Rat. E.M. X 8400. **1.** Nuclei of columnar cells. **2.** Granular endoplasmic reticulum. **3.** Mitochondria. **4.** Ribosomes. **5.** Golgi complexes. **6.** Secretory droplets.

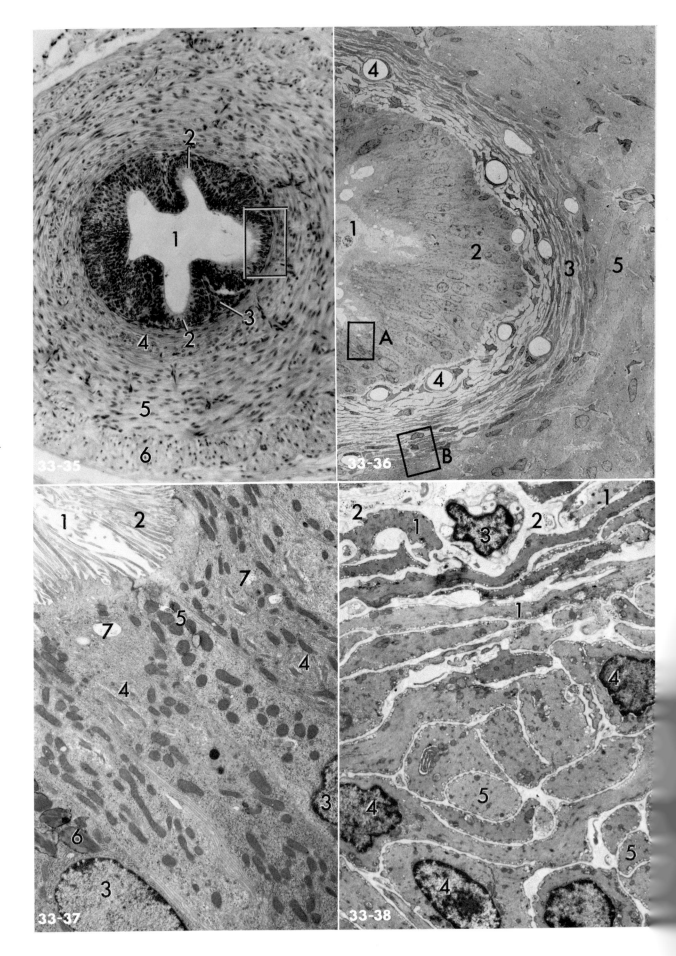

Fig. 33-35. Cross-sectioned ductus deferens. Monkey. L.M. X 130. **1.** Lumen. **2.** Pseudostratified columnar epithelium. **3.** Lamina propria. **4.** Inner longitudinal smooth muscle layer. **5.** Middle circular smooth muscle layer. **6.** Outer longitudinal smooth muscle layer.

Fig. 33-36. Enlargement of area similar to rectangle in Fig. 33-35. Ductus deferens. Rat. E.M. X 640. **1.** Lumen. **2.** Pseudostratified columnar epithelium. **3.** Lamina propria. **4.** Capillaries. **5.** Inner longitudinal smooth muscle layer.

Fig. 33-37. Enlargement of rectangle (A) in Fig. 33-36. Ductus deferens. Rat. E.M. X 4300. **1.** Lumen. **2.** Stereocilia. **3.** Nuclei. **4.** Golgi complexes. **5.** Mitochondria. **6.** Lipid droplets. **7.** Secretory droplets.

Fig. 33-38. Enlargement of area similar to rectangle (B) in Fig. 33-36. Ductus deferens. Rat. E.M. X 4500. **1.** Some of the cells in the lamina propria are smooth muscle cells, representing a kind of muscularis mucosae. **2.** Collagen of lamina propria. **3.** Nucleus of Schwann cell of non-myelinated nerve. **4.** Nuclei of smooth muscle cells in the inner longitudinal layer. **5.** Cross-sectioned peripheral parts of smooth muscle cell cytoplasm.

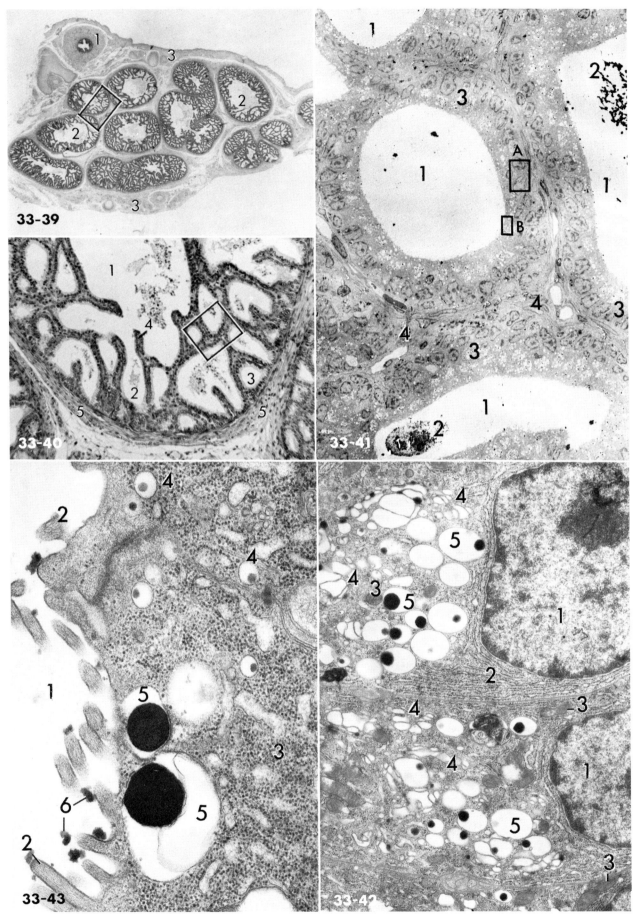

Fig. 33-39. Cross section of ductus deferens and seminal vesicle. Monkey. L.M. X 11.
1. Ductus deferens. **2.** Lumen of the coiled tube which constitutes the seminal vesicle.
3. Capsule.

Fig. 33-40. Enlargement of rectangle in Fig. 33-39. Seminal vesicle. Monkey. L.M. X 107.
1. Main lumen. **2.** Diverticulum. **3.** Crypt.
4. Ridge covered by epithelium. **5.** Lamina muscularis.

Fig. 33-41. Enlargement of area similar to rectangle in Fig. 33-40. Seminal vesicle. Rat. E.M. X 630. **1.** Lumina of diverticuli.
2. Accumulation of secretion. **3.** Simple columnar epithelium. **4.** Connective tissue with capillaries.

Fig. 33-42. Enlargement of area similar to rectangle (A) in Fig. 33-41. Seminal vesicle. Rat. E.M. X 10,000. **1.** Nuclei of epithelial cells. **2.** Granular endoplasmic reticulum.
3. Mitochondria. **4.** Golgi complexes.
5. Secretory granules, with and without electron-dense core.

Fig. 33-43. Enlargement of area similar to rectangle (B) in Fig. 33-41. Seminal vesicle. Rat. E.M. X 32,000. **1.** Lumen.
2. Microvilli. **3.** Ribosomes. **4.** Small secretory granules. **5.** Large secretory granules with dense core. **6.** Residue of discharged dense core of secretory granule.

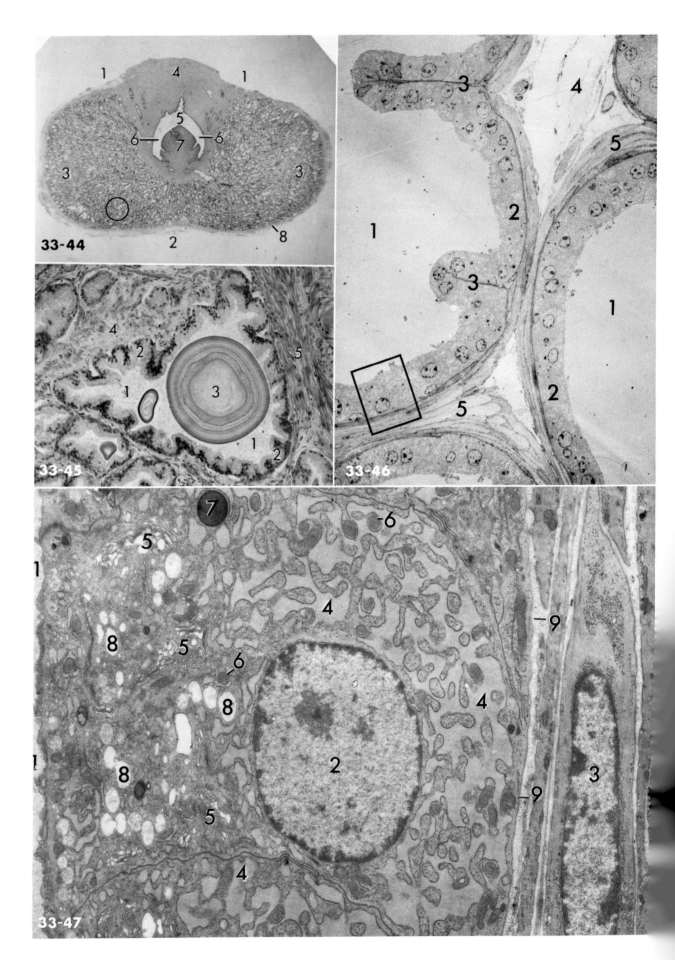

Fig. 33-44. Cross section of prostate gland. Monkey. L.M. X 5. **1.** Anterior (pubic) surface. **2.** Posterior (rectal) surface. **3.** Lateral lobes. **4.** Broad median septum. **5.** Prostatic urethra. **6.** Prostatic sinus. **7.** Colliculus seminalis of urethral crest. **8.** Capsule.

Fig. 33-45. Enlargement of area similar to circle in Fig. 33-44. Prostate. Human. L.M. X 125. **1.** Alveolar lumen. **2.** Glandular epithelium. **3.** Corpora amylacea. **4.** Connective tissue stroma. **5.** Smooth muscle cells.

Fig. 33-46. Survey of prostatic alveoli. Dorsal prostate. Rat. E.M. X 560. **1.** Alveolar lumen. **2.** Glandular epithelium. **3.** Epithelial folds. **4.** Connective tissue stroma. **5.** Smooth muscle cells.

Fig. 33-47. Enlargement of area similar to rectangle in Fig. 33-46. Dorsal prostate. Rat. E.M. X 8000. **1.** Lumen of gland. **2.** Nucleus of cuboidal epithelial cell. **3.** Nucleus of smooth muscle cell. **4.** Dilated cisternae of granular endoplasmic reticulum. **5.** Golgi complexes. **6.** Mitochondria. **7.** Lysosome. **8.** Secretory droplets. **9.** Thin basal lamina (not seen at this magnification).

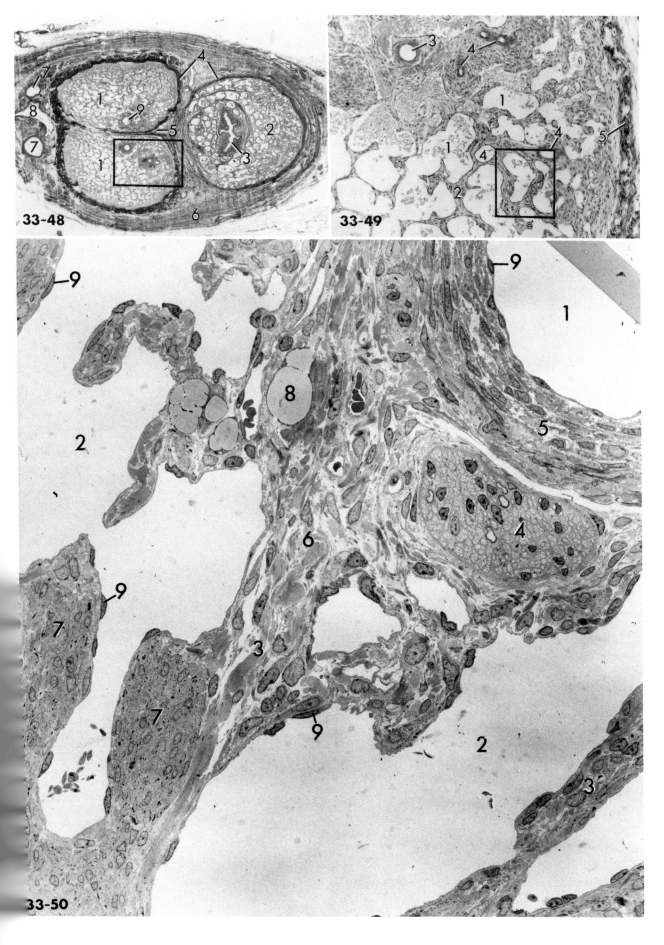

Fig. 33-48. Cross section of root of penis. Newborn child. L.M. X 13. **1.** Corpora cavernosa penis. **2.** Corpus cavernosum (spongiosum) urethrae. **3.** Urethra. **4.** Tunica albuginea. **5.** Septum penis. **6.** Fascia penis. **7.** Dorsal arteries. **8.** Dorsal vein. **9.** Central arteries.

Fig. 33-49. Enlargement of area similar to rectangle in Fig. 33-48. Penis. Newborn child. L.M. X 90. **1.** Lacunae (sinuses). **2.** Trabeculae. **3.** Central artery. **4.** Helicine arteries and arterioles. **5.** Tunica albuginea.

Fig. 33-50. Enlargement of area similar to square in Fig. 33-49. Penis. Rat. E.M. X 600. **1.** Lumen of helicine artery. **2.** Lacunae (sinuses). **3.** Trabeculae. **4.** Nerve bundle (only non-myelinated axons). **5.** Smooth muscle cells in media. **6.** Trabecula with collagenous bundles. **7.** Trabecula with smooth muscle bundles. **8.** Fat cell. **9.** Nuclei of endothelial cells.

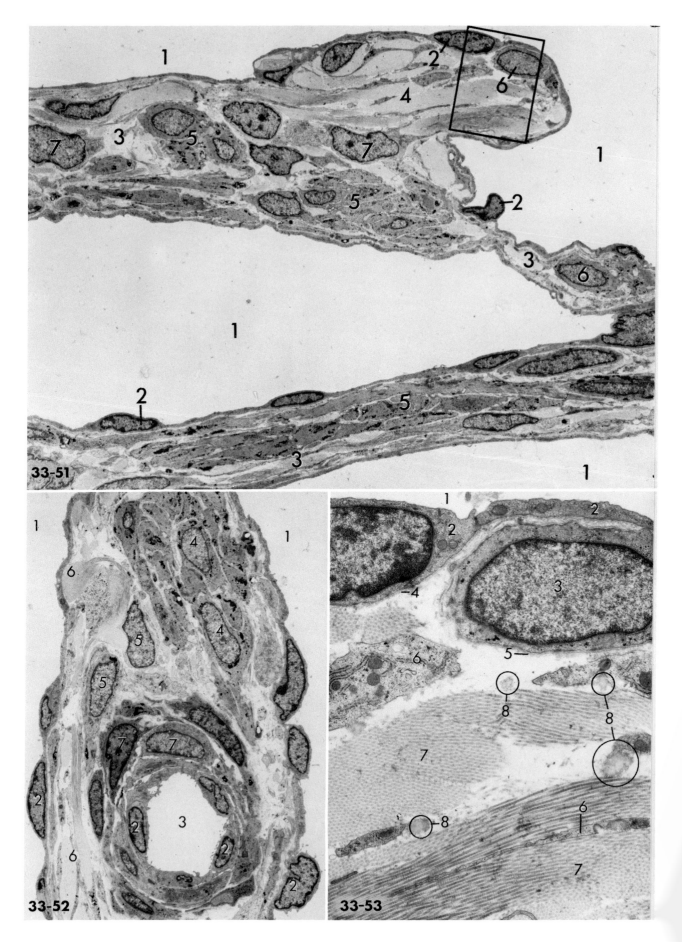

Fig. 33-51. Survey of cavernous tissue. Corpus cavernosum penis. Rat. E.M. X 1740. **1.** Lacunae (sinuses). **2.** Nuclei of endothelial cells. **3.** Trabeculae. **4.** Bundles of collagenous fibrils. **5.** Bundles of smooth muscle cells. **6.** Nuclei of singly occurring smooth muscle cells. **7.** Nuclei of fibroblasts.

Fig. 33-52. Trabecula. Corpus cavernosum penis. Rat. E.M. X 1800. **1.** Lacunae. **2.** Nuclei of endothelial cells. **3.** Lumen of cross-sectioned small helcine arteriole. Luminal diameter 10 μ. **4.** Nuclei of smooth muscle cells in a muscle bundle in the core of a trabecula. **5.** Nuclei of fibroblasts. **6.** Bundles of collagenous fibrils. **7.** Longitudinally oriented smooth muscle cells of the helcine arteriole.

Fig. 33-53. Enlargement of rectangle in Fig. 33-51. Corpus cavernosum penis. Rat. E.M. X 9000. **1.** Lacuna. **2.** Endothelium (non-fenestrated). **3.** Nucleus of smooth muscle cell. **4.** Basal lamina of endothelium. **5.** Basal (external) lamina of smooth muscle cell. **6.** Cytoplasmic strands of fibroblasts. **7.** Bundles of collagenous fibrils. **8.** Circles: cross-sectioned elastic fibrils.

398

References

TESTIS

Bawa, S. R. The fine structure of the Sertoli cell of the human testis. J. Ultrastruct. Res. *9*: 459–474 (1963).

Bedford, J. M. and Nicander, L. Ultrastructural changes in the acrosome and sperm membranes during maturation of spermatozoa in the testis and epididymis of the rabbit and monkey. J. Anat. *108*: 527–543 (1971).

Belt, W. D. and Cavazos, L. F. Fine structure of the interstitial cells of Leydig in the boar. Anat. Rec. *158*: 333–350 (1967).

Bishop, D. Sperm motility. Physiol. Rev. *42*: 1–59 (1962).

Burgos, M. H., Vitale-Calpe, R. and Aoki, A. Fine structure of the testis and its functional significance. *In:* The Testis. (Eds. A. D. Johnson, W. R. Gomes and N. L. Van Demark), Vol. I, pp. 551–649. Academic Press, New York, 1970.

Bröckelman, J. Fine structure of germ cells and Sertoli cells during the cycle of the seminiferous epithelium in rat. Z. Zellforsch. *59*: 820–850 (1963).

Christensen, A. K. and Fawcett, D. W. The fine structure of testicular interstitial cells in mice. Am. J. Anat. *118*: 551–572 (1966).

Clermont, Y. The cycle of the seminiferous epithelium in man. Am. J. Anat. *112*: 35–52 (1963).

de Kretser, D. M. The fine structure of the testicular interstitial cells in men of normal androgenic status. Z. Zellforsch. *80*: 594–609 (1967).

Dym, M. and Fawcett, D. W. The blood-testis barrier in the rat and the physiological compartmentation of the seminiferous epithelium. Biol. Reprod. *3*: 308–326 (1970).

Fawcett, D. W. The structure of the mammalian spermatozoon. Int. Rev. Cytol. *7*: 195–234 (1958).

Fawcett, D. W. The topographical relationship between the plane of the central pair of flagellar fibrils and the transverse axis of the head in guinea-pig spermatozoa. J. Cell Sci. *3*: 187–189 (1968).

Fawcett, D. W. and Ito, S. The fine structure of bat spermatozoa. Am. J. Anat. *116*: 567–610 (1965).

Flickinger, C. and Fawcett, D. W. The junctional specializations of Sertoli cells in the seminiferous epithelium. Anat. Rec. *158*: 207–222 (1967).

Mann, T. Biochemistry of Semen and of the Male Reproductive Tract. Wiley, New York, 1964.

Nicander, L. An electron microscopical study of cell contacts in the seminiferous tubules of some mammals. Z. Zellforsch. *83*: 375–397 (1967).

Roosen-Runge, E. C. The process of spermatogenesis in mammals. Biol. Rev. *37*: 343–377 (1962).

Ross, M. H. Contractile cells in human seminiferous tubules. Science *153*: 1271–1273 (1966).

Schmidt, F. C. Licht- und elektronenmikroskopische Untersuchungen am menschlichen Hoden und Nebenhoden. Z. Zellforsch. *63*: 707–729 (1964).

EPIDIDYMIS

Friend, D. S. Cytochemical staining of multivesicular body and Golgi vesicles. J. Cell Biol. *41*: 269–279 (1969).

Friend, D. S. and Farquhar, M. G.: Functions of coated vesicles during protein absorption in the rat vas deferens. J. Cell Biol. *35*: 357–376 (1967).

Hamilton, D. W., Jones, A. L. and Fawcett, D. W. Cholesterol biosynthesis in the mouse epididymis and ductus deferens: a biochemical and morphological study. Biol. Reprod. *1*: 167–184 (1969).

Horstmann, E. Elektronenmikroskopie des menschlichen Nebenhodenepithels. Z. Zellforsch. *57*: 692–718 (1962).

Ladman, A. J. The fine structure of the ductuli efferentes of the opossum. Anat. Rec. *157*: 559–576 (1967).

Ladman, A. J. and Young, W. C. An electron microscopic study of the ductuli efferentes and rete testis of the guinea pig. J. Biophys. Biochem. Cytol. *4*: 219–226 (1958).

Mason, K. E. and Shaver, S. L. Some functions of the caput epididymis. Ann. N.Y. Acad. Sci. *55*: 585–593 (1952).

Morita, I. Some observations on the fine structure of the human ductuli efferentes testis. Arch. Histol. Japon. *26*: 341–365 (1966).

Nicander, L. An electron microscopical study of absorbing cells in the posterior caput epididymidis of rabbits. Z. Zellforsch. *66*: 829–847 (1965).

Niemi, M. The fine structure and histochemistry of the epithelial cells of the rat vas deferens. Acta Anat. *60*: 207–219 (1965).

Orgebin-Crist, M. C. Studies on the function of the epididymis. Biol. Reprod. Suppl. 1: 155–175 (1969).

SEMINAL VESICLES

Deane, H. W. and Porter, K. R. A comparative study of cytoplasmic basophilia and the population density of ribosomes in the secretory cells of the mouse seminal vesicle. Z. Zellforsch. *52*: 697–711 (1960).

Riva, A. Fine structure of human seminal vesicle epithelium. J. Anat. *102*: 71–86 (1967).

PROSTATE

Brandes, D. The fine structure and histochemistry of prostatic glands in relation to sex hormones. Int. Rev. Cytol. *20*: 207–276 (1966).

Brandes, D. and Portela, A. The fine structure of the epithelial cells of the mouse prostate. I. Coagulating gland epithelium. J. Biophys. Biochem. Cytol. *7*: 505–510 (1960).

Brandes, D. and Portela, A. The fine structure of the epithelial cells of the mouse prostate. II. Ventral lobe epithelium. J. Biophys. Biochem. Cytol. *7*: 511–514 (1960).

Flickinger, C. J. The fine structure and development of the seminal vesicles and prostate in the fetal rat. Z. Zellforsch. *109*: 1–14 (1970).

Huggins, C. The prostatic secretion. Harvey Lectures *42*: 148–193 (1947).

PENIS

Leeson, T. S. and Leeson, C. R. The fine structure of cavernous tissue in the adult rat penis. Investig. Urology *3*: 144–154 (1965).

34 Female reproductive system

Fig. 34-1. Ovary. Cat. E.M. X 11. **1.** Cortex.
2. Medulla. **3.** Follicles. **4.** Corpora lutea.

Fig. 34-2. Enlargement of rectangle in Fig.
34-1. L.M. X 16. **1.** Primordial follicles.
2. Secondary follicle. **3.** Stroma. **4.** Corpus
luteum. **5.** Interstitial gland.

Fig. 34-3. Enlargement of area similar to
rectangle in Fig. 34-2. Rat. E.M. X 860.
1. Peritoneal cavity. **2.** Germinal epithelium.
3. Tunica albuginea with interstitial
fibroblasts. **4.** Primordial follicles. **5.** Oocyte
of secondary follicle. Nucleus is not in
plane of section. **6.** Zona pellucida.
7. Follicular cells. **8.** Basal lamina.
9. Theca folliculi. (interna). **10.** Theca
folliculi (externa). **11.** Capillaries.

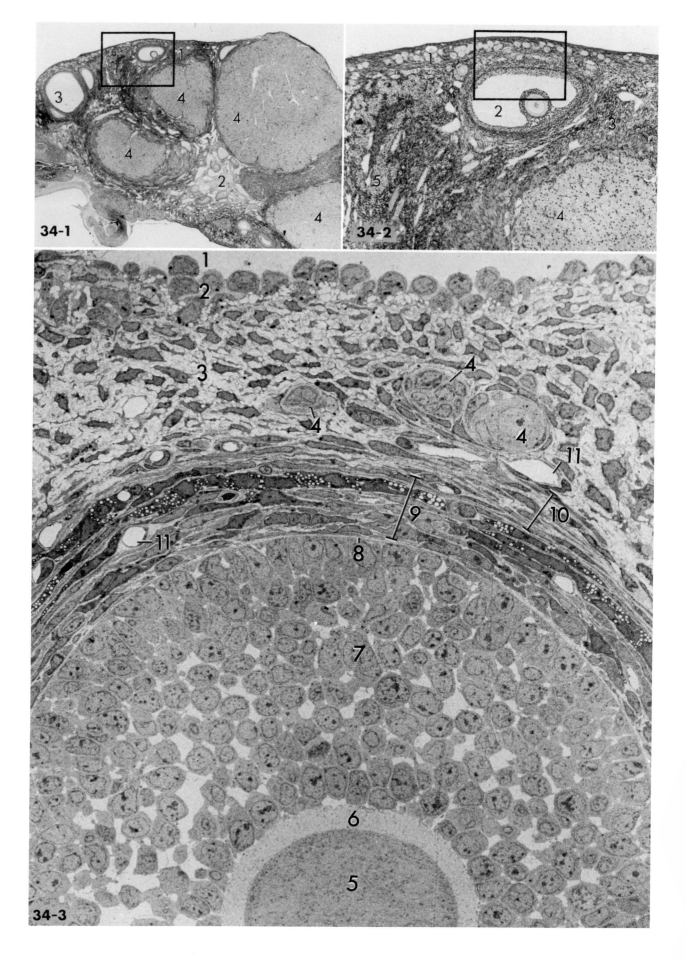

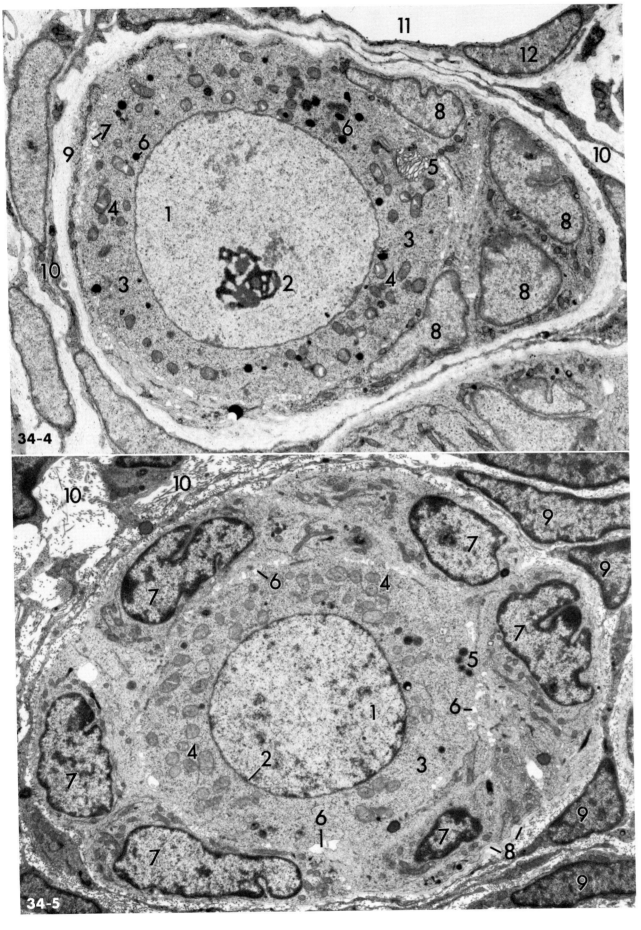

Fig. 34-4. Primordial follicle. Ovary. Rat. E.M. X 5400. **1.** Nucleus of primordial germ cell. **2.** Nucleolus in reticular form. **3.** Ooplasm. **4.** Mitochondria. **5.** Golgi complex. **6.** Cortical granules. **7.** Slightly ruffled surface of primordial germ cell. **8.** Nuclei of follicular cells. **9.** Thin cytoplasmic sheath of follicular cells, embracing the germ cell. **10.** Stromal cells. **11.** Lumen of capillary. **12.** Nucleus of endothelial cell.

Fig. 34-5. Primary follicle. Ovary. Rat. E.M. X 4400. **1.** Nucleus of primary oocyte. The nucleolus is not in the plane of section. **2.** Nuclear envelope. **3.** Ooplasm. **4.** Mitochondria. **5.** Cortical granules. **6.** Surface of oocyte. **7.** Nuclei of cuboidal follicular cells. **8.** Basal lamina. **9.** Nuclei of stromal cells. There is no theca folliculi formed as yet. **10.** Collagen of ovarian stroma.

403

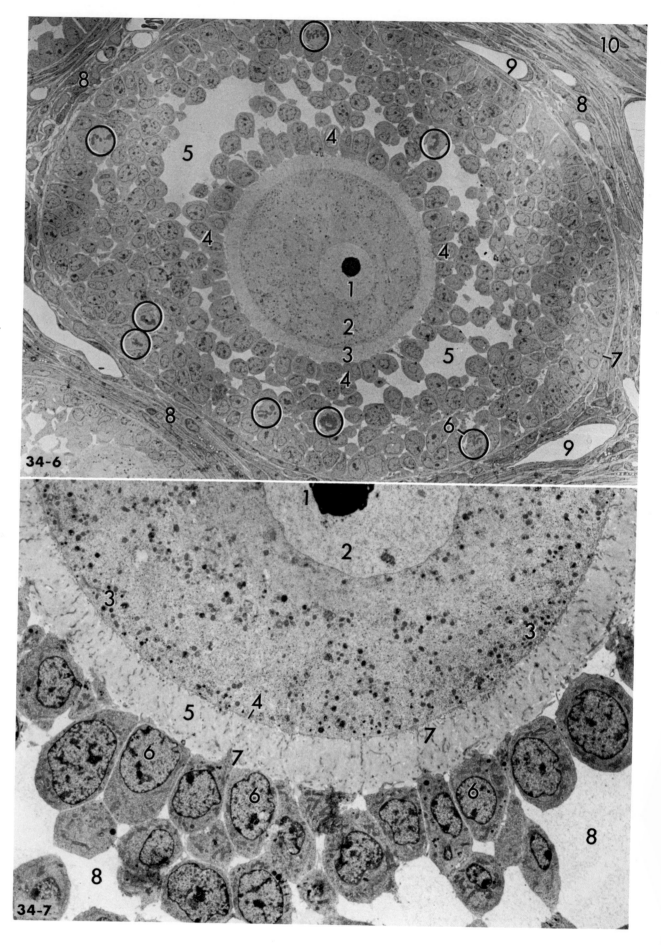

Fig. 34-6. Early secondary vesicular follicle.
Ovary. Rat. E.M. X 580. **1.** Nucleus.
2. Secondary oocyte. **3.** Zona pellucida.
4. Corona radiata. **5.** Antrum folliculi.
6. Cells of membrana granulosa, many of
which are in various stages of mitosis
(circles). **7.** Basal lamina (glassy membrane).
8. Thecae folliculi. **9.** Perifollicular
capillaries. **10.** Ovarian stroma.
Fig. 34-7. Part of early secondary vesicular
follicle. Ovary. Rat. E.M. X 1800.
1. Nucleolus. **2.** Nucleus of secondary oocyte.
3. Cortical granules. **4.** Surface oocyte.
5. Zona pellucida. **6.** Nuclei of the follicular
cells which make up the corona radiata.
7. Slender cell processes from the oocyte and
the corona radiata cells penerate the zona
pellucida. **8.** Antrum folliculi with precipitated
liquor folliculi.

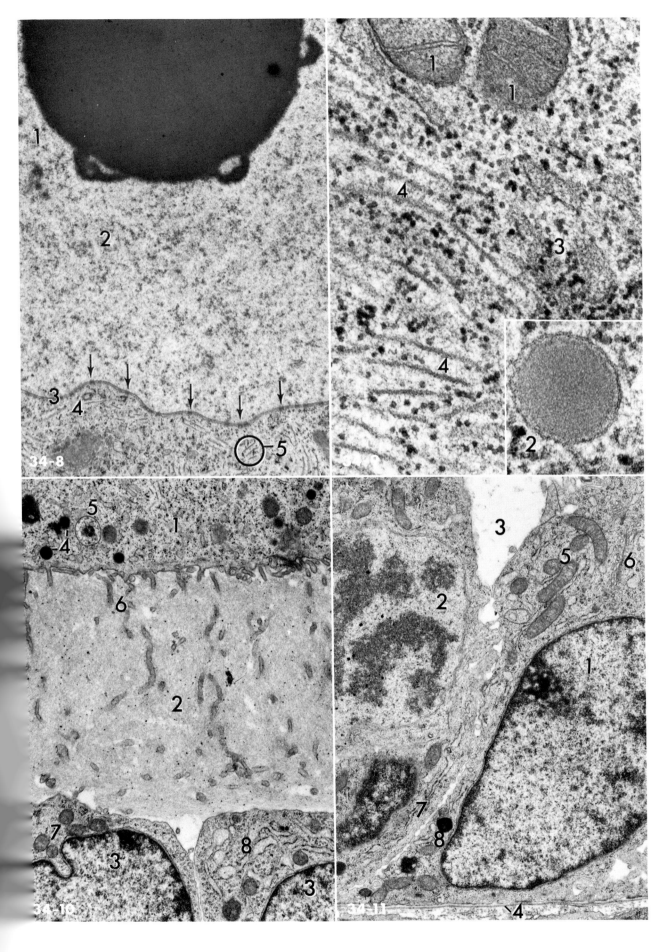

Fig. 34-8. Secondary follicle. Ovary. Rat. E.M. X 15,000. **1.** Nucleolus of oocyte is extremely electron-dense with only occasional peripheral threads. **2.** Nucleoplasm is finely granular. **3.** Nuclear envelope with numerous pores (arrows). **4.** Ooplasm. **5.** Crystalline bodies (plaques).

Fig. 34-9. Detail of the ooplasm of a secondary oocyte. Ovary. Rat. E.M. X 60,000. **1.** Mitochondria with membranous cristae. **2.** Inset: granule of the type classified as cortical granule; boundary membrane is of the single trilaminar type. (X 100,000). **3.** The majority of these dense dots are particulate glycogen; the smaller may be ribosomes. **4.** Crystalline bodies (plaques).

Fig. 34-10. Detail of secondary follicle. Ovary. Rat. E.M. X 13,000. **1.** Peripheral part of secondary oocyte. **2.** Zona pellucida with finely fibrillar substance. **3.** Nuclei of follicular cells of corona radiata. **4.** Cortical granules. **5.** Lysosome. **6.** Microvilli. **7.** Mitochondria. **8.** Granular endoplasmic reticulum.

Fig. 34-11. Detail of secondary follicle. Ovary. Rat. E.M. X 8000. **1.** Nucleus of membrana granulosa cell. **2.** Nucleus in late telophase. **3.** Intercellular space which communicates with antrum folliculi. **4.** Basal lamina. **5.** Mitochondria. **6.** Golgi complex. **7.** Granular endoplasmic reticulum. **8.** Lipid droplet.

Fig. 34-12. Section of part of wall of secondary follicle. Ovary. Rat. E.M. X 1800. **1.** Nuclei of follicular cells of membrana granulosa. **2.** Dividing follicular cell. **3** Plane of basal lamina (glassy membrane). The lamina itself is not discernible at this magnification. **4.** Nuclei of the cells which make up the theca interna. **5.** These cells are also part of the theca interna; their cytoplasm is filled with lipid droplets. **6.** Capillaries in theca interna. **7.** Nuclei of cells which make up the theca externa.

Fig. 34-13. Detail of cells in the theca interna of secondary follicle. Ovary. Rat. E.M. X 29,000. **1.** Nucleus. **2.** Golgi complex. **3.** Mitochondria. **4.** Cisternae of the granular endoplasmic reticulum. **5.** Ribosomes. **6.** Slender part of an adjacent cell with thin filaments in the cytoplasm. **7.** Lysosome. **8.** Intercellular space. **9.** Collagenous fibrils.

Fig. 34-14. Detail of cells in theca externa of secondary follicle. Ovary. Rat. E.M. X 9000. **1.** Nuclei. **2.** Major part of the cytoplasm is occupied by filaments. **3.** A minor part of the cytoplasm has granular endoplasmic reticulum. **4.** Particulate glycogen. **5.** Large intercellular spaces with a network of collagenous fibrils.

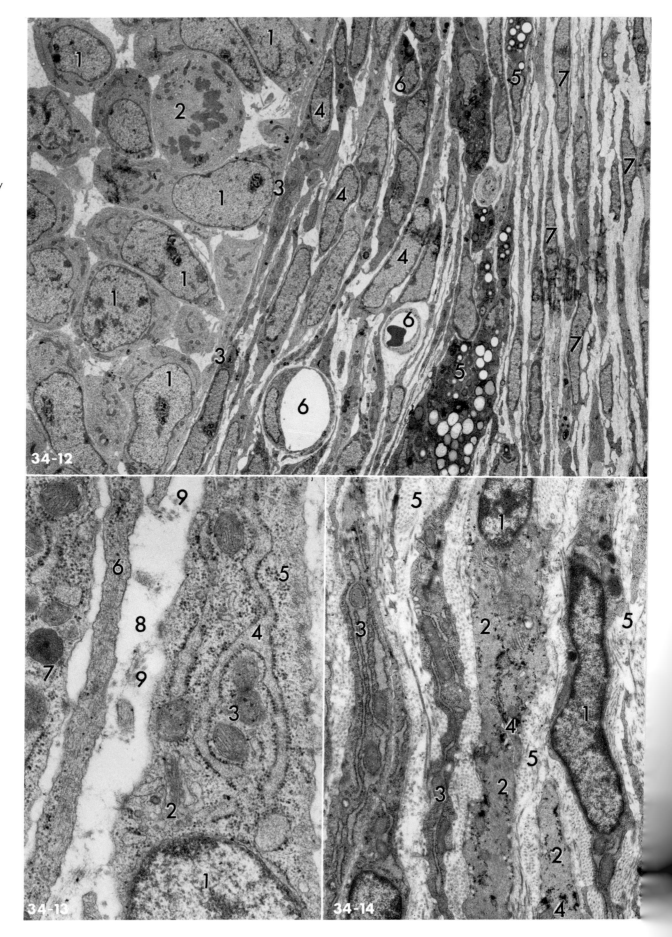

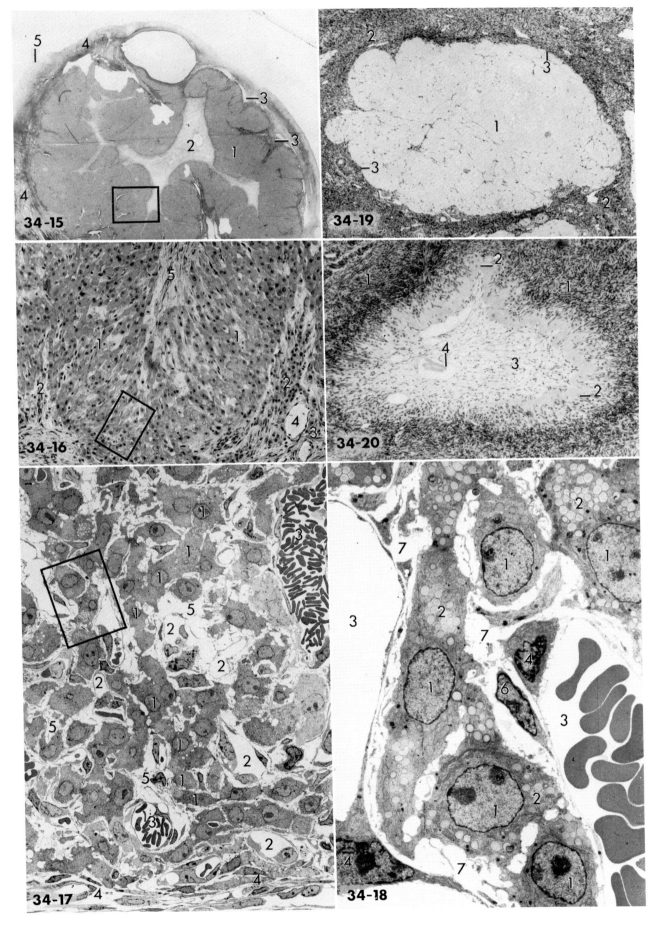

Fig. 34-15. Corpus luteum of pregnancy. Ovary. Human. L.M. X 5.5. **1.** Folded layer of granulosa lutein cells. **2.** Former follicular cavity. **3.** Wedges of theca lutein cells. **4.** Theca externa cells. **5.** Ovarian surface.

Fig. 34-16. Enlargement of area similar to rectangle in Fig. 34-15. Corpus luteum of pregnancy. Ovary. Human. L.M. X 100. **1.** Cords of granulosa lutein cells. **2.** Wedges of theca lutein cells. **3.** Theca externa cells. **4.** Capillary. **5.** Fibroblasts and loose connective tissue in former follicular antrum.

Fig. 34-17. Enlargement of area similar to rectangle in Fig. 34-16. Corpus luteum. Ovary. Rat. E.M. X 540. **1.** Cords of granulosa lutein cells. **2.** Capillaries. **3.** Large venous capillaries. **4.** Theca externa (barely seen). **5.** Intercellular spaces.

Fig. 34-18. Enlargement of area similar to rectangle in Fig. 34-17. Ovary. Rat. E.M. X 1700. **1.** Nuclei of granulosa lutein cells. **2.** Lipid droplets. **3.** Capillaries. **4.** Nuclei of endothelial cells. **5.** Erythrocytes. **6.** Pericyte. Note that theca lutein cells are missing in rats. **7.** Intercellular spaces.

Fig. 34-19. Corpus albicans. Ovary. Human. L.M. × 43. **1.** Corpus albicans is made up of extracellular hyaline masses and some residual cells of the former corpus luteum. **2.** Ovarian stroma. **3.** Border toward the ovarian stroma is sharp and the transition abrupt.

Fig. 34-20. Corpus atreticum. Ovary. Human. L.M. × 85. **1.** Ovarian stroma. **2.** Folded, thickened remnant of the glassy membrane. **3.** Former membrana granulosa, now highly disorganized. **4.** Residue of collapsed zona pellucida.

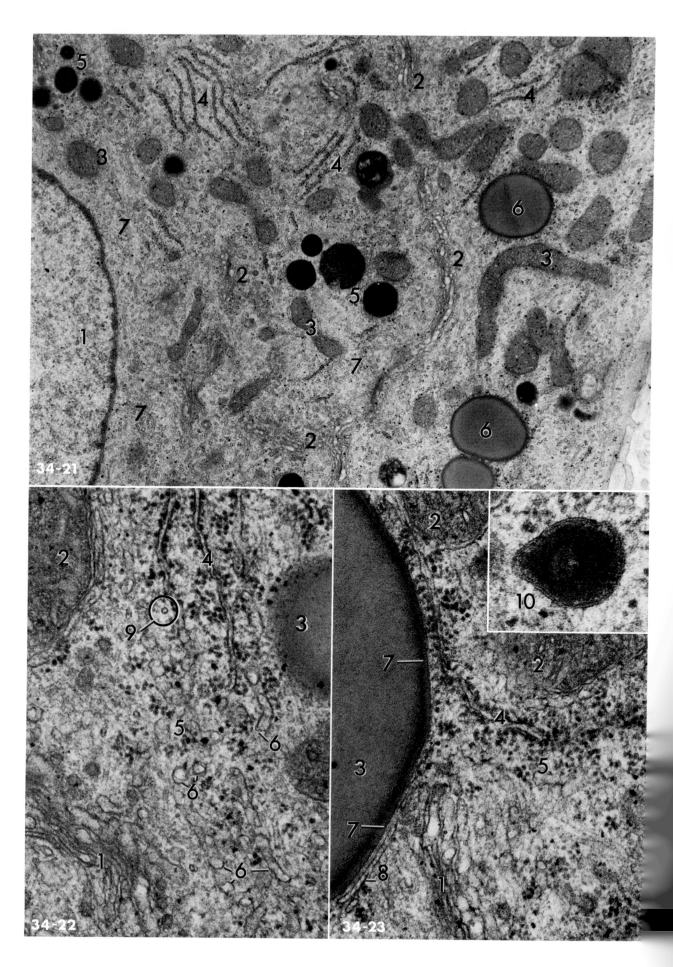

Fig. 34-21. Fine structural organization of granulosa lutein cell. Corpus luteum. Ovary. Rat. E.M. X 14,500. **1.** Nucleus. **2.** Golgi complexes. **3.** Mitochondria. **4.** Granular endoplasmic reticulum. **5.** Lipofuscin pigment granules (secondary lysosomes). **6.** Lipid droplets. **7.** The overall "busy" cytoplasmic background is occupied by vesicular and tubular profiles of the agranular endoplasmic reticulum.

Fig. 34-22 & 34-23. Details of granulosa lutein cell. Corpus luteum. Ovary. Rat. E.M. X 58,000. **1.** Golgi complex. **2.** Mitochondria. **3.** Lipid droplets. **4.** Granular endoplasmic reticulum. **5.** Ribsosomes. **6.** Agranular endoplasmic reticulum. **7.** Lipid droplet boundary membrane. **8.** Agranular endoplasmic reticulum closely apposed to lipid boundary membrane. **9.** Microtubule. **10.** Inset: lysosome with single trilaminar boundary membrane (X 100,000).

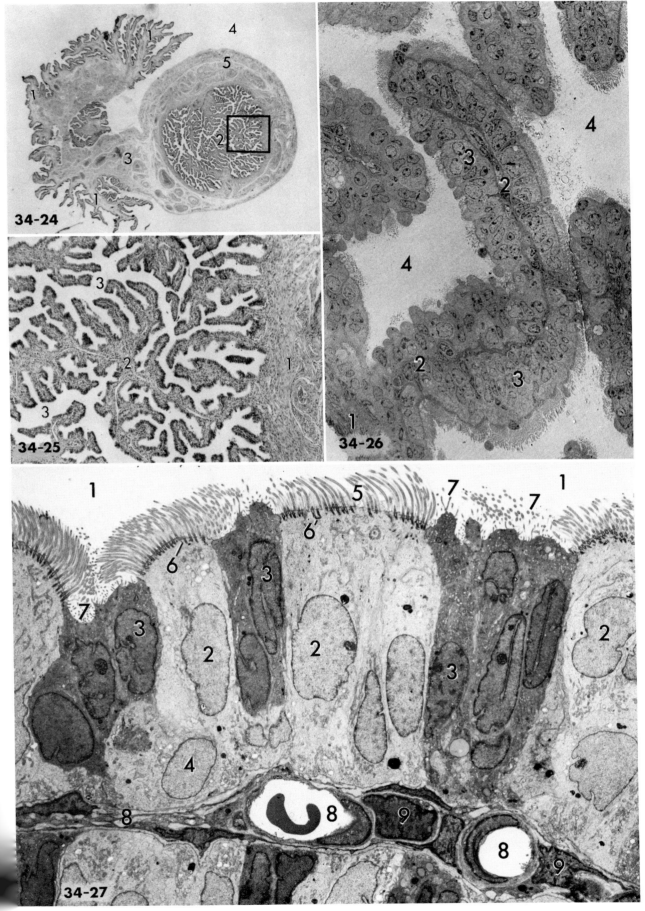

Fig. 34-24. Cross section of oviduct. Human. L.M. X 8. **1.** Fimbriae. **2.** Ampulla. **3.** Mesosalpinx. **4.** Peritoneal cavity. **5.** Muscularis.

Fig. 34-25. Enlargement of rectangle in Fig. 34-24. Human. L.M. X 44. **1.** Muscularis. **2.** Highly folded mucosa. **3.** Lumen of ampulla.

Fig. 34-26. Part of ampullary mucosa in oviduct. Mouse. E.M. X 560. **1.** Muscularis. **2.** Lamina propria of folded mucous membrane. **3.** Ciliated epithelium. **4.** Lumen of ampulla.

Fig. 34-27. Part of simple columnar ciliated epithelium in ampulla of oviduct. Rat. E.M. X 1750. **1.** Lumen of ampulla. **2.** Nuclei of ciliated cells. **3.** Nuclei of non-ciliated, secretory cells (peg-cells). **4.** Occasionally, basal cells occur. **5.** Cilia. **6.** Basal bodies. **7.** Microvilli. **8.** Capillary lumina. **9.** Fibroblasts in lamina propria.

Fig. 34-28. Section of wall of uterus. Proliferative phase. Human. L.M. X 7.
1. Uterine cavity. **2.** Endometrium. **3.** Myometrium. **4.** Functionalis of endometrium. **5.** Basalis of endometrium (between levels indicated by dashed lines).

Fig. 34-29. Endometrium in proliferative phase. Uterus. Human. L.M. X 30. **1.** Uterine cavity. **2.** Endometrial stroma. **3.** Straight uterine glands in functionalis. **4.** Slightly coiled uterine glands in basalis. **5.** Myometrium.

Fig. 34-30. Enlargement of area similar to rectangle in Fig. 34-29. Uterine gland. Proliferative phase. Human. E.M. X 540.
1. Lumen of uterine gland. **2.** Tall, columnar epithelial cells, some with short dome-like protrusions into the lumen. **3.** Epithelial cells in mitosis. **4.** Endometrial stroma.

Fig. 34-31. Enlargment of rectangle in Fig. 34-30. Detail of epithelium of uterine gland. Proliferative phase. Human. E.M. X 4500.
1. Lumen of uterine gland. **2.** Thin basal lamina. **3.** Nuclei of columnar epithelial cells. **4.** Nuclei in late telophase of mitosis. **5.** Plane of cell separation. **6.** Mitochondria. **7.** The high background electron density is due to numerous microsomes. **8.** Microvilli.

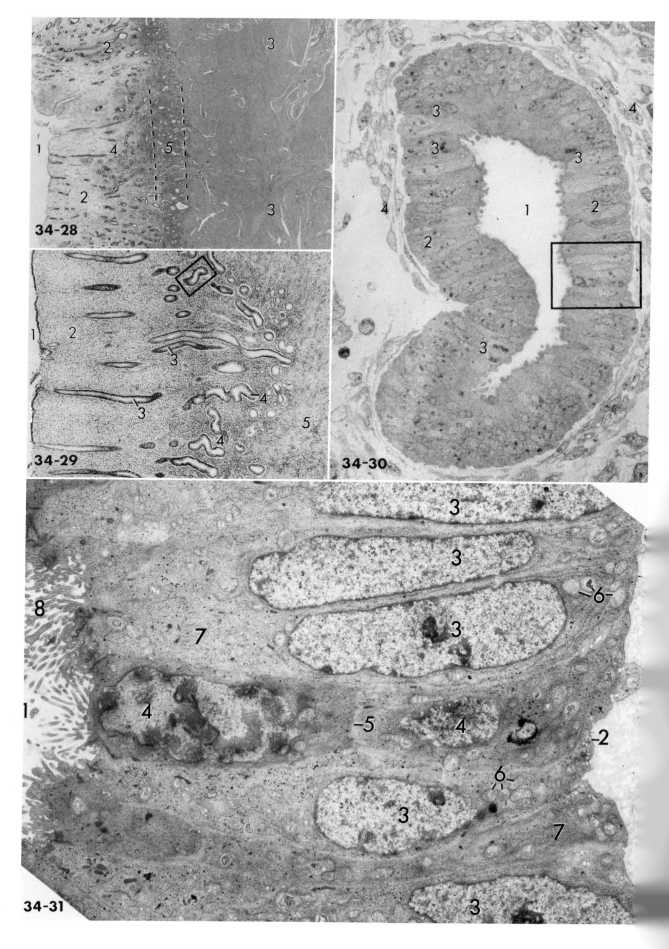

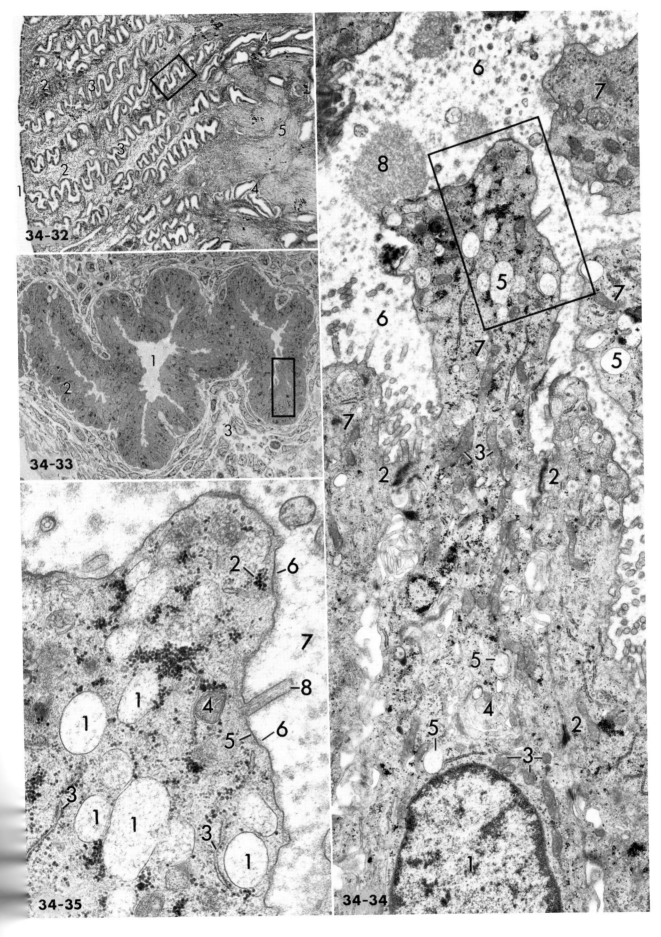

Fig. 34-32. Endometrium in late secretory phase. Uterus. Human. L.M. X 27. **1.** Uterine cavity. **2.** Endometrial stroma. **3.** Highly coiled uterine glands in functionalis. **4.** Slightly coiled uterine glands in basalis. **5.** Myometrium.

Fig. 34-33. Enlargement of area similar to rectangle in Fig. 34-32. Uterine gland. Late secretory phase. Human. E.M. X 480. **1.** Lumen of uterine gland. **2.** Medium high columnar epithelial cells, some with tall dome-like protrusions. **3.** Endometrial stroma.

Fig. 34-34. Enlargement of area similar to rectangle in Fig. 34-33. Detail of epithelial cell in uterine gland. Late secretory phase. Human. E.M. X 9500. **1.** Nucleus of epithelial cell in uterine gland. **2.** Junctional complexes. **3.** Mitochondria. **4.** Golgi zone. **5.** Secretory droplets. **6.** Lumen of uterine gland. **7.** Dome-like cell protrusions. **8.** Finely fibrillar masses of mucin.

Fig. 34-35. Enlargement of rectangle in Fig. 34-34. Tip of epithelial cell in uterine gland. Late secretory phase. Human. E.M. X 55,000. **1.** Secretory droplets. **2.** Particulate glycogen. **3.** Granular endoplasmic reticulum. **4.** Mitochondrion. **5.** Surface membrane. **6.** Glycocalyx or layer of mucin attached to the cell surface. **7.** Mucin free in the lumen. **8.** Microvillus.

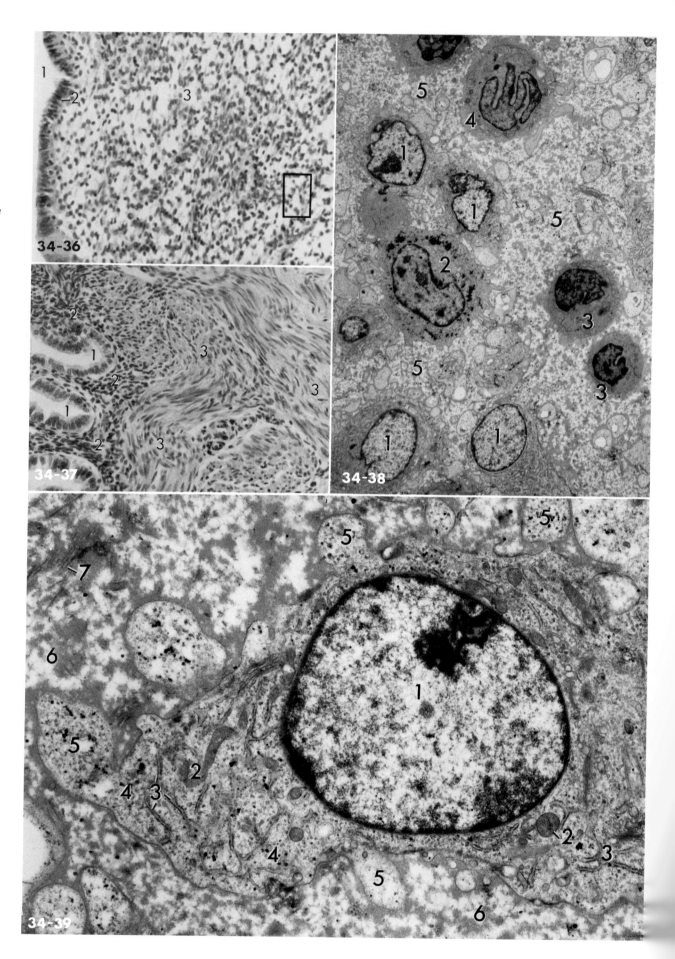

Fig. 34-36. Endometrial stroma. Late secretory phase. Uterus. Human. L.M. X 200. **1.** Uterine cavity. **2.** Surface epithelium. **3.** Loose endometrial stroma between uterine glands (glands not shown).

Fig. 34-37. Transitional zone between endometrium and myometrium. Late secretory phase. Uterus. Human. L.M. X 220. **1.** Lumen of uterine glands in basal layer of endometrium (basalis). **2.** Dense endometrial stroma. **3.** Smooth muscle cells of myometrium.

Fig. 34-38. Enlargemeent of area similar to rectangle in Fig. 34-36. Detail of endometrial stroma. Late secretory phase. Uterus. Human. E.M. X 1800. **1.** Nuclei of fibroblast-like stromal cells. **2.** Stromal cell with large glycogen accumulations. **3.** Lymphocytes. **4.** Monocytes. **5.** Intercellular space with mucoid material.

Fig. 34-39. Detail of fibroblast-like cell (stromal or decidual cell). Endometrial stroma. Late secretory phase. Uterus. Human. E.M. X 9000. **1.** Nucleus. **2.** Mitochondria. **3.** Granular endoplasmic reticulum. **4.** Free ribosomes. **5.** Bulbous cell processes (pseudopods). **6.** Mucoid masses in extracellular space. **7.** Fine collagenous fibrils.

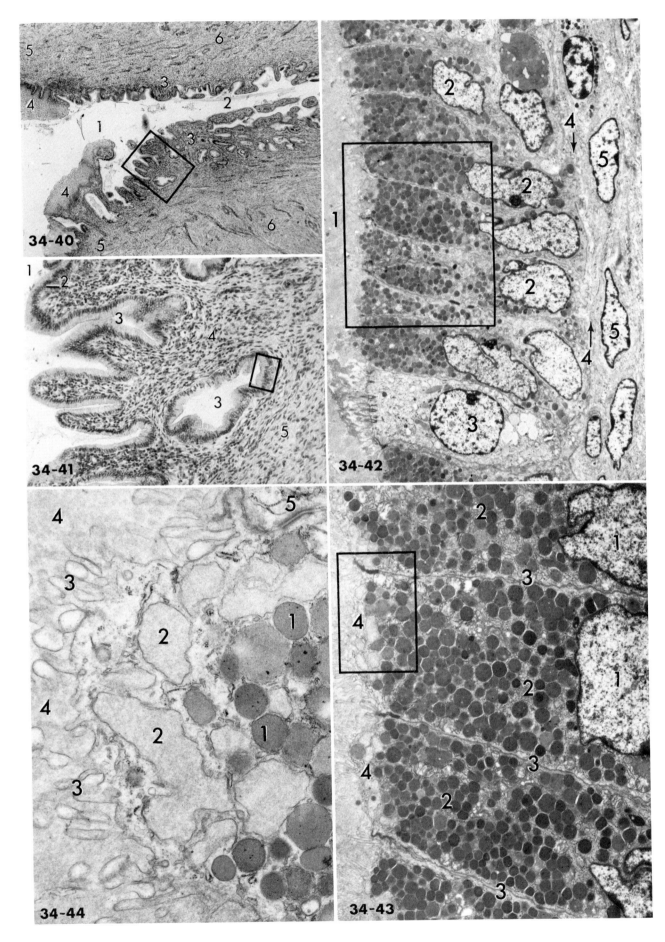

Fig. 34-40. Longitudinal section of cervix uteri. Human. L.M. X 24. **1.** External cervical os. **2.** Cervical canal. **3.** Endocervix. **4.** Exocervix. **5.** Portio vaginalis. **6.** Mixture of dense connective tissue and smooth muscle fibers.

Fig. 34-41. Enlargement of the rectangle in Fig. 34-40. Endometrium. Cervix uteri. Human. L.M. X 125. **1.** Cervical canal. **2.** Surface epithelium. **3.** Branched, tubular cervical glands. **4.** Dense endometrial connective tissue. **5.** Smooth muscle cells.

Fig. 34-42. Enlargement of area similar to rectangle in Fig. 34-41. Survey of glandular epithelium. Cervix uteri. Human. E.M. X 1800. **1.** Lumen of gland. **2.** Nucleus of mucous cell. **3.** Nucleus of ciliated cell. **4.** Level of basal lamina. **5.** Nuclei of fibroblasts in stroma.

Fig. 34-43. Enlargement of area similar to rectangle in Fig. 34-42. Glandular epithelium. Cervix uteri. Human. E.M. X 4400. **1.** Nuclei. **2.** Mucigen granules. **3.** Cell borders. **4.** Cell apex.

Fig. 34-44. Enlargement of area similar to rectangle in Fig. 34-43. Apex of epithelial cell. Cervical gland. Human. E.M. X 29,000. **1.** Highly electron-dense secretory (mucigen) granules. **2.** Secretory vacuoles. **3.** Microvilli. **4.** Lumen with mucoid masses. **5.** Junctional complex.

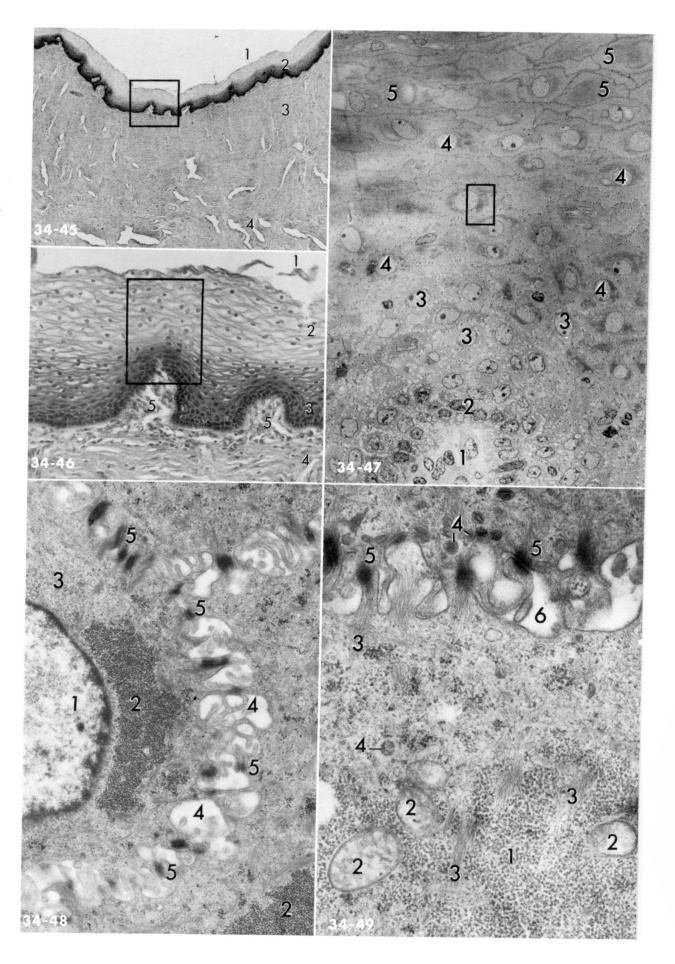

Fig. 34-45. Wall of vagina. Human. L.M. X 30.
1. Lumen of vagina. **2.** Stratified squamous epithelium. **3.** Lamina propria. **4.** Venous channels.

Fig. 34-46. Enlargement of rectangle in Fig. 34-45. Stratified squamous non-keratinized epithelium. Vagina. Human. L.M. X 200.
1. Lumen with some superficial squamous cells being shed. **2.** Intermediate cells.
3. Basal cells. **4.** Lamina propria.
5. Connective tissue papillae.

Fig. 34-47. Enlargement of area similar to rectangle in Fig. 34-46. Stratified squamous non-keratinized epithelium. Vagina. Human. E.M. X 600. **1.** Connective tissue papilla.
2. Cuboidal basal cells. **3.** Nuclei of cells in layers above basal cell layer. **4.** Cells in the middle of the epithelium starting to accumulate glycogen. **5.** Superficial cells with large accumulations of glycogen. These cells appear vacuolated in routine histological preparations.

Fig. 34-48. Enlargement of area similar to rectangle in Fig. 34-47. Epithelium of vagina. Human. E.M. X 10,000. **1.** Nucleus. **2.** Large glycogen accumulations. **3.** Ribosomes.
4. Intercellular space. **5.** Desmosomes.

Fig. 34-49. Detail of cell from middle layers of stratified squamous epithelium. Vagina. Human. E.M. X 43,000. **1.** Masses of particulate glycogen. **2.** Mitochondria.
3. Tonofilaments. **4.** Membrane-coating granules. **5.** Desmosomes. **6.** Intercellular space.

414

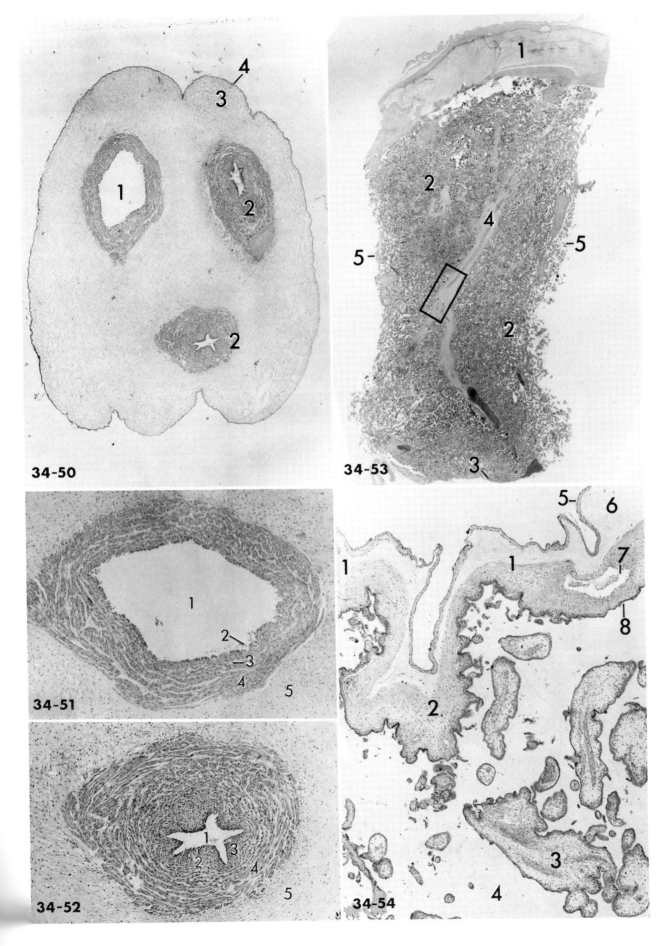

Fig. 34-50. Cross section of umbilical cord. Human. L.M. X 15. **1.** Umbilical vein. **2.** Umbilical arteries. **3.** Mucous connective tissue (Wharton's jelly). **4.** Amnion.

Fig. 34-51. Enlargement of vein in Fig. 34-50. Umbilical cord. Human. L.M. X 38. **1.** Lumen. **2.** Endothelium. **3.** Inner (thin) longitudinal layer of smooth muscle cells. **4.** Outer (thick) circular layer of smooth muscle cells. **5.** Mucous connective tissue.

Fig. 34-52. Enlargement of lower artery in Fig. 34-50. Umbilical cord. Human. L.M. X 44. **1.** Lumen. **2.** Endothelium (elastica interna missing). **3.** Inner (thick) longitudinal layer of smooth muscle cells. **4.** Outer circular layer of smooth muscle cells. **5.** Mucous connective tissue.

Fig. 34-53. Full term placenta. Human. L.M. X 6. **1.** Chorionic plate. **2.** Chorion frondosum. **3.** Surface detached from decidual (basal) plate. **4.** Main-stem villus. **5.** Cut surfaces.

Fig. 34-54. Part of placenta. Second month of gestation. Human. L.M. X 36. **1.** Chorionic plate. **2.** Main-stem villus. **3.** Terminal villi. **4.** Intervillous space. **5.** Amnion. **6.** Extra-embryonic mesoderm. **7.** Placental vein. **8.** Trophoblastic layer.

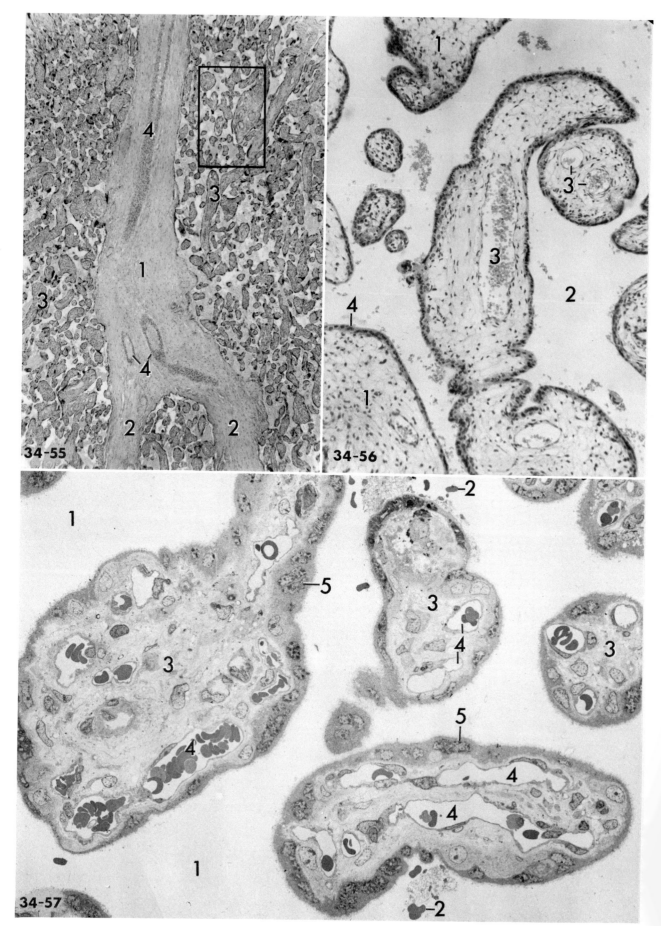

Fig. 34-55. Enlargement of rectangle in Fig. 34-53. Full term placenta. Human. L.M. X 31. **1.** Main-stem villus. **2.** Branching villus. **3.** Terminal villi. **4.** Arteries.

Fig. 34-56. Enlargement of area similar to rectangle in Fig. 34-55. Full term placenta. Human. L.M. X 130. **1.** Terminal villi of varying sizes. **2.** Intervillous space. **3.** Fetal blood vessels. **4.** Trophoblastic layers.

Fig. 34-57. Area similar to Fig. 34-56. Mid-pregnancy placenta. Human. E.M. X 600. **1.** Intervillous space. **2.** Maternal erythrocytes. **3.** Cores of terminal villi. **4.** Fetal blood vessels. **5.** Trophoblastic layers.

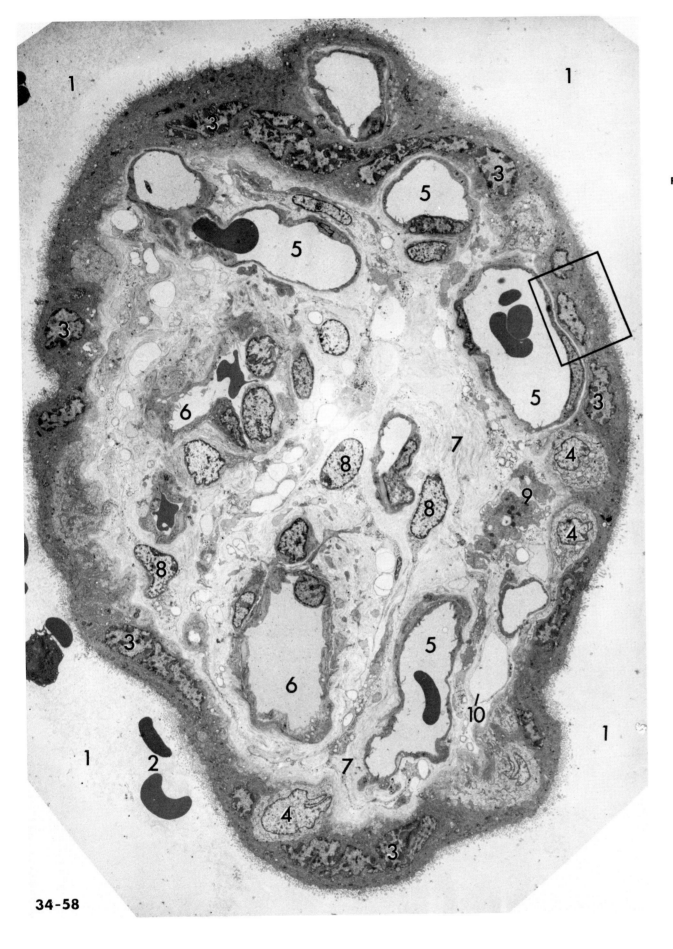

Fig. 34-58. Cross-sectioned terminal villus. Mid-pregnancy placenta. Human. E.M. X 2100. **1.** Intervillous space. **2.** Maternal erythrocytes. **3.** Nuclei of syncytiotrophoblastic layer. **4.** Nuclei of cytotrophoblasts (Langhans cells). **5.** Fetal blood capillaries. **6.** Arterioles. **7.** Bundles of collagenous fibrils in the mesenchymal connective tissue core of the villus. **8.** Mesenchymal cells (fibroblasts). **9.** Part of macrophage (Hofbauer cell). **10.** Lymph capillary.

34-58

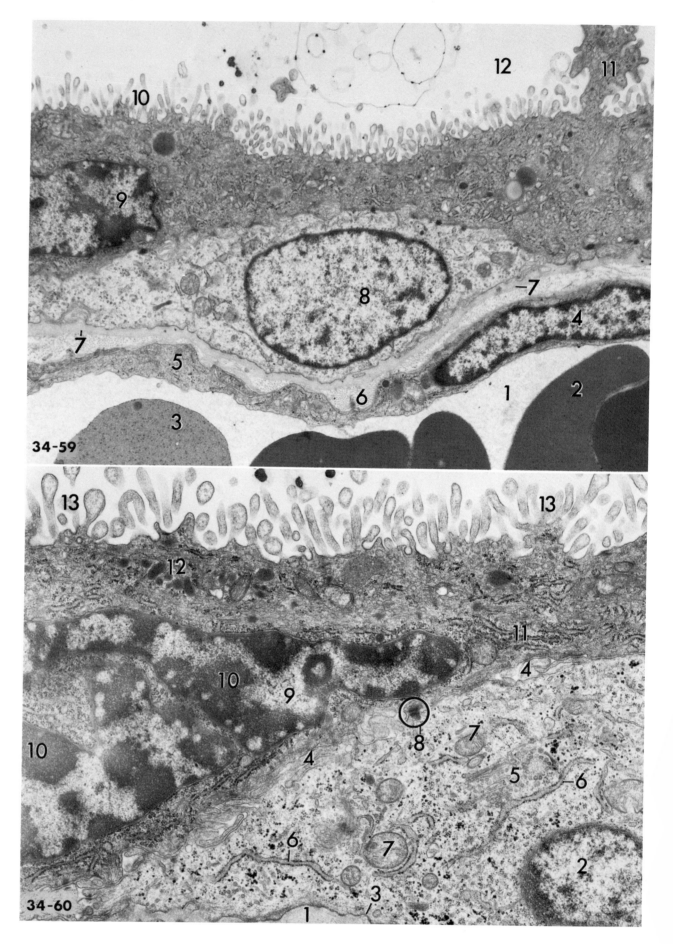

Fig. 34-59. Enlargement of area similar to rectangle in Fig. 34-58. General organization of placental barrier. Mid-pregnancy placenta. Human. E.M. X 9200. **1.** Lumen of fetal capillary. **2.** Erythrocytes. **3.** Reticulocyte. **4.** Nucleus of endothelial cell. **5.** Endothelial cytoplasm. **6.** Collagenous fibrils. **7.** Basal lamina. **8.** Nucleus of cytotrophoblast (Langhans cell). **9.** Nucleus of syncytiotrophoblastic layer. **10.** Microvilli. **11.** Club-shaped cytoplasmic protrusion. **12.** Intervillous space.

Fig. 34-60. Detail of placental barrier. Mid-pregnancy. Human. E.M. X 18,000. **1.** Basal lamina. **2.** Nucleus of cytotrophoblast. **3.** Basal cell membrane. **4.** Lateral cell membrane with narrow cytoplasmic processes. **5.** Golgi complex. **6.** Granular endoplasmic reticulum. **7.** Mitochondria. **8.** Circle: desmosome. **9.** Nucleus of syncytiotrophoblastic layer. **10.** Highly condensed chromatin. **11.** Granular endoplasmic reticulum. **12.** Primary lysosomes. **13.** Microvilli of varied shape.

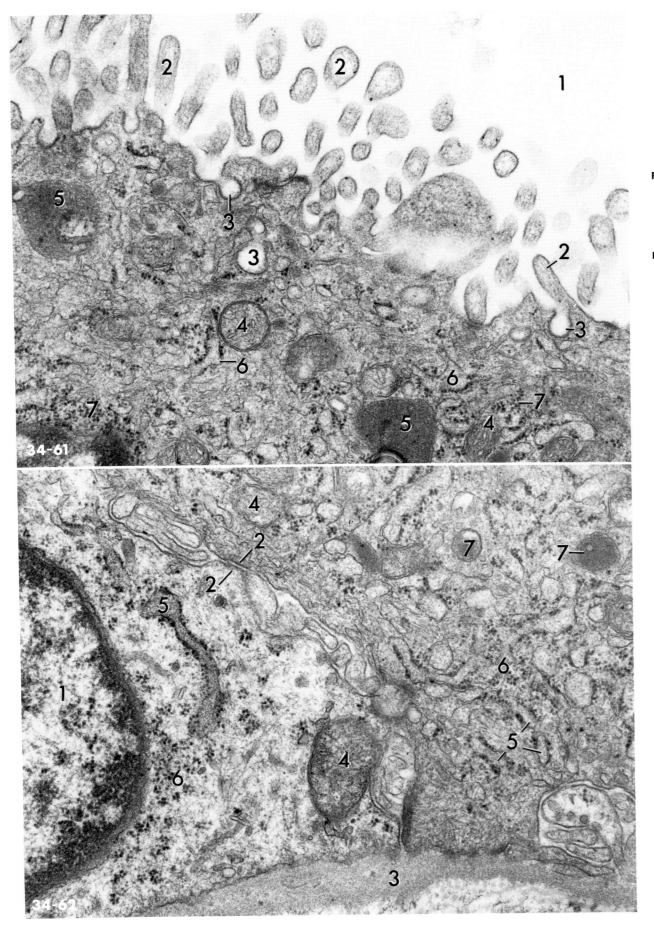

Fig. 34-61. Detail of apical part of syncytiotrophoblast. Placenta. Mid-pregnancy. Human. E.M. X 40,000. **1.** Intervillous space. **2.** Microvilli. **3.** Pinocytotic invaginations. **4.** Mitochondria. **5.** Lysosomes. **6.** Granular endoplasmic reticulum. **7.** Free ribosomes.

Fig. 34-62. Detail of base of placental barrier. Mid-pregnancy. Human. E.M. X 40,000. **1.** Nucleus of cytotrophoblast (Langhans cell). **2.** Adjoining membranes of cytotrophoblast and syncytiotrophoblast. The cytoplasm is highly electron-dense in the syncytiotrophoblast, and electron-lucent in in the cytotrophoblast. **3.** Basal lamina. **4.** Mitochondria. **5.** Granular endoplasmic reticulum. **6.** Free ribosomes. **7.** Lysosomes.

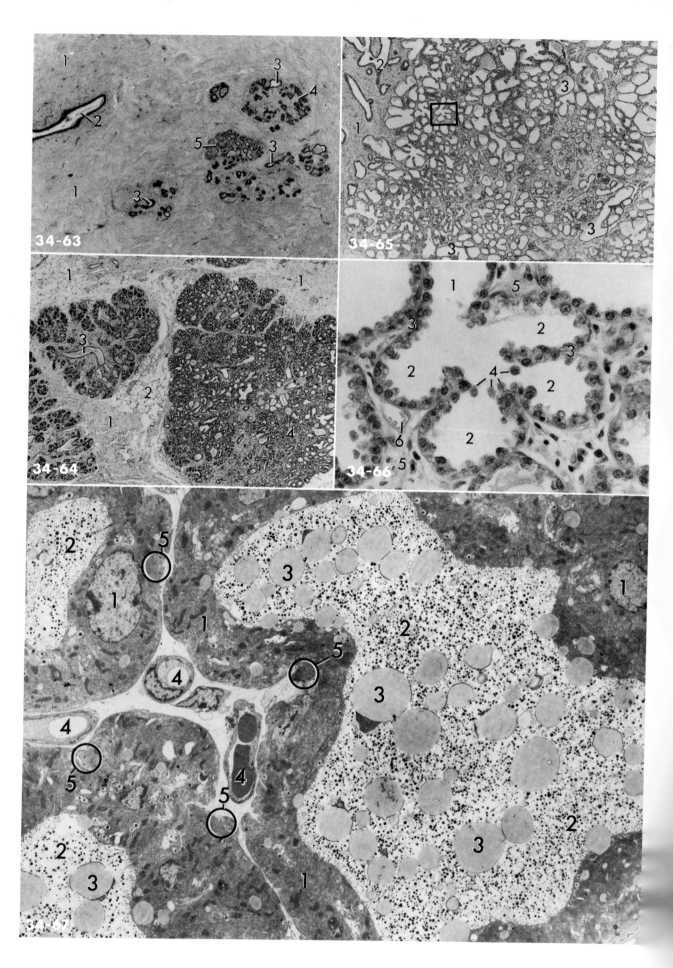

Fig. 34-63. Resting mammary gland of non-pregnant adult woman. L.M. X 30. **1.** Dense irregular connective tissue. **2.** Interlobar duct. **3.** Intralobular ducts. **4.** Branches of intralobular ducts. **5.** Remaining alveolar buds; present because of possible slight proliferation during latter part of menstrual cycle.

Fig. 34-64. Proliferating mammary gland toward end of pregnancy. Human. L.M. X 30. **1.** Interlobular connective tissue septa. **2.** Adipose tissue. **3.** Intralobular duct. **4.** Proliferating intralobular ducts with some collapsed and some distended alveoli.

Fig. 34-65. Lactating mammary gland. Human. L.M. X 30. **1.** Interlobular connective tissue septum. **2.** Interlobular ducts. **3.** Dilated secretory alveoli.

Fig. 34-66. Enlargement of rectangle in Fig. 34-65. Human. L.M. X 350. **1.** Branching of terminal duct. **2.** Alveoli. **3.** Simple cuboidal epithelium. **4.** Milk droplets. **5.** Intralobular loose connective tissue. **6.** Capillary.

Fig. 34-67. Alveoli of lactating mammary gland. Mouse. E.M. X 1800. **1.** Nuclei and cytoplasm of alveolar epithelial cells. **2.** Lumina of aveoli with small milk protein particles. **3.** Lipid droplets of milk. **4.** Perialveolar capillaries in loose connective tissue. **5.** Circles: sites where a cytoplasmic process of a myoepithelial cell is located.

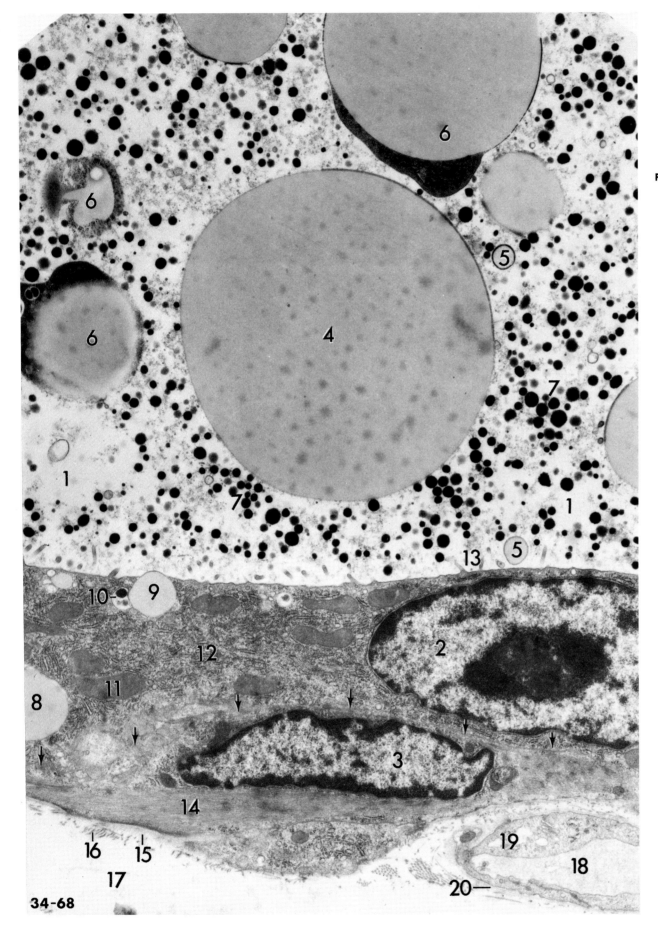

Fig. 34-68. Survey of secretory epithelium in alveolus of lactating mammary gland. Mouse. E.M. X 9500. **1.** Lumen of alveolus. **2.** Nucleus of secretory epithelial cell. **3.** Nucleus of myoepithelial cell. The cell borders of these two cells can be seen with some difficulty at the tip of the arrows. **4.** Large milk lipid droplet suspended in luminal fluid. **5.** Small milk lipid droplets. **6.** Lipid droplets retaining detached peripheral coat of cytoplasm. **7.** Milk protein particles. **8.** Lipid droplets in cell cytoplasm. **9.** Lipid droplet near cell surface. **10.** Protein particle in a vacuole. **11.** Mitochondrion. **12.** Short profiles of granular endoplasmic reticulum. **13.** Short microvilli. **14.** Bundle of myofilaments. **15.** Basal lamina. **16.** Reticular fibrils. **17.** Loose connective tissue. **18.** Lumen of blood capillary. **19.** Endothelium. **20.** Basal lamina of capillary.

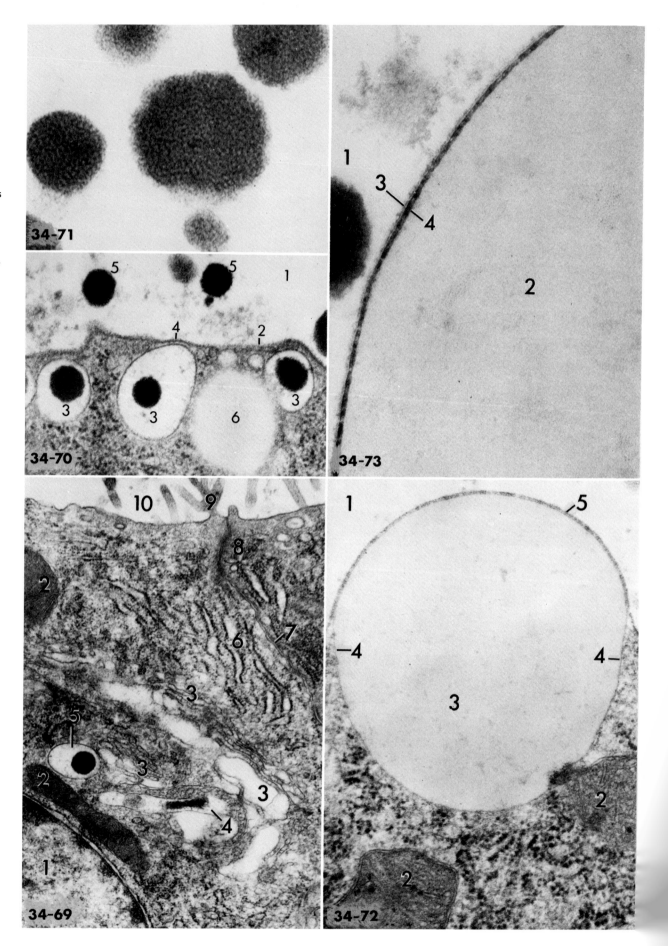

Fig. 34-69. Detail of epithelial cells in alveolus of lactating mammary gland. Mouse. E.M. X 29,000. **1.** Nucleus. **2.** Mitochondria. **3.** Golgi membranes and saccules. **4.** Early synthesis of core of protein particle in a Golgi saccule. **5.** Protein particle in vacuole, separating from the Golgi zone. **6.** Granular endoplasmic reticulum. **7.** Cell membrane. **8.** Junctional complex. **9.** Microvilli. **10.** Lumen of alveolus.

Fig. 34-70. Detail of apical surface of lactating epithelial cell. Mammary gland. Mouse. E.M. X 59,000. **1.** Lumen of alveolus. **2.** Surface membrane. **3.** Protein particles in vacuoles. **4.** Thin sheet of cytoplasm separates boundary membrane of vacuole from surface membrane. These two membranes fuse at the moment of particle discharge. **5.** Discharged milk protein particles. **6.** Lipid droplet sectioned tangentially

Fig. 34-71. Detail of discharged milk protein particles. Mammary gland. Mouse. E.M. X 172,000. The particles are not surrounded by a membrane. They are composed of minute globules, each about 25 Å in diameter, arranged in a crystalline array.

Fig. 34-72. Detail of apical surface of lactating epithelial cell. Mammary gland. Mouse. E.M. X 62,000. **1.** Lumen of alveolus. **2.** Mitochondria. **3.** Lipid droplet elevating the cell surface in the process of discharge. **4.** Thin boundary membrane at cytoplasm/droplet interface. **5.** Thin rim of cytoplasm.

Fig. 34-73. Highly enlarged detail of part of discharged milk lipid droplet. Mammary gland. Mouse. E.M. X 129,000. **1.** Alveolar lumen. **2.** Core of lipid droplet. **3.** Superficial leaflet of surface trilaminar membrane. **4.** Fusion of inner leaflet and lipid droplet boundary membrane.

422

References

OVARY

Adams, E. C. and Hertig, A. T. Studies on guinea pig oocytes. I. Electron microsccopic observations on the development of cytoplasmic organelles in oocytes of primordial and primary follicles. J. Cell Biol. *21*: 397–427 (1964).

Adams, E. C. and Hertig, A. T. Studies on the human corpus luteum. I. Observations on the ultrastructure of development and regression of the luteal cells during the menstrual cycle. J. Cell Biol. *41*: 696–715 (1969).

Adams, E. C. and Hertig, A. T. Studies on the human corpus luteum. II. Observations on the ultrastructure of luteal cells during pregnancy. J. Cell Biol. *41*: 716–735 (1969).

Baca, M. and Zamboni, L. The fine structure of human follicular oocytes. J. Ultrastruct. Res. *19*: 354–381 (1967).

Baker, T. G., Beaumont, H. M. and Franchi, L. L. The uptake of tritiated uridine and phenylalanine by the ovaries of rats and monkeys. J. Cell Sci. *4*: 655–675 (1969).

Baker, T. G. and Franchi, L. L. The fine structure of oogonia and oocytes in human ovaries. J. Cell Sci. *2*: 213–224 (1967).

Belt, W. D., Cavazos, L. F., Anderson, L. L. and Kraeling, R. R. Fine structure and progesterone levels in the corpus luteum of the pig during pregnancy and after hysterectomy. Biol. Reprod. *2*: 98–113 (1970).

Bjersing, L. On the morphology and endocrine function of granulosa cells in ovarian follicles and corpora lutea. Acta Endocrinol. Suppl. *125*: 1–23 (1967).

Bjersing, L. On the ultrastructure of granulosa lutein cells in porcine corpus luteum. With special reference to endoplasmic reticulum and steroid hormone synthesis. Z. Zellforsch. *82*: 187–211 (1967).

Blanchette, E. J. A study of the fine structure of the rabbit primary oocyte. J. Ultrastruct. Res. *5*: 349–363 (1961).

Blanchette, E. J. Ovarian steroid cells. I. Differentiation of the lutein cells from the granulosa follicle cell during the preovulatory stage and under the influence of exogenous gonadotrophins. J. Cell Biol. *31*: 501–516 (1966).

Blanchette, E. J. Ovarian steroid cells. II. The lutein cell. J. Cell Biol. *31*: 517–542 (1966).

Cavazos, L. F., Anderson, L. L., Belt, W. D., Henricks, D. M., Kraeling, R. R. and Melampy, R. M. Fine structure and progesterone levels in the corpus luteum of the pig during the estrous cycle. Biol. Reprod. *1*: 83–106 (1969).

Crisp. T. M. and Browning, H. C. The fine structure of corpora lutea in ovarian transplants of mice following luteotrophin stimulation. Am. J. Anat. *122*: 169–192 (1968).

Crisp, T. M., Dessouky, A. D. and Denys, F. R. The fine structure of the human corpus luteum of early pregnancy and during the progestational phase of the menstrual cycle. Am. J. Anat. *127*: 37–70 (1970).

Dahl, E. Studies of the fine structure of ovarian interstitial tissue. I. A comparative study of the fine structure of the ovarian interstitial tissue in the rat and the domestic fowl. J. Anat. *108*: 275–290 (1971).

Davies, J. and Broadus, C. D. Studies on the fine structure of ovarian steroid-secreting cells in the rabbit. I. The normal interstitial cells. Am. J. Anat. *123*: 441–474 (1968).

Delson, B., Lubin, S. and Reynolds, S. R. M. Vascular patterns in the human ovary. Am. J. Obstet. Gynecol. *57*: 842–853 (1949).

Enders, A. C. and Lyons, W. R. Observations on the fine structure of lutein cells. II. The effects of hypophysectomy and mammotrophic hormone in the rat. J. Cell Biol. *22*: 127–141 (1964).

Espey, L. L. Ultrastructure of the apex of the rabbit Graafian follicle during the ovulatory process. Endocrinology *81*: 267–276 (1967).

Gillim, S. W., Christensen, A. K. and McLennan, C. E. Fine structure of the human menstrual corpus luteum at its stage of maximum secretory activity. Am. J. Anat. *126*: 409–428 (1969).

Goecke, H. Die Endausbreitung des vegetativen Nervengewebes im menschlichen Ovarium und ihre Bedeutung für die Funktion des Ovariums. Arch. Gynäk. *166*: 187–189 (1938).

Hadek, R. The structure of the mammalian egg. Int. Rev. Cytol. *18*: 29–72 (1965).

Hertig, A. T. The primary human oocyte: some observations on the fine structure of Balbiani's vitelline body and the origin of the annulate lamellae. Am. J. Anat. *122*: 107–138 (1968).

Hertig, A. T. and Adams, E. C. Studies on the human oocyte and its follicle. I. Ultrastructural and histochemical observations on the primordial follicle stage. J. Cell Biol. *34*: 647–675 (1967).

Hisaw, F. L. The development of the Graafian follicle and ovulation. Physiol. Rev. *27*: 95–119 (1947).

Norrevang, A. Electron microscopic morphology of oogenesis. Int. Rev. Cytol. *23*: 114–186 (1968).

Odor, D. L. The ultrastructure of unilaminar follicles of the hamster ovary. Am. J. Anat. *116*: 493–522 (1965).

Odor, D. L. and Blandau, R. J. Ultrastructural studies on fetal and early postnatal mouse ovaries. Am. J. Anat. *124*: 163–186 (1969).

O'Shea, J. D. An ultrastructural study of smooth muscle-like cells in the theca externa of ovarian follicles in the rat. Anat. Rec. *167*: 127–140 (1970).

Osvaldo-Decima, L. Smooth muscle in ovary of the rat and monkey. J. Ultrastruct. Res. *29*: 218–237 (1970).

Papadaki, L. and Beilby, J. O. W. The fine structure of the surface epithelium of the human ovary. J. Cell Sci. *8*: 445–465 (1971).

Schlafke, S. and Enders, A. C. Cytological changes during cleavage and blastocyst formation in the rat. J. Anat. *102*: 13–32 (1967).

Short, R. V. Steroids in the follicular fluid and the corpus luteum of the mare. A "two-cell type" theory of ovarian steroid synthesis. J. Endocrin. *24*: 59–63 (1962).

Simkins, C. S. Development of the human ovary from birth to sexual maturity. Am. J. Anat. *51*: 465–505 (1932).

Szollosi, D. Development of cortical granules and the cortical reaction in rat and hamster eggs. Anat. Rec. *159*: 431–446 (1967).

Witschi, E. Migration of germ cells of human embryos from the yolk sac to the primitive gonadal folds. Contr. Embryol. *32*: 67–80 (1948).

OVIDUCT

Björkman, N. and Fredricsson, B. Ultrastructural features of the human oviduct epithelium. Int. J. Fertil. *7*: 259–266 (1962).

Clyman, M. J. Electron microscopy of the human fallopian tube. Fertil. & Steril. *17*: 281–301 (1966).

Novak, E. and Everett, H. S. Cyclical and other variations in the tubal epithelium. Am. J. Obstet. Gynecol. *16*: 499–530 (1928).

Nilsson, O. Electron microscopy of the fallopian tube epithelium of rabbit in oestrus. Exp. Cell Res. *14*: 341–354 (1958).

Snyder, F. F. Changes in the human oviduct during the menstrual cycle and pregnancy. Bull. Johns Hopkins Hosp. *35*: 141–146 (1924).

UTERUS

Albert, E. N. and Pease, D. C. An electron microscopic study of uterine arteries during pregnancy. Am. J. Anat. *123*: 165–194 (1968).

Bo, W. J., Odor, D. L. and Rothrock, M. L. The fine structure of uterine smooth muscle of the rat uterus at various time intervals following a single injection of estrogen. Am. J. Anat. *123*: 369–384 (1968).

Bo, W. J., Odor, D. L. and Rothrock, M. L. Ultrastructure of uterine smooth muscle following progesterone or progesterone-estrogen treatment. Anat. Rec. *163*: 121–132 (1969).

Borell, U., Nilsson, O. and Westman, A. The cyclical changes occurring in the epithelium lining the endometrial glands. An electron microscopic study in the human being. Acta Obstet. Gynecol. Scand. *38*: 364–377 (1959).

Cavazos, F., Green, J. A., Hall, D. G. and Lucas, F. V. Ultrastructure of the human endometrial glandular cell during the menstrual cycle. Am. J. Obstet. Gynecol. *99*: 833–854 (1967).

Colville, E. A. The ultrastructure of the human endometrium. J. Obstet. Gynaecol. Brit. Commonwealth *75*: 342–350 (1963).

Danforth, D. N. The fibrous nature of the human cervix, and its relation to the isthmic segment in gravid and non-gravid uteri. Am. J. Obstet. Gynecol. *53*: 541–560 (1947).

Daron, G. H. The arterial pattern of the tunica mucosa of the uterus in Macacus rhesus. Am. J. Anat. *58*: 349–419 (1936).

Enders, A. C. and Schlafke, S. Cytological aspects of trophoblast-uterine interaction in early implantation. Am. J. Anat. *125*: 1–30 (1969).

Enders, A. C. and Schlafke, S. Penetration of the uterine epithelium during implantation in the rabbit. Am. J. Anat. *132*: 219–240 (1971).

Goerttler, K. Die Architektur der Muskelwand des menschlichen Uterus und ihre funktionelle Bedeutung. Morphol. Jahrb. *65*: 45–128 (1930).

Gompel, C. The ultrastructure of the human endometrial cell studied by electron microscopy. Am. J. Obstet. Gynecol. *84*: 1000–1009 (1962).

Hinglais-Guillaud, N. L'ultrastructure de l'exocol normal de la femme (exocervix). Bulletin du Cancer *46*: 212–252 (1959).

Laguens, R. and Lagrutta, J. Fine structure of human

uterine muscle in pregnancy. Am. J. Obstet. Gynecol. *89*: 1040–1048 (1964).

Larkin, L. H. and Flickinger, C. J. Ultrastructure of the metrial gland cell in the pregnant rat. Am. J. Anat. *126*: 337–354 (1969).

Nilsson, O. Electron microscopy of the glandular epithelium in human uterus. I. Follicular phase. J. Ultrastruct. Res. *6*: 413–421 (1962).

Nilsson, O. Electron microscopy of the glandular epithelium in human uterus. II. Early and late luteal phase. J. Ultrastruct. Res. *6*: 422–431 (1962).

Ross, R. and Klebanoff, S. J. Fine structural changes in uterine smooth muscle and fibroblasts in response to estrogens. J. Cell Biol. *32*: 155–167 (1967).

Salvatore, C. A. The growth of human myometrium and endometrium. Studies of cytological aspects. Anat. Rec. *108*: 93–109 (1950).

Sengel, A. and Stoebner, P. Ultrastructure de l'endomètre humain normal. I. Le chorion cytogène. Z. Zellforsch. *109*: 245–259 (1970).

Sengel, A. and Stoebner, P. Ultrastructure de l'endomètre humain normal. II. Les glandes. Z. Zellforsch. *109*: 260–278 (1970).

Smith, L. J. Metrial gland and other glycogen containing cells in the mouse uterus following mating and through implantation of the embryo. Am. J. Anat. *119*: 15–23 (1966).

Themann, H. and Schünke, W. The fine structure of the glandular epithelium of the human endometrium, electron microscopic morphology. pp. 99–134. *In* The Normal Human Endometrium (Ed. H. Schmidt-Matthiesen). McGraw-Hill, New York, 1963.

Terzakis, J. A. The nucleolar channel system of human endometrium. J. Cell Biol. *27*: 293–304 (1965).

Wynn, R. M. and Harris, J. A. Ultrastructural cyclic changes in the human endometrium. I. Normal preovulatory phase. Fertil. & Steril. *18*: 632–648 (1967).

Wynn, R. M., Harris, J. A. and Wooley, R. S. Ultrastructural cyclic changes in the human endometrium. II. Normal postovulatory phase. Fertil. & Steril. *18*: 721–738 (1967).

UMBILICAL CORD

Hoyes, A. D. Ultrastructure of the epithelium of the human umbilical cord. J. Anat. *105*: 149–162 (1969).

Leeson, C. R. and Leeson, T. S. The fine structure of the rat umbilical cord at various times of gestation. Anat. Rec. *151*: 183–197 (1965).

Parry, E. W. Some electron microscope observations on the mesenchymal structures of full-term umbilical cord. J. Anat. *107*: 505–518 (1970).

PLACENTA

Boyd, J. D. and Hamilton, W. J. Development and structure of the human placenta from the end of the 3rd month of gestation. J. Obstet. Gynaecol. Brit. Commonwealth *74*: 161–226 (1967).

Enders, A. C. Formation of syncytium from cytotrophoblast in the human placenta. Obstet. Gynecol. *25*: 378–386 (1965).

Enders, A. C. Fine structure of anchoring villi of the human placenta. Am. J. Anat. *122*: 419–452 (1968).

Enders, A. C. and King, B. F. The cytology of Hofbauer cells. Anat. Rec. *167*: 231–252 (1970).

Hamilton, W. J. and Boyd, J. D. Development of the human placenta in the first three months of gestation. J. Anat. *94*: 297–328 (1960).

Rhodin, J. A. G. and Terzakis, J. The ultrastructure of the human full-term placenta. J. Ultrastruct. Res. *6*: 88–106 (1962).

Terzakis, J. A. The ultrastructure of normal human first trimester placenta. J. Ultrastruct. Res. *9*: 268–284 (1963).

Wislocki, G. B. and Dempsey, E. W. Electron microscopy of the human placenta. Anat. Rec. *123*: 133–168 (1955).

VAGINA

Cooper, R. A., Cardiff, R. D. and Wellings, S. R. Ultrastructure of vaginal keratinization in estrogen treated immature Balb/cCRGL mice. Z. Zellforsch. *77*: 377–403 (1967).

Eddy, E. M. and Walker, B. E. Cytoplasmic fine structure during hormonally controlled differentiation in vaginal epithelium (mouse). Anat. Rec. *164*: 205–218 (1969).

Gregoire, A. T., Kandil, O. and Ledger, W. J. The glycogen content of human vaginal epithelial tissue. Fertil. & Steril. *22*: 64–68 (1971).

Papanicolaou, G. N. The sexual cycle in the human female as revealed by vaginal smears. Am. J. Anat. *53*: 519–637 (1933).

Smith, B. G. and Brunner, E. K. The structure of the human vaginal mucosa in relation to the menstrual cycle and to pregnancy. Am. J. Anat. *54*: 27–86 (1934).

Stegner, H. and Iwata, M. Elektronenmikroskopische Untersuchungen am Scheidenepithel der Ratte. Mikr. Anat. Forsch. *76*: 491–508 (1967).

MAMMARY GLANDS

Bargmann, W. and Knoop, A. Über die Morphologie der Milchsekretion. Licht- und elektronenmikroskopische Studien an der Milchdrüse der Ratte. Z. Zellforsch. *49*: 344–388 (1959).

Helminen, H. J. and Ericsson, J. L. E. Studies on the mammary gland involution. I. On the ultrastructure of the lactating mammary gland. J. Ultrastruct. Res. *25*: 193–213 (1968).

Hollmann, K. H. Sur des aspects particuliers des protéines élaborées dans la glande mammaire. Étude au microscope électronique chez la lapine en lactation. Z. Zellforsch. *69*: 395–402 (1966).

Kurosumi, K., Kobayashi, Y. and Baba, N. The fine structure of the mammary glands of lactating rats, with special reference to the apocrine secretion. Exp. Cell Res. *50*: 177–192 (1968).

Wooding, F. B. P. The mechanism of secretion of the milk fat globule. J. Cell Sci. *9*: 805–821 (1971).

Wooding, F. B. P. The structure of the milk fat globule membrane. J. Ultrastruct. Res. *37*: 388–400 (1971).

35 Eye

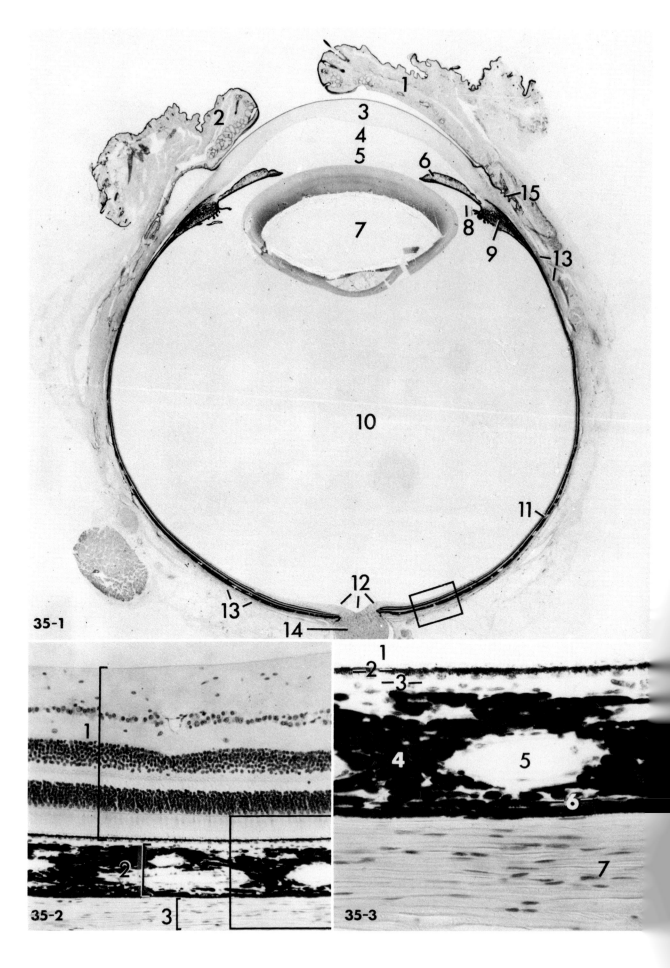

Fig. 35-1. Vertical meridional section of eyeball and eyelids through pupil and optic nerve. Monkey. L.M. X 7.5. **1.** Upper eyelid (enlarged in Fig. 35-39). **2.** Lower eyelid (enlarged in Fig. 35-42). **3.** Cornea. **4.** Anterior chamber. **5.** Pupil. **6.** Iris. **7.** Lens (center of lens removed by the preparation process). **8.** Posterior chamber. **9.** Ciliary body. **10.** Vitreous body. **11.** Retina. **12.** Optic disk and papilla. **13.** Sclera. **14.** Optic nerve (enlarged in Fig. 35-32). **15.** Fornix of conjunctival sac (enlarged in Fig. 35-43).

Fig. 35-2. Principal layers of wall of eyeball. Enlargement of area similar to rectangle in Fig. 35-1. Monkey. L.M. X 168. **1.** Retina (innermost layer). **2.** Choroid (middle layer). **3.** Sclera (outermost layer).

Fig. 35-3. Choroid and sclera. Enlargement of area similar to rectangle in Fig. 35-2. Monkey. L.M. X 435. **1.** Outer segments of rods and cones. **2.** Pigmented epithelium of retina. **3.** Choriocapillaris. **4.** Heavily pigmented stroma. **5.** Blood vessel. **6.** Suprachoroidea. **7.** Collagenous bundles and nuclei of fibroblasts in sclera.

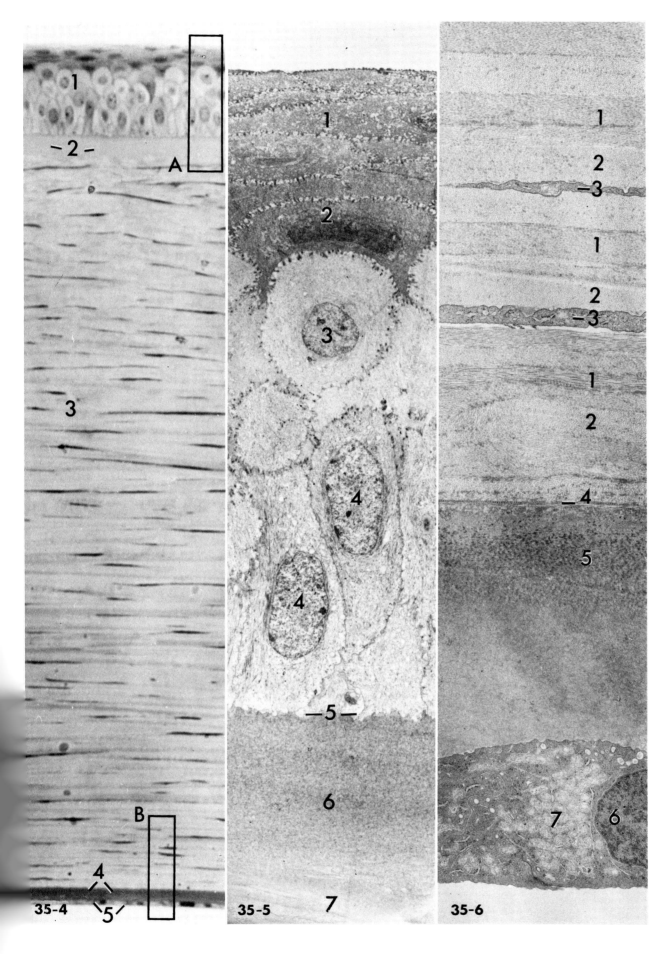

Fig. 35-4. Cornea. Human. L.M. X 184.
1. Stratified squamous non-keratinized
epithelium. **2.** Bowman's membrane. **3.** Stroma.
4. Descemet's membrane. **5.** Endothelium.

Fig. 35-5. Corneal epithelium. Enlargement of
area similar to rectangle (A) in Fig. 35-4.
Human. E.M. X 3200. **1.** Superficial squamous
cells. **2.** Wing cell with partly obscured
nucleus. **3.** Nucleus of polyhedral
intermediate cell. **4.** Nuclei of columnar cells.
5. Level of basal lamina (not resolved).
6. Bowman's membrane. **7.** Stromal connective
tissue elements.

Fig. 35-6. Corneal stroma and endothelium.
Enlargement of area similar to rectangle (B) in
Fig. 35-4. E.M. X 10,000. **1.** Longitudinally
sectioned collagenous fibrils of corneal stroma.
2. Cross-sectioned collagenous fibrils of
corneal stroma. **3.** Cytoplasmic extensions of
fibroblasts (keratocytes). **4.** Border zone
between corneal stroma and Descemet's
membrane. **5.** Descemet's membrane with
some faintly discernible periodicity.
6. Nucleus of endothelial cell. **7.** Numerous
mitochondria.

35-4   35-5   35-6

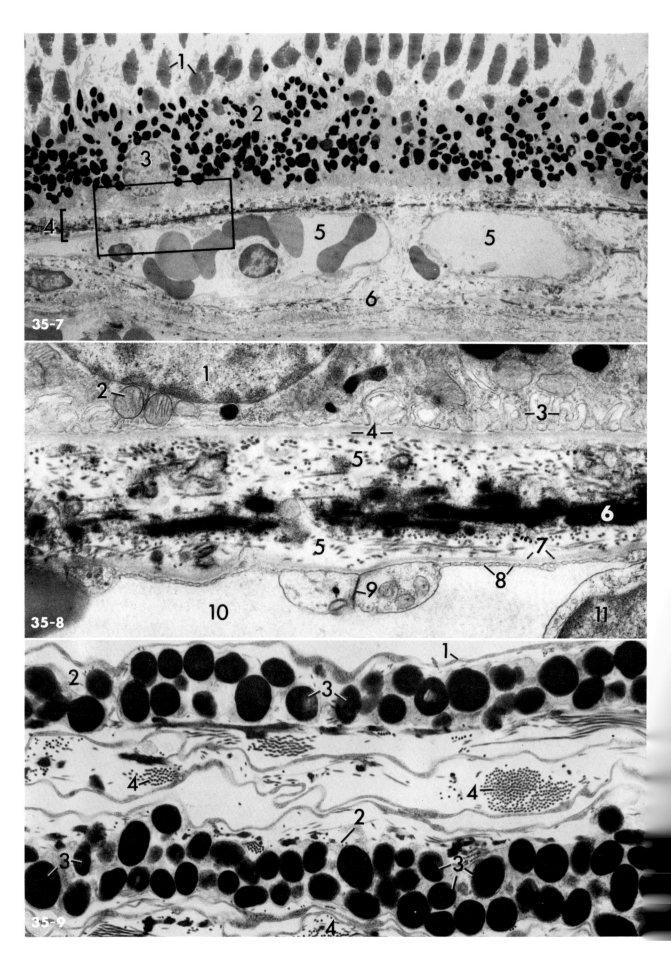

Fig. 35-7. Junctional area between retina and choroid. Rat. E.M. X 1900. **1.** Outer segments of rods and cones. **2.** Pigmented epithelium of retina. **3.** Nucleus of pigmented cell. **4.** Bruch's membrane. **5.** Lumina of blood capillaries of choriocapillaris. **6.** Connective tissue elements of choroid stroma.

Fig. 35-8. Bruch's membrane. Enlargement of area similar to rectangle in Fig. 35-7. Rat. E.M. X 15,000. **1.** Nucleus of pigmented epithelial cell of retina. **2.** Mitochondria. **3.** Base of epithelial cell with cell membrane folds. **4.** Basal lamina of retina. **5.** Collagenous fibrils of Bruch's membrane. **6.** Elastic fibers of Bruch's membrane. **7.** Basal lamina of blood capillary. **8.** Fenestrated endothelium. **9.** Junctional area of apposed endothelial cells. **10.** Capillary lumen. **11.** Nucleus of endothelial cell.

Fig. 35-9. Choroid stroma. Monkey. E.M. X 14,000. **1.** Melanocyte cell membrane. **2.** Melanocyte. **3.** Pigment granules. **4.** Bundles of collagenous fibrils.

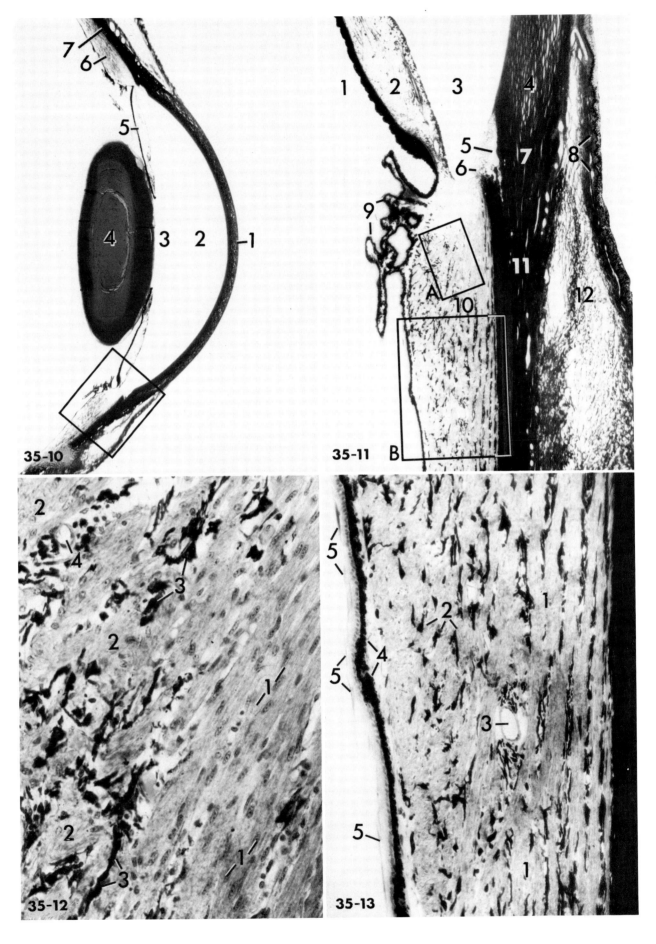

Fig. 35-10. Meridional section of anterior portion of the eye. Eyelids removed. Monkey. L.M. X 9. **1.** Cornea (appears dark with trichrome stain). **2.** Anterior chamber. **3.** Pupil. **4.** Lens. **5.** Iris. **6.** Ciliary body. **7.** Sclera (appears dark with trichrome stain).

Fig. 35-11. Root of iris. Enlargement of rectangle in Fig 35-10. Monkey. L.M. X 43. **1.** Posterior chamber. **2.** Iris. **3.** Anterior chamber. **4.** Cornea. **5.** Canal of Schlemm. **6.** Intertrabecular spaces. **7.** Limbus (sclero-corneal junction). **8.** Bulbar conjunctiva. **9.** Ciliary processes (pars plicata). **10.** Ciliary muscle. **11.** Sclera. **12.** Episclera.

Fig. 35-12. Ciliary muscle. Enlargement of area similar to rectangle (A) in Fig. 35-11. Monkey. L.M. X 320. **1.** Meridional-radial smooth muscle cells. **2.** Circular smooth muscle cells. **3.** Melanocytes. **4.** Small arteriole.

Fig. 35-13. Ciliary body. Pars plana. Enlargement of rectangle (B) in Fig. 35-11. Monkey. L.M. X 120. **1.** Smooth muscle cells of ciliary body. **2.** Melanocytes. **3.** Small artery. **4.** Ciliary epithelium. **5.** Zonules.

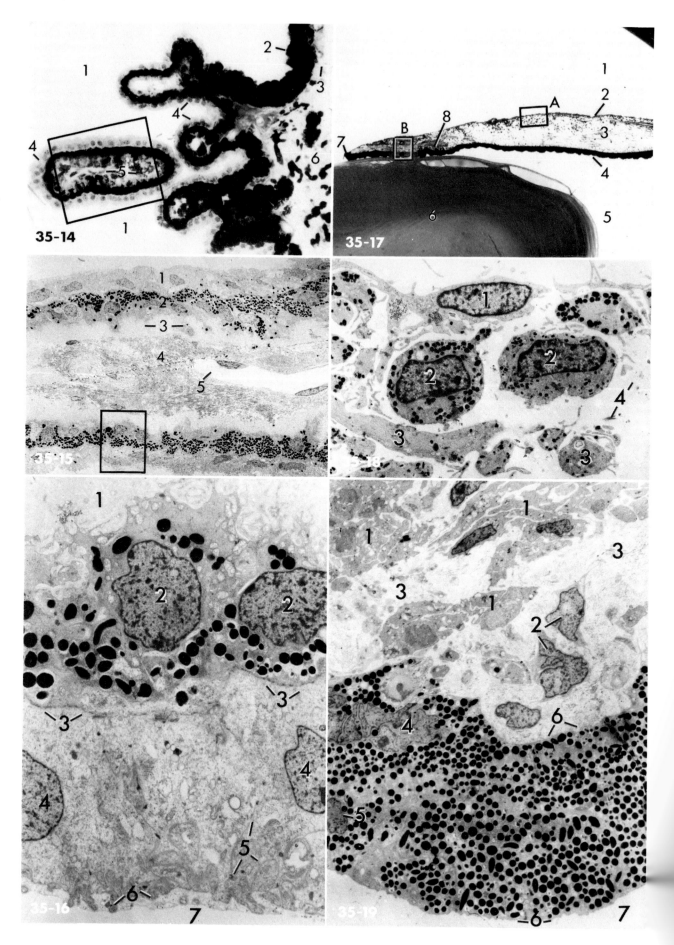

Fig. 35-14. Ciliary body. Pars plicata. Monkey. L.M. X 200. **1.** Posterior chamber. **2.** Posterior surface epithelium of iris. **3.** Root of iris. **4.** Ciliary processes covered by ciliary epithelium. **5.** Ciliary stroma with blood capillaries. **6.** Melanocytes.

Fig. 35-15. Ciliary process. Enlargement of area similar to rectangle in Fig. 35-14. Human. E.M. X 600. **1.** Inner non-pigmented epithelium. **2.** Outer pigmented epithelium. **3.** Basement membrane, increased in thickness as part of aging changes. **4.** Ciliary stroma. **5.** Blood capillary.

Fig. 35-16. Ciliary epithelium. Enlargement of area similar to rectangle in Fig. 35-15. Human. E.M. X 3500. **1.** Basement membrane. **2.** Nuclei of pigmented cells. **3.** Junctional complexes of apposed cell membranes. **4.** Nuclei of non-pigmented cells. **5.** Interlocking of highly folded cell membranes. **6.** Level of inner limiting membrane (basal lamina). **7.** Posterior chamber.

Fig. 35-17. Iris. Monkey. L.M. X 33. **1.** Anterior chamber. **2.** Anterior surface of iris. **3.** Stroma. **4.** Posterior surface of iris. **5.** Posterior chamber. **6.** Lens. **7.** Pupillary border of iris. **8.** Sphincter muscle.

Fig. 35-18. Iris. Anterior surface. Enlargement of area similar to rectangle (A) in Fig. 35-17. Human. E.M. X 4000. **1.** Nucleus of fibroblast. **2.** Nuclei of melanocytes. **3.** Cell processes of melanocytes in stroma. **4.** Delicate bundles of collagenous fibrils.

Fig. 35-19. Iris. Pupillary border zone. Enlargement of area similar to rectangle (B) in Fig. 35-17. Human. E.M. X 1600. **1.** Smooth muscle cells of pupillary sphincter. **2.** Nuclei of fibroblasts. **3.** Collagenous fibrils in stroma of iris. **4.** Nuclei of anterior pigmented epithelial cells. **5.** Nucleus of posterior pigmented epithelial cell. **6.** Levels of basal laminae. **7.** Posterior chamber.

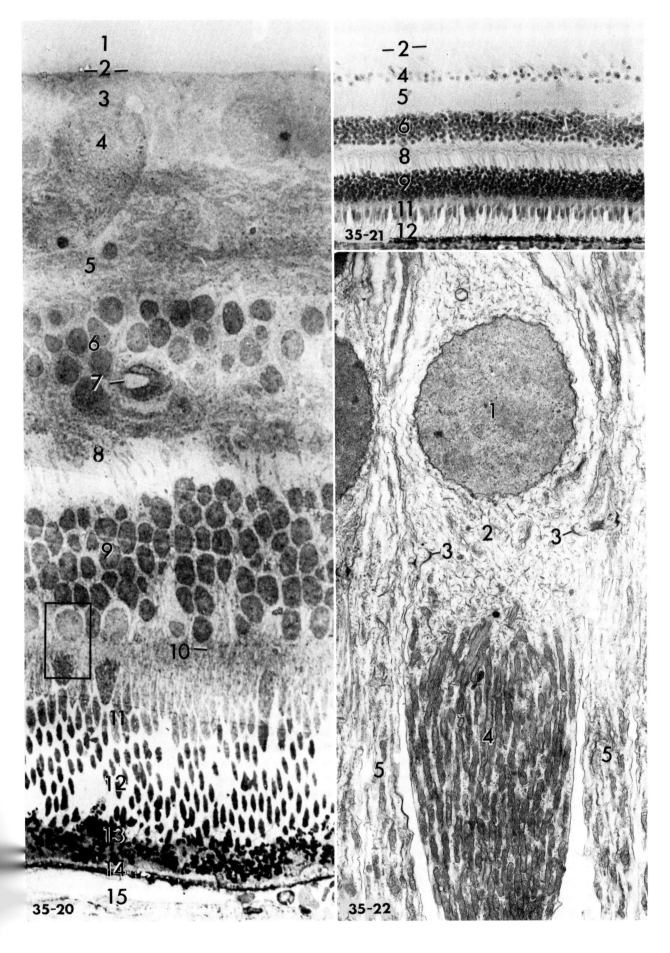

Fig. 35-20. Retina. Rat. E.M. X 840.

Fig. 35-21. Retina. Monkey. L.M. X 200.

1. Vitreous body. 2. Inner limiting membrane. 3. Nerve fiber layer. 4. Ganglion cells. 5. Inner plexiform (synaptic) layer. 6. Inner nuclear layer of bipolar cells. 7. Blood vessel. 8. Outer plexiform (synaptic) layer. 9. Outer nuclear layer of rods and cones. 10. Outer limiting membrane of zonulae adhaerentes. 11. Inner segments of rods and cones. 12. Outer segments of rods and cones. 13. Pigmented epithelium. 14. Bruch's membrane. 15. Choriocapillaris.

Fig. 35-22. Cone cell. Enlargement of area similar to rectangle in Fig. 35-20. Retina. Rat. E.M. X 6500. 1. Nucleus of cone cell. 2. Cytoplasm (finely filamentous). 3. Inner cone segment (ellipsoid) filled with elongated mitochondria. 4. Zonulae adhaerentes forming outer limiting membrane. 5. Inner segments of rod cells.

Fig. 35-23. Inner and outer segments of rods. Retina. Monkey. E.M. X 10,000. **1.** Inner segments of rods (ellipsoids) filled with long mitochondria. **2.** Outer segments. **3.** Connecting region. Section does not traverse plane of connecting cilium.

Fig. 35-24. Connecting region of inner and outer rod segments. Retina. Cat. E.M. X 19,000. **1.** Mitochondria of inner segment of rod. **2.** Basal body of cilium. **3.** Connecting cilium. **4.** Rod cell membrane. **5.** Outer segment with rod disks.

Fig. 35-25. Rod outer segment. Retina. Rat. E.M. X 31,000. **1.** Rod disks. **2.** Rod cell membrane. **3.** Microvilli of pigment epithelium. **4.** Pigment granules. **5.** Area of contact between rod outer segment and pigment epithelium.

Fig. 35-26. Pyramidal synaptic termination of cone cell (pedicle). Retina. Cat. E.M. X 28,000. **1.** Dendritic branches of bipolar neurons and horizontal cells in outer plexiform layer. **2.** Synaptic ribbons. **3.** Synaptic vesicles of cone pedicle. **4.** Mitochondria. **5.** Narrow part of cone cell, continuous with its perinuclear cytoplasm. **6.** Adjacent oval terminations of rod cells (spherules).

Fig. 35-27. Rod cell. Nuclear region. Inner nuclear layer. Retina. Rat. E.M. X 9000. **1.** Nuclei of rod cells. **2.** Perinuclear cytoplasm (perikaryon). **3.** Narrow part of rod cell cytoplasm.

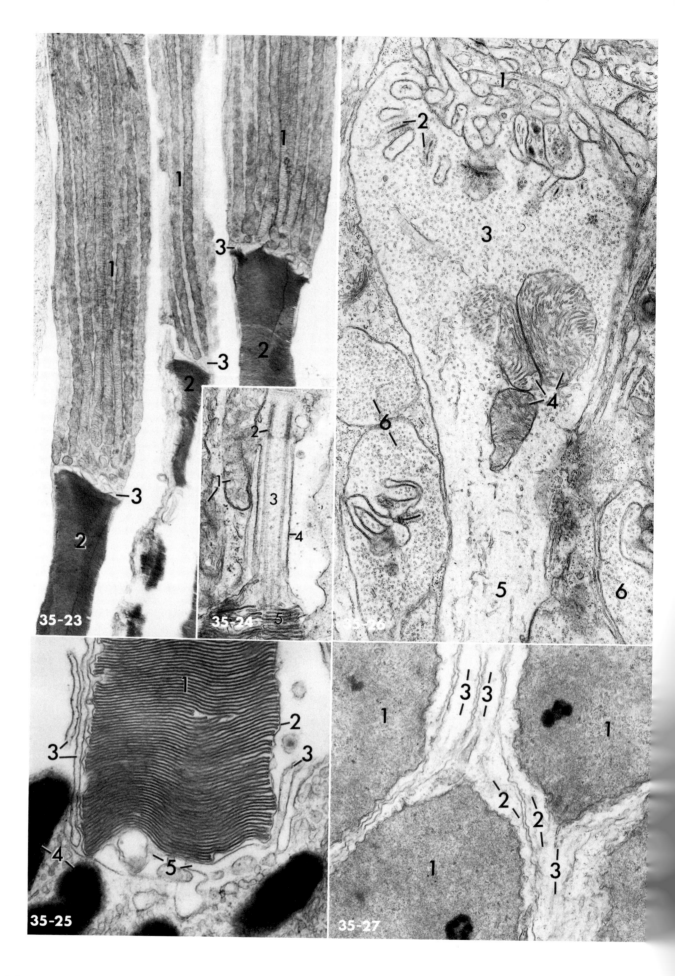

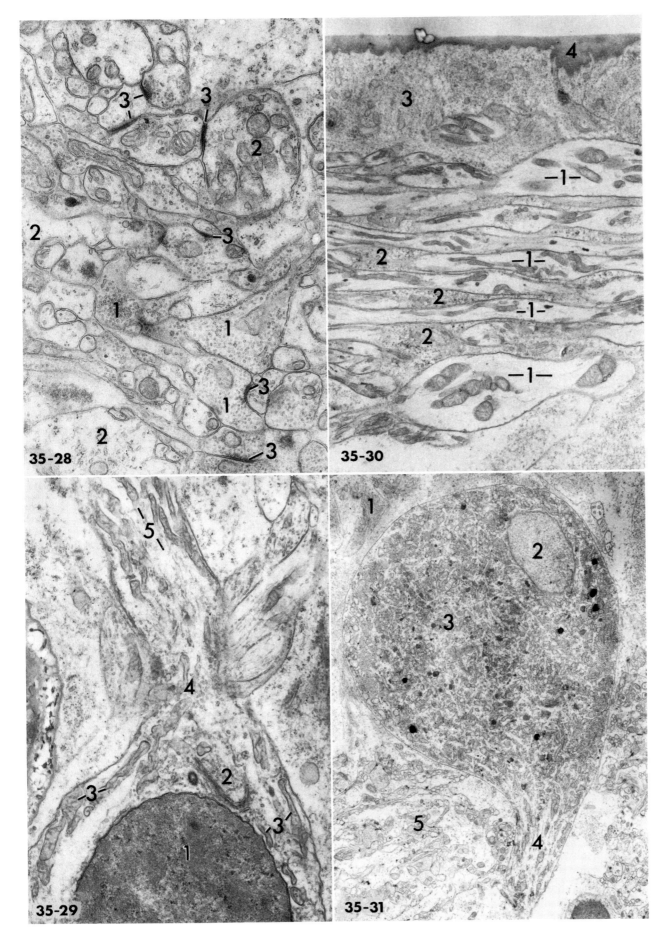

Fig. 35-28. Inner plexiform (synaptic) layer. Retina. Rat. E.M. X 19,000. **1.** Axonal endings of bipolar cells with synaptic vesicles. **2.** Ganglion cell processes. **3.** Synaptic junctions.

Fig. 35-29. Axon hillock of bipolar neuron. Retina. Rat. E.M. X 9000. **1.** Nucleus of bipolar neuron. **2.** Golgi apparatus. **3.** Mitochondria. **4.** Axon hillock. **5.** Axon.

Fig. 35-30. Nerve fiber layer. Retina. Rat. E.M. X 5000. **1.** Axons of retinal ganglion cells with mitochondria. **2.** Cytoplasm of glial cells. **3.** Cytoplasm of Müller cells. **4.** Internal limiting membrane.

Fig. 35-31. Ganglion cell. Retina. Rat. E.M. X 2700. **1.** Nerve fiber layer. **2.** Nucleus of ganglion cell. **3.** Voluminous perikaryon with numerous Nissl bodies, mitochondria and secondary lysosomes (dark bodies). **4.** Dendrite. **5.** Inner plexiform layer.

Fig. 35-32. Meridional section of optic disk and optic nerve. Monkey. L.M. X 32. **1.** Optic disk. **2.** Optic papilla (annular ridge). **3.** Retina. **4.** Sclera. **5.** Lamina cribrosa with intraocular part of optic nerve. **6.** Orbital part of optic nerve.

Fig. 35-33. Orbital part of optic nerve. Cross section. Monkey. L.M. X 24. **1.** Meninges. **2.** Vaginal spaces. **3.** Septal tissue. **4.** Nerve fascicles. **5.** Central blood vessels.

Fig. 35-34. Optic nerve. Cross section. Enlargement of area similar to rectangle in Fig. 35-33. Rat. E.M. X 620. **1.** Pia mater. **2.** Each nerve fascicle contains numerous myelinated nerve axons. **3.** Blood vessels.

Fig. 35-35. Optic nerve. Cross section. Enlargement of area similar to rectangle in Fig. 35-34. Rat. E.M. X 1900. **1.** Blood vessel in pia mater. **2.** Capillary in nerve fascicle. **3.** Myelinated axons. **4.** Astrocytic (glial) cytoplasm. **5.** Nucleus of astrocyte. **6.** Nuclei of oligodendrocytes.

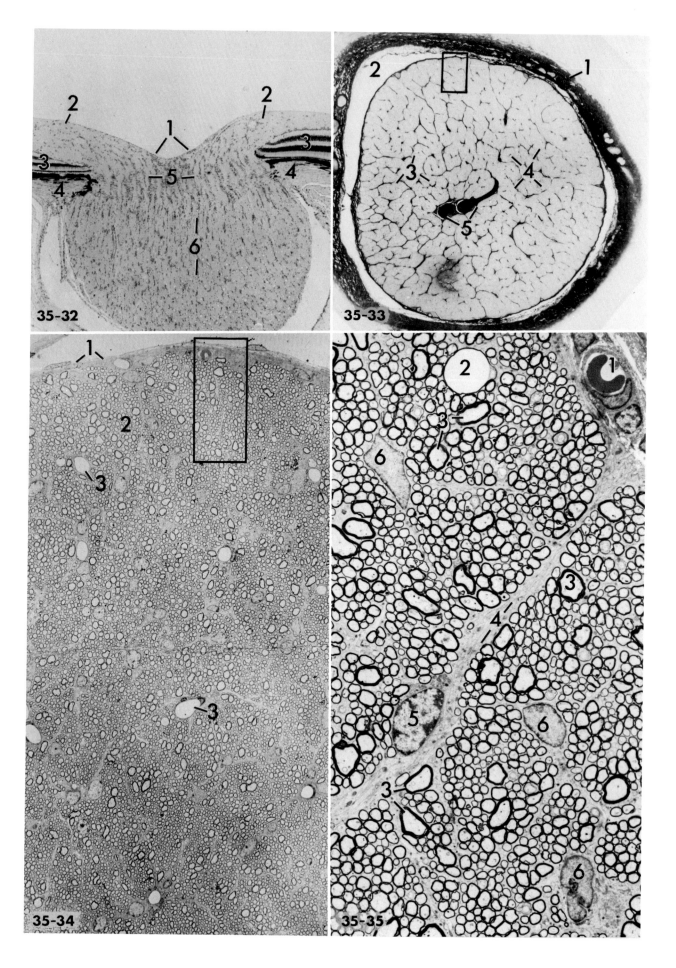

35-32

35-33

35-34

35-35

434

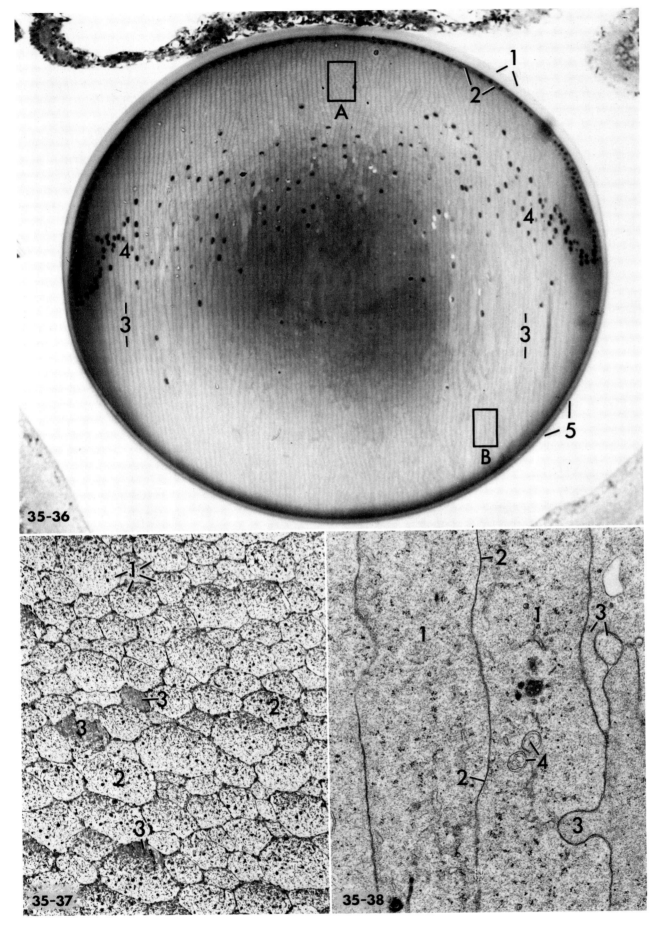

Fig. 35-36. Lens. Mouse. Adult. L.M. X 136.
1. Anterior lens capsule. **2.** Cuboidal epithelial cell. **3.** Lens fibers. **4.** Nuclei of lens fibers. **5.** Posterior lens capsule.

Fig. 35-37. Lens fibers (cells). Cross section. Enlargement of area similar to rectangle (A) in Fig. 35-36. Rat. E.M. X 1700. **1.** Hexagonal profiles of cross-sectioned lens fibers are quite apparent. **2.** Small dense dots represent mitochondria. **3.** Dense accumulations of fibrillar material. Nuclei are not present at level of this section.

Fig. 35-38. Lens fibers. Longitudinal section. Rat. E.M. X 20,000. **1.** Finely granular and filamentous cytoplasm. **2.** Zonulae occludentes of apposed cell membranes. **3.** Interdigitations. **4.** Mitochondria.

Fig. 35-39. Upper eyelid. Enlarged from Fig. 35-1. Monkey. L.M. X 28. **1.** Epidermis. **2.** Orbicularis oculi muscle. **3.** Tarsal plate. **4.** Conjunctiva. **5.** Cornea. **6.** Tarsal glands. **7.** Eyelashes (cilia).

Fig. 35-40. Upper eyelid. Enlargement of rectangle (A) in Fig. 35-39. L.M. X 130. **1.** Orbicularis oculi muscle. **2.** Connective tissue. **3.** Tarsal plate. **4.** Tarsal glands. **5.** Conjunctiva.

Fig. 35-41. Upper eyelid. Enlargement of rectangle (B) in Fig. 35-39. L.M. X 120. **1.** Ciliary sweat glands of Moll. **2.** Hair follicles. **3.** Sebaceous glands of Zeiss.

Fig. 35-42. Lower eyelid. Tarsal glands of Meibom. Monkey. L.M. X 110. **1.** Saccules of modified sebaceous gland cells. **2.** Excretory duct. **3.** Dense connective tissue.

Fig. 35-43. Area of upper fornix of conjunctival sac. Direct continuation of Fig. 35-39 and enlarged from Fig. 35-1. Monkey. L.M. X 52. **1.** Fornix of conjunctival sac. **2.** Bulbar conjunctiva. **3.** Sclera. **4.** Limbus (corneoscleral junction). **5.** Cornea. **6.** Ciliary body. **7.** Iris. **8.** Anterior chamber. **9.** Posterior chamber. **10.** Ciliary processes.

Fig. 35-44. Conjunctival sac. Enlargement of rectangle in Fig. 35-43. L.M. X 185. **1.** Connective tissue of upper-eyelid. **2.** Conjunctival epithelium with numerous mucous (goblet) cells lining posterior surface of upper eyelid. **3.** Stratified squamous, non-keratinized epithelium of bulbar conjunctiva.

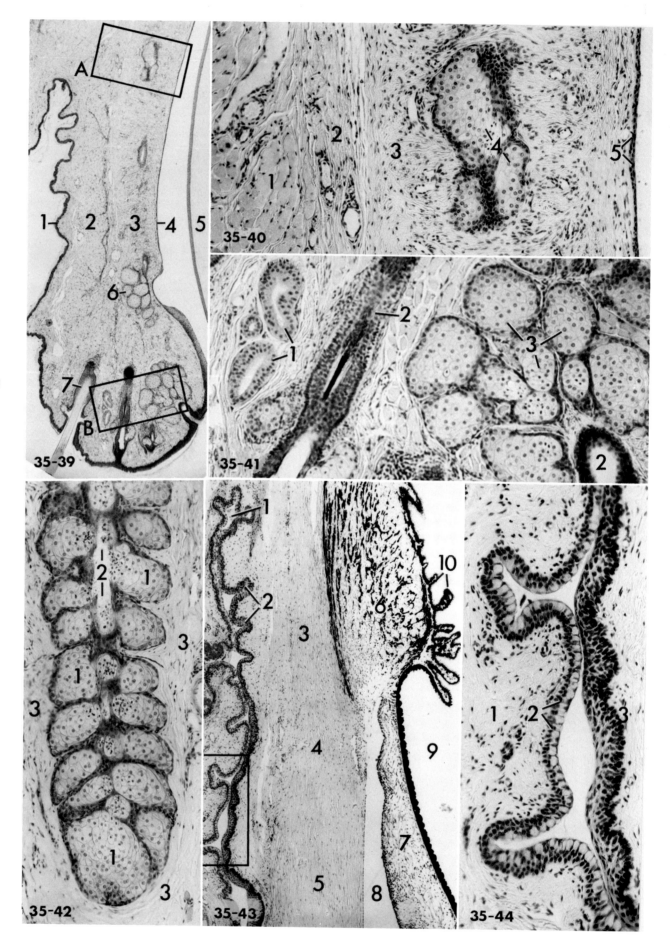

References

EYE

Cohen, A. I. Vertebrate retinal cells and their organization. Biol. Rev. *8*: 427–459 (1963).

Davson, H. (Ed.). The Eye. Vols. 1–4. Academic Press, New York, 1962.

Dowling, J. E. Organization of vertebrate retinas. Invest. Ophthal. *9*: 665–680 (1970).

Fine, B. S. and Yanoff, M. Ocular Histology. Harper & Row, New York, 1972.

Hogan, M. J., Alvarado, J. A., and Weddell, J. E. Histology of the Human Eye. Saunders, Philadelphia, 1971.

Orzalesi, N., Riva, A. and Testa, F. Fine structure of human lacrimal gland. I. The normal gland. J. Submicroscop. Cytol. *3*: 283–296 (1971).

Rohen, J. W. Das Auge und seine Hilfsorgane. Handbuch mikr. Anat. Menschen. W. Möllendorff and W. Bargmann (Eds.), Vol. 3, Part 4. Springer-Verlag, Berlin, 1964.

Smelser, G. K. (Ed.). The Structure of the Eye. Academic Press, New York, 1961.

Villegas, G. M. Ultrastructure of the human retina. J. Anat. *98*: 501–513 (1964).

36 Ear

Fig. 36-1. Greatly schematized representation of the outer, middle, and inner ear to assist in forming a concept of the general topography of this region. 1. Auricle of external ear. 2. Lobule. 3. Cartilage. 4. External auditory meatus. 5. Tympanic membrane. 6. Tympanic cavity. 7. Malleus. 8. Incus. 9. Stapes. 10. Oval window. 11. Facial nerve (cross-sectioned). 12. Vestibule. 13. Utricle with macula. 14. Lateral (horizontal) semicircular canal and duct with ampulla and crista. 15. Anterior (vertical) semicircular canal and duct with ampulla and crista. 16. Posterior (vertical) semicircular canal and duct with ampulla and crista. 17. Endolymphatic duct. 18. Endolymphatic sac. 19. Saccule with macula. 20. Ductus reuniens. 21. Cochlea. 22. Cochlear aqueduct. 23. Round window. 24. Internal auditory meatus. 25. Dura mater. 26. Cranial cavity. 27. Auditory (Eustachian) tube. 28. Parotid gland. 29. Temporal bone.

Fig. 36-2. Cochlea. Axial section. Guinea pig. L.M. X 29. 1. Modiolus. 2. Space in modiolus for the cochlear nerve. 3. Bony shell of guinea pig cochlea. 4. Scala tympani. 5. Cochlear duct. 6. Scala vestibuli. 7. Helicotrema.

Fig. 36-3. Cochlea. Enlargement of area similar to rectangle in Fig. 36-2. L.M. X 52. 1. Scala vestibuli. 2. Cochlear duct. 3. Scala tympani. 4. Spiral ligament. 5. Organ of Corti; rectangle enlarged in Fig. 36-4. 6. Bony spiral lamina. 7. Spiral ganglion. 8. Cochlear nerve. 9. Temporal bone.

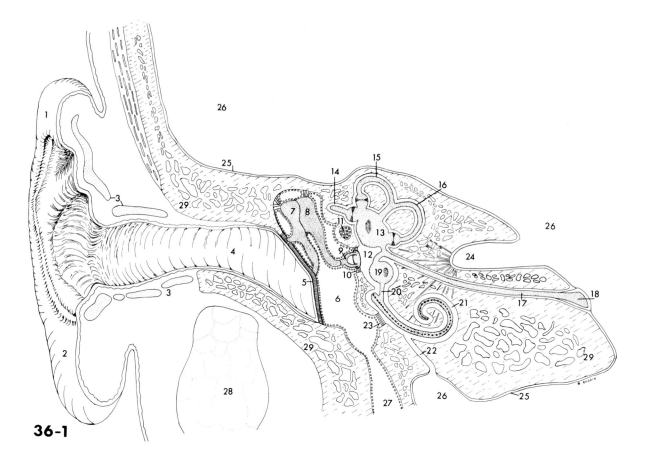

36-1

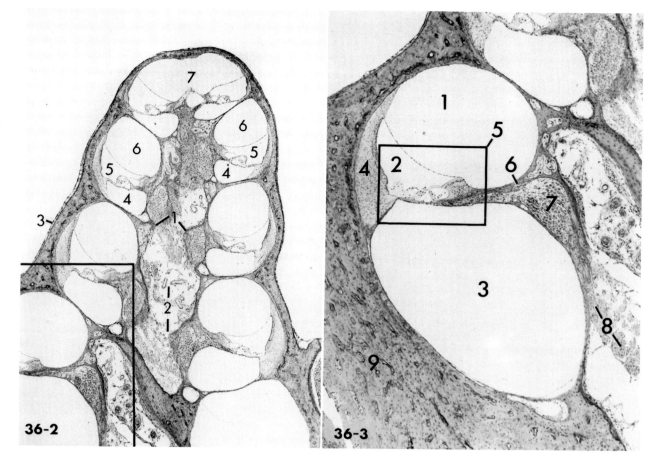

36-2

36-3

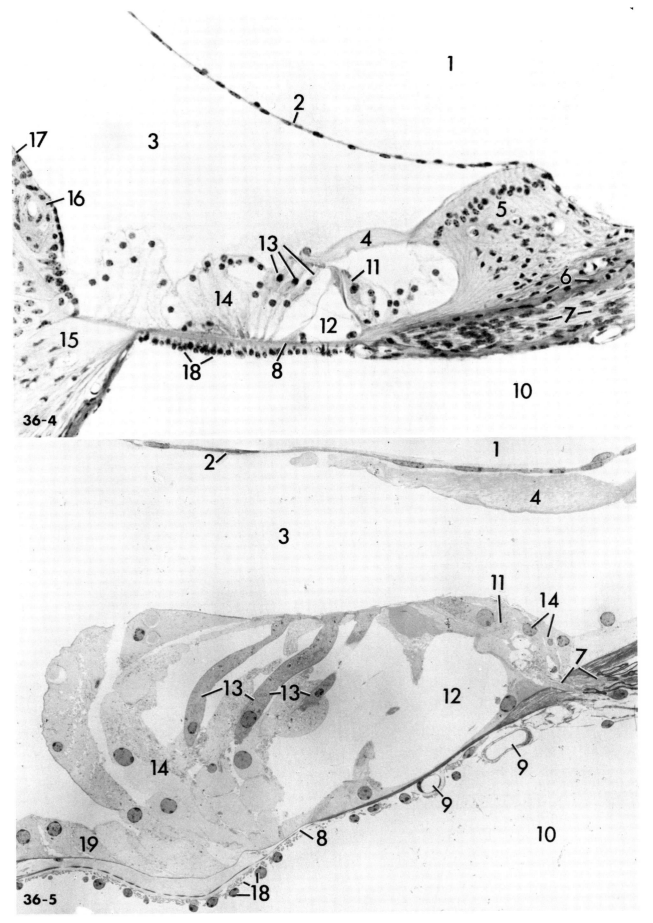

Fig. 36-4. Organ of Corti. Guinea pig. L.M. X 300.
Fig. 36-5. Organ of Corti. Guinea pig. E.M. X 600.
  1. Scala vestibuli (containing perilymph).
  2. Vestibular (Reissner's) membrane.
  3. Cochlear duct (containing endolymph).
  4. Tectorial membrane. **5.** Limbus. **6.** Osseous spiral lamina. **7.** Cochlear nerve. **8.** Basilar membrane. **9.** Capillaries. **10.** Scala tympani (containing perilymph). **11.** Inner hair cells. **12.** Inner tunnel (of Corti) between inner and outer pillar cells. **13.** Outer hair cells. **14.** Supporting cells. **15.** Spiral ligament. **16.** Spiral prominence. **17.** Stria vascularis. **18.** Epithelial cells. **19.** Cells of Claudius.

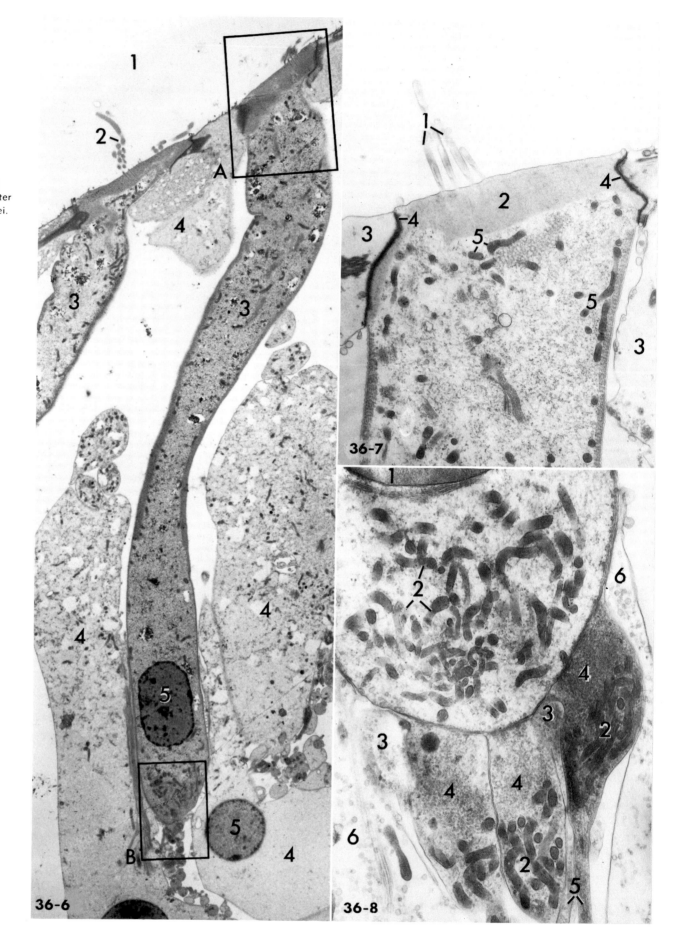

Fig. 36-6. Organ of Corti. Guinea pig. E.M. X 2300. **1.** Cochlear duct. **2.** Stereocilia. **3.** Outer hair cells. **4.** Outer phalangeal cells. **5.** Nuclei.

Fig. 36-7. Apical part of outer hair cell. Enlargement of area similar to rectangle (A) in Fig. 36-6. Guinea pig. E.M. X 9000. **1.** Stereocilia of outer hair cell. **2.** Cuticular cell plate. **3.** Outer phalangeal cells. **4.** Junctional complexes. **5.** Mitochondria.

Fig. 36-8. Basal end of outer hair cell. Enlargement of area similar to rectangle (B) in Fig. 36-6. Guinea pig. E.M. X 15,000. **1.** Part of nucleus of inner hair cell. **2.** Mitochondria. **3.** Afferent nerve endings. **4.** Efferent nerve endings with numerous synaptic vesicles. **5.** Nerve processes. **6.** Phalangeal cells.

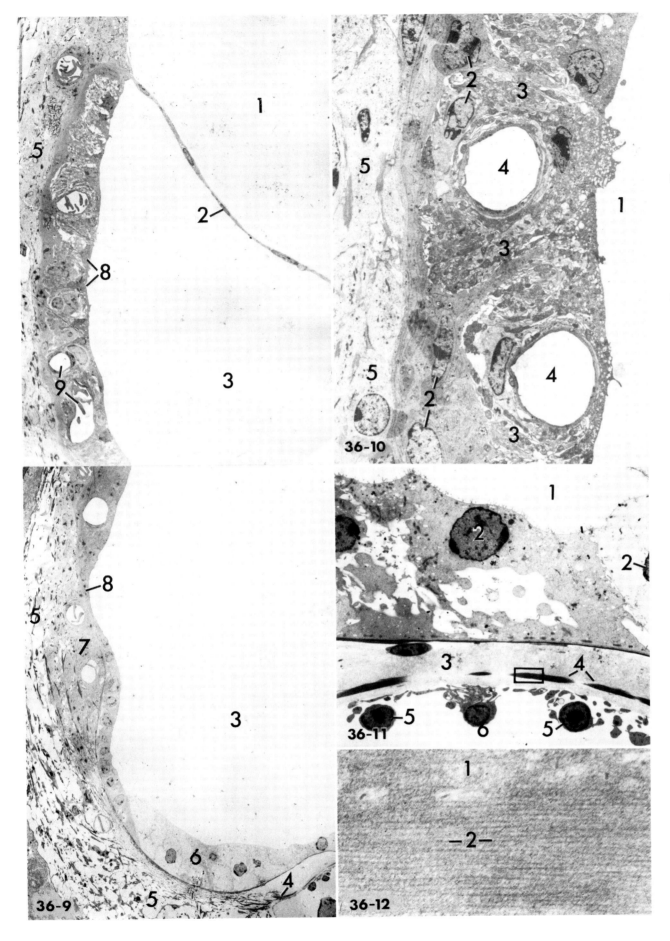

Fig. 36-9. Topography of the external (lateral) wall of the cochlear duct. Guinea pig. E.M. X 500. **1.** Scala vestibuli. **2.** Vestibular (Reissner's) membrane. **3.** Cochlear duct. **4.** Attachment of basilar membrane to the spiral ligament. **5.** Spiral ligament. **6.** Cells of Claudius. **7.** Spiral prominence. **8.** Epithelium of stria vascularis. **9.** Intraepithelial capillaries.

Fig. 36-10. Survey of epithelium of stria vascularis. Guinea pig. E.M. X 1900. **1.** Lumen of cochlear duct. **2.** Nuclei of epithelial cells. **3.** Numerous mitochondria and an intricate system of interlocking cell membranes. **4.** Lumina of intraepithelial capillaries. **5.** Epithelial cells of scala tympani.

Fig. 36-11. Survey of basilar membrane, peripheral to the organ of Corti. Guinea pig. E.M. X 1900. **1.** Lumen of cochlear duct. **2.** Nuclei of Claudius' cells. **3.** Amorphous substance of basilar membrane. **4.** Auditory strings. **5.** Epithelial cells of scala tympani. **6.** Lumen of scala tympani.

Fig. 36-12. Auditory string. Longitudinal section of basilar membrane. Enlargement of area similar to rectangle in Fig. 36-11. Guinea pig. E.M. X 64,000. **1.** Amorphous substance of basilar membrane. **2.** Filaments of auditory strings.

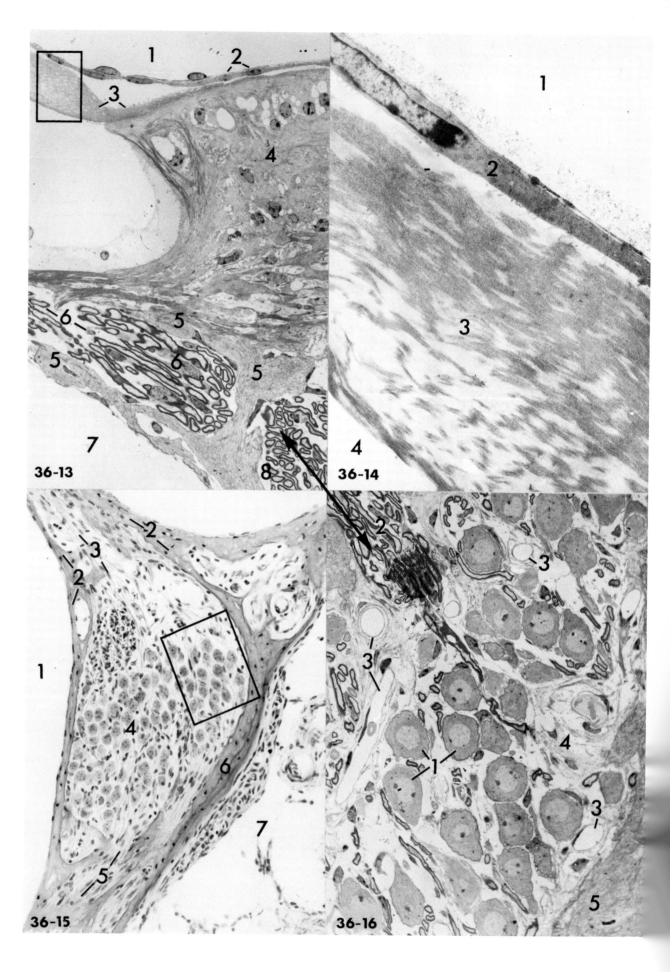

Fig. 36-13. Topography of the inner (medial) wall of the cochlear duct. Guinea pig. E.M. X 5000. **1.** Lumen of scala vestibuli. **2.** Vestibular membrane. **3.** Origin of tectorial membrane. **4.** Limbus. **5.** Osseus spiral lamina. **6.** Myelinated cochlear nerve fibers in bony canal. **7.** Lumen of scala tympani. **8.** Arrow indicates continuity with structures in Fig. 36-16.

Fig. 36-14. Tectorial membrane. Enlargement of area similar to rectangle in Fig. 36-13. Guinea pig. E.M. X 4500. **1.** Scala vestibuli. **2.** Vestibular membrane consists of two squamous epithelia. **3.** Bundles of delicate filaments embedded in an amorphous substance form the tectorial membrane. **4.** Lumen of cochlear duct.

Fig. 36-15. Spiral ganglion. Cochlea. Guinea pig. L.M. X 220. **1.** Scala tympani. **2.** Osseous spiral lamina. **3.** Peripheral nerve processes of bipolar ganglion cells. **4.** Bipolar nerve cells of spiral ganglion. **5.** Central nerve processes of bipolar ganglion cells. **6.** Bony frame of modiolus. **7.** Hollow center of modiolus.

Fig. 36-16. Survey of bipolar ganglion cells of spiral ganglion. Cochlea. Enlargement of area similar to rectangle in Fig. 36-15. Guinea pig. E.M. X 620. **1.** Bipolar ganglion cells. **2.** Arrow. Peripheral myelinated nerve fibers are directly continuous with those seen at arrow in Fig. 36-13. **3.** Blood capillaries. **4.** Loose connective tissue. **5.** Bone matrix.

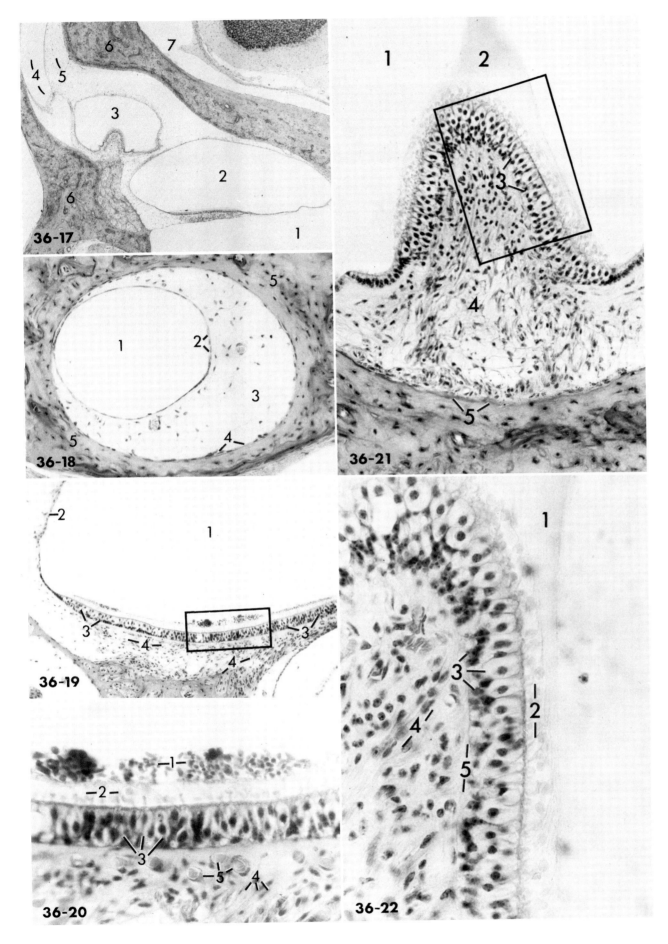

Fig. 36-17. Inner ear. Vestibular labyrinth. Guinea pig. L.M. X 29. **1.** Vestibule. **2.** Saccule with macula. **3.** Ampulla of semicircular canal with crista ampullaris. **4.** Semicircular duct. **5.** Semicircular canal. **6.** Temporal bone. **7.** Cranial cavity.

Fig. 36-18. Cross section of semicircular canal and duct. Guinea pig. L.M. X 171. **1.** Semicircular duct (containing endolymph). **2.** Wall of duct. **3.** Semicircular canal (containing perilymph). **4.** Endosteum. **5.** Temporal bone.

Fig. 36-19. Part of saccule. Vestibular labyrinth. Guinea pig. L.M. X 115. **1.** Cavity of saccule (containing endolymph). **2.** Wall of saccule. **3.** Macula. **4.** Vestibular nerve fibers.

Fig. 36-20. Part of macula of saccule. Enlargement of rectangle in Fig. 36-19. L.M. X 460. **1.** Otolithic membrane with otoconia. **2.** Stereocilia. **3.** Hair cells and supporting cells. **4.** Vestibular nerve fibers. **5.** Capillaries.

Fig. 36-21. Crista ampullaris. Semicircular duct. Guinea pig. L.M. X 220. **1.** Lumen of semicircular duct (containing endolymph). **2.** Cupula. **3.** Hair cells. **4.** Connective tissue of crista. **5.** Edge of bone, marking the extent of the bony ampulla.

Fig. 36-22. Crista ampullaris. Enlargement of area similar to rectangle in Fig. 36-21. L.M. X 506. **1.** Part of cupula. **2.** Stereocilia. **3.** Hair cells and supporting cells. **4.** Nerve fibers. **5.** Level of basal lamina.

References

EAR

Davis, H. Biophysics and physiology of the inner ear. Physiol. Rev. *37*: 1–49 (1957).

de Lorento, A. J. D. (Ed.). Vascular Disorders and Hearing Defects. University Park Press, Baltimore, 1973.

Engström, H. and Wersäll, J. Structure and innervation of the inner ear sensory epithelia. Int. Rev. Cytol. *7*: 535–585 (1958).

Engström, H. and Ades, H. W. (Eds.). Inner ear studies. Acta Otolaryng. Suppl. 301 (1973).

Engström, H., Ades, H. and Anderson, A. Structural Pattern of the Organ of Corti. Almquist and Wiksell, Stockholm, 1966.

Flock, Å. Structure of the macula utriculi with special reference to directional interplay of sensory response as revealed by morphological polarization. J. Cell Biol. *22*: 413–431 (1964).

Hinojosa, R. and Rodriquez-Echandia, E. L. The fine structure of the stria vascularis of the cat inner ear. Am. J. Anat. *118*: 631–664 (1966).

Iurato, S. (Ed.). Submicroscopic Structure of the Inner Ear. Pergamon Press, New York, 1967.

Johnson, F. R., McMinn, R. M. H. and Atfield, G. N. Ultrastructural and biochemical observations on the tympanic membrane. J. Anat. *103*: 297–310 (1968).

Kawabata, I. and Paparella, M. M. Ultrastructure of normal human middle ear mucosa. Ann. Otol. Rhin. Laryngol. *78*: 125–137 (1968).

Kimura, R. S., Schuknecht, H. F. and Sando, I. Fine morphology of the sensory cells in the organ of Corti of man. Acta Otolaryngol. *58*: 390–408 (1965).

Lundquist, P.-G. The endolymphatic duct and sac in the guinea pig. An electron microscopic and experimental investigation. Acta Otolaryngol. Suppl. 201 (1965).

Nakai, Y. and Hilding, D. Vestibular and endolymph-producing epithelium. Electron microscopic study of the development and histochemistry of the dark cells of the crista ampullaris. Acta Otolaryngol. *66*: 120–128 (1968).

Smith, C. A. Electron microscopy of the inner ear. Ann. Otol. Rhin. Laryngol. *77*: 629–643 (1968).

Smith, C. A. and Sjöstrand, F. S. Structure of the nerve endings on the external hair cells of the guinea pig cochlea as studied by serial sections. J. Ultrastruct. Res. *5*: 523–556 (1961).

Spoendlin, H. H. Organization of the sensory hairs in the gravity receptors in utricle and saccule of the squirrel monkey. Z. Zellforsch. *62*: 701–716 (1964).

Spoendlin, H. H. The organization of the cochlear receptor. *In* Advances in Oto-Rhino-Laryngology, Vol. 13, S. Karger, Basel, 1966.

Wersäll, J. Studies on the structure and innervation of the sensory epithelium of the cristae ampullares in the guinea pig. Acta Otolaryngol. Suppl. 126 (1956).

Index